Pathology of Small Mammal Pets

Pathology of Small Mammal Pets

Patricia V. Turner, Marina L. Brash, and Dale A. Smith

WILEY Blackwell

This edition first published 2018
© 2018 John Wiley & Sons, Inc.

The right of Patricia V. Turner, Marina L. Brash and Dale A. Smith to be identified as the author(s) of this work has been asserted in accordance with law.

Registered Office
John Wiley & Sons, Inc., 111 River Street, Hoboken, NJ 07030, USA

Editorial Office
John Wiley & Sons, Inc., 111 River Street, Hoboken, NJ 07030, USA

For details of our global editorial offices, customer services, and more information about Wiley products visit us at www.wiley.com.

Wiley also publishes its books in a variety of electronic formats and by print-on-demand. Some content that appears in standard print versions of this book may not be available in other formats.

Library of Congress Cataloging-in-Publication Data

Names: Turner, Patricia V., author. | Brash, Marina L., author. | Smith, Dale A.
  (Dale Alison), 1956- author.
Title: Pathology of small mammal pets / Patricia V. Turner, Marina L. Brash,
  Dale A. Smith.
Description: Hoboken, NJ : John Wiley & Sons Inc., 2018. | Includes
  bibliographical references and index. |
Identifiers: LCCN 2017002361 (print) | LCCN 2017026818 (ebook) | ISBN
  9781118969595 (Adobe PDF) | ISBN 9781118969588 (ePub) | ISBN 9780813818313
  (cloth)
Subjects: LCSH: Ruminants--Diseases--Diagnosis. |
  Rabbits--Diseases--Diagnosis. | MESH: Rodent Diseases--pathology | Rabbits
  | Animal Diseases--pathology | Pets | Ferrets | Hedgehogs
Classification: LCC SF997.5.R64 (ebook) | LCC SF997.5.R64 T87 2018 (print) |
  NLM SF 997.5.R64 | DDC 636.935--dc23
LC record available at https://lccn.loc.gov/2017002361

Cover Design: Wiley
Cover Images: (Left) © GK Hart/Vikki Hart/Gettyimages; (Center and Right) Courtesy of Patricia V. Turner, Marina L. Brash and Dale A. Smith

Set in 10/12pt Warnock by SPi Global, Chennai, India
Printed and bound in Singapore by Markono Print Media Pte Ltd

10 9 8 7 6 5 4 3 2 1

Contents

Preface

Pathology of Small Mammal Pets provides current information on congenital abnormalities, spontaneous and infectious diseases, degenerative and neoplastic conditions, and incidental findings for a range of popular small mammal pets. We have not attempted to be exhaustive in content, since there are excellent, well-established resources available already for laboratory rabbits, ferrets, and rodents, but instead have taken a practical, systems approach to conditions likely to be seen predominantly in companion animal settings. We have supplemented this with relevant information for breeding operations, including pet store suppliers as well as facilities breeding small mammals for food for other species, and, in the case of rabbits, for commercial meat rabbit production, as it is next to impossible for veterinarians to find information on these groups of animals in traditional veterinary medicine and pathology publications. Where information is available, we have also addressed herd or colony management strategies for various conditions, again, recognizing that it is often not enough to have a diagnosis in hand to provide optimal client support and patient care. Veterinary expertise in animal health management can readily be transferred following a review of species-specific information found in this book. It goes without saying that the public health responsibilities of veterinarians and veterinary pathologists extend to these small mammals in all the settings in which they are commonly encountered.

This book is intended primarily for veterinarians, veterinary pathologists, veterinary technicians, and veterinary students, but it may also be of interest to animal owners, breeders, and producers. Although there is much more work to be done in this field of practice, knowledge of small mammal diseases, interest in small mammal medicine, and availability of high quality veterinary care for these species have grown exponentially over the past decade. The increased popularity of small mammals as pets may reflect increased urban dwelling and a need for people to engage with animals in a more compact environment. Small mammal clients are often very knowledgeable about their animals and have high expectations for quality veterinary support to improve animal care and well-being.

We were inspired to take on this project close to a decade ago by a colleague and mentor, Dean H. Percy, who reminded us on more than one occasion of the glaring gap in the literature. As is typical for many books, what began as a casual hallway conversation morphed into a full-fledged effort. It has been a long and interesting journey, and we hope that the information gathered within this volume will be of use to fellow veterinary colleagues. Small mammals are charming and fascinating animals to work with and we hope that this resource will be used as a means to enhance their care. Despite our best efforts and given the continuing evolution of knowledge in this field, we know that there will be errors and omissions, and we invite readers to provide suggestions for correcting and improving this work.

Acknowledgments

We are grateful to our colleagues who work in veterinary practice, diagnostic laboratories, and as private consultants for sharing their expertise during the preparation of this book. Small mammal pathology cases are not seen routinely in many diagnostic laboratories thus it can be difficult to develop clinicopathologic correlates to ensure continued learning for veterinary clinicians and pathologists alike. Publication of case reports in meetings proceedings and journals is essential for improving the quality of care for patients and service to clients. Case reports are often not credited sufficiently in academic settings, however, without these publications many conditions affecting small mammal pets would not be formally documented.

We would especially like to recognize the support given to us by our families. We owe a special debt to Fabio, Allan and Betty, Ken, and Brian who have indulged us repeatedly over the years to make time for this project. Their enduring patience, encouragement, and sense of humor have inspired us to see this book through to completion. We thank Erica Judisch and Susan Engelken at Wiley who have patiently monitored our progress and provided gentle nudges and support at every turn. We would also like to thank Peggy Chiappetta, Janessa Price, and Adriana Rodriguez for pulling blocks, organizing histology slides, and conducting literature searches along the way; Deirdre Stuart and Zenya Brown for indexing assistance; Kristine Smith for scanning neglected boxes of kodachromes; Beverly McEwen for endless database searches; Grant Maxie for advice, support, and encouragement; and Josepha DeLay and the AHL Histotechnology team for immunohistochemistry expertise and a willingness to try their antibody magic in new and untested territory. This group has also been endlessly patient with our requests to find blocks, pull slides, prepare recuts, and conduct many special stains.

While many have shared images with us, in particular, our colleagues Hugues Beaufrère and Michael Taylor from the Ontario Veterinary College, Colette Wheler from the University of Saskatchewan, Rick Axelson and Evan Mavromatis at The Links Road Animal and Bird Clinic, Mike Ritter at the New Hamburg Veterinary Clinic, and Markus Luckwaldt of Luckwaldt Mobile Veterinary Services have all provided numerous high quality images for us to use for this book (or found others to supply the images) over the years and we are indebted to these individuals for these visual records. In addition, Dean Percy, John Harkness, Colette Wheler, and Hugues Beaufrère provided valuable comments and edits to the text of the book during its preparation. Many of our current and past colleagues and graduate students at the Animal Health Laboratory and within the Department of Pathobiology, University of Guelph have contributed small mammal necropsy and clinical photographs to the OVC Pathology repository for which we are very grateful.

Image Credits

Every effort has been made to attribute photographs and photomicrographs to their rightful owners and we apologize in advance if we have inadvertently missed any contributor. We are deeply appreciative of the following individuals for providing permissions to use images in this book, for sending good cases our way, and for assisting with enhancing the AHL/OVC Pathobiology image repository:

Calgary Avian and Exotic Pet Clinic: Kerry Korber
Canadian Food Inspection Agency: Carissa Embury-Hyatt
Carleton University: Kerri Nielsen
Louisiana State University: Joao Brandao
Luckwaldt Mobile Veterinary Services: Markus Luckwaldt
New Hamburg Veterinary Clinic: Mike Ritter
Oklahoma State University: Ian Kanda
Penn State University: Timothy Cooper
Rat Fancy Club: Debbie Ducommun
Seoul National University: Jae Hak Park

The Links Road Animal and Bird Clinic: Rick Axelson, Evan Mavromatis
University of Calgary: Jennifer Davies
University of Guelph/Animal Health Laboratory: Hibret Adissu, Tara Arndt, Hugues Beaufrère, Laura Bassal, Brian Binnington, Emily Brouwer, Jeff Caswell, Bridget Lee Chow, Nicole Compo, Rebecca Egan, David Eshar, Robert Foster, Bob Hampson, Elein Hernandez, David Hobson, Joelle Ingrao, Doran Kirkbright, Jennifer Kylie, Brandon Lillie, Emily Martin, Dean Percy, Chris Pinelli, Anil Puttaswamy, Leah Schutt, Hein Snyman, Janet Sunohara-Neilson, W. Michael Taylor, Laetitia Tatiersky, Jessica Walsh, Krishna Yekkala.
University Health Network: Alyssa Goldstein, Janet Sunohara-Neilson
University of Montreal: Pierre Hélie
University of Saskatchewan: Colette Wheler
Yale University: Amanda Beck

1

Rabbits

1.1 Introduction

Domestic rabbits (*Oryctolagus cuniculus*) are descendants of wild European rabbits that were originally found on the Iberian Peninsula by the Phoenicians. Rabbits have been kept by humans for over 3,000 years, largely as a self-replicating source of food, but also for their pelts and later, as pets. Roman writings describe leporaria, walled yards, to keep rabbits contained for hunting. Rabbits were later kept in warrens, courtyards, and islands for breeding and food production, and breeding pairs were released on various islands and in newly discovered lands by naval circumnavigators to ensure a source of fresh meat was available on subsequent visits. In approximately 600 CE, a papal decree declared that unhaired newborn rabbits (laurices) were not meat but instead aquatic species and could be consumed during Lent, leading to a surge of rabbit breeding and domestication in monasteries throughout the Middle Ages. Selective breeding in monasteries gave rise to many of the coat color variants and breeds in existence today. Rabbit breeding for hunting and meat production was initially controlled by seigneurial privilege but with the rise of the middle classes in Europe, raising rabbits became very popular and increasing numbers of animals were kept as pets. Intensification of rabbit farming occurred in parts of Europe and Asia in the early part of the twentieth century, and later, in the early 1950s, in North America. Rabbit breeder associations and specialty hobbyist clubs have been in existence in Europe and North America for over 100 years. Rabbits make gentle and inquisitive pets and are popular with children and adults alike.

When considering rabbit disease, it is important to know the age of the animal and the typical life cycle, be it commercial or pet. The natural lifespan will vary depending upon the size of the rabbit, with larger breeds, such as Flemish giant and New Zealand white rabbits living between 7 and 9 years, while dwarf breeds will live longer; 10–14 years. Rabbits bred for commercial meat purposes in North America tend to be of New Zealand white or Californian background, both of which produce large,

fast-growing animals with a high muscle to bone ratio. The white pelts harvested from these animals are used as a by-product for fur trim and felt production. Various spotted and colored hybrid animals may be seen on different farms; however, and other breeds are sporadically introduced from Europe to improve disease resistance and to provide hybrid vigor. In North America, breeding does and bucks kept in commercial meat operations are culled at 2–3 years of age (earlier in Europe) and young rabbits (fryers) are sent to market between 8–14 weeks of age, depending on the efficiency of the operation. Artificial insemination is used in some commercial operations to better manage disease, reproductive cycles, and parturition (i.e., "all in, all out" management systems). Many commercial rabbit breeders also breed or sell rabbits for the pet trade, either dealing directly with pet stores or distributors or by selling animals at the farm gate. While increasing numbers of commercial operations are more selective about barn entry and on-farm biosecurity practices are improving, significant gastrointestinal and respiratory diseases are still present on most of these farms in North America. Many pet rabbits, and there are over 48 breeds recognized by the American Rabbit Breeder Association, come from breeding operations that are not raising animals for meat. These breeding operations may or may not provide routine antimicrobial preventive medications to animals, and the patterns of disease seen in rabbits originating from these sources can be quite different than for commercial meat rabbit operations. Finally, fewer pet rabbits, usually New Zealand white or Dutch-belted breeds, may be adopted directly from research facilities. These rabbits usually originate in commercial laboratory animal breeding facilities and have a very high health status, often being free of gastrointestinal and respiratory infections, which are common in conventionally bred animals. Pet rabbits adopted from rabbit rescue agencies or animal shelters have unknown health backgrounds and may have come from situations of severe neglect. Thus, the types of diseases and conditions that are seen in rabbits will vary considerably, depending on the source.

Pathology of Small Mammal Pets, First Edition. Patricia V. Turner, Marina L. Brash and Dale A. Smith.
© 2018 John Wiley & Sons, Inc. Published 2018 by John Wiley & Sons, Inc.

Pet rabbits are often neutered at sexual maturity, which occurs between 3–6 months of age, with smaller breeds maturing more rapidly. Neutering is done to manage or prevent behavioral problems as well as to reduce the risk of certain age-related neoplastic conditions. Rabbits coming from research facilities as well as some commercial or show breeding operations may be identified by a tattoo inside one ear. Increasingly, pet rabbits receive micro-chip implants for identification purposes.

Depending on where the rabbit originates, it may be euthanatized by the producer or a veterinary clinic for post-mortem evaluation. Currently accepted on-farm euthanasia practices include blunt force trauma applied to the back of the head, nonpenetrating captive bolt, cervical dislocation, and carbon dioxide inhalation. Animals killed by physical methods may demonstrate oronasal blood staining at post-mortem. Pen mates often cannibalize animals dying on farm and this type of trauma may be recognized by a lack of associated hemorrhage or inflammation. Sedation followed by intravenous or intracardiac barbiturate overdose or anesthetic inhalant gas overdose are more commonly used as euthanasia methods for pet rabbits by veterinary clinics. Because of very rapid tissue deterioration after death, when dealing with investigations of gastrointestinal disease in rabbits coming from commercial operations, it is highly recommended to have the client submit several live affected animals. Post-mortem examination and tissue sampling should occur as rapidly as possible after death.

1.2 Integument Conditions

Rabbit skin is thin and fragile compared with the skin of other species and the pelage consists of a dense undercoat of secondary hairs as well as larger, longer primary guard hairs. Rex rabbits have a defect in the hair growth cycle, resulting in a plush, short, velvety coat lacking the long guard hairs of other breeds. Rabbit hair normally undergoes periods of cyclic and seasonal growth and molting, which may influence hair regrowth patterns following clipping for surgical or other procedures. Regrowth does not occur evenly over the body with independent cycles noted for the dorsum and ventrum. Hair growth cycles also differ among breeds. For example, Angora rabbit hair follicles have been reported to have a growth phase of 14 weeks compared to a 5-week cycle in New Zealand white rabbits, as well as having a higher follicular growth rate. Both these factors likely contribute to the long hairs produced by the Angora breed.

Rabbits have numerous sebaceous glands associated with clusters of hair follicles on their chin (submental gland), feet, and prepuce, which are used for scent-marking (chinning) novel and familiar objects and spaces by sexually mature animals. Modified sebaceous glands are also found in the genital area, and within the rectum. Rabbits are not thought to possess sweat glands but do have modified apocrine glands within the ear (ceruminous apocrine gland), in the perineal area of both sexes, and in the submandibular area. Although mammary glands are not part of the integument, they are discussed in this section because of their cutaneous association.

The external ears of rabbits have only a vertical canal, i.e., they lack a horizontal canal, thus differing from those of other small companion animals, and the vasculature of the ears has an important function in thermoregulation, providing for counter-current heat exchange.

Healthy rabbits are fastidious in their habits and groom their pelage frequently, thus a poor quality, staring hair coat is a sign of poor health. Interestingly, rabbits with orodental disease have a 63 times greater risk of subsequently developing dermatologic disease. This is postulated to be due to decreased nutrition and poor body condition, matting from drooling or other discharge, and decreased grooming in unthrifty or painful animals secondary to chronic dental disease and abscesses.

Skin conditions represent almost 30% of pet rabbit primary care presentations. The most commonly reported conditions include pododermatitis, abscesses, alopecia, parasites, cutaneous masses, and moist dermatitis.

1.2.1 Alopecia

Focal or diffuse alopecia or hair loss is a common presenting condition and there are many potential causes for simple alopecia in rabbits, some of which may be physiologic. Rabbits typically undergo at least two cycles of hair growth and shedding annually and some breeds will undergo four or more cycles. Nutritional and disease status, hormone levels, age, and sex will all influence pelage quality, as well as growth and shedding patterns.

1.2.1.1 Presenting Clinical Signs
Uncomplicated alopecia may present as areas of focal to patchy to generalized hair loss. Owners may report over-grooming, hair pulling or chewing (barbering) or excessive shedding. The skin is intact in these cases unless there are lesions associated with trauma or fighting. Both long guard hairs and secondary hairs may be affected. Alopecia secondary to various endocrinopathies may be associated with vulvar swelling and thinning of the skin in does.

1.2.1.2 Pathology
An infectious etiology should be suspected if hair loss is accompanied by scaliness, pruritus, moist dermatitis or abscessation (see Section 1.2.2 Bacterial Dermatitis). The pattern and distribution of alopecia may provide

clues as to the underlying cause. Hair loss around the muzzle or face may be associated with mechanical abrasion from rough edges on caging or feeders. Similarly, hair loss on the palmar surface of the feet is seen with wire bottom caging (see Section 1.27). Fur chewing can be detected readily on skin biopsy by identification of normal, intact hair follicles and hair shafts that are broken off at the epithelial surface. Simple alopecia related to seasonal, stress-induced or endocrine-related shedding will be detected histologically by complete loss of hair in affected areas with dormant follicles, typically with minimal to no accompanying inflammation and no epithelial scaling or crusting.

Undulating epithelium with disorganized hair follicles and hyperkeratosis has been reported in rabbits with congenital hypotrichosis. Thickening of the skin and ears with crusting, conjunctivitis, and alopecia can be seen in rabbits with severe vitamin B6 deficiency, in conjunction with neurologic signs, such as seizures.

1.2.1.3 Laboratory Diagnostics
Skin biopsies, skin scrapings, microbiologic culture and sensitivity, and circulating steroid hormone and thyroxin levels may be evaluated to differentiate noninfectious from infectious causes of hair loss. It is important to recognize that epithelial thickness will vary markedly depending on the site sampled and control tissues must be sampled from a similar site as affected tissues. Some diagnostic laboratories can determine circulating steroid hormone levels for rabbits, which may be used to support the diagnosis of alopecia-associated endocrinopathy. These levels are not evaluated routinely, however, and appropriate age- and sex-matched reference intervals must be available for comparison. Alopecia has not been reported in association with diabetes mellitus in rabbits.

1.2.1.4 Differential Diagnoses
Normal seasonal shedding and regrowth of the pelage should be differentiated from changes induced by behavioral problems, trauma, adverse stress, inappropriate diet, insufficient dietary fiber content, pregnancy or pseudopregnancy, and mechanical wear from feeders or rough edges on cages. Mechanical abrasion often results in alopecia localized to the nose or face. Behaviorally-induced alopecia is common and may be initiated by boredom (fur chewing), low fiber diets, aggression or other maladjustment syndromes.

Bilaterally symmetrical alopecia in intact does may be associated with hyperestrogenism secondary to ovarian or uterine disease, or other endocrinopathies, including adrenal gland disorders. Pregnant or pseudopregnant does normally will pull hair from their dewlap, forelegs, ventrum, and other parts of their body to line a nest prior to kindling, which may result in thinning of the coat in these places. In pregnant does, the hair loosens up to two weeks prepartum, facilitating nest building. Does exhibiting early to midgestational hair loss and nest-building behaviors are assumed to be pseudopregnant. Hypothyroidism with bilaterally symmetrical alopecia and skin thinning has also been reported in rabbits.

Certain chemotherapeutic medications, such as doxorubicin and adriamycin, as well as radiation therapy, may induce hair loss and clients should be forewarned prior to treatment with these medications or therapies of potential side effects, including alopecia. Sudden psychological or physical stress may also induce focal or generalized hair loss (telogen effluvium). In research settings, strains of autosomal recessive hairless rabbits may be found but congenital hypotrichosis is otherwise rare in pet and commercial meat rabbits. Alopecia has also been reported in rabbits with underlying thymoma (see Section 1.3 Endocrine Conditions).

1.2.1.5 Group or Herd Management
Careful evaluation of housing and husbandry conditions should be implemented for noninfectious causes of alopecia. Dietary adequacy should be ascertained and animal caging should be inspected for surface irregularities if mechanically-induced alopecia is suspected. Co-housed animals may need to be separated to evaluate overgrooming and barbering. Finally, ovariectomy may be recommended in nonbreeding does to prevent pseudopregnancy and associated nest-building behaviors.

1.2.2 Bacterial Dermatitis and Abscesses

Bacterial dermatitis and abscesses may result from local skin or wound contamination or trauma, or systemic distribution of bacteria with secondary skin colonization (Figure 1.1). Abscesses may be single or multiple, and generally contain thick purulent material. Facial abscesses are often associated with dental disease and may fistulate with resulting intraoral or external tracts.

1.2.2.1 Presenting Clinical Signs
All ages, breeds and both sexes may be affected with bacterial dermatitis and abscesses. Affected areas may be erythematous with superficial scaling, induration, alopecia, exudation and ulceration. Cellulitis may develop if subcuticular tissues are involved. In these cases, rabbits may present with pyrexia, anorexia, and depression and may guard the affected area. Moist dermatitis and cellulitis may be malodorous and can become secondarily infested with larvae from *Calliphorid* flies (secondary myiasis, see Section 1.2.4).

The clinical history and distribution of lesions may provide hints as to the etiopathogenesis of the condition.

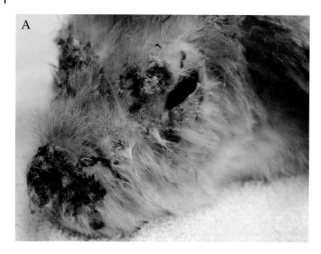
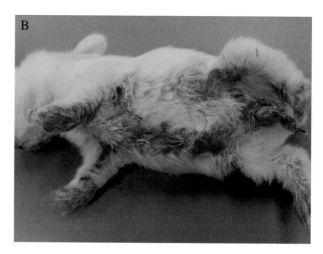

Figure 1.1 A: Fighting wounds in a pet rabbit inflicted by a cagemate, with secondary bacterial infection. B: Staphylococcal pyoderma in a preweaned kit presenting with erythema, patchy hair loss, and exudative dermatitis. Many kits from the same barn were dying with similar skin lesions, which were related to rough nestbox flooring and wet shavings used as nesting material, both of which created dermal microabrasions, predisposing to bacterial infection. *Source:* A: Courtesy of The Links Road Animal and Bird Clinic.

Bacterial dermatitis is usually secondary to other conditions, such as minor trauma, fighting injuries, systemic staphylococcal infections in young kits, abrasions from feeders or caging, poor husbandry with persistent wet or dirty conditions, or urine dribbling or scalding with secondary perineal or ventral abdominal dermatitis and ulceration. Biting and fighting lesions with secondary abscessation are common in pair or group-housed animals, especially if animals are introduced following sexual maturation. Finally, rabbits with impaired mobility or obese animals may be unable to groom effectively, leading to accumulations of urine and feces on the perineal skin with secondary dermal irritation and infection.

1.2.2.2 Pathology

Several well-described bacterial agents and cutaneous disease conditions are recognized in rabbits and are detailed further below. In general, abscesses in rabbits are caused by *Staphylococcus aureus*, *Pasteurella multocida*, *Pseudomonas aeruginosa*, or less commonly, by *Proteus* sp., *Bacteroides* sp., and other bacteria. Maxillary and mandibular abscesses arising within the oral cavity may be related to oral or gingival trauma with secondary infection by *Fusobacterium* sp., *Streptococcus* spp., *Actinomyces* sp., or *Arcanobacterium* sp. (Figure 1.2). Rarely, *Francisella tularensis*, the agent of tularemia, will induce cutaneous abscesses in wild cottontail rabbits. Animals infected with this agent usually demonstrate systemic illness and depression, and may die peracutely.

1.2.2.3 Staphylococcosis

The most common agent isolated from lapine abscesses and cases of suppurative dermatitis or cellulitis is *Staphylococcus aureus*, a Gram-positive coccoid bacterium. In addition, *S. aureus* is commonly associated with cases of mastitis (blue breast), pododermatitis (sore hocks), visceral abscessation, metritis, respiratory disease, conjunctivitis, and septicemia in rabbits (see Sections 1.2.5 and 1.2.7). Staphylococcal dermatitis lesions vary with age, sex, and virulence of infecting bacteria. The bacterium is a common opportunistic agent carried on the skin and within the nasal passages and oropharynx of rabbits and their human caregivers.

There are at least five known biotypes of *S. aureus*, based on biochemical properties, and 23 or more phage types, all of which can reassort to create strains of differing virulence, which largely determine the severity of *S. aureus*-induced disease. Low virulence strains induce isolated abscesses and mild dermatitis in rabbits while high virulence strains may induce disease outbreaks with high mortality. Some isolates appear to be host-specific while some are transmissible between species, for example, humans and rabbits. It is not uncommon for animals to be concurrently infected with more than one biotype. In general, rabbit-specific strains of *S. aureus* are susceptible to most antibiotics. However, there have been reports of pet rabbits infected with methicillin-resistant *S. aureus* (MRSA).

Typical superficial lesions caused by *Staphylococcus aureus* include localized, soft to firm nonpainful fluctuant swellings (abscesses) or focal to locally extensive mild to ulcerative exudative dermatitis (Figure 1.2B). Generalized pustular dermatitis with secondary septicemia, internal organ abscessation, and mortality has been noted in young rabbits from affected herds. Multifocal suppurative lesions may be found upon the surface and within the parenchyma of the spleen, liver, kidney, heart,

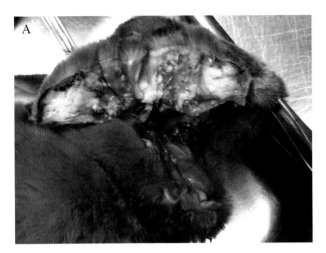 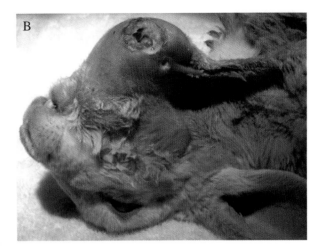

Figure 1.2 A: Multiple facial abscesses in sectioned skin. *Source:* A: Courtesy of M. Luckwaldt. B: Ulcerated submandibular abscess secondary to chronic dental disease. *Source:* B: Courtesy of The Links Road Animal and Bird Clinic.

and lung. Abscesses may be isolated, multifocal, or miliary. Depending on the age of the lesion, marked, predominantly neutrophilic infiltrates may be seen histologically and dense Gram-positive coccoid bacterial colonies are typically abundant around and within lesions, including abscesses. As for other animals, PAS-positive Splendore-Hoeppli material may sometimes be present around dense multifocal aggregates of bacterial colonies (botryomycosis). In peracute cases of staphylococcal septicemia, numerous bacterial colonies may be observed in tissues without significant leukocytic infiltrates or other inflammatory reaction. Death in these cases is presumed to occur from exotoxin-mediated shock. In more chronic lesions with abscessation, a thick fibrous capsule surrounds the necrotic foci, which are comprised of mature and degenerate neutrophils, bacterial colonies, and cellular debris. Edema, granulation tissue, plump fibroblasts, macrophages and multinucleate giant cells may be present in tissues surrounding the abscess.

1.2.2.4 Cutaneous Necrobacillosis
Necrobacillosis (Schmorl's disease) in rabbits is caused by *Fusobacterium necrophorum*, a Gram-negative, anaerobic, non-motile, non-spore-forming, pleomorphic bacterium that is normally found within the gastrointestinal tract and feces of many animals, including rabbits. There are several subspecies of *F. necrophorum*, which may contribute to varying virulence and morphology (e.g., filamentous to rod-shaped). The most significant virulence factors contributing to dermal necrosis and disease are leukotoxin and the lipopolysaccharide found in the bacterial cell wall. Bacterial infection is presumed to occur following fecal contamination of traumatized skin or oral lesions, which may readily occur in a coprophagic animal such as the rabbit. Lesions of mild exudative to deep necrosuppurative dermatitis with induration, erythema, and inflammation may appear around the head, face, neck, and feet. Necrotizing fasciitis, osteomyelitis, septicemia, thromboembolism, and visceral abscessation and necrosis have also been reported in chronic and severe cases.

1.2.2.5 Pseudomoniasis
Pseudomonas aeruginosa is a ubiquitous aerobic, non-spore-forming, Gram-negative, rod-shaped bacterium that causes opportunistic disease in a range of hosts. The bacterium is found in the environment in soil and water and may colonize the skin. Bacterial colonies often have a mucoid phenotype in culture because of prolific bacterial production of surface polysaccharides. These polysaccharides form biofilms that protect the bacteria from common disinfectants, inhibit antibiotic penetration, and in some cases, are linked to genes conferring antibiotic resistance.

In rabbits, *P. aeruginosa* infections may produce moist or ulcerative dermatitis, or cutaneous or visceral abscesses. Moist dermatitis occurs most commonly on the face or forelimbs of animals with malocclusion and secondary ptyalism, and in animals that are maintained in wet housing conditions, or under the dewlap or between cutaneous folds in heavy rabbits. Moist dermatitis is characterized by serous to serosuppurative exudates with erythema, alopecia, and matting of hair around the lesion. Chronic lesions may ulcerate. The purulent debris and hair surrounding these lesions may be malodorous and have a characteristic bluish-green cast, caused by bacterial expression of pyocyanin, an exopigment and virulence factor.

1.2.2.6 Cutaneous Spirochetosis
Treponematosis (venereal spirochetosis, rabbit syphilis, vent disease) is caused by a Gram-negative

spirochete, *Treponema paraluiscuniculi*. The condition is not zoonotic and occurs sporadically in breeding and pet rabbits. The spirochete is transmitted horizontally to kits during suckling and during breeding in adult animals. Lesions develop 3–6 weeks following exposure and are most prominent on the mucocutaneous junctions of the genitalia, perianal skin, nose, mouth, and eyelids. The lesions begin as foci of erythema and edema and progress to papules or vesicles, followed by focal ulceration with crusting, and scaling or hyperkeratosis (Figure 1.3). Histologically, skin lesions may have moderate acanthosis, spongiosis, and orthokeratotic hyperkeratosis, with multifocal areas of erosion and ulceration. Typical argyrophilic long slender spirochetes may be seen within the serocellular crust with a Warthin-Starry stain.

Mild or subclinical disease is most common, but *T. paraluiscuniculi* infection has also been associated with abortion, metritis, and infertility in breeding does. This condition may present with similar cutaneous manifestations as for *Pasteurella multocida* infection (i.e., moist nasal dermatitis, cheilitis, conjunctivitis, and rhinitis). It is an important differential to consider as spirochetosis may be readily treated, whereas chronic pasteurellosis often requires repeated treatment and is rarely cured.

1.2.2.7 Laboratory Diagnostics

Bacterial dermatitis and abscesses are diagnosed via culture and sensitivity of lesions or exudate, cytology and/or skin biopsy. In-toto removal of abscesses is recommended to minimize environmental contamination. Increases in total white blood cell counts may not be seen with severe bacterial infections in rabbits; however, marked increases in relative neutrophil (heterophil) numbers may be noted. Most laboratories do not routinely

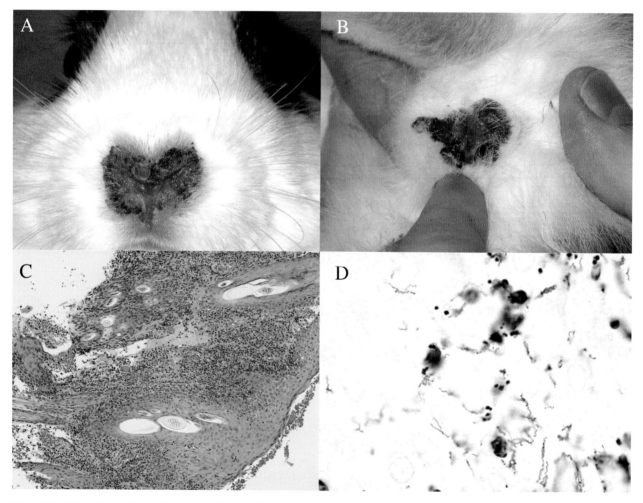

Figure 1.3 A: Focal ulceration and crusting of the nasal skin in a rabbit with cutaneous treponematosis. B: Venereal lesions on the same animal. C: Infection with *Treponema paraluiscuniculi* results in focal erosion with acanthosis, crusting, and moderate mixed, predominantly neutrophilic infiltrates. D: A Warthin-Starry stain demonstrates long, slender *T. cuniculi* spirochetes. *Source:* A and B: Courtesy of The Links Road Animal and Bird Clinic.

conduct phage typing for *S. aureus*, however, phage typing may be necessary to determine root causes of disease outbreaks.

The appearance and distribution of gross lesions of rabbit syphilis are often diagnostic. Diagnosis of *Treponema* sp. in formalin-fixed tissue sections requires Warthin-Starry silver staining to visualize the spirochetes, which may be few in number. Dark field microscopy of fresh scrapings of lesions and serological tests, including a hemagglutination test, fluorescent *Treponema* antigen preparation (FTA) and the Rapid Plasma Reagin (RPR) test, may be employed to aid in the diagnosis of this disease. However, anti-*Treponema* antibodies are slow to develop, requiring 5–6 weeks from the time lesions appear, suggesting that serology is less effective for diagnosing active cases.

1.2.2.8 Differential Diagnoses
Other possible causes of dermatitis include dermatophytosis, ectoparasitism, and contact allergy. Differential diagnoses for abscesses include cutaneous cysts, lipomas, cuterebriasis, hematoma, or neoplasia, such as lymphosarcoma. *Yersinia pestis* infection with cutaneous swellings ("bubos") occurs rarely in wild cottontail rabbits in the United States and may be transmitted to humans during handling of sick animals or carcass dressing.

1.2.2.9 Group or Herd Management
Staphylococcosis is a major cause of carcass condemnation at abattoirs, and induces significant morbidity, culling, and mortality in enzootically infected commercial rabbit meat operations due to visceral and cutaneous abscesses, and reproductive failure. Herd infection rates of up to 70% have been reported. In these situations, eradication via test and cull procedures and repopulation with clean animals is the only proven method of eliminating the agent from a herd. Interspecies transmission of *S. aureus* may occur, and appropriate hand-washing procedures should be in place after handling animals with suspect lesions.

Rabbit spirochetosis tends to be self-limiting, with spontaneous regression of lesions usually occurring within several weeks. Untreated rabbits can remain seropositive, suggesting a carrier state, possibly due to maintenance of the organism in regional lymph nodes. For these reasons, treatment of affected rabbits and other in-contact rabbits is the preferred method of control.

1.2.3 Dermatophytosis

Dermatophytosis (ringworm) is a superficial fungal infection of keratinized structures such as the hair, skin, and nails, and is a common clinical and subclinical entity in pet and commercial production rabbits. Disease is typically mild; however, the chronic treatment required for eradication, potential for cross-species transmission, including to humans, and persistence of spores in the environment makes this an agent of concern whenever it is diagnosed. *Trichophyton mentagrophytes* is the organism isolated most commonly from rabbits; however, *Microsporum* spp. may also infect rabbits. Young age, suboptimal housing environments, poor nutrition, and intercurrent disease may predispose animals to clinical disease. A carrier state is common in otherwise healthy rabbits with a reported prevalence rate of 4–36%.

Other types of deep or systemic mycoses or yeast infections in rabbits are rare. *Malassezia cuniculi* is a newly identified yeast cultured from the ear canal and inguinal areas of otherwise healthy rabbits but the organism has not been associated with clinical disease in the absence of predisposing factors, such as immunocompromise.

1.2.3.1 Presenting Clinical Signs
Typical presenting signs of dermatophytosis include non-pruritic or mildly pruritic, focal to patchy alopecia with erythema, and scaling of skin around the margins of the lesion. Surrounding hair shafts may be broken, with a stubbled appearance. Lesions are usually present on the face, extremities, and nail beds although they can be found anywhere on the body.

1.2.3.2 Pathology
Histologically, there is hyperkeratosis, epidermal and follicular acanthosis with mild neutrophilic to pyogranulomatous perivascular and intraepithelial dermatitis and folliculitis of affected skin. Arthroconidia and septate fungal hyphae are present in skin sections and may be visualized better following periodic acid-Schiff or Gomori's methenamine silver staining of sections.

1.2.3.3 Laboratory Diagnostics
Definitive diagnosis of dermatophytosis may be made from fungal culture of skin scrapings and debris, growth in Dermatophyte Medium (DTM), and microscopic evaluation of skin biopsies. Species-specific identification of the infecting organism requires culture and, possibly, molecular diagnostic methods.

1.2.3.4 Differential Diagnoses
Barbering or overgrooming, mechanical trauma, contact allergies, and external parasitism are potential differential diagnoses for dermatophytosis.

1.2.3.5 Group or Herd Management
Transmission of arthroconidia occurs by direct contact and via fomites. Infections are readily transmitted between animals that live in close proximity or that are

housed indoors at high densities. Because infectious material may remain viable in the environment for several years, environmental sanitation is as important as individual animal treatment for managing this disease. Dermatophyte infections are potentially zoonotic and may be spread to humans and other animals in the household or on premises. Appropriate hand-washing regimes should be in place after handling animals. Young, pregnant, or immunosuppressed animals or humans may be at increased risk of contracting the disease.

1.2.4 External Parasites

There are a number of important ectoparasitic infestations of rabbits, including fur and ear mites, fleas, lice, and myiasis, which may induce pruritus, alopecia, and dermatitis. Infestations with ectoparasites are usually readily identified during careful gross examination of the pelage and microscopic evaluation of skin biopsies may not be necessary. Presenting signs, pathology, and other diagnostic information for the most important external parasites of rabbits are detailed below.

1.2.4.1 Fur Mites

Fur mites are common in wild, pet, and commercial rabbits, and *Cheyletiella parasitovorax* ("walking dandruff") is isolated most frequently. It is a nonburrowing, actively moving mite with a broad host range, including humans, that lives on superficial debris and lymph secretions obtained by piercing the skin with chelicerae (paired piercing mouthparts). All life forms (i.e., larvae, nymph and adult) may be found on the host; however, the adult female mite may survive off the host for a week or longer. Presenting signs may include mild pruritus, flaking, scaling skin, seborrhea, and alopecia anywhere on the body, although many animals will be asymptomatic. Mites are pale yellowish-white, up to 0.54 mm long, and can be visualized moving around at the base of hair shafts with the unaided eye when the hair coat is parted (Figure 1.4). Diagnosis of an infestation is achieved best by direct observation or microscopic evaluation of a cellophane tape impression of the pelage. Characteristic morphologic features of adults include four pairs of legs each with a distal comb, instead of a claw. Histologic examination of skin biopsies may be nondiagnostic, and may show only orthokeratotic hyperkeratosis and mild acanthosis with superficial perivascular dermatitis.

Leporacarus gibbus (*Listrophorus gibbus*) is another common non-burrowing fur mite of wild and domestic rabbits that can be found on the dorsal flank, extremities, or almost anywhere on the pelage. It spends its entire life cycle on the host. Although widely considered to be nonpathogenic, the mite may induce mild pruritus, scaling, moist dermatitis, and alopecia in infested animals and

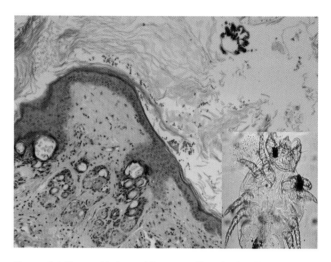

Figure 1.4 Dermatitis in a rabbit caused by *Cheyletiella parasitovorax*. Significant scaling dermatitis is present and there is minimal dermal inflammation. An adult mite can be seen in the superficial scale. Inset: Wet mount of *C. parasitovorax* mite. *Source:* Courtesy of C. Wheler.

may be diagnosed via methods as described above. It is readily seen, with the unaided eye or with a hand lens, as 0.2–0.5 mm long brown specks attached to the hair shaft. The mite is motile, brown, and laterally compressed with four pairs of legs and a projection from the head over the mouth parts. *L. gibbus* has specially adapted legs that allow it to cling to hair shafts. Human infestations resulting in erythematous and pruritic, papular dermatitis have also been reported.

1.2.4.2 Ear Mites

Otitis externa secondary to ear mite infestations is common in pet and meat-producing rabbits and is caused by *Psoroptes cuniculi*, a large, white, ovoid, highly motile, non-burrowing mite that is up to 0.7 mm long. *Psoroptes* sp. feed on lymph and cellular debris and pierce the skin with their mouthparts. Both mechanical trauma and hypersensitivity to mite feces are thought to induce irritation and inflammation. Early infestations may be inapparent, although experimental studies of acute and chronic *Psoroptes* infestations in rabbits have demonstrated decreased activity levels, chinning, and other abnormal behaviors. Heavy infestations lead to head shaking, ear drooping, intense pruritus with secondary excoriations, hyperemia, induration, serous exudation, and ulceration along with decreased food intake and body weight losses. A dense gray-brown serocellular crust may be visible within the ear canal (Figure 1.5). *Psoroptes* sp. are seen readily in scrapings of ear canal debris collected in mineral oil. Mite species should be verified to rule out sarcoptic and notoedric

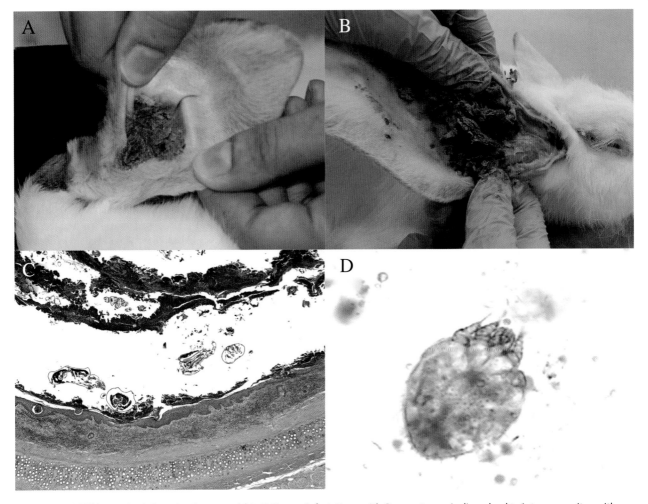

Figure 1.5 A: Mild ear mite infestation in a pet rabbit. B: Severe infestations with *Psorpoptes cuniculi* can lead to intense pruritus with excoriations and secondary bacterial infections, as in this rabbit with secondary dermatitis. C: Mites are readily noted feeding on the surface of the ear canal in microscopic section. D: A *Psoroptes cuniculi* mite from an ear swab. *Source:* A: Courtesy of The Links Road Animal and Bird Clinic.

mange, which may have more serious implications. Ectopic psoroptic dermatitis of the face and ventrum has been reported. Lesions include the appearance of thick serocellular crusts with erythematous borders, exudative dermatitis with matted hair, and accompanying alopecia.

Environmental treatment is critical with this agent as female mites can live off the host for several weeks, leading to re-infestation. *Psoroptes cuniculi* has a scrupulous host range and is not zoonotic.

1.2.4.3 Other Mites

Sarcoptic (*Sarcoptes scabiei var. cuniculi*) and notoedric (*Notoedres cati*) mange are uncommon in pet and commercial rabbits. Both of these burrowing arthropods are round with short stubby legs that do not project beyond the body margins, and blunt mouth parts. They are seen in less well-haired areas of the skin, including the face, legs, and ear canal, and induce an intense pruritus with marked inflammation, exudation, ulceration, secondary pyoderma, and anorexia. They can be detected only with deep skin scrapings or skin biopsy. Histologic features include parakeratotic hyperkeratosis and acanthosis, with epidermal neutrophilic infiltrates. Cross-sections of mites are present within the stratum corneum and demonstrate a thick chitinous cuticle with short appendages, skeletal muscle and a body cavity with gastrointestinal and reproductive tracts. Both mite species may infest human handlers.

Demodex cuniculi is rarely reported as a cause of clinical signs in rabbits, presenting as mild pruritus, seborrhea and focal to patchy alopecia. Mites have a typical narrow, elongated appearance and are present in the hair follicles, as per other *Demodex* spp. Whereas the prevalence of infestation is unknown, the pathologic significance is thought to be minor.

1.2.4.4 Cutaneous Myiasis

Both primary and secondary myiasis (fly strike) may occur in rabbits. Primary myiasis occurs when larvae penetrate living tissue to feed and develop (obligate host life cycle), whereas secondary myiasis occurs when flies that feed and develop on decomposing organic matter lay eggs on soiled or necrotic tissue of animals, with subsequent larval development (opportunistic host life cycle). Primary myiasis occurs in rabbits of all ages and health status, whereas secondary myiasis typically is seen in neglected or debilitated animals with open sores, moist dermatitis, or fecal or urine soiling of the hind end.

In North America, primary myiasis in rabbits is caused by botfly larvae (*Cuterebra* spp.) and wild and domestic species are susceptible. Human botfly (*Dermatobia hominis*) infestation of rabbits is seen in neotropical areas where this parasite is endemic. Rabbits that are housed or exercised outdoors are more likely to be infested with *Cuterebra* spp. larvae, and most infestations occur at hot, humid times of the year. Flies lay eggs on the tips of grasses at the entrance to the burrow or near the nest or cage. After hatching, larvae attach to the pelage of a passing host and are subsequently ingested during normal grooming. Most larvae migrate through the body to subcutaneous sites for further development, but they may also migrate to aberrant locations anywhere in the body. Presenting signs will depend on the migration site and number of larvae, but lesions generally appear as large, nonpainful fistulous swellings, approximately 1–3 cm diameter on the neck, dorsum, axillary, or inguinal areas (Figure 1.6). Each swelling contains a single larva and upon close examination, a breathing pore is present in the surface of the swelling. Larvae are white, cream or black with prominent spines over their body surface.

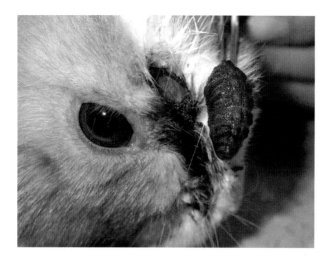

Figure 1.6 *Cuterebra* spp. larva being removed from the head of a rabbit. *Source:* Courtesy of The Links Road Animal and Bird Clinic.

A serosuppurative discharge may be present around the breathing pore with matting of the surrounding hair. Young rabbits with heavy infestations may become debilitated and anorexic, and death of a larva can lead to rapid shock and death of the host. Surgical removal of the larvae is curative. Left untreated, larvae will complete development in 1–2 months and emerge spontaneously from the cyst to pupate. Aberrant migration of larvae has been reported in the brains of pet rabbits housed outdoors during warm weather, with subsequent death. Larval migration tracts in the brain and spinal cord of these animals contained localized areas of malacia, necrosis, and hemorrhage with moderate mixed leukocytic infiltrates.

Secondary myiasis occurs when species of *Calliphorid* flies (blow flies) are attracted to oviposit on feces- or urine-stained matted hair or open, untreated wounds or areas of exudative dermatitis. Affected animals may be debilitated, obese, or suffer from diarrhea, neglect, or other conditions that hamper normal grooming, including malocclusion. Animals housed indoors or outdoors may be infested and warm, humid environments promote fly and larval development. Larvae (maggots) hatch within 24 hours or less and feed on superficial debris and necrotic tissue, contributing to a fetid odor. Larvae are visible grossly once matted hair and necrotic tissue are removed and debrided. Secondary bacterial infection of the necrotic, infested areas may occur and animals may die of shock or sepsis, regardless of treatment.

1.2.4.5 Fleas

Flea species infesting rabbits include *Cediopsylla simplex* and *Spilospyllus cuniculi*. In households with dogs or cats, indoor pet rabbits are more likely to be infested with *Ctenocephalides canis* or *C. felis*. Fleas and their feces (flea dirt) may be found on the face, ears, or within the pelage, particularly over the dorsal trunk, and animals may present with pruritus, alopecia, focal erythema, and scaling at the flea bite sites. Hypersensitivity to flea saliva has been reported in rabbits. Environmental decontamination and treatment of other susceptible household pets are important for eradication. In geographical areas where the diseases are prevalent, fleas can serve as a vector for myxomatosis, tularemia, and plague.

1.2.4.6 Lice

Haemodipsus ventricosus, the rabbit louse, is a sucking louse that affects domestic and wild rabbits, and wild hares. Infestation of pet and commercial rabbits is rare and associated with neglect or conditions of poor husbandry. The dorsal trunk is affected more commonly and presenting signs may include pruritus, alopecia, erythematous papules, anemia, weakness, and, if infestations are heavy, death. Lice are up to 2.5 mm in length and can be seen by the unaided eye. A diagnosis of pediculosis is usually possible following careful gross examination of the pelage. Lice will migrate away from the skin when the pelt is cooled and can be detected post-mortem on the tips of hairs after chilling the carcass for 30 minutes in a plastic bag. The eggs are large and ovoid and are cemented to the base of the hairs and are readily apparent. Transmission is by direct contact between animals or with contaminated bedding. As with fleas, lice can serve as a vector for myxomatosis, tularemia, and plague.

1.2.4.7 Ticks
Several species of ticks can parasitize pet and commercial rabbits. The rabbit tick, *Haemaphysalis leporispalustris*, is common in wild rabbits and may harbor various zoonotic bacteria and spirochetes, including *Borrelia burgdorferi*, as well as *Francisella tularensis*. Rabbit ticks rarely bite humans or other mammals. Severe infestations may lead to marked anemia and weakness.

1.2.4.8 Laboratory Diagnostics
In most instances, diagnosis of external parasitism is obvious in live animals or on gross examination of the carcass. Definitive diagnosis of sarcoptic, notoedric, or demodectic mange requires skin biopsy or deep skin scrapings. Speciation of mites, in particular, is important, as some are zoonotic or may infest other household pets.

1.2.4.8 Group or Herd Management
Quarantine of new arrivals should occur for at least two weeks before introducing new rabbits into a herd or household with other rabbits to minimize transmission of ectoparasites or other diseases to naive animals. Individual treatment of pet animals may be possible for mite and flea infestations. However, treatment and subsequent eradication of fur or ear mites from large breeding herds are difficult. Meat withdrawal times must be specified for any therapeutics given to meat-producing rabbits, and caution should be exercised when extrapolating ectoparasite treatments from other species. Organophosphate toxicity has been reported in rabbits associated with malathion dipping for mites. Environmental decontamination is important for all external parasites to minimize re-infestation of rabbits or other species. Owners should be educated regarding protecting pet rabbits from parasite transmission when rabbits are housed or exercised outside, and informed about potentially zoonotic diseases, including rabbit ectoparasites and diseases that they may transmit. Owners should be advised to seek medical attention if they experience any consistent signs of disease such as pruritus. Cases of suspect animal neglect, characterized by severe, untreated ectoparasitism, may require further investigation by local anti-cruelty agencies.

1.2.5 Mastitis
In commercial rabbit herds, mastitis (blue breast) is a significant cause of economic loss and suffering, and culling of breeding does, and may occur at any time during lactation. The common name for this condition arises from the cyanosis and necrosis seen in affected glands. Mastitis may occur also in pet or commercial pseudopregnant does.

1.2.5.1 Presenting Clinical Signs
Does with mastitis may present with one or more indurated, erythematous mammary glands that are painful. Animals may be depressed, lethargic, and pyrexic, and some animals will die acutely. Agalactia can occur and does may refuse to nurse kits, both factors resulting in subsequent kit mortality. Recrudescence of mastitis may occur in later lactations in does that recover and are rebred.

1.2.5.2 Pathology
Both acute gangrenous mastitis and chronic suppurative mastitis with secondary abscessation may occur, the differences in presentation likely attributable to bacterial virulence factors and host immunity. *Staphylococcus aureus* is isolated in the vast majority of cases, and *Pasteurella multocida* and *Streptococcus* spp. are less common. Enterotoxin from high virulence strains of *S. aureus* may induce immunosuppression in the host. Both the bacterial biotype and presence of various phages contribute to bacterial virulence.

The acute gangrenous form of mastitis is less common and gross signs include hemorrhage, edema, and cyanosis of the affected glands. In the more chronic form, glands are firm, with edema, necrosis, and purulent exudate noted on cut section. Teats overlying affected glands may become swollen and cyanotic, and a purulent to brown discharge may be present. Subcutaneous abscesses, pododermatitis, and pyometra also may be present in affected animals. The etiopathogenesis of the condition is unknown and may occur through trauma to the teats or glands, autoinoculation during grooming, or from kits, as kits from infected does have been demonstrated to infect naive does during suckling.

Histologically, there are marked neutrophilic infiltrates within the stroma of the affected gland, with lesser numbers of lymphocytes, plasma cells, and macrophages. Edema, hemorrhage, and necrosis may be present. Discrete abscesses and dense colonies of Gram-positive cocci are generally present in the affected areas. There may be full thickness necrosis of the overlying skin.

1.2.5.3 Laboratory Diagnostics
Bacterial cultures of draining fluid or biopsied or post mortem tissue should be conducted to confirm the

infectious agent. Cultures may be sterile, however, suggesting that exotoxins may be important in disease pathogenesis. Bacterial biotype and phage typing are not routinely performed on submitted samples and should be specifically requested, if needed.

1.2.5.4 Differential Diagnoses

Cutaneous myiasis, subcutaneous abscesses, and benign and malignant tumors should be considered as potential differential diagnoses in mature does with ventral cutaneous swellings.

1.2.5.5 Group or Herd Management

Because of the significant impact on overall operation, commercial breeding does with mastitis should be culled to minimize bacterial burden in the environment. Cages should be examined for rough edges or points, which may induce trauma. New entries into the herd should be quarantined for at least two weeks to minimize spread of infectious agents to naive animals. There is currently no vaccine available to prevent staphylococcosis in rabbits.

1.2.6 Cutaneous Masses and Neoplasia

While commercial laboratory and meat rabbits are usually relatively short-lived, various cutaneous masses are seen with increasing frequency in aged pet animals. Some tumors are virally mediated, and it is helpful for prognosis to classify masses based on malignant behavior and viral induction. Non-viral, benign neoplastic masses seen with regularity in rabbits include collagen hamartoma (sometimes reported as dermal fibrosis), collagenous nevus, cutaneous xanthoma, trichoblastoma, trichoepithelioma, fibroma, lipoma, and nonviral papilloma. Other cutaneous masses that are not virus-associated include squamous cell carcinomas (Figure 1.7A), basal cell tumors (Figure 1.7B), piloleiomyomas and piloleiomyosarcomas (Figure 1.8), keratoacanthomas, soft tissue sarcomas (Figure 1.9), fibrosarcomas, cutaneous lymphomas, and malignant melanomas. Melanomas are highly uncommon in pet rabbits, although both amelanotic and pigmented forms have been described. Viral-mediated non-malignant masses and lesions include Shope fibroma, cottontail rabbit papilloma, oral papillomatosis, leporid herpesvirus-4-induced lesions (LeHV-4; see Respiratory-LeHV4), and myxomatosis.

Invasive and recurrent post-vaccinal interscapular fibrosarcoma has been reported in a pet rabbit in Europe following vaccination with commercial products for myxoma virus and rabbit hemorrhagic disease virus. Tumor characteristics included marked proliferation of pleomorphic neoplastic fibroblasts amidst a background of multinucleated giant cells and infiltrating lymphocytes.

Various cutaneous glandular tumors are seen on occasion, including Meibomian gland adenoma, submandibular apocrine gland hyperplasia, adenoma and adenocarcinoma, mammary gland adenocarcinoma, and sebaceous adenocarcinoma of the external auditory ear canal. Some authors have reported rare cases of mesenchymal tumors in rabbits with cutaneous manifestations, such as myxosarcoma, giant cell sarcoma, eosinophil granulocytic sarcoma, osteosarcoma, leiomyosarcoma, or rhabdomyosarcoma (Figure 1.10), but these are uncommon. Stromal myxoid differentiation is reported frequently with anaplastic sarcomas and this has been

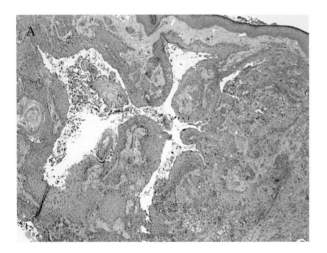 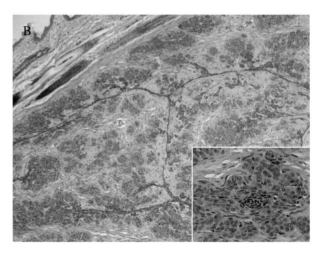

Figure 1.7 A: Invasive squamous cell carcinoma with disordered epithelial maturation and formation of keratin pearls in the pinna of a rabbit. B: A well-differentiated basal cell tumor from the neck of a rabbit. Inset: The tumor is moderately cellular, well-demarcated, multilobular, unencapsulated, and composed of basilar cells arranged in variably sized islands, separated by a moderately dense fibrous stroma.

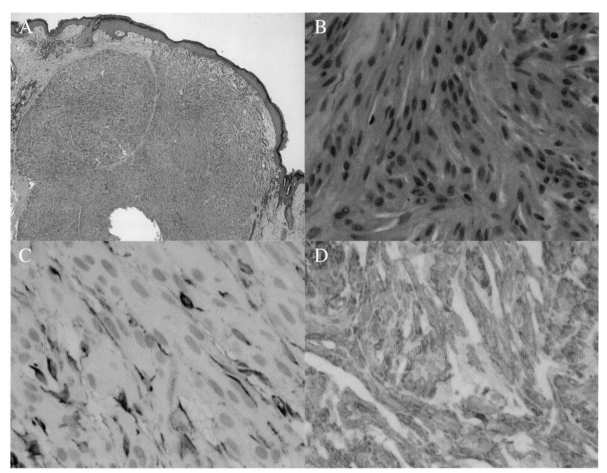

Figure 1.8 A: Cutaneous mass from a 9-year-old neutered female rabbit. The mass is round, raised, and circumscribed but not encapsulated, and composed of plump eosinophilic interweaving spindle to strap-like cells resembling smooth muscle cells. B: The strap-like tumor cells resemble the arrector pili muscles associated with the nearby hair follicles. Nuclei within these strap-like cells are round to ovoid to rectangular with mild anisokaryosis and no mitotic figures are seen. C: Tumor cells are positively labelled for vimentin. D: Tumor cells have strongly positive cytoplasmic labeling for smooth muscle actin, consistent with a diagnosis of piloleiomyoma.

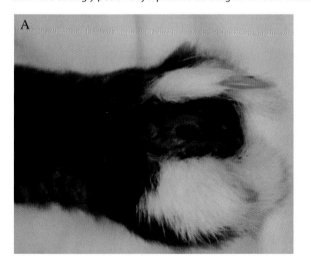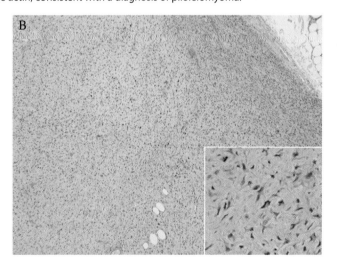

Figure 1.9 A: An invasive soft tissue sarcoma of the foot of a rabbit. B: Tissue from a large, lobulated scapular mass in a 9 year-old male rabbit. Smaller nodules were present in the lung and aorta. The mass is composed of a monotypic population of spindle cells within an abundant fibrovascular stroma. Inset: The cells have indistinct cellular borders, abundant eosinophilic fibrillar cytoplasm, convoluted angular nuclei, and there is 4-fold anisocytosis and anisokaryosis, with rare mitoses. A poorly differentiated sarcoma was diagnosed.
Source: A: Courtesy of The Links Road Animal and Bird Clinic.

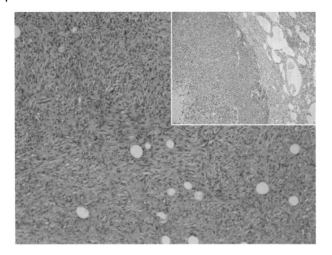

Figure 1.10 Rhabdomyosarcoma of the heart, skin (depicted) and lung (inset). Multiple variably-sized nodules of spindle cells forming whorls and clusters are seen within the dermis. The neoplastic cells have variably-sized nuclei, a strap-like appearance, and up to 5 mitoses/400x field. Immunohistochemistry of the tumor demonstrated positive cytoplasmic labeling for vimentin (inset: lung mass, counterstain: Mayer's hematoxylin) and muscle actin, but the tumor was negative for S100 and smooth muscle actin.

suggested as a rabbit-specific phenotypic characteristic. All tumor types have similar characteristics to those seen in other companion animal species and the long-term prognosis is based on adequacy of resection of tumor margins, cellular atypia, necrosis, pleiomorphism, mitoses, and metastases. Masses that are more common or that are specific to rabbits are discussed in greater detail below.

1.2.6.1 Laboratory Diagnostics

Fine needle aspirates and surgical or excisional biopsies are highly recommended when cutaneous masses are noted in rabbits to differentiate between infectious and neoplastic diseases. Additional testing may be required to confirm suspected viral infections, including serology, virus isolation, electron microscopy, and immunohistochemistry.

1.2.6.2 Collagen Hamartoma

Collagenous hamartoma (collagen nevus) is a very common nonneoplastic proliferative lesion seen in most breeds and both sexes of rabbits. Usually, masses are noted by the owner on the ventral abdomen or dorsum and present as nonpainful firm discrete masses or plaques, sometimes with sparse overlying hair or alopecia (Figure 1.11). Histologically, they are bland in appearance, consisting of localized dense collagen aggregates and scattered fibroblasts within the dermis with no evidence of dermal inflammation. The overlying epithelium and adnexal structures may be mildly attenuated and atrophic.

1.2.6.3 Trichoblastoma

Trichoblastoma is one of the most common tumor types seen in rabbits and these tumors are usually benign and slow-growing. Solitary masses may be found anywhere on the body, and are seen equally in males and females. Historically, many of these masses were identified as basal cell tumors; however, because of morphologic similarities to tumors seen in dogs and cats, they are identified more correctly as trichoblastomas. The tumor is thought to derive from primitive follicular cells within the dermis and there are several subclassifications, based

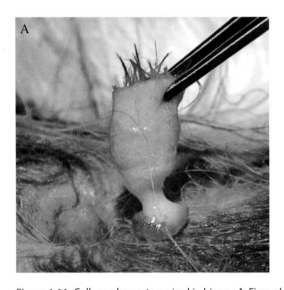
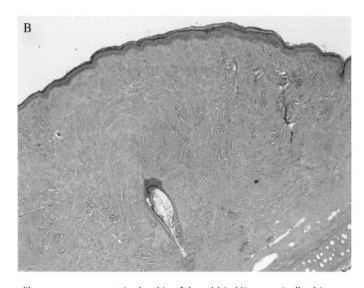

Figure 1.11 Collagen hamartoma in skin biopsy. A: Firm, plaque-like mass was present in the skin of the rabbit. Microscopically, this mass consisted of dense collagen aggregates. B: Tissue from a firm, raised, white mass on a rabbit ear. The dermis is expanded by dense hypocellular bundles of mature connective tissue containing remnants of follicular structures and is covered by mildly hyperplastic epithelium, consistent with a collagen nevus (hamartoma). *Source:* A: Courtesy of The Links Road Animal and Bird Clinic.

on the microscopic appearance. Grossly, nodules may be exophytic or ulcerated and vary in size. On cut section, they are often multilobular and are distinguished readily from the surrounding epithelial and dermal tissue. Histologically, a mild to moderate collagenous stroma supports expansile lobules, ribbons, and trabeculae of basophilic neoplastic cells. Squamous differentiation may be present. Cells at the periphery of lobules may have a palisading appearance. Tumors are not transmissible and surgical resection is curative.

1.2.6.4 Cutaneous Lymphoma

Cutaneous lymphoma is reported rarely in rabbits and may occur in association with systemic lymphosarcoma (B cell-mediated; nonepitheliotropic lymphoma) or be limited to the skin (T cell-mediated; epitheliotropic lymphosarcoma or mycosis fungoides). Animals may present with alopecic plaques or nodules of thickened, erythematous skin with superficial ulcers and crusting. The lesion may be mildly pruritic and can occur on any part of the body. Histologically, there is focal edema and marked infiltration of the epidermis and superficial and deep dermis with neoplastic lymphocytes, and, in some cases, superficial ulceration with a serous crust. Small clusters of neoplastic lymphocytes may be seen within the epithelium (Pautrier's microabscesses) or surrounding hair follicle epithelium. Epitheliotropic lymphoma is described typically as being of T cell origin in humans and animals. Immunophenotyping of tumor cells with CD3 markers has not been performed routinely in rabbits, hindering comparisons with similar tumors in other companion animals.

1.2.6.5 Giant Cell Sarcoma

Giant cell sarcomas are an uncommon tumor of rabbits. In humans, they are thought to originate from the bone but they are poorly characterized in rabbits and the origin is unknown. All breeds may be affected and masses are most frequently noted in older rabbits. These isolated cutaneous tumors may be found anywhere on the body but are seen most commonly on a limb. The microscopic appearance is consistent with a highly anaplastic sarcoma with poorly demarcated boundaries. Tumors consist of dense streams of spindloid to stellate cells within a myxoid stroma and with scattered multinucleated giant cells. There is marked anisocytosis and anisokaryosis of neoplastic cells and mitoses are abundant. Metastases have been reported and local recurrence may be seen with incomplete resection. Using immunohistochemical labeling, neoplastic cells typically demonstrate positive cytoplasmic labeling for vimentin and smooth muscle actin but are negative for S-100 and desmin.

A vimentin-positive, multilobular and cystic invasive synovial myxoma has been reported on the caudal thigh of a pet rabbit. Multinucleated giant cells were not a feature of this tumor; lobules of neoplastic tissue were surrounded by reactive bone and neoplastic cells induced a marked plasmacytic inflammation.

1.2.6.6 Papillomas

Papillomas are superficial, nonpainful, usually benign verrucoid or hornlike growths that occur generally on haired skin or in and around the oral cavity of rabbits. Several variants of papillomas are recognized, at least two of which are virally-induced. Spontaneously regressing nonviral papillomas occur in rabbits and present as solitary polypoid masses with a smooth or exophytic surface (Figure 1.12). Occasionally, rectoanal papillomas are reported that protrude from the anus, leading to tenesmus and frank hemorrhage, if the tissue is friable. Complete surgical excision is curative (Figure 1.13)

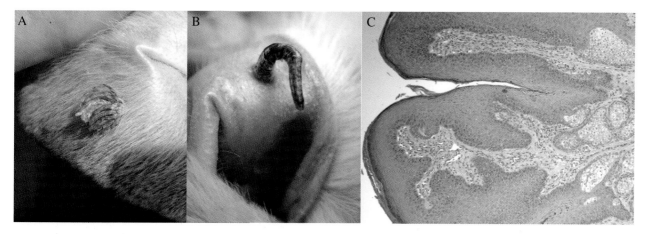

Figure 1.12 A: A verrucoid papilloma on the ear of a rabbit. B: A more keratinized papilloma on a rabbit ear. Papillomas can occur anywhere on the body but are more common on the head and face. C: Oral papilloma from the external surface of the lip of a rabbit, demonstrating sebaceous differentiation. *Source:* A: Courtesy of The Links Road Animal and Bird Clinic.

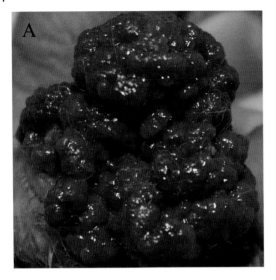
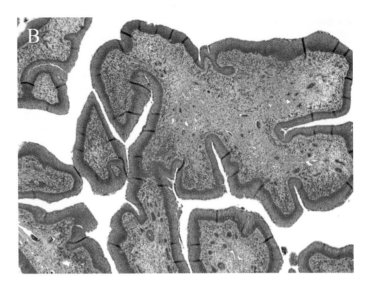

Figure 1.13 A: A rectoanal papilloma in a rabbit presenting with tenesmus. B: Microscopically, there is moderate acanthosis and folding of the epithelium and a dense fibrovascular underlying matrix with a mild, mixed, predominantly neutrophilic dermal infiltrate. *Source:* A: Courtesy of The Links Road Animal and Bird Clinic.

Rabbit oral papilloma virus (ROPV), a double-stranded DNA virus within the family Papillomaviridae, may induce oral lesions in young rabbits up to 18 months of age. Lesions present as multiple non-ulcerated exophytic masses on the gingiva, around the teeth, and under the tongue. The frequency of viral infection may approach 33% in some herds. Conjunctival papillomas have also been reported in a Flemish giant rabbit that may have been immunocompromised by other disease. Histologically, masses are well demarcated, do not involve the dermis, and are characterized by marked hyperkeratosis and acanthosis with spongiosis and epithelial cytoplasmic vacuolation. Basophilic intranuclear inclusion bodies may be present within vacuolated cells of the stratum spinosum and viral particles can be demonstrated by electron microscopy. Regressing masses may additionally demonstrate moderate lymphocytic infiltrates. Tumors regress spontaneously, a process dependent upon cell-mediated immunity, and lifelong immunity is conferred.

Cottontail rabbit papilloma virus (CRPV; Shope papilloma) induces benign papillomas in the eastern cottontail species (*Sylvilagus floridanus*) that spontaneously regress with development of virus-directed cell-mediated immunity. The virus was used extensively as a model for human papilloma vaccine development. CRPV may be transmitted to domestic rabbits (*Oryctolagus cuniculus*) by arthropod vectors or direct contact with cottontail rabbits; however, the agent does not appear to be transmissible between domestic rabbits. In the domestic rabbit, the virus may induce multifocal, firm, dry horny growths on the head and face. In some animals, malignant

induction occurs with progression to in situ squamous cell carcinoma. Transformation may be exacerbated by ultraviolet light exposure, because the virus is thought to inhibit DNA repair induced by ultraviolet damage.

1.2.6.7 Myxomatosis

Myxomatosis is a systemic viral disease with primary cutaneous manifestations. It is caused by a large double-stranded, enveloped DNA poxvirus that persists in the environment. The disease is more common in summer months, being spread passively by arthropod vectors, such as biting flies, fleas, and mosquitoes, or by direct contact of infected objects or surfaces with open wounds or other cutaneous lesions. The virus is enzootic in many wild rabbit populations (*Sylvilagus* spp.), in which clinical signs are generally localized and self-limiting, appearing as a cutaneous fibroma, but the virus induces severe disease with high mortality in domestic rabbits. The virus was introduced into the wild Australian rabbit population in 1950 in an attempt to biologically control the burgeoning population and was initially effective, inducing significant mortality. However, the virus has since become host-adapted and enzootic. The virus may predispose infected animals to acquire other bacterial and viral infections because of immunosuppressant effects.

Myxomatosis is not a disease generally seen in North American pet or commercial rabbits, although it is enzootic in the wild rabbit population in northern California. The condition remains an important cause of morbidity and loss in commercial and pet rabbits in South America, Europe, Asia, and Australia. Disease control in these countries is achieved by vaccination with a live attenuated Shope fibroma virus product. Vaccine immunity is reportedly short-lived. Control of arthropod vectors is also important for minimizing disease occurrence.

Presenting Clinical Signs Many viral strains have been identified and there are at least two clinical forms of myxomatosis that are recognized: the classical myxomatous form and the amyxomatous form. In the more common myxomatous form, animals present with depression, anorexia, pyrexia, lethargy, generalized swelling of the face and eyelids, purulent nasal discharge and conjunctivitis, and with firm subcutaneous plaques or discrete nodules. Death usually ensues in 20–100% of affected animals within 10 days to three weeks, due to severe virus-induced immunosuppression with overwhelming secondary Gram-negative bacterial sepsis and multi-organ failure. Death can be peracute because of severe pulmonary edema and systemic shock. In the amyxomatous form, the major presenting signs are respiratory disease and conjunctivitis; viral transmission appears to be by aerosol, and mortality is higher, killing >85% of affected animals.

Pathology In the myxomatous form of the disease, the cutaneous plaques and nodules have a mucoid appearance on cut section. Microscopically, they are bland looking, consisting of streams of mesenchymal cells within a loose, pale, basophilic, edematous, and myxomatous stroma with associated nonsuppurative inflammation. The overlying epidermis may be hyperplastic or ulcerated and crusted. Eosinophilic intracytoplasmic inclusion bodies may be seen within the epidermis or follicular cells, in addition to syncytial cells. Viral replication occurs in local lymph nodes, leading to lympholysis and depletion, and the virus disseminates to other internal organs. There are few to no cutaneous signs in the atypical form and lesions are those of severe pneumonia, often compounded by pre-existing bacterial bronchopneumonia.

Histologically, if no viral inclusion bodies are present, single cutaneous masses can be difficult to distinguish from those caused by infection with Shope fibroma virus or a myxosarcoma. Other ancillary tests including virus isolation, PCR, or electron microscopy may be indicated to confirm a diagnosis.

1.2.6.7 Shope Fibromatosis
Shope fibromatosis is induced by a rabbit poxvirus (Shope fibroma virus), which is antigenically distinct from myxoma virus that is enzootic within cottontail populations in North America. Sporadic outbreaks of the virus are reported in domestic rabbits with outdoor access. In the natural host, the virus induces benign, raised plaque-like subcutaneous fibrous proliferations

on the trunk, legs, feet, and head, which regress spontaneously with development of cell-mediated immunity. Histologically, tumors consist of marked fibroblast aggregations within a dense collagenous or myxomatous stroma with moderate nonsuppurative inflammation. Rare eosinophilic intracytoplasmic inclusion bodies may be seen within fibroblasts. There is moderate overlying hyperkeratosis, downgrowth of rete pegs, ballooning degeneration of epithelial cells, and prominent keratohyalin granules. The virus may be transmitted to domestic rabbits via mosquitoes and biting flies, where it induces similar lesions. Systemic and lethal disease may occur in very young rabbits infected with this virus. A differential diagnosis for this infection is a spindle cell tumor.

1.2.6.8 Mammary Gland Tumors
Mammary gland hyperplasia (both cystic and noncystic forms), dysplasia, adenoma, adenocarcinoma, and matrix-producing carcinomas are seen periodically in intact aging does. Although rare, mammary tumors may also occur in intact bucks. Lesions are seen typically in animals at least 5 years of age and present as one or more nonpainful enlarged glands with clear to brown discharge. The teat associated with the affected gland may be discolored or enlarged. In does, mammary gland abnormalities are often seen in conjunction with endometrial hyperplasia, uterine adenocarcinoma (in approximately 30% of does in one study) or prolactin-secreting pituitary adenoma (see also Sections 1.3.1 and 1.9.6). In rabbits with pituitary adenomas, serum levels of prolactin in affected animals are reported to be 10- to 1000-fold greater than normal. It is not known whether mammary tumors are associated with hormonal imbalances or other disease in males. Cyclosporine-induced mammary gland hyperplasia and atypia is reported in both male and female rabbits and hyperplasia is exacerbated by co-treatment with methylprednisolone, a potent immunosuppressant in rabbits. Cyclosporine interferes with prolactin binding and may contribute to hyperprolactinemia in affected animals, which may induce mammary hyperplasia. Rabbits have more prolactin receptors in their mammary glands than do other species, which may predispose them to this treatment effect.

Histologically, mammary tumors may be firm with either or both a cystic or solid appearance (Figure 1.14). In cystic hyperplasia, multiple coalescing nodules may be present in solid, tubular or papillary arrangements supported by a fine to moderate fibrovascular stroma, with central secretion of proteinaceous fluid containing sloughed epithelial cells and macrophages. In solid neoplastic masses, lobules are hypercellular and contain nests and cords of neoplastic epithelial cells, often arranged as tubules or acini, set within in a dense

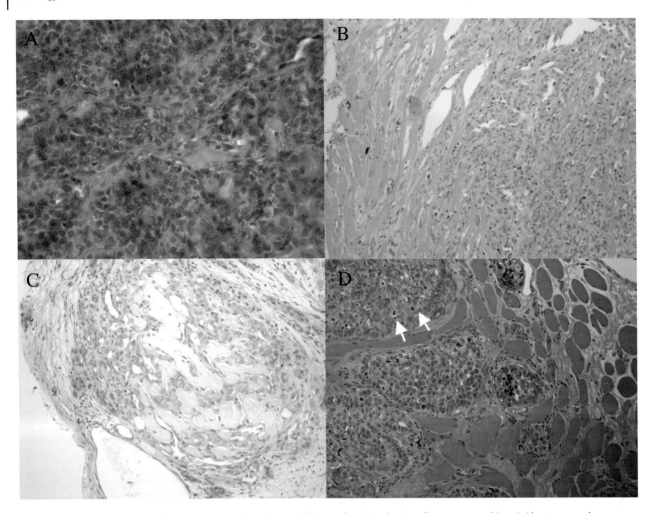

Figure 1.14 A: Mammary gland adenocarcinoma in a 4-year-old intact doe. Neoplastic cells are arranged in acini but are poorly differentiated and there is jumbling of layers. Mitoses are 8-10/400x field. B: This tumor had metastasized widely to the heart (B) and lungs, with local seeding of inguinal tissues (C). D: Mammary tumors in bucks are often highly aggressive, as seen with this mass, which is invading the subcutis and associated muscle (arrows point to abundant mitotic figures).

fibrovascular stroma. Neoplastic cells may be polygonal with distinct cell borders and contain a central nucleus and variable numbers of nucleoli. Acini may contain proteinaceous material. A myxoid stroma may be seen in matrix-producing tumors. Mitoses vary with the aggressiveness of the neoplasm, more aggressive tumors may also contain hemorrhagic and necrotic areas. Larger masses may ulcerate, and metastasis to local lymph nodes and lungs is seen late in the course of the disease. In one study, invasive tumors with high mitotic rates and containing myoepithelial differentiation had a 17% recurrence rate after surgical removal. Metastatic tumors may also occur in bucks, and in one case, led to severe dyspnea and death from pulmonary metastases 6 months after the primary mammary tumor was resected. Immunohistochemistry with both calponin (a cytoplasmic marker) and p63 (a nuclear marker) may be helpful in distinguishing noninvasive tumors from more invasive ones. Both will label nonneoplastic myoepithelial cells surrounding ductal structures; these cells are generally not present in more invasive carcinomas.

Fibromatous mammary gland hyperplasia has been reported in male and female rabbits treated with cyclosporine. Lesions reverse spontaneously with cessation of drug administration.

1.2.7 Pododermatitis

The undersides of rabbit feet lack footpads and are covered with dense fur. Chronic ulcerative and granulomatous or pyogranulomatous lesions (sore hocks) of varying size can sometimes be found on the plantar surfaces of the skin overlying the metatarsal bones of the feet (Figure 1.15). Lesion development is generally attributed to obesity, genetics, and breed predisposition, e.g., Rex rabbits, wire flooring, trauma to the feet or wet or dirty bedding.

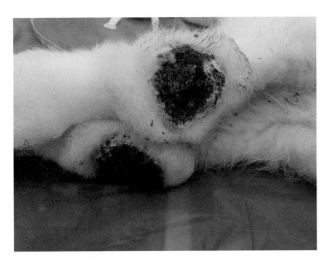

Figure 1.15 Bilateral, chronic, ulcerative pododermatitis in a breeding doe housed in a wire bottom cage.

Prevalence of pododermatitis is higher in neutered adult female rabbits and bedding rabbits on hay seems to reduce the risk of developing the condition. Animals presenting with pododermatitis may be very painful and reluctant to move. This condition is a significant cause of morbidity and culling in commercial breeding operations.

1.2.7.1 Pathology

Lesions begin as focal patches of hyperkeratosis of the skin overlying the epiphyses of the metatarsal bones and will progress eventually to ischemic cutaneous necrosis and ulceration, which may become secondarily infected with bacteria, typically *Staphylococcus aureus.* Suppuration may be present under a superficial crust. Well-established lesions may not resolve, even with aggressive debridement, and tendonitis and osteomyelitis may be seen as sequelae.

1.2.7.2 Group or Herd Management

This condition is largely preventable by ensuring that animals are housed in large enough enclosures that permit free movement; that enclosures are kept well bedded, clean and dry; that flooring is atraumatic, and that animal weight is managed by an appropriate diet.

1.2.8 Other Skin Conditions

1.2.8.1 Fur Chewing

Fur chewing (barbering) may be seen in both males and females and may occur anywhere on the body of the rabbit or may result from the actions of a conspecific cagemate. This is an abnormal behavior, and potential causes include boredom, dietary insufficiencies, inadequate fiber, overcrowding, or other types of behavioral maladjustments. If skin biopsies are taken, the hair

follicles and shafts within the dermis are seen to be intact, with the hair shaft broken off at the epidermis. There is usually no to minimal inflammation of the surrounding epidermis.

1.2.8.2 Sebaceous Adenitis

Sebaceous adenitis (exfoliative dermatosis) is a nonpruritic, sporadic, dermatologic condition seen predominantly in older adults resulting in patchy to generalized areas of alopecia and scaling, surrounded by an erythematous border. Early lesions consist of hyperkeratosis and pyogranulomatous inflammation centered on sebaceous glands, but in more chronic lesions, mixed infiltrates of lymphocytes, plasma cells, and macrophages predominate and sebaceous glands may no longer be present. Lymphocytic folliculitis and interface dermatitis have also been reported in some rabbits chronically affected with this condition. Some cases have been associated with underlying thymoma. The etiology is thought to be immune-mediated based on T cell infiltration around sebaceous glands and hair follicles, and good clinical response to cyclosporine therapy; however, further investigation is required as disease triggers are unknown. Differential diagnoses for this condition include fungal infections, nutritional disorders, ectoparasite infestation, and epitheliotropic lymphoma.

1.2.8.3 Contact Dermatitis

Rabbit skin is sensitive and rabbits may develop hypersensitivity to environmental allergens in a manner similar to other species. Animals may present with focal pruritus, alopecia, and scaling dermatitis. Most reports are anecdotal.

1.2.8.4 Frostbite

Frostbite is reported occasionally in pet rabbits. Typically, this condition results in ischemic necrosis and sloughing of the distal ear tips but toes may also be affected. Differentials for frostbite include trauma, intraspecific aggression (Figure 1.16A) and perivascular injections of irritating substances.

1.2.8.5 Cutaneous Asthenia

Cutaneous asthenia (Ehlers-Danlos-like syndrome, dermatosparaxis) has been reported rarely in pet rabbits. Animals with this condition may present with multifocal nonpruritic and nonhealing wounds. Tearing of the skin may occur during attempts to gently restrain animals or evaluate dermal hydration (Figure 1.17). The condition refers to a genetically transmitted connective tissue disorder, often secondary to a deficiency in procollagen N-peptidase, leading to marked skin fragility and abnormal elasticity. Recognizable microscopic alterations may not be visible in affected skin when compared to skin from unaffected animals. Decreased dermal thickness may be

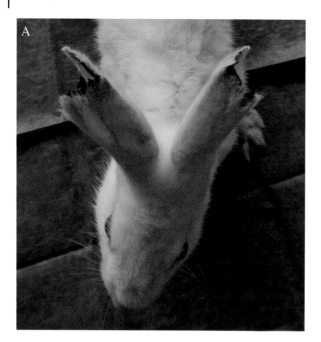

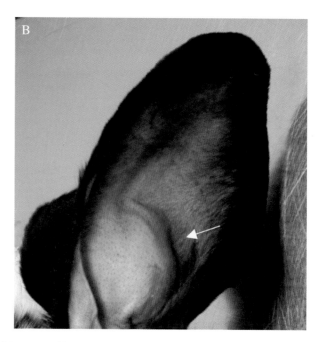

Figure 1.16 A: Ear trauma from cagemates in a young preweaned rabbit. B: Aural hematoma in a rabbit. *Source:* B: Courtesy of The Links Road Animal and Bird Clinic.

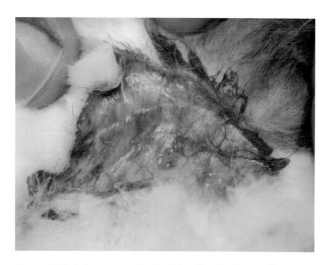

Figure 1.17 Cutaneous asthenia (Ehlers-Danlos-like syndrome) in a young rabbit with very fragile skin that tore easily. *Source:* Courtesy of The Links Road Animal and Bird Clinic.

evident microscopically, although this may be difficult to gauge, depending upon the area of skin evaluated. Ultrastructural and immunohistochemical studies may be needed to demonstrate abnormal collagen content and fibril orientation. In humans, at least 10 subtypes of Ehlers-Danlos-like syndrome are recognized, some with autosomal dominant, autosomal recessive and X-linked recessive transmission. The mode of disease transmission is unknown in rabbits.

1.2.8.6 Actinic Keratosis

Actinic keratosis has been reported sporadically in rabbits and may result from excessive exposure to UVB radiation. The condition presents as epidermal scaling, crusting, and erythema, particularly in nonpigmented and less haired areas, such as the pinnae. Orthokeratotic hyperkeratosis, dermal fibrosis, and basal cell dysplasia may be seen in sections of affected skin. Corneal damage (photokeratitis) may also be present in affected rabbits. Differential diagnoses for the nonpruritic scaling, crusting, and erythema include thymoma and hypersensitivity reactions. Rabbits exposed to environmental allergens may develop hot, swollen, erythematous ears with secondary overgrooming (presumably because of the irritation), and self-induced trauma, leading to crusting.

1.2.8.7 Lyme Borreliosis

Natural infections with *Borrelia burgdorferi* infections have not been reported to date in domestic rabbits; however, wild rabbits are a natural reservoir for the spirochete, which is transmitted by the rabbit tick, *Haemaphysalis leporispalustris.* In experimental studies, classic cutaneous Lyme disease lesions were induced in New Zealand white rabbits and consisted of localized erythema and induration of injection sites. Numerous spirochetes were readily visible in cutaneous biopsies of the affected areas. Pet rabbits that spend time outdoors in direct contact with grass in regions in which the tick and spirochete are prevalent may be at risk.

1.3 Endocrine Conditions

There are very few reports of spontaneous endocrine disorders in rabbits. Disorders related to imbalances in calcium homeostasis are common and the pathologist should be aware of metabolic differences in the rabbit compared with other domestic animal species (see Eckerman-Ross, 2008 for a detailed review).

Calcium homeostasis is predominantly under the control of parathyroid hormone (PTH), calcitonin, and vitamin D. In rabbits, in contrast to other species, uptake of calcium from the gastrointestinal tract is largely unregulated and is proportional to the level of the calcium in the diet. Calcium is absorbed by passive diffusion whereas absorption of dietary phosphorus is under the control of vitamin D_3. Plasma levels of calcium may be higher than for other species, and urinary excretion of calcium is proportional to dietary intake rather than metabolic need. Up to 60% of ingested calcium may be excreted in the urine as calcium carbonate monohydrate and anhydrous calcium carbonate, and together with ammonium magnesium phosphate crystals lead to a thick, opaque color and consistency. Changes in urine pH may lead to urolithiasis (see Section 1.8.1.3 for further information). PTH levels are detectable in rabbits even at high serum calcium concentrations, and are thought to function to increase calcium reabsorption from the distal nephron and bone. Intestinal calcium absorption is largely independent of serum vitamin D_3 levels, however, vitamin D deficiency results in decreased renal excretion of phosphorus and calcium. Vitamin D-dependent active transcellular transport of calcium from the intestine does occur when dietary calcium levels are low.

1.3.1 Other Endocrine Conditions

A colony of spontaneously diabetic New Zealand white rabbits was bred for research use for several decades in the United States. Histologically, these animals displayed hypergranulation of β-cells within pancreatic islets, suggestive of a defect in insulin secretion rather than a lack of insulin production, but no other morphologic changes were noted.

Adrenal gland masses have been reported in two neutered male pet rabbits. In both cases, animals became aggressive before clinical presentation and had elevated serum testosterone levels compared with rabbits without adrenal gland masses. Unilaterally enlarged adrenal glands were noted during laparotomy and reported to be consistent with adrenal gland hyperplasia and carcinoma, respectively.

Several reports exist for **prolactin-secreting pituitary adenomas** in does. Cystic mammary gland hyperplasia and dysplasia with teat enlargement and discoloration are often the first clinical signs noted in affected animals. Affected animals may present additionally with thinning of the pelage. Prolactin levels in affected animals ranged from 22 ng/mL to 2.2 µg/mL (reference range 1.7–2.7 ng/mL) and more mammary glands may be affected with increasing serum prolactin levels. Pituitary glands were enlarged up to 10-fold by acidophil adenomas, consisting of encapsulated cords and trabeculae of neoplastic cells with few mitoses supported by a fine fibrovascular stroma, which compressed the surrounding normal parenchyma.

No spontaneous tumors have been described for the thyroid or parathyroid glands of rabbits.

1.4 Respiratory Conditions

Rabbits are obligate nose breathers since the epiglottis is engaged over the caudal margin of the soft palate, and they have an acute sense of smell. A longitudinal septum divides the nasal cavities into two and the ventromedial nasal meatus extends the nasal cavities into the oropharynx. The nasolacrimal duct passes on each side through the orbital fossa to connect medially to the nasal cavity. There are three lobes to each lung; cranial, middle and caudal. Subclinical or clinical respiratory disease is very common in pet and commercial meat rabbits and may predispose these animals to sudden death during handling or anesthetic induction. Transfer of fomites and infectious particles between animals is further aggravated by the high density under which these animals are housed in commercial operations, especially if the ventilation is suboptimal. Further, because of the very close apposition of dental structures to nasal and paranasal sinuses in the rabbit, severe dental disease can impinge upon nasal structures.

Rabbits have a small thorax for their size and abundant abdominal viscera such that when they are anesthetized and placed in dorsal recumbency for surgery, it may be difficult for animals to ventilate spontaneously, especially if there is underlying intercurrent respiratory disease. Thus, hypoxemia and subsequent sudden death may be seen following anesthesia if animals have not been adequately ventilated.

1.4.1 Pasteurellosis

Pasteurellosis remains a very significant clinical and subclinical respiratory condition largely of domestic rabbits, although the bacterium has also been cultured from wild eastern cottontails (*Sylvilagus* sp.). It is frequently carried as an inapparent infection by rabbits and has an estimated prevalence of infection of up to 94%. Pasteurellosis is a significant cause of culling of breeding does and production loss in commercial settings. Although strains of

Pasteurella multocida are typically species-specific, similar strains have been detected between rabbits and co-housed sheep, poultry, and cats. Bacterial pathogenicity is conferred by various enzymes and toxins released by the bacteria, including hyaluronidase, neuraminidase, dermato- and osteolysins, and endotoxin, as well as fimbriae that enhance adherence to cell surfaces. Various subspecies of *P. multocida* exist but are rarely characterized by diagnostic labs further than initial speciation. One European study reported that *Pasteurella canis* was cultured from 5% of suspect *Pasteurella* cases received.

1.4.1.1 Presenting Clinical Signs

Rabbits affected with *P. multocida* may present with sneezing and mucopurulent discharge or crusting around the nares, and exudate may be present on the forepaws as a consequence of grooming (Figure 1.18). The nasolacrimal duct is often blocked resulting in chronic epiphora and conjunctivitis and clinical or subclinical uni- or bilateral otitis media/interna may be present. Whereas the respiratory form of pasteurellosis predominates, peracute septicemia, reproductive failure and abortions, and superficial or deep abscessation may occur, and these conditions will present according to the system affected. Sudden death following anesthetic induction is a very common presenting sign for both clinically and subclinically affected pet rabbits.

1.4.1.2 Pathology

Pasteurellosis may occur in several forms, including epizootics of peracute pneumonia with high mortality; chronic respiratory disease with fibrinopurulent bronchopneumonia, conjunctivitis and otitis media; local or systemic abscesses; and metritis or orchitis. Miliary hepatic necrosis may be seen in septicemia cases. The tympanic bullae should always be inspected when pasteurellosis is suspected. Chronically infected animals with rhinitis may have turbinate atrophy and lysis of the tympanic bullae as a result of bacterial osteolytic toxin production and concurrent inhibition of osteoblast activity. Acute fibrinous pleuropneumonia is characterized by fibrinohemorrhagic lobar pneumonia and pleuritis, frequently with concurrent hemipyothorax and pericarditis (Figure 1.19). In females with genital infections, vaginal exudate is typically purulent, thick, and gray to yellow. Localized abscesses may affect various tissues including myocardium, brain, testes, muscle, and subcutis, and tend to be well encapsulated and contain thick, white, purulent material. Chronic abscessation involving the mandible is a particular problem, because of lysis of the underlying alveolar bone, leading to pathologic fracture. In peracute septicemic forms, gross lesions may be few, and include wet, congested lungs and a dark, enlarged spleen.

In animals with chronic rhinitis, the nasal mucosal epithelium may become hyperplastic with goblet cell hypertrophy, loss of cilia, and abundant infiltrating neutrophils and lymphocytes. Sloughed epithelial cells, degenerate neutrophils, and other cell debris may accumulate within the nasal passages. Turbinates may become atrophied and irregular in appearance with periosteal fibroplasia. Enzootic bronchopneumonia is characterized by consolidation of the anteroventral lung lobes, atelectasis, mucopurulent bronchitis, hyperplastic bronchiolar epithelium with loss of cilia, and

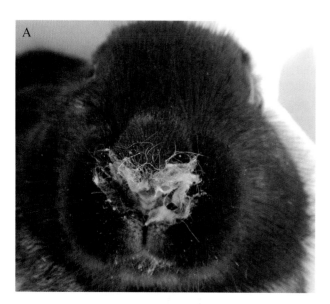
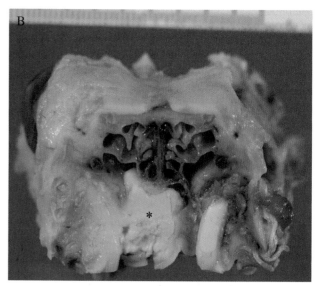

Figure 1.18 A: *Pasteurella*-induced mucopurulent rhinitis in a rabbit. B: Abscessation and erosion of the palate (*) contributing to mucopurulent discharge in a rabbit with pasteurellosis. Atrophic rhinitis may also be present.

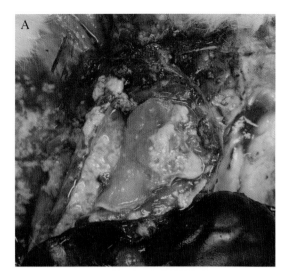
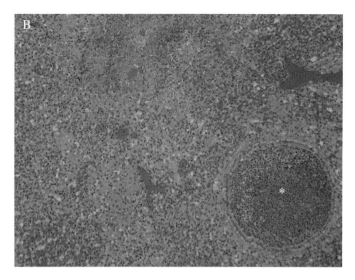

Figure 1.19   A: Fibrinopurulent pleuropneumonia in a rabbit with pasteurellosis. B: There is often marked alveolar consolidation and necrosis in cases of pasteurellosis and airways (*) are filled with neutrophils and cellular debris.

peribronchial lymphocytic cuffing. Acute hemorrhage, microvascular fibrin thrombi, and pulmonary edema may be seen in peracute respiratory and septicemic forms of the disease.

1.4.1.3   Laboratory Diagnostics

Pasteurella multocida is a Gram-negative nonmotile, non-spore-forming, facultative anaerobic coccobacillus. It can be classified further based on capsular and somatic serotypes or molecular fingerprint. Capsular type A is most common and adheres closely to respiratory mucosa, while capsular types D and F are the next most common. Serologically, somatic serotypes 1, 3, and 12 are most common. For any given serotype; however, there may be significant interbreed differences in susceptibility to disease. For example, Flemish giant rabbits may be more susceptible to disease following exposure to some strains of *P. multocida* compared with New Zealand white rabbits. This difference is attributed to suppression of macrophage function in the former breed by the bacterium. PCR and ELISA assays may be used to detect exposure and infection. Deep nasal swabs collected under sedation or general anesthesia may be required for accurate culture and isolation of the organism.

1.4.1.4   Differential Diagnoses

Other causes of rhinitis and bacterial bronchopneumonia in rabbits include *Bordetella bronchiseptica*, *Streptococcus agalactiae*, and *Klebsiella pneumoniae* (Figure 1.20A). Both *Bordetella* sp. and *Klebsiella* sp. may be cultured from the oropharynx of otherwise normal rabbits, suggesting that these bacteria are secondary or opportunistic pathogens in rabbits. *Bordetella* sp. infection may induce ciliostasis and macrophage dysfunction in rabbits, further exacerbating the course of disease. The agent has also been isolated in pure culture from sick rabbits, making its role as a primary vs secondary pathogen controversial. *Mycobacterium genavense* has been reported as a cause of pleural effusion and granulomatous pneumonia in a young dwarf rabbit with *Encephalitozoon* sp. co-infection. Histologic evaluation should readily distinguish the associated pulmonary lesions, including abundant foamy alveolar macrophages containing intracellular acid-fast bacilli, from those induced by *Pasteurella*.

Nasal exudate or crusting and mild rhinitis may be seen with infections caused by *Treponema paraluiscuniculi*. Severe maxillary dental disease with tooth root abscessation may present as chronic facial fistulas or mucopurulent nasal discharge. Other agents inducing abscesses include *Staphylococcus aureus* (Figure 1.18B) and *Pseudomonas* spp. Causes of head tilt include encephalitozoonosis, ear mite infestation, and visceral larval migrans. Rabbit viral hemorrhagic disease may mimic the peracute form of pasteurellosis, however, generally a large number of rabbits are affected during a VHD outbreak.

1.4.1.5   Group or Herd Management

Transmission of *P. multocida* between rabbits likely occurs by direct contact with an infected animal or by contact with contaminated fomites. Aerosol transmission is less common except in cases of acute infection when more infective particles are shed into the

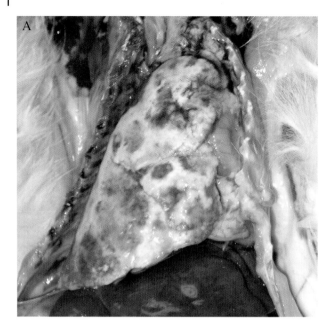

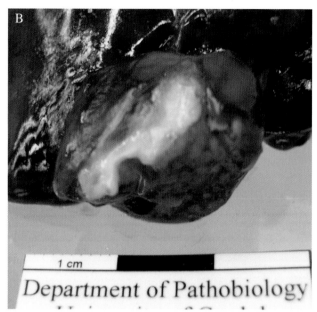

Figure 1.20 A: Mixed bacterial infection (*Pasteurella multocida* and *Bordetella bronchiseptica*) resulting in pneumonia and pulmonary consolidation in this rabbit. B: Streptococcal abscesses can also be seen sporadically in the lungs and other tissues of rabbits.

environment. Separation of cages to prevent nose-to-nose contact may be beneficial in reducing the spread of bacteria between animals. Infection with *P. multocida* may occur at birth or within the first few months of life, although clinical disease is typically not apparent until weanlings are seven to eight weeks of age. Segregated early weaning-medication practices and Caesarian red-erivation with fostering onto clean does are two methods that have been used successfully to eradicate *P. multocida* from rabbit herds. A *Pasteurella*-free herd must be managed on a closed-herd principle (no entry of foreign animals allowed) or with entry restricted to rabbits from herds known to be free of the organism. Once the infection is established, antibiotic treatment is generally intermittent and palliative. Poor hygiene, including high ammonia levels, and dusty bedding or hay may exacerbate underlying disease in rabbits. *P. multocida* may be transmitted to human caregivers, and there are rare reports of meningitis in children following handling of infected pet rabbits. Hand hygiene is an important preventive after handling potentially infected rabbits.

1.4.2 Bordetellosis

Bordetella bronchiseptica is a small, motile, Gram-negative coccobacillus that is transmitted by direct contact with clinically affected animals, carrier hosts, contaminated fomites, and respiratory aerosols. Although many animals eventually develop immunity and eliminate the infection, carrier rabbits are common.

1.4.2.1 Presenting Clinical Signs

Rabbits may harbor *B. bronchiseptica* in their upper respiratory passages, including the paranasal sinuses, and subclinical infection is common. The usual consequence of infection with this agent, through ciliary and epithelial damage, is a predisposition to other infections, particularly pasteurellosis, although primary *B. bronchiseptica* rhinitis is noted occasionally.

1.4.2.2 Pathology

Rabbits are much less likely to develop primary disease from *Bordetella* sp. infection compared with guinea pigs. Mucopurulent nasal exudate and rhinitis may be seen with or without bronchopneumonia.

1.4.2.3 Laboratory Diagnostics

A definitive diagnosis is based on clinical signs and culture of *B. bronchiseptica* from exudate of the nasopharynx, trachea, bronchial lumen, or middle ear. When nasal swabs are used to screen animal colonies for carriers, MacConkey agar is the preferred culture medium because it retards growth of contaminants.

1.4.3 Cilia-Associated Respiratory Bacillus Infection

Naturally occurring infections by the cilia-associated respiratory bacillus (CARB) have been reported in rabbits, with high prevalence (30–100%) in one study of commercial rabbitries in Europe. CARB is a Gram-negative gliding bacterium and pathogenicity is correlated highly with the strain origin (i.e., rat or rabbit), as host-adapted strains will be more pathogenic than nonhomologous strains. Transmission is by direct contact, and the bacilli are transmitted poorly by fomites. No gross lesions are seen in rabbits although, histologically, mild hypertrophy and hyperplasia of the trachea and bronchi may occur, accompanied by a mild, mixed inflammatory cell infiltrate. Bacilli interdigitate between cilia in respiratory epithelium and interfere with the mucociliary apparatus, predisposing to other bacterial infections. The bacilli are argyrophilic and may be detected with a Warthin-Starry stain.

1.4.4 Viral Hemorrhagic Disease

Viral or rabbit hemorrhagic disease (RHD) is a peracute viral infection of domestic rabbits (*Oryctolagus cuniculus*). A closely related virus causes a similar hemorrhagic disease syndrome in wild European hares, known as the European brown hare syndrome (EBHS). Rabbit hemorrhagic disease is caused by a nonenveloped, single-stranded, positive-sense RNA lagovirus, known as rabbit hemorrhagic disease virus or RHDV, within the Caliciviridae family. Outbreaks of the disease have occurred in commercial rabbitries around the world and RHD is a reportable disease in the United States and Canada. In many parts of the world, pet and commercial meat rabbits are vaccinated against this infection, although newer virus strains (RHDV2) have arisen recently that induce disease and death in vaccinated rabbits, suggesting poor antibody cross-reactivity. RHD is enzootic in wild rabbit populations in Australia, New Zealand, and parts of Europe and recently some species of hares in Europe have demonstrated susceptibility to virulent strains.

Nonpathogenic strains of rabbit calicivirus and moderately pathogenic strains have also been identified.

1.4.4.1 Presenting Clinical Signs

In kits from vaccinated does, susceptibility begins 5–6 weeks after birth. The hallmark of the disease is sudden death with very high morbidity and mortality (80–100%). Animals may be lethargic and pyrexic and die within 24–72 hours. Other signs include depression, anorexia, dyspnea, hematuria, convulsions, and epistaxis. Because death is acute, affected animals are often in good body condition. The acute form is seen primarily in epizootic outbreaks. Subacute cases with milder symptoms are seen in the later and enzootic stages of infection. Although most animals that survive are resistant to reinfection, some of those that are serologically positive may still carry and shed the virus intermittently. Chronic nonclinical infection is rare because seroconversion usually affords complete protection. Animals less than one month of age are resistant to infection.

1.4.4.2 Pathology

Blood-tinged nasal discharge, hepatomegaly, splenomegaly, and serosal ecchymoses are typical findings at necropsy (Figure 1.21). Pulmonary edema and hemorrhage, hepatic necrosis, intestinal crypt necrosis, and lympholysis have also been described.

Histologically, there is multifocal to coalescing hepatic necrosis with little associated inflammation (Figure 1.22). Microinfarctions due to disseminated intravascular coagulation may be seen scattered throughout the myocardium, pulmonary parenchyma, kidneys, and other organs. Microscopic changes in the spleen include necrosis and the presence of microthrombi in small

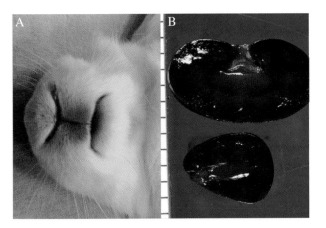
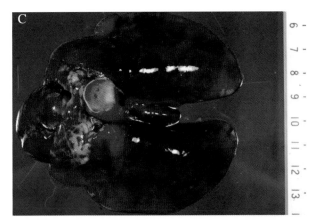

Figure 1.21 A: Blood-tinged nasal discharge in a rabbit dying acutely of rabbit hemorrhagic disease virus (RHDV). B: Acute bilateral renal hemorrhage and necrosis in a rabbit infected with RHDV. C: Massive pulmonary hemorrhage and necrosis in a rabbit with acute RHDV. *Source*: A: Courtesy of C. Embury-Hyatt. B and C: Courtesy of J.H. Park.

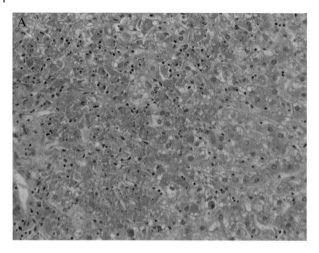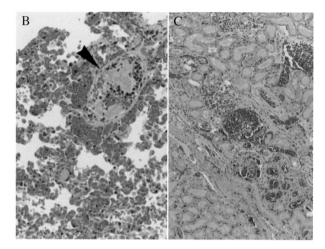

Figure 1.22 A: Massive hepatic necrosis in a rabbit infected with rabbit hemorrhagic disease virus (RHDV). B: Fibrin thrombi (arrowhead) are present in pulmonary vessels in addition to hemorrhage and congestion of parenchyma. C: Multifocal renal infarcts are a common finding in rabbits dying of RHD. *Source:* A, B and C: Courtesy of J.H. Park.

vessels. Central nervous system changes, such as microthrombosis, may be found, but are less common than in the other organs.

1.4.4.3 Laboratory Diagnostics

Diagnosis is based typically on the peracute nature of the disease combined with characteristic gross and histopathology findings. Virus isolation, hemagglutination assays, PCR, and immunohistochemistry are the methods used to confirm infection. Nucleic acid sequencing coupled with phylogenetic analyses may be required to completely identify isolates.

1.4.4.4 Differential Diagnoses

Leporid herpesvirus-4 may present with acute signs of lethargy, pyrexia, anorexia, epistaxis, and dyspnea; however, the clinical course of the disease is not usually peracute. Septicemic forms of pasteurellosis may mimic VHD. Epistaxis may be induced by nasal foreign bodies and tumors.

1.4.4.5 Group or Herd Management

There is no treatment for this condition and vaccination is not permitted in either Canada or the United States. The condition is reportable in both countries.

1.4.5 Herpesvirus Pneumonia (LeHV-4)

Leporid herpesvirus-4 is a recently identified rabbit alphaherpesvirus, which has been implicated in a number of small disease outbreaks in commercial and pet rabbits in Canada and the United States. Naturally occurring species-specific herpesvirus infections are rare in domestic rabbits; infections with known domestic and cottontail rabbit gammaherpesviruses are typically asymptomatic.

1.4.5.1 Presenting Clinical Signs

Affected animals present with focal cutaneous ulcers with crusting, subcutaneous swellings, lethargy, respiratory distress, and abortion. In the few reported outbreaks, all age groups have been susceptible to infection with high morbidity (>50%) and moderate mortality (>25%). Intercurrent bacterial respiratory infections may augment the clinical signs, leading to a poor outcome.

1.4.5.2 Pathology

Grossly, multifocal facial cutaneous swellings and necrosis with crusting can be present. Multifocal to generalized hemorrhage may be present throughout the lungs and viscera in acute cases, with focal gray areas of necrosis. Microscopically, a marked, generalized necrotizing and hemorrhagic bronchopneumonia with denuding of airways and severe generalized alveolar flooding with fluid, fibrin, and infiltrating neutrophils and macrophages is seen (Figure 1.23). Prominent glassy eosinophilic intranuclear viral inclusions are present, especially in nasal and bronchiolar epithelium, and there may be fibrinoid necrosis and thrombosis of arterioles. Similar massive fibrinohemorrhagic necrosis is seen in the spleen and liver with intranuclear inclusions in endothelial and stromal cells (Figure 1.24). Frank hemorrhage into the intestine may be seen and brain lesions are variably present.

1.4.5.3 Laboratory Diagnostics

This is an emerging disease within rabbits and different substrains of the virus may produce slightly different patterns of disease. Clinical signs are most severe within 7–10 days post-infection, with nasal shedding of virus detected as early as 2 days post infection. The disease

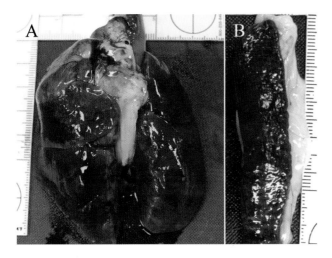

Figure 1.23 A: Marked, multifocal to coalescing pulmonary hemorrhage and necrosis in a rabbit infected with leporid herpesvirus-4. B: This rabbit also had massive, multifocal splenic necrosis.

may be diagnosed based on the severity of clinical signs combined with the microscopic findings of typical herpetic glassy, pale eosinophilic intranuclear inclusion bodies. A specific virus neutralization assay is available at a limited number of diagnostic laboratories.

1.4.5.4   Differential Diagnoses
Human herpes simplex virus (human herpesvirus-1) may infect rabbits, but clinical signs and pathologic findings are usually limited to encephalitis. Viral hemorrhagic disease produces similar clinical findings of dyspnea, epistaxis, and pyrexia, but the time course of the disease following infection is generally more acute and inclusion bodies are not present. Myxoma virus infection may produce similar cutaneous and respiratory signs, but is readily distinguishable microscopically by the presence of poxvirus inclusions. Other causes of respiratory disease, including *Pasteurella multocida*, epistaxis due to foreign bodies, or nasal tumors may induce similar presenting signs. Adenoviral intranuclear inclusion bodies may be seen sporadically within upper respiratory epithelial cells of young pre-weaned rabbits but the clinical significance of this agent in rabbits is unknown (Figure 1.25).

1.4.5.5   Group or Herd Management
Relatively little is known about LeHV-4 in domestic rabbits, although transmission is likely by aerosol or direct contact, with respiratory and systemic dissemination, as for other herpesviruses. In multi-rabbit households or in commercial settings, sick animals should be isolated well away from unaffected animals. There is no specific treatment or vaccine available for this disease. The potential for cross-species transmission is unknown.

1.4.6   Pneumocystosis
Pneumocystis oryctolagi is a host-specific fungal organism that is ubiquitous in the environment. Little is known about rabbit-specific strains, however, most rabbits (pet, commercial, and research) are typically infected 1 month after birth, and appear to clear the infection within 3–4 weeks, although subclinical infection may persist. Multiparous pregnant does have been reported to transmit the fungus to offspring transplacentally. Mild focal pulmonary infiltrates containing eosinophils and plasma cells may be seen histologically, and the organisms, both trophic and cyst forms, are adherent to the alveolar epithelium. *Pneumocystis*-infected rabbits do not demonstrate the typical foamy alveolar macrophages

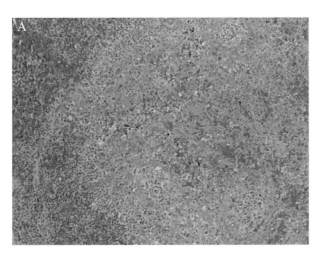

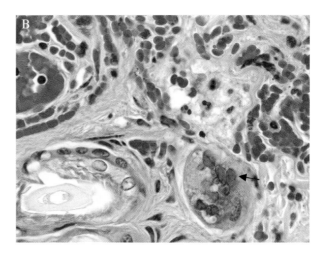

Figure 1.24   A: Microscopically, lungs from rabbits infected with leporid herpesvirus-4 (LeHV-4) demonstrate marked necrohemorrhagic bronchopneumonia. B: Syncytial cells with prominent glassy, pale eosinophilic intranuclear inclusion bodies (arrow) can be found in the skin (depicted) and bronchiolar epithelium in the early stages of LeHV-4 disease.

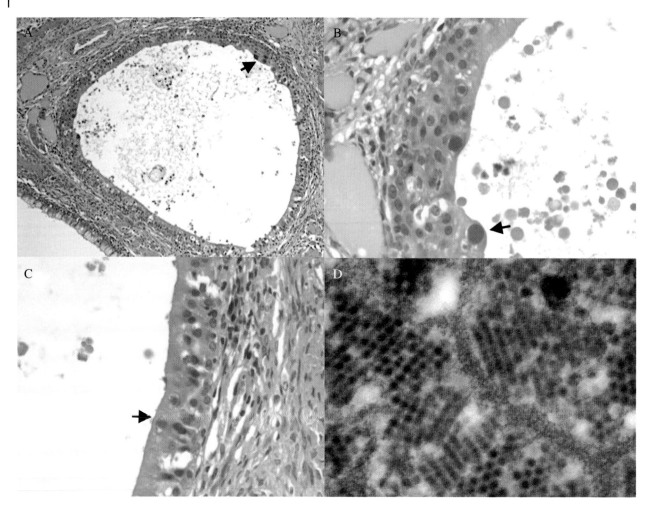

Figure 1.25 A: Adenoviral rhinitis in a young pre-weaned rabbit from a farm with marked, ongoing losses of pre-weaned kits from skin lesions. Animals were febrile with sneezing and serous nasal discharge in addition to skin lesions. Nasal epithelial cells with large basophilic intranuclear inclusion bodies (arrows) can be seen in multiple nasal sections (B) and (C). No inclusions were noted in tissues from adult rabbits on the same farm. D: Electron microscopy demonstrates virus particle arrays of a shape and size consistent with adenovirus. No other infectious agent was isolated from these kits and there were no other gross or microscopic lesions noted.

seen in mice and other species infected with *Pneumocystis* sp. The organisms may be visualized better with a Gomori's methenamine-silver stain. In mice, animals with previously resolved pneumocystosis may be susceptible to subsequent pulmonary hypertension. Microscopic evidence of pulmonary hypertension is not uncommon in rabbits and it is interesting to speculate whether the condition is associated with previous *P. oryctolagi* infection.

1.4.7 Neoplasia

Primary nasal and pulmonary tumors are very uncommon in rabbits. Lymphosarcoma, fibrosarcoma (Figure 1.26), thymoma (see Section 1.10), and pulmonary metastases of uterine and mammary gland tumors may occur with resultant dyspnea. Nasal carcinomas and adenocarcinomas have

been reported in pet rabbits leading to stertorous breathing if the nasal septum becomes deviated or if the rhinopharynx becomes obstructed by the mass.

1.4.8 Other Causes of Respiratory Disorders

Dust, **high ammonia** levels, and **irritant volatile oils**, such as pinene in softwood chip bedding, may induce irritation of the nasal mucosa, leading to rhinitis and sneezing. Chronic irritation and inflammation of the nasal passages may predispose animals to bacterial infections.

Allergic rhinitis has only been reported anecdotally in rabbits and has not been well characterized as a discrete clinical condition. **Elongated molar roots** may impinge upon the nasal cavity, resulting in stertorous breathing. At necropsy, the nasal sinuses of rabbits should always be opened and evaluated closely. **High**

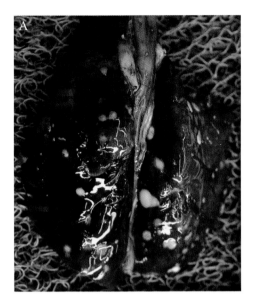 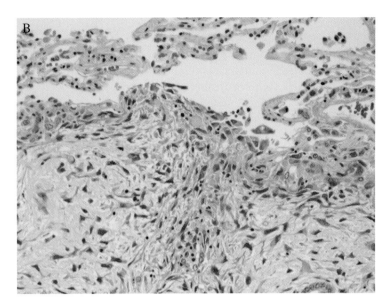

Figure 1.26 A: Anaplastic carcinoma metastatic to lungs in a 2-year-old female neutered rabbit with a history of paresis and seizures. B: A monotypic population of spindle cells form irregular interlacing streams, with each cell separated by abundant amphophilic fibrillar stroma. The cells have indistinct cellular borders, eosinophilic cytoplasm, and mitoses are 2/400x field.

ambient temperature may induce mild rhinitis. **Nasal foreign bodies**, for example, grass awns, may become impacted and inflamed, leading to a chronic mucopurulent discharge and intranasal foreign body reaction (Figure 1.27). **Cardiac disease** may result in pulmonary edema and pleural effusion, either of which may culminate in dyspnea and cyanosis. Several cases of **respiratory mycobacteriosis** with destruction of the nasal epithelium and multifocal pulmonary abscesses have been reported in pet rabbits due to *Mycobacterium* sp. infection. **Pulmonary aspergillosis** has also been reported in rabbits as an incidental finding. Multifocal

white nodules were noted throughout the parenchyma at necropsy, correlating with characteristic PAS-positive, dichotomously branched, septate hyphae in areas of granulomatous inflammation.

Post-anesthetic tracheal injury, ulceration, and stenosis can be seen in rabbits following endotracheal tube intubation (Figure 1.28). Affected animals may present with exertional cyanosis, respiratory stridor, serosan-

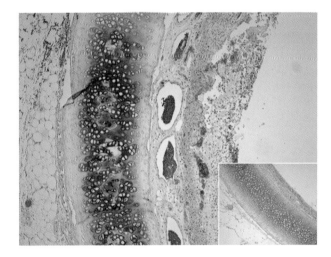

Figure 1.28 Tracheal stenosis in a 5-month-old rabbit intubated twice for isoflurane anesthesia at a 3-week interval. The animal became dyspneic one week after the second anesthesia and was euthanized. There is marked mucosal erosion with a dense serocellular exudate and marked submucosal congestion, mixed, predominantly neutrophilic leukocytic infiltrates, and fibrosis. Inset: normal trachea.

Figure 1.27 Foreign body (arrow) lodged in the nasopharynx of a rabbit with marked respiratory distress.

guinous oral or nasal exudate or sudden death. The injury is likely traumatic in origin, and lesions are seen in the proximal trachea, just distal to the larynx. Locally extensive to circumferential areas of epithelial attenuation and loss of cilia with or without erosion or ulceration, serofibrinous exudate admixed with superficial necrotic cellular debris, mixed leukocytic infiltrates, and marked submucosal congestion and edema are present. Acute injury may progress to fibrosis, stenosis, and complete tracheal obstruction in rabbits with repeated intubations, leading to sudden death. Similarly, over inflation of laryngeal mask airways can lead to pharyngeal edema and necrosis (Figure 1.29).

1.5 Musculoskeletal Conditions

Rabbits have a light skeleton, compared with other mammals of similar size, which represents approximately 8% of their body weight. Pet rabbits may be long-lived and may develop the typical age-related bone and joint degenerative conditions that are noted in other companion animal species. Musculoskeletal problems in rabbits are often complicated by obesity, muscle atrophy, and decreased bony mineralization, the latter two conditions occurring more commonly in animals fed a calcium-deficient diet or housed primarily in cages and given little opportunity for exercise.

When considering differential diagnoses for musculoskeletal disorders, it is important to note that any condition inducing anemia, malnutrition, inanition, cardiac disease, central nervous system disease, toxicity or pain may result in a clinical presentation of paresis and immobility. Further, animals with musculoskeletal disorders may present with other nonspecific signs related to decreased mobility, flexibility, and pain, including lack of grooming, urine scalding, fecal staining, and anorexia. A thorough post-mortem examination of all systems is necessary to definitively characterize the cause of clinical signs suggestive of musculoskeletal disease.

1.5.1 Dysplastic and Degenerative Disease

1.5.1.1 Splayleg

Splayleg is the common name for a clinical presentation in which a rabbit cannot adduct one or both hind limbs, resulting in decreased ambulation, paresis, or paralysis. The condition is transmitted as a complex recessive pattern of inheritance but there also appears to be a significant environmental component, as genetically normal rabbits may develop hip dysplasia, with a similar clinical outcome as in splayleg, when housed on smooth or slippery surfaces (Figure 1.30). Rabbits with acquired splayleg may in addition develop an inability to adduct one or both forelimbs. Obese animals and heavily pregnant does may present with postural abnormalities resembling splayleg; however, affected does typically return to normal postures post-kindling. On gross examination of rabbits with splayleg, femoral head torsion is noted in the affected limb(s) with thickening of the coxofemoral joint capsule, with or without lateral patellar luxation, valgus deformity, and tibial bowing. Muscular atrophy may be noted in affected limbs. Histologically, affected animals may have reduced myofiber size but there is no indication of peripheral nerve degeneration.

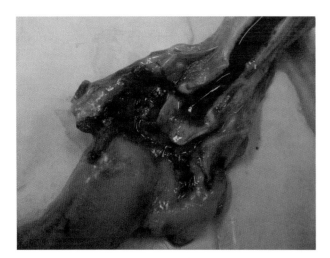

Figure 1.29 Pharyngeal hemorrhage and necrosis following repeated laryngeal mask airway (LMA) use for isoflurane anesthetic maintenance in a 5-month-old rabbit. Blood was noted in the LMA device following the final anesthetic session. Marked circumferential pharyngeal necrosis is seen. Overinflation of the device cuff can result in ischemic necrosis of pharyngeal tissues. *Source:* Courtesy of A. Goldstein.

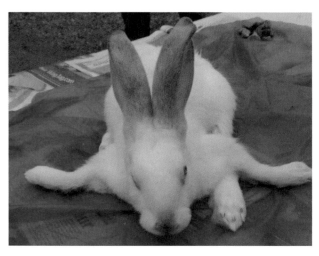

Figure 1.30 Splayleg in a young weaned rabbit. This animal was unable to abduct any leg.

1.5.1.2 Osteoarthritis and Vertebral Spondylosis

Osteoarthritis (degenerative joint disease) and vertebral spondylosis are increasingly recognized conditions in aging pet rabbits and are compounded by inactivity and obesity. In other species, osteoarthritis is typically multifactorial, but it is unknown whether there may be a hereditary component underlying disease initiation in rabbits. Animals with degenerative joint disease of the appendicular skeleton present with progressive joint stiffness and decreased activity, with or without pain and inflammation. Vertebral spondylosis may result following development of bridging vertebral osteophytes. Generally, the lumbar vertebrae are involved, leading finally to fusion and immobility of the vertebral bodies.

Gross and histologic changes with osteoarthritis will depend on the severity and duration of the condition. Fibrous thickening of articular cartilage with cartilaginous fibrillation, joint effusion, and mixed inflammatory cell infiltrates are noted early in the course of disease. In chronic cases, bony proliferation (osteophyte production) may occur at the junction of the joint capsule attachment and along the articular margins.

1.5.1.3 Intervertebral Disk Disease

Intervertebral disk rupture may occur following trauma or develop as a degenerative condition associated with aging. There is no clear association between the development of intervertebral disk disease and spondylosis in rabbits. Thoracic disks may be affected more commonly, but rupture can occur anywhere along the spinal column. The nucleus pulposus may become mineralized, and eventually extrude through rupture of the annulus fibrosis, leading to spinal cord compression and clinical signs of paresis or paralysis.

1.5.1.4 Nutritional Myopathies

Rabbits are very sensitive to vitamin E levels within their diet and because of this are used as animal models of vitamin E deficiency-induced myodegeneration. Affected kits and young weanlings present with signs of muscular dystrophy, and present with muscle pallor, severe muscle atrophy, weakness, inability to adduct limbs (i.e., acquired splayleg), and general unthriftiness. Reproductive failure may be noted in does fed vitamin E-deficient diets. Typically, a level of 40 mg/kg of vitamin E in the diet is sufficient to meet animal needs, although it may take several months for a dietary deficiency to be detected clinically.

High levels of vitamin A intake by rabbits may reduce the uptake of vitamin E from the diet, resulting in a functional deficiency. A definitive diagnosis requires characterization of serum and tissue levels of vitamin E. Normal adult rabbit serum levels for vitamin E are reported as 3–5 ug/mL, whereas normal liver levels range from 66–100 ug/g (wet weight). Normal vitamin A levels in adult rabbit serum are 700–1000 ng/mL, whereas liver levels of vitamin A range from 50–500 ng/g (wet weight).

Hypervitaminosis D may lead to mineralization of arterial media in multiple organs, as well as calcification of the gastric muscularis. Periosteal and endosteal mineral deposition may also be seen.

1.5.2 Neoplasia

Spontaneous bone neoplasia is reported uncommonly in rabbits. Of those cases reported, osteosarcoma is the most common diagnosis, with primary tumors reported in the femur, tarsus, humerus, rib, skull, maxilla, and lip, the latter case being diagnosed as an extraskeletal fibroblastic osteosarcoma. There is no clear association between large breed size and osteosarcoma, as is seen in other companion animal species; however, affected animals tend to be middle-aged or older. One case report exists of cutaneous osteosarcoma in a one year-old dwarf rabbit that was metastatic to the lungs. Animals with osteosarcoma may present with pyrexia, lameness (if a limb is involved), and induration around the affected site. Pathologic fractures may also be present. Proliferative and necrotizing lesions are seen histologically, and are typically highly cellular and pleomorphic, with poorly characterized spindle to stellate cells that produce an osteoid matrix (Figure 1.31). Osteocalcin immunohistochemistry has been used to characterize osteoblast-like activity within these tumors. Local infiltration of soft tissue, joint bridging, and pulmonary metastases with pleural effusion have been reported in rabbits with osteosarcoma. Thoracic radiography should be used to complement histopathology of the primary mass when determining a prognosis for a surgical biopsy case.

Pathologic fractures may also occur in rabbits secondary to metastasis, proliferation, and necrosis induced by other neoplasms (Figure 1.32 and Figure 1.33). Lymphosarcoma is a very common tumor in rabbits, and spinal lymphosarcoma with pathologic vertebral fracture and cord compression has been reported (see Section 1.10). Uterine adenocarcinoma, the most common tumor of intact does, has also been reported to metastasize to the femur with resultant osteolytic lesions and pathologic fracture (see Section 1.8).

1.5.3 Trauma

Fractures and luxations of the legs and vertebral column occur occasionally in pet rabbits when animals are inadvertently dropped, struggle during restraint or jump from a height (Figure 1.34A). Fracture of the sixth or seventh lumbar vertebrae is relatively common in such

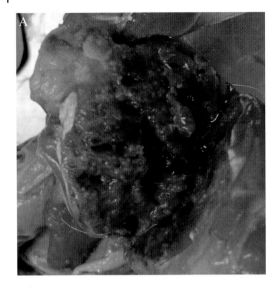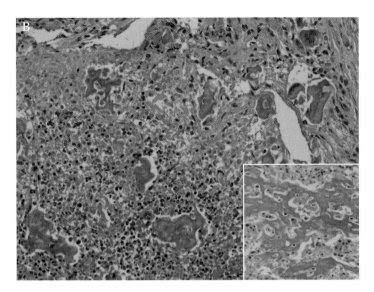

Figure 1.31 A: Scapular osteosarcoma in a 7 year-old Netherland dwarf rabbit. B: Microscopically, the mass is poorly circumscribed and consists of spindle-shaped neoplastic cells with moderate amounts of cytoplasm and elongate nuclei arranged in streams and whorls, embedded in a moderate fibrovascular matrix. Bone spicules are present throughout the mass (inset). Necrosis was apparent centrally, and there were up to 10 mitoses/400x field.

cases, with subsequent compression of the spinal cord. Both carry a poor prognosis and may result in urine retention because of damage to the visceral efferent lower motor neurons.

Fractures and luxations of other bones and joints may occur following trauma or inadvertent entrapment and are usually grossly evident. Animals with mandibular fractures may present with anorexia, asymmetrical facial swelling, and associated crepitus. Rabbits without access to regular physical exercise may be at increased risk for fractures because of reduced bony mineralization.

1.5.4 Other Musculoskeletal Conditions

Metabolic bone disease (secondary nutritional hyperparathyroidism) is recognized in other small mammals as a pathologic condition resulting from a dietary imbalance of calcium and phosphorus. Although rabbits have atypical processes for calcium absorption, regulation, and excretion, compared with other domestic mammals (see Section 1.3), it is likely that inappropriate dietary calcium/phosphorus content underlies at least some of the dental disease seen. Rapid dental growth, up to 0.25 cm/incisor per week, places a heavy demand on continuous bone mineralization processes. A recent survey found reduced serum levels of calcium and albumin and increased levels of serum parathyroid hormone in rabbits with advanced dental disease when compared to unaffected rabbits that were provided with outdoor exercise opportunities. This provides circumstantial support for metabolic bone disease as an underlying etiology for dental disease.

Osteomyelitis is a common sequela to mandibular, dental, and deep bacterial abscesses, and may result in pain, inanition, and pathologic fractures, depending on the location. Abscesses in rabbits are caused by *Staphylococcus aureus*, *Pasteurella multocida*, *Pseudomonas aeruginosa*, or less commonly by *Proteus* sp., *Bacteroides* sp., and other bacteria. Maxillary and mandibular abscesses arising from the oral cavity may be related to oral or gingival trauma with secondary infection by *Fusobacterium* spp., *Streptococcus* spp., *Actinomyces* sp., or *Arcanobacterium* sp. (Figure 1.34B).

Osteoporosis is seen primarily in rabbits that do not receive enough dietary calcium. Loss of alveolar bone and demineralization of teeth may result in root elongation and malocclusion, part of the acquired dental disease syndrome (see Section 1.6 Gastrointestinal Tract Conditions–Dental Disease for further information). In severe cases, root resorption and fractures may result, exacerbating inanition.

Mandibular odontogenic cysts in rabbits can arise secondary to trauma or inflammation and must be differentiated from abscesses, trauma, or neoplasia.

Iatrogenic injection-induced **myonecrosis** with subsequent paresis and pain can be seen following intramuscular treatment with irritating substances, such as acidic antibiotics, for example, trimethoprim-sulfa, and injectable anesthetic agents, such as ketamine. Small animal formulations, oral dosing procedures, and minimum injection volumes should be used to reduce this risk.

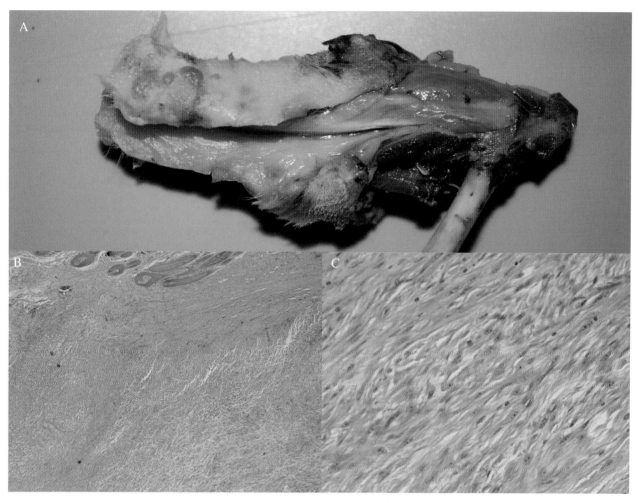

Figure 1.32 A: Fibrosarcoma of the skin and foreleg in a surgical biopsy from an 8 year-old male neutered rabbit. B: Immediately below the dermal-epidermal junction, the dermis is expanded by densely woven interlacing streams of spindle cells that are sometimes widely spaced in places as a result of deposition of pale basophilic ground substance and variable amounts of collagen. The cells are expanding and filling the dermis and extend to the dermal-epidermal junction. C: There is marked loss of lamellar bone, proliferation of small amounts of woven bone, and infiltration by neoplastic spindle cells with moderate numbers of mitoses. *Source:* A: Courtesy of M. Luckwaldt.

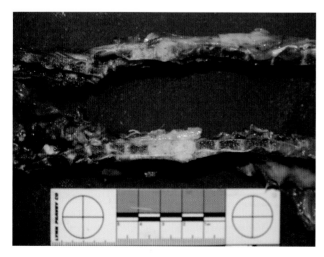

Figure 1.33 Vertebral neoplasia in a young, female, neutered rabbit with progressive paralysis. An undifferentiated sarcoma infiltrated the vertebrae at T4-T6, compressing the spinal cord.

Inadvertent ionophore intoxication has been reported in rabbits following exposure to several ionophores in the feed, including narasin, salinomycin, and the highly toxic maduramicin. Lesions reported include skeletal and cardiac myofibre degeneration and necrosis with mononuclear leukocytic infiltrates.

Fluoride-induced hyperostosis with painful firm thickening of the distal extremities and mandible developed rapidly in rabbits inadvertently fed excessive levels of dietary fluoride. Animals had severe periosteal and endosteal thickening in addition to multifocal gastric ulceration and adenomatous gastroduodenal proliferation. The normal dietary level of fluoride for rabbits is 150 mg/kg whereas in this report, animals were fed 300 mg/kg or greater due to a feed mill mixing error.

Vertebral synovial cysts leading to extradural cord compression were determined to underpin an acute

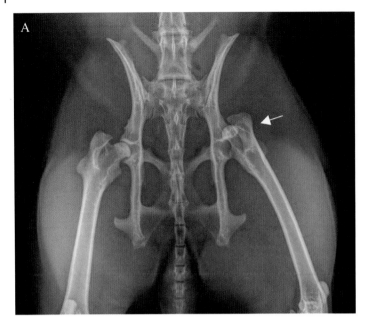 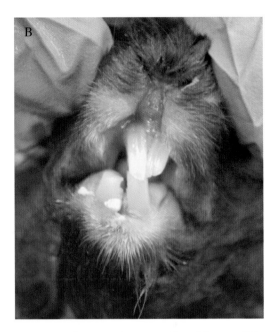

Figure 1.34 A: Radiograph demonstrating traumatic hip luxation (arrow) in a rabbit. B: Dental abscess and osteomyelitis of the mandible. Swelling and purulent exudate can be seen around the lower right incisor.

progressive posterior paresis in a young miniature lop rabbit. Cysts were thin-walled and lined by synoviocytes and were associated with the articular facets at the level of T12-L1. Given the young age of the animal (8 months), it is likely that the cysts were congenital in nature.

Rabbits are susceptible to **rabies virus** and may present with paresis or paralysis following infection. A history of outdoor housing with proximity to raccoons is typical in reported cases (see Section 1.9.3 for a complete description). This disease is both zoonotic and reportable in North America.

1.6 Gastrointestinal Conditions

Gastrointestinal conditions are very common in companion and commercial meat rabbits and are related primarily to aspects of management, diet, and husbandry. Rabbits have open-rooted incisors, premolars, and molars, and have a dental formula of 2(I:2/1, C:0/0, P:3/2, and M:3/3) for a total of 28 teeth, although some rabbits do not have a second pair of upper incisors (peg teeth). When present, the peg teeth are found immediately behind the primary incisors on the maxillary arcade. Premolar and molar teeth are indistinguishable, except by position, and are collectively referred to as cheek teeth. The occlusion of the upper and lower incisors allows them to be constantly sharpened. Rabbits have a limited ability to open their mouth wide, although there

is considerable side to side movement that occurs naturally during chewing.

Rabbits have a large, thin-walled simple glandular stomach that normally contains some ingested hair and that terminates in a muscular pylorus. They do not vomit. Pancreatic and bile ducts enter the duodenum at separate locations and the small intestine is relatively short compared to other companion animal species. Rabbits are hind gut fermenters with an ample thin-walled, coiled cecum. Peyer's patches are prominent in the mid to distal jejunum and ileum. Rabbits have a fleshy lymphoid dilatation at the ileocecal junction, the sacculus rotundus, as well as a long fleshy lymphoid vermiform appendix forming the blind end of the cecum. Up to 50% of the lymphoid tissue in the rabbit may be found in the gastrointestinal tract. The proximal colon is sacculated and contains the fusus coli, which regulates fecal and fluid movement. Multinucleated giant cells are seen commonly in the appendix of clinically normal rabbits and may contain refractile foreign material. Similarly, dense infiltrates of well differentiated plasma cells can be noted in the small and large intestinal mucosa of otherwise healthy New Zealand white and Dutch belted rabbits kept for research purposes. The significance of these infiltrates is unknown.

Young rabbits acquire gut flora through consumption of cecotrophs from the dam. The primary flora of the juvenile rabbit is composed of *Bacteroides* spp., and recent fecal microbiome studies suggest that it changes to predominantly *Firmicutes* (specifically, *Lachnospiraceae* and *Ruminococcaceae* families) and *Verrucomicrobia* taxa later in life, although some variation in flora will occur with diet, enrichment, and use of antimicrobial agents. Cecotroph ingestion occurs two or more times daily, approximately 4 to 8 hours after meals, and is thought to provide rabbits with additional vitamins and proteins. The total gastrointestinal transit time for a rabbit may be up to 20 hours.

1.6.1 Oral Conditions

1.6.1.1 Dental Disease

Dental conditions are very common in pet rabbits and the oral cavity should always be examined carefully by

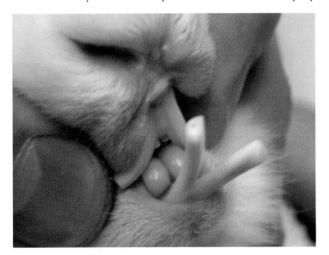

Figure 1.35 Severe incisor malocclusion in a young rabbit. *Source:* Courtesy of The Links Road Animal and Bird Clinic.

the pathologist for signs of incisor or cheek tooth malocclusion, with subsequent laceration of the lingual or buccal mucosa. Clinical presentation may include vague signs of anorexia, recent weight loss, decreased fecal pellets, salivation, inability to apprehend food, or bruxism (grinding of the teeth).

A genetic predisposition to incisor malocclusion due to mandibular prognathism or absence of one or more incisors or peg teeth (leading to malocclusion) may be seen in dwarf and small breeds of rabbits (Figure 1.35). Cheek tooth malocclusion often arises because of insufficient dietary fiber, which prevents normal dental wear and chewing motions of the jaw, and insufficient dietary calcium, which leads to alveolar bone mobilization, elongation of tooth roots, loosening of periodontal ligaments, and crown elongation (see Section 1.3, for a more complete description of calcium homeostasis). Migration of apical molar tooth roots may result in mandibular and maxillary exostoses and impaction (Figure 1.36). Dental caries may be seen in elongated teeth resulting from lack of wear.

Periapical tooth root abscesses are common sequelae and may be found in intraoral, facial, or retrobulbar locations with or without fistulation. Common agents cultured from oral abscesses in rabbits include a mixture of Gram positive and negative aerobic and anaerobic bacteria, including *Fusobacterium* spp., *Streptococcus* spp., *Actinomyces* sp. or *Arcanobacterium* sp. Osteomyelitis and pathologic fracture of the mandible may occur in chronic cases as well as inadvertent iatrogenic mandibular fracture when veterinary clinicians

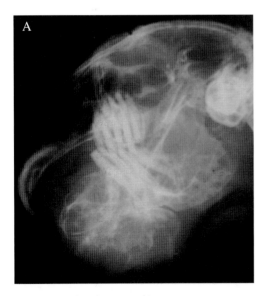
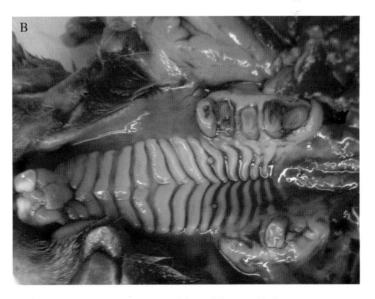

Figure 1.36 A: Radiograph demonstrating severe cheek teeth malocclusion in an aged rabbit with loss of the mandibular incisors, severe bony reaction, and significant calcium loss. B: Dental abnormalities in a rabbit with hemilateral failure of tooth eruption. This was an incidental finding at necropsy. *Source:* A: Courtesy of The Links Road Animal and Bird Clinic.

attempt to debride abscesses with significant bony involvement.

1.6.1.2 Oral Neoplasia

Oral papillomatosis, squamous cell carcinoma, and mandibular osteosarcoma are seen occasionally in the oral cavity of rabbits. (See Section 1.4.7, for a fuller description of oral papillomatosis and squamous cell carcinoma.) Other tumors are uncommon (Figure 1.37).

1.6.1.3 Other Oral Conditions

Enamel hypoplasia is occasionally seen in juvenile animals, although the etiopathogenesis is unknown. Acquired enamel hypomineralization may be seen with dietary hypocalcemia, resulting in mottling and discoloration of tooth surfaces and fine superficial ridge formation. Oral foreign bodies occur, some of which may penetrate the mucosa, initiating abscesses. Head trauma may result in incisor, mandibular or, less commonly, maxillary **fractures**. Dietary **zinc deficiencies** induce oral parakeratotic hyperkeratosis in growing rabbits, as well as other skin abnormalities. Normal dietary zinc levels are approximately 170 ug/g of diet.

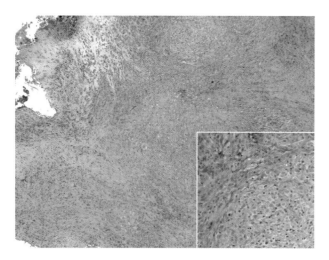

Figure 1.37 Ulcerated gingival mass from a 10 year-old male neutered rabbit. The lamina propria is edematous and contains poorly delineated nodules, clusters and whorls of fleshy ovoid to angular cells (inset) with large, single to multiple vesicular nuclei and vacuolated cytoplasm separated by rippling eosinophilic fibrillar matrix. Infrequent mitotic figures are seen (<1/400x field). Neoplastic cells were negative for pancytokeratin and anti-Melan A immunohistochemistry; however, 60% of the neoplastic cells demonstrated cytoplasmic labeling with PNL2 antibody. In dogs, melanomas can demonstrate variable expression of antigens identified by these two antibodies, and staining with either or both supports a diagnosis. The mass was diagnosed as an amelanotic melanoma.

Sialoadenitis is seen rarely in rabbits and may present as fluctuant to firm salivary gland swellings. Microscopically, mixed inflammatory cell infiltrates and necrosis may be present. Unilateral **necrotizing sialometaplasia** of the left submandibular salivary gland was reported in a young New Zealand white rabbit with a concurrent comminuted mandibular fracture. The salivary gland infarction in this case was attributed to local trauma and disruption of the blood supply. **Parotid gland adenocarcinoma** leading to head tilt, inanition, and wasting has been reported in a mature Rex rabbit. The mass compressed the trigeminal and facial nerves and resulted in osteolysis of the tympanic bullae and the mandibular ramus on the affected side.

1.6.2 Gastric Conditions

Whereas mechanical gastric impaction may occur sporadically, a much more common condition of pet rabbits resulting in gastric accumulation of hair or other material is gastrointestinal stasis, resulting in defective gastric and intestinal emptying. The etiology is complex and is thought to involve insufficient dietary fiber, excessive dietary carbohydrates, insufficient exercise, dehydration or lead toxicity. Clinical signs in affected animals may include inappetence, anorexia, abdominal discomfort, bruxism, and reduced size or number of fecal pellets. Animals with this condition present grossly with a large, firm, mucous-covered mass of hair admixed with other ingesta in the stomach. The condition is indistinguishable from mechanical gastric impaction and examination for intragastric foreign bodies, such as carpet, plastic, or rubber, within the pyloric region is necessary for differentiation

Gastric dilatation and rupture occur in rabbits and must be distinguished from post-mortem bloat with rupture or ruptured gastric ulcers (Figure 1.38A). The pathogenesis may involve gastric obstruction or fermentation of carbohydrates with excessive gas production.

Gastric ulcers with or without perforation and peritonitis are seen with moderate frequency at necropsy and are usually secondary to physiologic stress or systemic disease, including pasteurellosis, enterocolitis, and intussusception (Figure 1.38B).

Dystrophic mineralization of the gastric submucosa is seen in rabbits with chronic renal disease or with hypervitaminosis D. In these cases, soft tissue mineralization may also be present in the aortic intima, kidney, and myocardium.

Helicobacter heilmannii and several other *Helicobacter* species have been isolated in scant numbers from the stomachs of rabbits. It is unknown whether these are true pathogens for rabbits, as the majority of animals from which *Helicobacter* spp. are isolated have no clinical

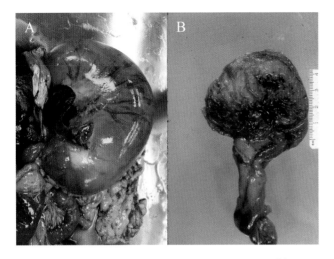

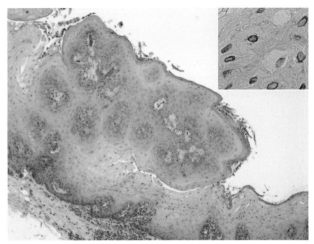

Figure 1.38 A: Gastric dilatation and acute rupture in a rabbit. B: Gastric ulceration is common in commercial meat rabbits and ulcers can perforate, resulting in sudden death.

Figure 1.39 Exophytic esophageal papilloma from a young rabbit. These masses are virus-induced and pale, eosinophilic intranuclear inclusion bodies can be seen in infected epithelial cells (inset).

signs of disease and no significant gross or microscopic changes. Some of the animals have mild to moderate lymphoplasmacytic antral infiltrates.

Gastric neoplasia is uncommon in rabbits. Gastric lymphosarcoma is seen sporadically as a manifestation of multicentric disease and consists of typical mucosal, submucosal, or intramuscular infiltrates of small neoplastic lymphocytes with scattered macrophages, sometimes with mucosal ulceration. Metastatic hemangiosarcoma has been reported, as well as gastric adenocarcinoma and gastric leiomyoma. Gastric and esophageal papillomas are seen sporadically and are likely virally-induced (Figure 1.39).

1.6.3 Enteric Conditions

Enteritis complex, resulting in diarrhea (Figure 1.40) is seen frequently in rabbits and often is related to husbandry or dietary management issues. As a hindgut fermenter, the rabbit has a complex cecal bacterial flora with 10^9 or more organisms per g of feces. Any condition or disorder that results in a prolonged reduction in food intake or intestinal motility or that alters gastric or intestinal pH may alter the flora, resulting in dysbiosis and diarrhea. Dysbiosis may be iatrogenic and follow oral treatment of rabbits with narrow spectrum antibiotics, such as penicillins, cephalosporins, macrolides, and lincosamides, resulting

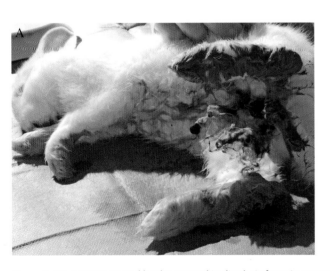

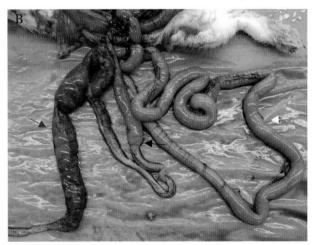

Figure 1.40 A: Ventrum and hocks covered in diarrheic feces in a young growing meat rabbit. B: Enteric disease in rabbits is often segmental. The jejunum and ileum of this animal are gassy and fluid-filled (white arrow), the cecum contains watery hemorrhagic content (red arrow), and the proximal colon contains mucinous material (black arrow). It is important to sample at all levels to determine the underlying etiopathogenesis.

in elimination of resident anaerobic flora and lumenal pH change. Enteritis contributes to significant morbidity and mortality in commercial rabbits, and can be seen as both enzootic disease with ongoing losses and culling of fryers and epizootic outbreaks with high mortality. Weanling and juvenile rabbits are particularly sensitive to developing enteritis at the time when their diet and gut flora change from being primarily lactose-based to cellulose-based. At this time, the gastric pH of weanlings drops from 5–6.5 to 1–2. Enteritis is generally multifactorial, involving the complex interplay between two or more agents or factors. Bacterial enteritis may be induced by *Escherichia coli*, *Clostridium spiroforme*, *C. difficile*, *C. perfringens*, *C. piliforme*, *Lawsonia intracellularis* or *Enterococcus* sp. Viral enteritis may be induced by several agents, including rotavirus, coronavirus, and astrovirus, and protozoal enteritis is induced by various *Eimeria* spp. Mucoid enteropathy is also seen as part of the enteritis complex but the pathogenesis is poorly understood.

In all cases, following infection with pathogenic infectious agents, a combination of increased mucosal permeability (e.g., from enterotoxemia or direct mucosal injury in coccidiosis), hypersecretion (enterotoxemia), and malabsorption (viruses) results in diarrhea. Death may ensue from loss of electrolytes and water, acidosis, and from the manifold systemic effects of toxins.

1.6.3.1 Coliform Enteritis

Escherichia coli is the most common etiologic agent of diarrhea in rabbits as in other mammals. The bacterium may be isolated from feces of normal rabbits and may proliferate during disease or post-mortem, when intestinal pH changes. Thus, isolation of *E. coli* must always be interpreted in context with other microbiologic and pathology findings, including strain and virulence factors, density of colonization, other agents isolated, and associated histologic changes. In North America and Europe, *E. coli* is a significant cause of culling and death in commercial rabbitries, but is less commonly isolated from pet and laboratory rabbits.

E. coli is a Gram-negative, pleomorphic rod-shaped bacterium that is nonmotile and non-spore-forming. There are seven classes of pathogenic *E. coli* including: enteropathogenic *E. coli* (EPEC), enterohemorrhagic *E. coli* (EHEC), enteroinvasive *E. coli* (EIEC), enterotoxigenic *E. coli* (ETEC), enteroaggregative *E. coli* (EAEC), diarrhea-associated hemolytic *E. coli* (DHEC), and cyto-lethal descending toxin (CDT)-producing *E. coli*. Many pathogenic *E. coli* are capable of producing heat stabile and labile toxins; the heat labile toxin closely resembles cholera toxin. The toxins are elaborated directly into the cytoplasm of the cell, where they induce a cAMP-activated increase in cell permeability, leading to cell death. Different strains have other virulence factors and adhesin

repertoires. For example, EPEC strains secrete a collection of intimins (adhesin proteins), enterocyte effacement proteins, and transcriptional regulators that interfere with the host cell metabolism. ETEC strains produce enterotoxins that cause cell death and a secretory diarrhea. EIEC strains invade and multiply in enterocytes, causing exudative enteritis and endotoxemia. EHEC strains are thought to have evolved from EPEC strains and embed in enterocyte cytoplasmic membranes, efface microvilli, and produce a Shiga-like toxin, with resultant damage to mucosa, leading to hemorrhage and diarrhea. Thus, disease manifestation is highly dependent upon strain.

Presenting Clinical Signs The clinical signs associated with pathogenic coliform infection; severe watery to hemorrhagic (less common) diarrhea with anorexia and wasting, may be attributable solely to the organism, but frequently other microorganisms are involved in the disease process. For example, an outbreak of diarrhea in suckling or weanling animals may be attributable only to infection with EPEC (Figure 1.41) or there may be two or more pathogens acting together to produce clinical disease. Concurrent infections with a pathogenic strain of *E. coli* have been shown to have an additive effect in animals infected with rotavirus, intestinal coccidiosis, and *L. intracellularis*. All ages may be affected; however, infection in suckling or weanling animals is more common.

Pathology Grossly, animals present with dilated loops of gut and fecal staining of the perineum and hind end. Depending on the strain of *E. coli* involved, lesions may be confined primarily to the small or large intestine, and disease severity is highly variable. Microscopically, bacilli may be evident blanketing the mucosal surface in close apposition to the microvilli and there may be swelling and sloughing of enterocytes in affected regions (Figure 1.42). Effacement of the mucosa, villus atrophy, and fusion of villi are typically seen, with marked neutrophilic and lymphoplasmacytic mucosal and submucosal infiltrates, and submucosal edema.

Laboratory Diagnostics Culture, serotyping, and toxin isolation may be used to definitively identify pathogenic *E. coli* although, typically, histopathology and culture are used for routine diagnostic cases.

Differential Diagnoses Viral, protozoal, and other bacterial agents can induce enteritis; multiple concurrent agents should be suspected.

Group or Herd Management *E. coli* is transmitted by the fecal-oral route and is difficult to eliminate from commercial rabbitries, once established, but the disease

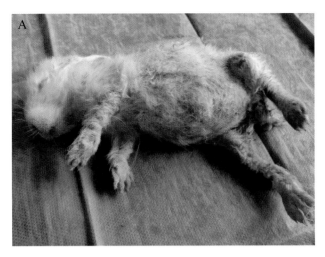
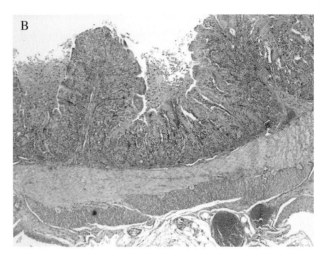

Figure 1.41 A: Coliform diarrhea in a suckling rabbit. B: Enteropathogenic *E. coli* (EPEC) in a rabbit kit. There is marked sloughing of small intestinal enterocytes with villus atrophy and fusion.

may be kept at manageable levels with good hygiene and nutritional management. Sufficient levels of vitamin E in the diet may ensure an adequate immune response when low level bacterial challenges occur. The same serotypes that are pathogenic for rabbits may infect other mammalian species, including pigs and chickens. Multispecies farms that include commercial rabbit production are common and surveys evaluating cross-species populations of pathogenic bacteria are lacking. It is important to note that EHEC is considered to be an emerging human pathogen and rabbits from pet and commercial sources are reported to be reservoirs of this bacterium. Rabbits may carry EHEC subclinically. Experimental infection of rabbits with EHEC has led to renal hypoxia and damage, similar to the condition of hemolytic uremic syndrome in humans.

1.6.3.2 Clostridial Enteritis

Clostridial infections are important causes of intestinal disorders of rabbits. There are several predisposing factors that contribute to the development of clinical disease from these Gram-positive, anaerobic, spore-forming pathogens, particularly events that disrupt the normal microbial population. These include inappropriate antibiotic administration and rapid dietary and environmental changes. Oral treatment with antimicrobial agents directed primarily against Gram-positive bacteria (e.g., penicillins, cephalosporins, macrolides, and lincosamides) has been associated with enteric dysbiosis and overgrowth of *C. difficile* in rabbits. The essential virulence factors of *C. difficile* are toxin A (a potent enterotoxin) and B (a potent cytotoxin). The disease may manifest with a neural component, as well, caused by

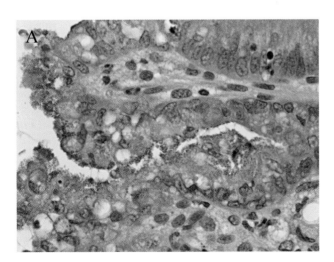
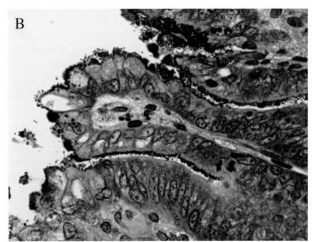

Figure 1.42 A: Attaching and effacing *E. coli* in the jejunum of a rabbit. B: Gram staining demonstrates dense blanketing of enterocytes by short Gram-negative rods.

release of substance P and subsequent mast cell degranulation. Bacterial spores are present in the cecum of normal animals but usually proliferate only after disruption of the normal gut flora, which competitively limits growth of *C. difficile* in healthy individuals. Colonization of the jejunum can result in peracute death.

In rabbits fed a high carbohydrate diet, clostridial enteropathy has been attributed to infection with either *C. perfringens* or *C. spiroforme*, however, *C. spiroforme* may be the more important clostridial pathogen in this species. *C. perfringens* is classified into five types; A, B, C, D, and E, based on production of one or more of the four major toxins (alpha, beta, epsilon, and iota). The disease syndrome following infection typically involves enterotoxemia and enteritis, usually involving the proximal gastrointestinal tract. Detection of enterotoxin in the feces of affected animals is the most sensitive means of confirming infection. *C. spiroforme* production of iota toxin, usually in the cecum, results in enterotoxemia

Presenting Clinical Signs   Animals present typically with dehydration, anorexia, and watery to hemorrhagic diarrhea. All ages may be affected, and animals may die peracutely with good body condition.

Pathology   There is little distinction between the signs and lesions induced by different clostridial species, although multifocal hepatic necrosis may also be seen in rabbits infected with *C. perfringens.* and multifocal hepatic necrosis, typhlocolitis, and myocarditis may be seen following infection with *C. piliforme.* On gross examination, distension of intestines with watery to hemorrhagic content occurs, typically involving the cecum, ileum, or proximal colon, accompanied by green to black fecal staining of the hind end. Ecchymoses may be present on the serosal surface of the cecum, and a fibrinous pseudomembrane may overlie an ulcerated mucosa. Microscopically, there is marked mucosal erosion and ulceration with frank hemorrhage into the lumen and, occasionally, a mat of fibrin admixed with degenerate neutrophils and cellular debris is adherent to the ulcerated surface (Figure 1.43). Mucosal edema and hemorrhage may be seen and bacterial organisms are typically present in the lumen, close to the mucosal surface.

Laboratory Diagnostics   Identification of the typical Gram-positive coiled or curved *C. spiroforme* on direct smear of the terminal ileum or cecum may assist with confirming a diagnosis (Figure 1.44). Strict anaerobic culture is required when culturing for these agents. Because low levels of clostridial species may be cultured from normal rabbits, demonstration of specific toxin elaboration by ELISA or PCR is needed for definitive diagnosis of *C. perfringens* and *C. difficile* enteritis.

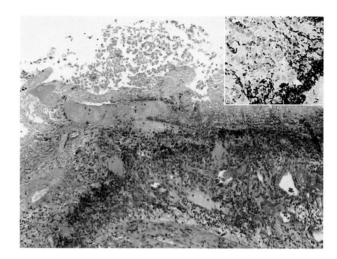

Figure 1.43   Marked necrohemorrhagic enteritis in a young rabbit co-infected with *C. perfringens* and *E. coli*. Inset: A Brown and Brenn stain demonstrates abundant Gram-positive rods on the lumenal surface, consistent with *C. perfringens*. *E. coli* was identified on culture.

Group or Herd Management   Outbreaks of clostridial enteropathy with mortality are common in commercial rabbitries, and occur occasionally in the research environment. Increasing the fiber content of the feed may result in a reduced incidence of the disease.

1.6.3.3   Proliferative Enteritis

Proliferative enteritis is caused by infection with *Lawsonia intracellularis*, a Gram-negative, obligate, intracellular nonmotile argyrophilic organism that occurs as curved to straight, short rods. The bacterium is transmitted by the oral-fecal route and there is no subspecies specificity.

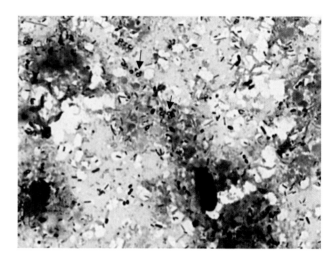

Figure 1.44   A: *Clostridium spiroforme* organisms identified in a Gram-stained cecal smear from a rabbit with enterocolitis. Numerous Gram-positive, coiled, and C-shaped bacteria are present (arrows).

Young growing animals and mature does and bucks are susceptible to infection.

Presenting Clinical Signs The clinical presentation may vary from acute onset with profuse diarrhea and dehydration resulting in high mortality; to an asymptomatic carrier state; to animals with chronic diarrhea, weight loss, and variable mortality.

Pathology At necropsy, fluid intestinal contents are present, and there may be mild to moderate mucosal thickening, particularly in the terminal small intestine and cecum, with enlargement of mesenteric lymph nodes.

Microscopic features include mucosal and cryptal hyperplasia with lymphohistiocytic infiltrates into the lamina propria, and in more chronic cases, erosion with mucosal and submucosal edema and sometimes dilatation of lacteals. In silver-stained (Steiner or Warthin-Starry) sections of affected cecum or ileum, large numbers of slightly curved, rod-shaped bacilli are usually aligned within the apical cytoplasm of enterocytes, with sparing of the microvillus border (Figure 1.45).

Laboratory Diagnostics The disease is diagnosed based on the characteristic microscopic findings, enhanced with silver stains or immunohistochemistry. ELISA and PCR assays are also available.

Group or Herd Management As for other causes of enteritis in rabbits, good dietary management and hygiene practices are critical for minimizing disease induced by this organism. *L. intracellularis* affects pigs as well as other domestic animal species; however, cross-species transfer from rabbits to other animals has not been evaluated.

1.6.3.4 Rotaviral Enteritis

Rotaviruses are species-specific enveloped RNA viruses that produce significant intestinal disease in a variety of young hosts. Rotaviruses are important agents implicated in diarrhea with mortality in 4–6-week-old animals from commercial rabbitries, an age at which maternal antibodies are declining. Older rabbits, including naïve adults, are susceptible to infection but are usually asymptomatic and may act as reservoirs, shedding virus for short periods into the environment. Serologic surveys of commercial rabbitries suggest a prevalence of 10% to 60%. Transmission is by the fecal-oral or airborne routes; post exposure, the virus replicates in enterocytes throughout the intestinal tract and may escape the intestine to infect extraintestinal tissues. In the small intestine, rotaviruses replicate selectively in enterocytes lining the tips of villi. The increased susceptibility of neonatal animals to clinical disease appears to be due in part to the reduced kinetic rate of enterocyte turnover in very young animals and the longer portion of the small intestine that is affected. Neonatal animals are unable to replace damaged epithelial cells quickly, resulting in collapse of villi and diarrhea. They are also less efficient at absorbing fluid from the large intestine than are older rabbits. Rotaviral infection may have an additive effect with concurrent *E. coli* infections in rabbits.

Presenting Clinical Signs Typical clinical signs in young animals include semi-fluid to watery green diarrhea with perianal soiling and dehydration. Animals may present with lethargy and suckle poorly. More severely dehydrated kits can die.

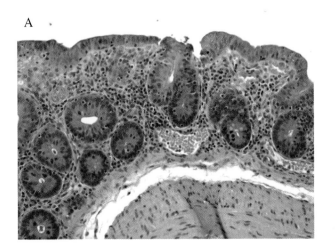
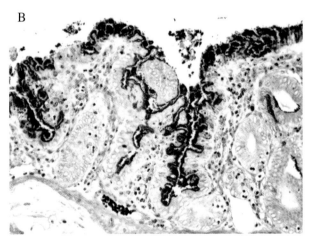

Figure 1.45 A: *Lawsonia intracellularis* infection in the cecum of a diarrheic rabbit. There is marked glandular hyperplasia and coiling, and numerous mitotic figures are present. B: Small, argyrophilic, rod-shaped bacteria are present within the apical cytoplasm of enterocytes, Warthin-Starry.

Pathology On gross examination, loops of small intestine and cecum are dilated with watery green content. Microscopically, blunting and fusion of villi are seen with attenuation of the mucosa, vacuolation of epithelial cells, and edema and mononuclear cell infiltrates within the lamina propria and submucosa. Focal epithelial cell degeneration may also be present throughout the large intestine.

Laboratory Diagnostics Detection of fecal viral particles by PCR or transmission electron microscopy, and serology are common means of confirming infection.

Coronaviral Enteritis Coronavirus infections occur naturally in rabbits and may play a role in enzootic enteritis in this species. The prevalence of antibodies to the virus in commercial rabbitries ranges from 3–33%. Clinical signs of enteric coronavirus infection include a passive, secretory, watery diarrhea, anorexia, and sudden death. Microscopic changes are similar to those seen for rotavirus and include marked blunting and necrosis of intestinal villi. The enveloped RNA virus is transmitted by the fecal-oral or airborne routes. The agent likely induces disease concurrently with other infections in the rabbit, as disease severity is highly variable. Carrier animals have been identified and may contribute to persistence of the infection in some rabbitries, in which there is a high incidence of mortality due to enteritis. Diagnosis is confirmed by recognition of the presence of viral particles in the feces of affected animals using transmission electron microscopy.

1.6.3.5 Enteric Coccidiosis

Enteric coccidiosis is an important diarrheal disease of rabbits. Infection may be reflected only by unthriftiness and poor feed conversion ratios. There are numerous species of coccidia that infect rabbits; however, the most common and pathogenic organisms include *Eimeria magna, E. piriformis, E. flavescens, E. irresidua,* and *E. intestinalis.* Transmission occurs by ingestion of sporulated oocysts; time for sporulation varies by *Eimeria* species from approximately 20–70 hours at 20°C. Sporozoite invasion of epithelial cells of the gut is followed by multiplication (schizogony, gametogony, and sporogony). Parasitized epithelial cells eventually rupture, resulting in release of organisms. The prepatent period is usually 5–9 days, depending on the species.

Coccidia can act as co-pathogens with a range of bacterial and viral agents. Animals may be infected with more than one strain of *Eimeria* sp., each living segmentally within a specific niche within the intestinal mucosa. In rabbits, immunity to one species of *Eimeria* is unlikely to confer immunity to other species. Infection induces marked oxidative stress and local and systemic immune modulation, which may predispose animals to other infections.

Presenting Clinical Signs The intensity of clinical signs may vary from inapparent infection to acute, profuse watery green to hemorrhagic diarrhea, with dehydration and death. Deaths most frequently occur during the weaning period. Depending on the species of infecting coccidia, lesions and organisms are present in small and large intestine.

Pathology Microscopically, numerous sexual and asexual phases of coccidial development are readily visible within enterocytes, and abundant numbers of thin-walled oocysts are present in the intestinal lumen (Figure 1.46). There is initially hyperplasia of villi,

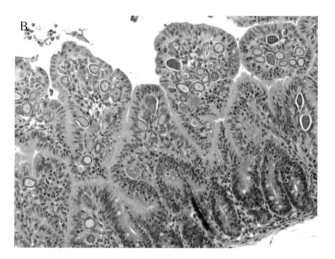

Figure 1.46 A: Ileum of a rabbit with severe coccidial enteritis. The small, multifocal white patches on the serosal surface (black arrows) correspond to underlying areas of mucosal necrosis. B: Numerous sexual and asexual stages of coccidial replication are seen in this intestinal section from a young rabbit with enteric coccidiosis.

followed by sloughing of epithelial cells and blunting and fusion of villi. Moderate mixed leukocytic infiltrates are present in the lamina propria, consisting of neutrophils, eosinophils, and lymphocytes.

Laboratory Diagnostics Oocysts are readily identified with fecal smears or flotation. Speciation is rarely carried out and is not needed to develop an effective treatment plan.

Group or Herd Management Because sporulation takes up to several days to occur, appropriate environmental hygiene practices should be in place to remove pre-infective oocysts from the environment of susceptible animals. The disease is typically self-limiting in older animals but separation of young susceptible animals from older animals shedding oocysts will help to limit disease spread.

1.6.3.6 Mucoid Enteropathy
Mucoid enteropathy is an unusual condition of unknown pathogenesis that occurs in juvenile (older fryers) and adult rabbits. The condition is seen with moderate frequency in commercial rabbits but is reported only rarely in pet and laboratory rabbits. Affected animals present with depression, anorexia, bruxism, gradual weight loss, and, on occasion, abdominal distension. Chronically affected animals may become constipated. The defining character of mucoid enteropathy is production of copious mucus in the absence of fecal pellets. The condition may occur in association with provision of diets low in fiber and high in carbohydrates, and may also be seen post-infection with a variety of enteric pathogens.

At post-mortem, the condition is found to be segmental, affecting the distal ileum, cecum, or colon most commonly (Figure 1.47). Opened sections of gut reveal a

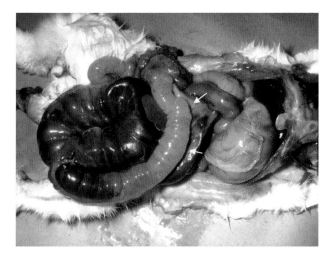

Figure 1.47 Segmental intestinal dilatation in a rabbit with marked mucoid enteropathy and typhlocolitis.

colorless semi-fluid to mucoid content with an absence of digesta. Some admixture of bile pigments may be present. In chronically affected animals, a mucoid mass may become inspissated resulting in obstruction and constipation. Microscopically, there is minimal mucosal inflammation and marked goblet cell hypertrophy within colonic glands and throughout the mucosa. Diagnosis is by gross and microscopic examination, using a process of elimination to rule out other enteric conditions.

1.6.3.7 Other Enteric Conditions
Salmonella **spp.** can be isolated infrequently from both symptomatic and asymptomatic commercial rabbits, often representing cross-contamination from another species. Most *Salmonella* spp. are zoonotic agents and their presence serves as a reminder that hand hygiene after handling rabbits or their tissues is essential. *Providentia vermicola*-induced septicemia was reported recently in an adult rabbit found dead with no premonitory signs. The large intestine was devoid of content and there were multifocal fibrinosuppurative serosal lesions. *Klebsiella oxytoca*-induced hemorrhagic enterocolitis with hepatic necrosis has also been reported from a rabbitry in Hungary. This condition was associated with prolonged use of antibiotic in the water to manage *S. aureus* infections, and may represent an example of bacterial selection.

Cryptosporidiosis has been reported in rabbits, and, in one case, waterborne human cryptosporidiosis was linked to contamination from a wild rabbit. Rabbit-derived cryptosporidia are typically not speciated further but the reported prevalence of infection in rabbits can be up to 7%. Little is known about the natural course of infection, but clinical signs include mild diarrhea and are self-limiting, except in weanling animals, in which more severe diarrhea and death may occur.

Oxyuriasis occurs in rabbits due to infection with the rabbit pinworm, *Passalurus ambiguus*. The parasite is nonpathogenic, even with heavy burdens, and characteristic nematode profiles may be seen incidentally in tissue sections of the anterior colon (Figure 1.48A).

Rabbits are the intermediate host for a number of carnivore **tapeworms**, and larval stages include *Cysticercus pisiformis* and *Coenuris serialis*, as well as infections with *Echinococcus granulosus*. Cysts may be found on the surface of the liver and elsewhere within the abdominal and pelvic cavities of rabbits. Animals with cysts are usually asymptomatic, but clinical signs will depend on the extent of space-occupying lesions induced by the cysts. Microscopically, oncospheres are segregated from hepatic parenchyma by a fibrous capsule and there may be focal granulomatous infiltration with degeneration of scattered local hepatocytes. Gross lesions of superficial linear scarring on the capsular surface of the liver should

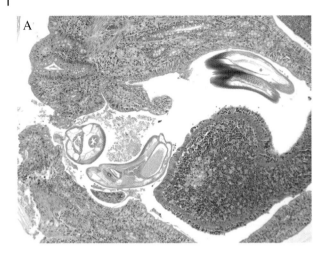
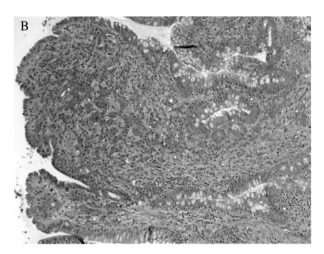

Figure 1.48 A: Multiple sections of pinworm (*Passaluris ambiguus*) in the ileum of a rabbit. This was an incidental finding. B: Section of ileocecocolic junction taken from a surgical biopsy from a 7-year-old neutered male rabbit with partial intestinal obstruction. Intestinal lymphoma was identified.

be differentiated from hepatic coccidiosis. Transmission occurs through contamination of bedding, food, or water by carnivore feces containing tapeworm eggs.

A novel **astrovirus** has recently been isolated from European and American commercial meat rabbits with enteritis complex, as well as from asymptomatic Canadian commercial meat rabbits. Astroviruses are small, single-stranded, non-enveloped RNA viruses within the genus Mamastrovirus and are highly prevalent in human infants with diarrhea. While the virus has been found in both symptomatic and asymptomatic rabbits, the prevalence is much higher in animals with diarrhea. More information is needed to understand the full epidemiology, clinical signs, and pathology associated with infections. There are currently no commercial diagnostic assays for this agent.

The role of **aflatoxins** in rabbit enteropathy is controversial. Rabbits are very sensitive to dietary levels with 2 ppm of the toxin reported to induce clinical signs. Higher levels result in reduced growth, feed refusal, anorexia, and depression. Focal hepatic necrosis with biliary hyperplasia and periportal fibrosis and lymphoplasmacytic infiltration may be seen in experimental animals chronically fed high levels of aflatoxins. Most rabbits with suspect subclinical or clinical aflatoxicosis have concurrent enteric infections, and it is difficult to define the contribution of each to the clinical condition noted. The recommended maximum aflatoxin content in rabbit food is no greater than 0.02 mg/kg in a diet with 12% moisture. Other mycotoxins, such as fumonisin B1 and B2, ochratoxin A, zearalenone, and deoxynivalenol, are tolerated at much higher levels in rabbit feed than aflatoxins.

Lead intoxication is anecdotally reported in pet rabbits with unsupervised access to furniture or building materials coated in lead paint. Rabbits often present with neurologic signs but weight loss, anorexia and gastrointestinal stasis may also be present. Basophilic stippling of erythrocytes may be seen on peripheral blood smears and blood lead levels in excess of 0.48 μmol/L are consistent with intoxication.

Colonic obstruction has been reported secondary to fibrous adhesions and intestinal stenosis or inadvertent suture penetrations that occurred following ovariohysterectomy in several pet rabbits. Animals presented with anorexia, gastrointestinal distension, and intestinal radiographic abnormalities were detected.

Intestinal and colonic **intussusception** and other intestinal accidents are reported rarely in rabbits. Intussusception is often associated with enteritis resulting from an underlying parasitic or bacterial infection. **Imperforate anus** with a rectovaginal fistula was seen in a young Netherland dwarf rabbit and assumed to be congenital in origin. Anecdotal reports are given for **intermittent ileus** following laparotomy or ovariohysterectomy in rabbits, presumably secondary to adhesion development.

Acquired dysautonomia with cecal impaction has been reported in hares (*Lepus* sp.) and domestic rabbits in the UK. The condition resembles grass sickness of horses and is characterized by neuronal chromatolysis without axonal degeneration or gliosis in sympathetic ganglia and neurons of the small intestinal myenteric and submucosal plexi as well as the brainstem. The etiopathogenesis is suggested to be a form of *Clostridium botulinum* intoxication, similar to grass sickness in horses.

Lymphosarcoma of the intestine, as a manifestation of multicentric disease, is seen in rabbits (Figure 1.48B). Other enteric tumors are very rare; however, anorectal papillomas are seen occasionally (see Section 1.4.7, for a more complete description of this condition).

1.6.4 Hepatobiliary Conditions

The rabbit liver has five lobes consisting of a left medial and lateral, right lateral, a quadrate, and caudate lobe. Rabbits have a gall bladder.

1.6.4.1 Hepatic Coccidiosis

Hepatic coccidiosis is caused by a single species, *Eimeria stiedae*, and is an important economic disease of commercial rabbitries. Following ingestion of sporulated oocysts, sporozoites penetrate epithelial cells of the intestine, and are transported to the liver via the portal circulation or lymphatics. There, sporozoites invade the bile duct epithelial cells, initiating schizogony. Following gametogony, epithelial cells rupture, releasing oocysts into the bile ducts, where they may infect other cells or pass via the bile into the intestine, where they are shed in the feces. The prepatent period is approximately two to four weeks with sporulation occurring within three days of oocyst shedding.

Presenting Clinical Signs Although virtually all rabbits raised under conventional conditions are exposed to *E. stiedae*, clinical disease is most common in young rabbits during the nursing and post-weaning period. Animals present with nonspecific signs of unthriftiness, distended abdomen, diarrhea, and anorexia. In heavy infestations, animals may present with jaundice.

Pathology Macroscopically, the liver is enlarged with raised, bosselated, firm, yellow-white lesions on the surface, which, upon cut section, are seen to represent enlarged and fibrotic bile ducts filled with yellow inspissated bile and necrotic debris (Figure 1.49). Microscopically, there is hyperplasia of bile duct epithelium leading to enlargement of bile ducts, and papillomatous projections into the lumen. Periductal and periportal fibrosis and mixed lymphohistiocytic infiltrates are common findings. Asexual and sexual coccidial stages are present within the bile duct epithelium, and smooth, thin-walled oocysts, approximately 30 μm × 20 μm, are demonstrated readily within affected bile ducts.

Laboratory Diagnostics Microscopic findings are pathognomonic. Demonstration of oocysts via fecal flotation is not diagnostic unless oocysts can be speciated and differentiated from intestinal coccidial species. Oocysts are also demonstrated readily in wet mount preparations of bile. Because enteritis and hepatitis in rabbits may be multifactorial, routine bacterial cultures (both aerobic and anaerobic) should be carried out to

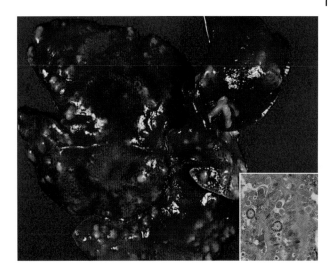

Figure 1.49 Hepatic coccidiosis is caused by *Eimeria stiedae* in rabbits. Linear to serpentine lesions are seen on the surface of the liver. Inset: Abundant sexual and asexual stages of *E. stiedae* are present within proliferative gall bladder epithelium. Oocytes are shed in the bile. *Source:* Courtesy of J.H. Park.

determine whether bacterial pathogens may be contributing to the clinical signs of disease.

Differential Diagnoses Clinical signs are nonspecific with hepatic coccidiosis. More common agents of enteritis should be considered if diarrhea is seen, as well as systemic disease with common bacteria, such as *P. multocida*, *S. aureus* or *L. monocytogenes*. *Clostridium piliforme*, in subclinically affected rabbits, and aflatoxicosis or other hepatic toxicants may induce similar clinical signs. *Fasciola hepatica*, the liver fluke, is seen sporadically within bile ducts of rabbits. Characteristic yellow-brown, ovoid, single operculate eggs that measure approximately 135 μm × 80 μm are seen with *F. hepatica* infections, and are differentiated readily from coccidial oocysts. Differential diagnoses for hepatic necrosis include *P. multocida*, *S. aureus*, *C. piliforme*, and *L. monocytogenes*.

Group or Herd Management Hepatic coccidiosis remains a significant disease in backyard breeder herds and organic commercial rabbitries, and is seen rarely in pet rabbits. Segregation of susceptible young from older, subclinically shedding animals and strict environmental and personnel hygiene practices will assist with disease management and eradication. Coccidia may act together with other opportunistic pathogens, such as *E. coli*, to produce clinical outbreaks of diarrhea.

1.6.4.2 Tyzzer's Disease

Tyzzer's disease is induced by *Clostridium piliforme*, a spore-forming, motile, rod-shaped, obligate, Gram-negative intracellular organism, which is transmitted by the fecal-oral route. Spores may persist for years within the environment. Bacterial subspecies are host-specific and thus the rabbit bacterium is not considered to be a zoonotic agent. Disease is initiated following a stressor, such as transportation or intercurrent disease.

Presenting Clinical Signs Infected animals, particularly weanlings or young adults, may die peracutely or present with nonspecific signs of depression, lethargy, and anorexia, with or without watery diarrhea. Older animals may be infected subclinically.

Pathology Classically, Tyzzer's disease presents with a triad of lesions: multifocal hepatic and myocardial necrosis and typhlocolitis. Within the ileum, cecum, and colon, lesions consist of acute segmental and transmural mucosal necrosis and edema with fibrinohemorrhagic exudate. Typical intracellular bacilli may be present within enterocytes and muscular layers of the affected ileum and cecum, and visualization is enhanced by silver (Steiner or Warthin-Starry) staining (Figure 1.50A). Within the liver, in more chronic infections, there are multifocal areas of coagulation necrosis with neutrophilic and histiocytic infiltrates and multinucleated giant cells. In rabbits, a careful search may be required to identify the characteristic bundles of bacilli in viable hepatocytes adjacent to foci of necrosis. Within the heart, there is focal to segmental myocardial degeneration with mononuclear cell infiltration and subsequent interstitial fibrosis.

Laboratory Diagnostics The disease is diagnosed based on the characteristic microscopic findings, enhanced

with silver stains. ELISA and PCR assays are also available.

Group or Herd Management Clostridial spores are resistant to common disinfectants such as alcohol and quaternary ammonium solutions; however, spores may be killed with 0.5% hypochlorite solutions. It is difficult to adequately sanitize environments post-infection, and spores remain infective for years. Tyzzer's disease is reported as a subclinical infection in wild cottontail rabbits and it may be that fecal spores from wild animals can contaminate hay grasses used as forage for domestic rabbits. In research settings, hay is usually autoclaved before being fed.

1.6.4.3 Hepatic Abscesses

Multifocal hepatic abscesses may be seen following infection with a number of bacterial agents in rabbits. Definitive diagnosis requires culture and sensitivity. More common agents include *P. multocida, S. aureus, L. monocytogenes, Salmonella* spp., and *Yersinia pseudotuberculosis* (Figure 1.51). Tularemia, caused by *Franciscella tularensis*, may occur in enzootic areas, where rabbits are housed outside and in contact with wild rabbits. Gloves should always be worn when handling or skinning wild rabbits because of the zoonotic risk potential.

1.6.4.4 Other Hepatobiliary Conditions

Viral hemorrhagic disease, also known as rabbit hemorrhagic disease or RHD, caused by the rabbit calicivirus may induce acute necrohemorrhagic hepatitis and peracute death with epistaxis, multi-organ failure, and disseminated intravascular coagulation (see Section 1.4.4,

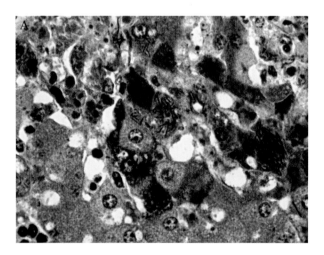
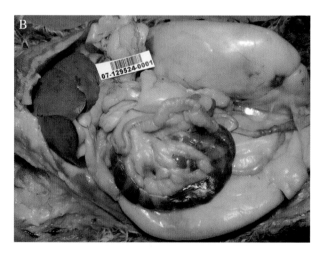

Figure 1.50 A: Liver from a rabbit with Tyzzer's disease (*Clostridium piliforme* infection). Numerous intracellular aggregates of long, stick-like, argyrophilic bacteria are seen in hepatocytes surrounding necrotic areas. Warthin-Starry. B: Marked hepatic lipidosis and extensive adipose stores in a mature rabbit. Severely obese animals are at risk of developing ketosis following changes in food intake.

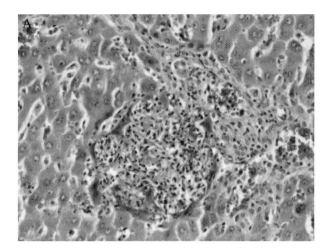 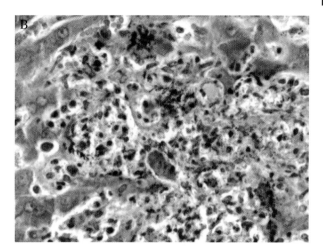

Figure 1.51 A: Multifocal hepatic necrosis in a doe with acute listeriosis. An increase in abortions was noted on this farm concurrently. B: Gram stain on liver tissue from this doe demonstrating short Gram-positive rods, consistent with *L. monocytogenes*. Bacterial culture was used to confirm the diagnosis.

for a more complete description). Similarly, **leporid herpesvirus-4** (see Section 1.45) may induce multifocal hepatic necrosis, pneumonia, and cutaneous swelling, ulceration, epistaxis, and death. Definitive diagnosis for both diseases relies on virus isolation or specific PCR, ELISA or VN assays.

Hepatitis E viruses are recently identified small, non-enveloped, positive-sense, single-stranded RNA viruses that are members of *Hepeviridae*. Novel hepatitis E virus serotypes (rbHEV) have been isolated from asymptomatic farmed rabbits in China and the United States, in wild and farmed rabbits in France with moderately high prevalence, as well as in clinically and subclinically infected pet rabbits in Italy and Canada, respectively. Viral antibodies have also been reported in asymptomatic specific pathogen free Dutch belted laboratory rabbits in North America, although viral serotype was not characterized. Hepatitis E viruses are found in a number of other species. Serotype 3 is most commonly isolated from naturally infected rabbits, a strain with potential to cross infect other species, including humans and pigs. Rabbits may also be infected with human serotypes and virus isolates should be sequenced to confirm the species of origin. Minimal clinical signs or pathology are reported in infected animals; however, detailed information is lacking on the epidemiology and the time course of infection. In the single clinical case in an adult pet rabbit reported in Italy, the animal was found dead and the cause of death was attributed to a severe *Pasteurella* pulmonary infection. Serum hepatocellular enzyme levels may be elevated in infected animals. Transmission occurs by fecal-oral and bloodborne routes. There are currently no commercial diagnostic assays available to monitor infections of rabbits with this agent.

Hepatic lipidosis is a common finding in obese bucks and does or does with metabolic acidosis in advanced pregnancy. A large greasy, pale liver is seen grossly, with marked macrovesicular hepatocellular lipidosis present microscopically (Figure 1.50B). The underlying cause(s) of metabolic acidosis are yet to be resolved and may involve dietary issues or intercurrent disease. Hepatic lipidosis is also commonly seen in anorexic adults undergoing fat mobilization to meet their metabolic energy requirements.

Rabbits are commonly used to evaluate **hepatic toxicants** in experimental settings and hundreds of common household and garden products are potentially toxic to them. Owners should be instructed to bring suspect plant or chemical toxicants when submitting animals for post mortem evaluation. Common intoxicants include aflatoxins, rodenticides, organophosphates, and various plants, such as avocado. Fumonisin B_1, a common mycotoxin contaminant of inadequately dried corn, induces hepatic necrosis in rabbits when present in the feed at levels exceeding 5 mg/kg.

Chronic copper intoxication resulting in acute hemoglobinuric nephrosis and severe hepatocellular necrosis has been reported in New Zealand white rabbits experiencing post-transportation anorexia. Animals had been fed a high copper diet at the commercial supplier to enhance growth (317 ppm; greater than 30x the recommended maintenance level for rabbits) but were clinically normal. It was hypothesized that the rabbits had chronic copper toxicosis that was subclinical until the transportation stress and resulting anorexia that developed from a sudden diet change led to hepatic lysosomal rupture and systemic release of toxic amounts of copper. Animals exhibited depression, anorexia, and icterus

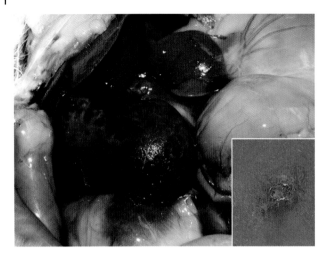

Figure 1.52 Liver lobe torsion in an 8-year-old rabbit. Inset: There is marked ischemic necrosis of the affected lobe. *Source:* Courtesy of The Links Road Animal and Bird Clinic.

prior to death. Hepatic copper concentrations in affected animals were approximately 317–995 ppm wet weight (4–6 ppm, reference range).

Liver lobe torsion occurs sporadically in rabbits and appears unrelated to breed, size, age, or sex. Unrelieved torsions may present as anorexia, lethargy, decreased fecal production or sudden death, although animals may survive for a considerable time after incomplete torsion. Anemia, thrombocytopenia and elevated serum levels of alanine aminotransferase, aspartate aminotransferase, and alkaline phosphatase may be detected ante mortem. The caudate lobe is most commonly affected and at post mortem will be dark red and friable, with microscopic evidence of acute ischemic necrosis (Figure 1.52).

Animals with more chronic disease may demonstrate capsular fibrosis surrounding the infarcted liver tissue. The etiopathogenesis for this condition is unknown although previous gastric dilatation with stretching of the left triangular ligament has been hypothesized.

Toxoplasmosis is rarely described in pet rabbits. Multifocal hepatic necrosis and coalescing areas of splenic necrosis have been consistently seen in individual cases, sometimes with myocarditis (Figure 1.53). Tachyzoites are abundant in affected tissues. Rabbits are likely infected by consuming water or feed contaminated with cat excreta containing *T. gondii* oocysts. Rabbit food should be stored in closed containers to minimize contamination and their water changed frequently. *T. gondii* can also be transmitted vertically in infected does.

Bile duct adenoma, biliary cystadenoma, cholangiocarcinoma (Figure 1.54), and **hepatic adenocarcinoma** are relatively uncommon spontaneous tumors in rabbits. Adenomas are composed of cords and nests of well differentiated biliary epithelium within an abundant fibrovascular stroma, and occasionally contain cystic dilatations. It is unknown whether hepatobiliary inflammation associated with *E. stiedae* infection predisposes animals to hyperplastic lesions, including adenomas and carcinomas, although in two cases, hepatic coccidiosis was also present. Other hepatobiliary tumors are very rare in rabbits.

1.7 Cardiovascular Conditions

Anatomically, both rabbit atrioventricular valves are bicuspid, and rabbits have poor collateral coronary arterial circulation, which may predispose the myocardium to

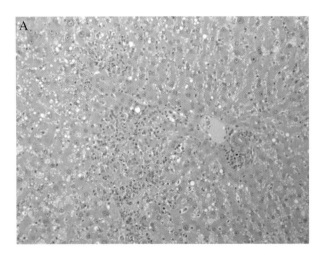
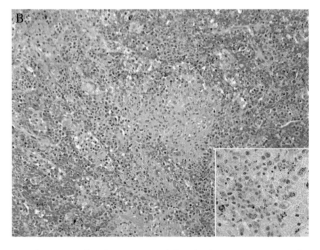

Figure 1.53 A: Multifocal hepatic necrosis in a 3-year-old rabbit due to *Toxoplasma gondii* infection. B: Multifocal splenic necrosis was also seen in this rabbit and numerous intracellular *Toxoplasma* cysts and zoites are positively labelled with immunohistochemistry. Inset: counter stain: Mayer's hematoxylin.

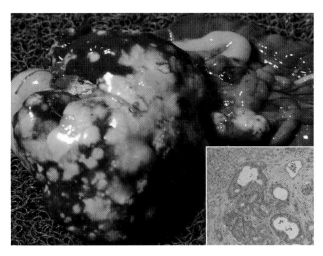

Figure 1.54 Cholangiocarcinoma in a 9-year-old neutered, male, Netherland dwarf rabbit presenting with dehydration, hypothermia, and ileus. Numerous metastases were present in other tissues, including lung and kidney. Inset: Neoplastic epithelial cells form acini and are supported by a dense fibrovascular stroma. The cells have indistinct cell borders and contain moderate to abundant eosinophilic cytoplasm, a large round to ovoid to vesicular nucleus and there is up to 6-fold anisocytosis and anisokaryosis as well as 15 mitoses/400x field.

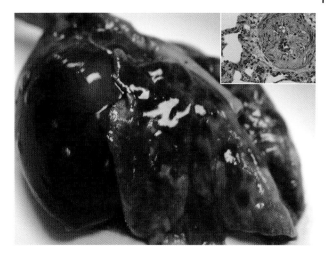

Figure 1.55 Congestive heart failure and pulmonary hypertension in an aged rabbit with dyspnea. The heart is enlarged and rounded and the lungs were wet and heavy. Inset: The pulmonary arteriolar tunica media is thickened with mild fibrinoid necrosis. Perivascular edema is moderate.
Source: Courtesy of H. Snyman.

hypoxemia and subsequent ischemic damage. Cardiac myocytes are approximately 20 μm in diameter and 100 μm long.

The true prevalence of cardiovascular disease is unknown in pet rabbits, as there are few reports in the literature. As per other clinical conditions, as rabbits receive better veterinary care and live longer, increasing numbers of degenerative cardiovascular cases may be reported. Significant differences in basal blood pressure exist between strains of rabbits, but whether this contributes to cardiovascular disease is unknown.

1.7.1 Cardiomyopathy

Dyspnea with sudden death may occur in rabbits and is thought to be due to persistent coronary arterial vasoconstriction following sudden catecholamine release, with resultant marked hypoxemia and infarction. Myocardial degeneration and early fibrosis can be seen several days following experimental dosing of rabbits with norepinephrine equivalent to naturally found levels. This circumstantially corroborates the clinical impression that rabbits are highly sensitive to environmental and physiologic stress.

Both dilated and hypertrophic cardiomyopathies have been reported to occur spontaneously in older rabbits and are associated with pleural effusion, biatrial enlargement, myofiber degeneration, and dissecting fibrosis (Figure 1.55). Incidental minimal to mild histopathologic

evidence of cardiomyopathy was reported in 32% of older New Zealand white rabbits in one study. In one animal, concurrent left atrial thrombosis was also noted. Valvular insufficiency and endocardiosis have been reported clinically in rabbits and may contribute to the condition. Rabbits have a naturally thin-walled right ventricle, a finding that should not be misdiagnosed as an abnormality at necropsy.

Post-anesthetic cardiomyopathy with myofiber necrosis, nonsuppurative inflammation, dissecting fibrosis, and death has been reported following anesthesia of rabbits with alpha-2 adrenergic agonists, specifically detomidine and xylazine (Figure 1.56A). There has been speculation that this form of cardiomyopathy occurs as an indirect toxic effect following persistent, drug-induced, coronary artery vasoconstriction with resultant myocardial hypoxemia, as animals provided with supplemental oxygen during general anesthesia induced by these agents do not develop the lesion.

As for skeletal muscle, dietary deficiency of vitamin E may result in a nutritional myocardial dystrophy, characterized by myofiber loss and degeneration, mineralization, and mononuclear leukocyte infiltration. Lesions may be visible grossly as patchy areas of pallor on the epicardial surface that extend into the underlying myocardium. Congestive heart failure may develop in animals that survive.

1.7.2 Myocarditis

Myocarditis has been reported in rabbits following systemic infection with a number of bacterial, parasitic, and viral

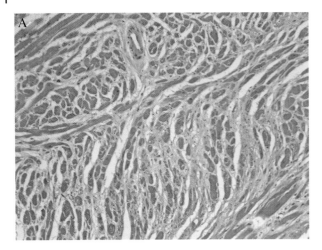
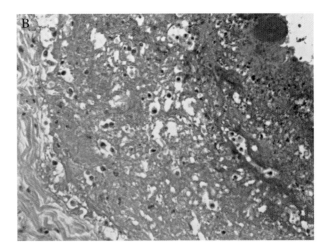

Figure 1.56 A: Dissecting myocardial fibrosis may develop in rabbits following anesthesia with alpha₂ agonists, such as xylazine and dexmedetomidine. B: Fibrinous epicarditis in a rabbit infected systemically with pasteurellosis. Dense bacterial colonies of short bacilli can be seen embedded in the fibrin.

agents, including *Pasteurella multocida* (Figure 1.56B), *Salmonella* spp. *Clostridium piliforme, Staphylococcus aureus, Toxoplasma gondii*, and *Encephalitozoon cuniculi* (Figure 1.57). As the heart is generally one of several tissues affected in each of these infections, special histologic stains on paraffin-embedded tissues, tissue culture and sensitivity, serology, and immunohistochemistry may be used to diagnose definitively the infection, in conjunction with gross and histologic findings from other tissues.

A coronavirus-induced generalized myocarditis with necrosis and pulmonary effusion has been reported in experimentally infected rabbits. Fragmentation and hyalinization of myofibers were prominent with local infiltration of multinucleated giant cells. Multi-organ necrosis was also described. The virus isolated was anti-

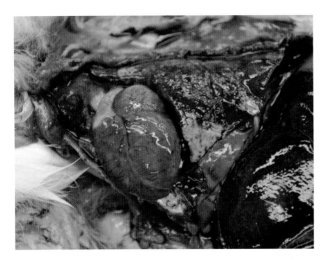

Figure 1.57 Endocarditis and myocarditis in a rabbit with septicemia as sequelae to dental abscessation with *Trueperella pyogenes*. The heart is enlarged and rounded, and areas of pallor are seen corresponding to underlying myocarditis.

genically similar to a human isolate and no further reports have been documented.

Valvular endocarditis and atrial thrombosis were reported in an experimental rabbit following inadvertent introduction of the Gram-negative opportunistic bacterium, *Achromobacter xylosoxidans*, during surgery. Strict aseptic technique should be maintained during any surgical procedure to minimize bacterial contamination of body cavities.

1.7.3 Myocardial Toxicity

Direct myocardial intoxication with subsequent necrosis may be seen following inadvertent administration of ionophores in the diet. Typically, this is a condition noted in commercial rabbits resulting from feed mill mixing or on-farm feeding errors. Maduramicin is particularly cardiotoxic to rabbits inducing acute epicardial hemorrhages, myocardial edema with myocyte hyalinization and necrosis, and sudden death. The underlying mechanism involves massive intracellular calcium release with subsequent cell swelling and death.

Similar myocardial intoxication may be seen in rabbits following treatment with anthracycline antibiotics, such as doxorubicin, or inadvertent ingestion of avocado leaves. Renal and hepatic necrosis and hydrothorax were reported following avocado leaf ingestion in rabbits. Persin, a poorly characterized fatty acid contained within the leaves, skin, bark, and pit of the avocado is thought to underlie the toxic response and similar toxicity has been reported in other domestic species.

1.7.4 Other Cardiovascular Conditions

Dystrophic calcification with medial mineralization of the aorta and other large vessels may be seen sporadi-

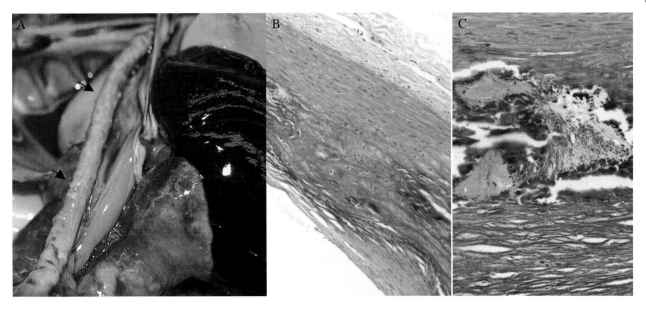

Figure 1.58 A: Aortic mineralization (arrows) resulting in a rigid vessel. This animal had underlying renal disease. B and C: Near circumferential mineralized medial plaques contributed to tissue rigidity.

cally in rabbits with chronic renal disease or in those inadvertently fed an excess of dietary vitamin D (Figure 1.58).

Congenital cardiovascular anomalies are reported rarely in rabbits. **Pulmonary hypertension** secondary to a ventricular septal defect (Eisenmenger's syndrome) has been reported in a New Zealand white rabbit. Other reported congenital anomalies in rabbits include vestigial pulmonary arterial trunks and pulmonic stenosis. These may be transmitted genetically as autosomal recessive conditions.

Hemangiosarcoma is a malignant endothelial cell tumor that is uncommon in rabbits. It has been reported in cutaneous, ovarian, and hepatic sites, with multiple metastases to the lungs and other organs. Abdominal tumors and implants may be friable and rupture, leading to hemoperitoneum and death. Tumors consist of anaplastic spindle cells surrounding irregular blood-filled channels. Immunohistochemical labeling with von Willebrand's factor is commonly used to confirm tumor identity in veterinary diagnostic laboratories; however, often a rabbit polyclonal antibody is used for this purpose, which leads to unacceptably high background levels of labeling in tumors in rabbits.

1.8 Genitourinary Conditions

1.8.1 Urinary Tract Conditions

Conditions of the urinary tract may affect any age, breed or sex of rabbit, with microsporidial disease and neoplasia being more common in older animals. Rabbit urine color may change with diet and season and may appear more or less pigmented and opaque, ranging from clear to cloudy to deep orange-red based on diet composition and amount of calcium sediment present (see Section 1.3, for a further discussion). A urinalysis is necessary to diagnose normal urine from hematuria. The smaller diameter of the male urethra makes male rabbits more prone to urolithiasis-related obstruction. Urine scalding and an associated moist dermatitis of the ventrum may be seen in animals housed in unhygienic conditions, animals unable to groom for any variety of reasons, animals unable to stand and assume appropriate micturition postures because of skeletal or neurologic conditions affecting the legs or spinal cord, and animals with renal disease (Figure 1.59). Again, a thorough investigation is indicated to determine the affected system. Finally, uterine disease in intact does may result in a sanguineous discharge that appears as hematuria.

1.8.1.1 Encephalitozoonosis
Encephalitozoon cuniculi is a Gram-positive, obligate intracellular, microsporidial parasite, which has a predilection for the kidney, eye, and central nervous system. Infections are common in rabbits in all settings and ante-mortem definitive diagnosis of the condition may be challenging.

Presenting Clinical Signs Infections with this agent are typically chronic, and clinical signs may range from none to sudden death. The kidney and brain are the most severely affected tissues, and renal failure and vestibular disease and paresis may be seen in infected animals in severe cases, either alone or in combination. Some

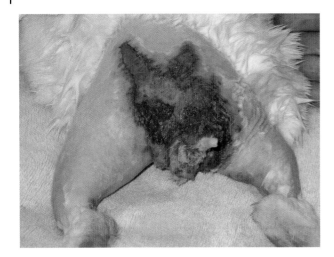

Figure 1.59 Severe urine scalding and moist dermatitis in a rabbit with chronic renal disease. *Source:* Courtesy of The Links Road Animal and Bird Clinic.

Microscopic lesions include focal to generalized granulomatous interstitial nephritis, sometimes with interstitial fibrosis. Organisms may be seen within renal tubular epithelial cells and collecting tubules. Focal interstitial pyogranulomatous to lymphocytic aggregates may be seen, with fibrosis in more chronic cases. In the brain and spinal cord, organisms may be encysted and quiescent with no signs of host reactivity. More active lesions are evidenced by pyogranulomatous inflammation and necrosis within the cerebral parenchyma with lymphoplasmacytic perivascular cuffing. Organisms are similar to coccobacilli in appearance, being approximately 1.5 x 2 μm, and are birefringent under polarized light. A Gram stain (Gram-positive) assists with visualization of parasitophorous vacuoles within lesions or in the parenchyma, unassociated with inflammation. Giemsa and carbol fuchsin stains may also be used to identify trophozoites. A granulomatous myocarditis may also be seen incidentally in affected animals at necropsy.

animals may clear the disease with no or few residual lesions. Dwarf rabbits are more susceptible to severe disease manifestations with this parasite. Phacoclastic uveitis is reported in dwarf rabbits, and may be uni- or bilateral (see Section 1.11 for more information).

Pathology In the more acute stages of the disease, the kidneys may be enlarged with grossly apparent small white foci distributed randomly throughout the cortex. Chronic renal infection is evidenced by generalized cortical surface pitting (Figure 1.60). Cerebral lesions are not evident grossly. The granulomatous brain lesions and renal pitting, caused by tissue destruction and scarring, persist for the life of the animal.

Laboratory Diagnostics Diagnosis may be challenging in live animals, as the disease may be subclinical and shedding of spores in the urine is intermittent. Serology is variably useful, detecting less than 50% of subclinical cases in one study. Further, a positive reaction and the presence of IgG only indicate exposure to the organism and not current infection. PCR assays may not always be accurate in ante mortem specimens. Histology with special stains or electron microscopy is diagnostic when lesions are present in brain sections, but can only be used on post mortem specimens.

Differential Diagnoses Potential differential diagnoses for renal disease include non-parasite-induced chronic renal

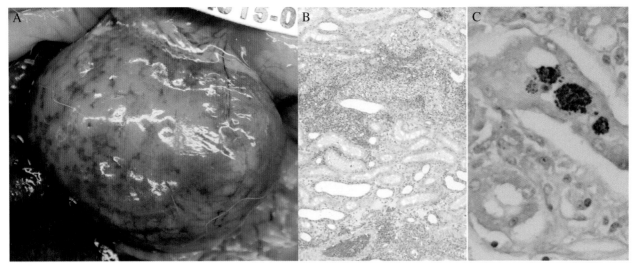

Figure 1.60 A: Renal pitting caused by *Encephalitozoon cuniculi* infection. B: There is a multifocal, nonsuppurative interstitial nephritis. C: Intratubular *E. cuniculi* trophozoites are Gram-positive.

failure and urolithiasis. Differentials for vestibular disease, paresis, and head tilt in the rabbit may include trauma, brain tumor, abscess, bacterial infection, idiopathic granulomatous encephalitis, and otitis media/interna. For phacoclastic uveitis, important differential diagnoses include bacterial uveitis or trauma.

Group or Herd Management Vertical transmission of spores may result in intraocular disease in offspring. *E. cuniculi* is capable of infecting other domestic mammals, including other companion animal species and immunocompromised humans. Cross-species transmission occurs by environmental contamination with spores in the urine or direct contact, thus careful hand hygiene is necessary after handling rabbits.

1.8.1.2 Chronic Renal Disease

Chronic renal disease is a common finding in older rabbits and animals may present acutely with anorexia, polyuria, polydipsia, azotemia, weight loss, and urine scalding (Figure 1.61). Lesions may consist of patchy to generalized nonsuppurative interstitial inflammation and fibrosis with or without renal tubular degeneration and regeneration, and multifocal renal tubular dilatation with proteinaceous or mineralized casts. Renal amyloidosis has been reported in two animals with chronic renal disease, confirmed with a Congo red stain and polarized light (apple green birefringence). An etiology may be difficult to determine and lesions may be related to past or subclinical microsporidial or bacterial infections, urolithiasis or inappropriate diet (e.g., hypercalcemia). Renal tubular mineralization or calcium deposition in other soft tissues may also be noted with severe renal damage and in cases of hypervitaminosis D.

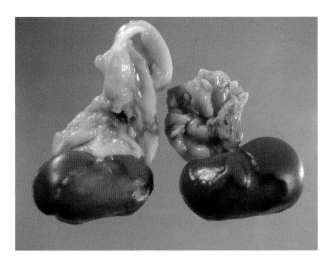

Figure 1.61 Chronic renal infarction. The kidneys were negative for *E. cuniculi* antigen.

1.8.1.3 Urolithiasis

In the rabbit, uroliths may be found anywhere within the urogenital tract from the renal pelvis, through to the distal urethra (Figure 1.62). Uroliths may be discrete or may present as fine calcium crystal precipitates in the urinary bladder ("sludge"). Clinical signs will depend upon the location of the urolith, the chronicity, and the degree of obstruction. Animals may present with lethargy, anorexia, urine scalding, hunched posture, bruxism, hematuria, and stranguria. Hydroureter and hydronephrosis may occur in severe cases with complete urine outflow obstruction. Renal or urinary bladder inflammation secondary to encephalitozoonosis or bacterial infection may alter urine pH, predisposing to calcium salt precipitation, as may dehydration, although factors predisposing animals to urolithiasis are incompletely understood. Urinary pH also may be affected by diet, leading to salt precipitation (see Section 1.3 for a more complete discussion of calcium metabolism in the rabbit). Typical rabbit urine pH ranges from 8–9, while calcium and phosphate may precipitate as crystals at pH 8.5–9.5.

1.8.1.4 Renal Neoplasia

Renal neoplasms reported in rabbits include nephroblastoma, lymphosarcoma, renal cell carcinoma, and hamartoma. Nephroblastoma (embryonal nephroma or Wilm's tumor) is relatively common in young rabbits and presents as a uni- or bilateral increase in kidney size, which may be grossly palpable, with lethargy and decreased urine and fecal output. Tumors arise from the primitive nephrogenic blastema and are typically moderately cellular, composed of a disorganized mixture of epithelial, mesenchymal, and blastemal cell populations, forming primitive glomeruli and tubules, supported and separated by a moderate fibrovascular stroma (Figure 1.63).

Renal cell carcinomas may arise from the pole of one kidney, and the pattern of growth may be solid to trabecular, papillary, or tubular. Clear cell variants occur in rabbits, as in other species.

Lymphosarcoma is the most common tumor of rabbits and one or both kidneys may be affected. Grossly, multifocal firm, raised, white masses may be seen on the cortical surfaces extending into the parenchyma on cut section. Histologically, tumor sections are seen to be composed of dense infiltrates of neoplastic lymphocytes. Tumors are often multicentric in nature, although rabbits rarely are leukemic.

1.8.1.5 Lead Intoxication

Lead intoxication is the most common toxicosis in rabbits and occurs following exposure and chewing of surfaces covered with lead-based paint. Animals may present with nonspecific signs of lethargy, anorexia, hematuria, blindness, and seizures, and anemia with

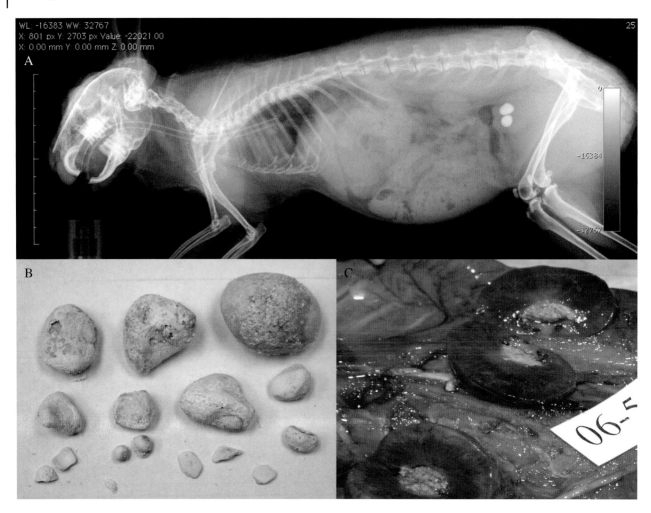

Figure 1.62 A: Lateral radiograph of an adult rabbit demonstrating 2 uroliths within the urinary bladder. B: Uroliths of varying sizes from rabbits. C: Uroliths may also be found within the renal pelvis as fine particles, as in this case, or as large staghorn concretions. *Source:* B: Courtesy of The Links Road Animal and Bird Clinic.

basophilic erythrocyte stippling may be seen on examination of blood smears. Renal tubular degeneration and necrosis with mineralization and intratubal hemoglobin casts are seen histologically, as well as other systemic effects, including myocardial and hepatocellular degeneration and necrosis. Lead concentrations in peripheral or heart blood greater than 0.48 umol/L are strongly suggestive of lead intoxication.

Other chemicals and toxicants will also induce acute renal failure in rabbits. The anesthetic combination of tiletamine/zolazepam induces acute renal tubular necrosis in rabbits and is contraindicated.

1.8.1.6 Other Renal Conditions

Bacterial cystitis and **pyelonephritis** are relatively common in pet rabbits and may result in renal abscessation, infarction, and failure in severe cases. Typical isolates include *S. aureus*, *E. coli*, *P. multocida*, and *K. pneumoniae*.

Polycystic kidney disease is seen sporadically in New Zealand white rabbits. Affected animals may or not present with clinical signs and the diagnosis may be incidental at necropsy. Cystic areas are variably-sized, single or multiple, and are seen as dilatations of tubules and/or glomeruli with loose mesenchymal interstitial expansion. Cysts are likely congenital in origin; however, the mode of inheritance has not been characterized. Other congenital defects reported for the urogenital tract include unilateral renal agenesis.

Inguinal herniation of the urinary bladder with incarceration by the inguinal ring was reported in one doe. **Inguinal/scrotal herniation of the urinary bladder** has been infrequently reported in bucks. Affected animals present with unilateral scrotal swelling and it is postulated that the open inguinal canal may predispose bucks to this condition. While incarceration of the urinary bladder may occur, these animals typically respond well to inguinal herniorrhaphy repair.

Lapine parvovirus has been recovered from the kidneys of naturally infected rabbits. The virus may be relatively nonpathogenic as experimental inoculation of young kits only results in transient loss of appetite.

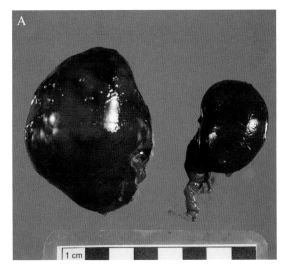
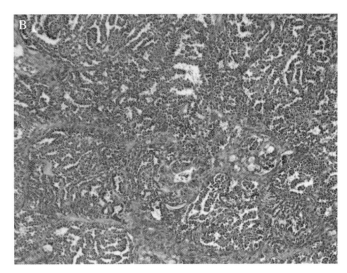

Figure 1.63 A: Nephroblastoma in a 1-year-old male rabbit. The enlarged kidney was palpable ante-mortem. B: The neoplastic tissue is highly cellular and the tumor is composed of a mixture of primitive glomeruli and abortive tubules within a moderate fibrovascular stroma.

1.8.2 Reproductive Tract Conditions

Does have duplex cervices leading into separate uterine horns. They reach puberty by about 6–8 months of age, slightly earlier in dwarf breeds. Does are induced ovulators and do not have an estrus cycle, thus vaginal smears are not useful for predicting reproductive cycle intervals in this species. Does generally ovulate approximately 10 hours post coitus and the gestation period is 30–35 days. Pseudopregnancy can occur following unsuccessful mating or following mounting by other females. The condition may manifest as mammary gland enlargement, hair plucking, and nest-building in the nonpregnant doe; however, signs will usually resolve within 18 days of breeding. Corpora lutea can be seen in the ovaries of pseudopregnant does. Dystocia due to fetal oversize or uterine inertia is moderately uncommon in rabbits. Kits are relatively precocious at birth, nursing only once daily, and they are weaned at 4–6 weeks of age.

In the buck, the testes descend at 8–12 weeks of age although the inguinal ring remains open in the buck throughout its life. Intestinal or bladder herniation may occur via this route if the inguinal rings are left open post-castration. Spermatozoa are produced by approximately 110 days of age, but bucks are not used for regular breeding until they are 135–140 days old. The spermatogenic cycle requires 45–60 days for completion.

1.8.2.1 Listeriosis

Listeriosis is a sporadic disease of rabbits, inducing sudden death of individuals or epizootics, particularly in pregnant animals. The disease is caused by *Listeria monocytogenes*, a Gram-positive, motile nonspore-forming rod.

Presenting Clinical Signs Because of a predilection of the bacterium for the gravid uterus and placenta, clinical signs are noted most commonly in pregnant does. Affected animals may show nonspecific signs of anorexia and bruxism, and late term abortions are common. Central nervous system signs of ataxia and blindness are unusual. Sudden death may occur.

Pathology Multifocal hepatic and splenic necrosis with lymphadenopathy, uterine hemorrhage and distension with fetal death and maceration (if not expelled), hydrothorax, and ascites may be seen grossly. Histologically, transmural necrosuppurative metritis and placentitis with abundant bacteria are present. Hepatic lesions consist of multifocal coagulative necrosis with marked neutrophilic infiltrates.

Laboratory Diagnostics A presumptive diagnosis may be made from the classic gross findings and clinical history. The organism is cultured readily from affected tissues using cold enrichment techniques and can also be demonstrated in tissue sections with a Gram stain.

Differential Diagnoses Listeriosis commonly results in late term abortions in rabbits. Other common causes of suppurative metritis in does include *Staphylococcus aureus* and *Pasteurella multocida*. Abortions may be induced with certain intoxications, including hypervitaminosis A, as well as by hyperthermia and stress.

Group or Herd Management Listeriosis may be transmitted by direct contact with clinically affected or subclinically infected carrier animals, by infected fomites, or via contaminated food, such as hay, or water. Sick animals should always be isolated from healthy animals. *Listeria monocytogenes* is a zoonotic agent, and appropriate hand hygiene is always important after handling rabbits.

1.8.2.2 Other Causes of Pyometra and Abortion

Pyometra and reduced reproductive performance are important sources of culling of breeding does in commercial herds. *P. multocida* and *S. aureus* are isolated frequently from affected animals and infection rates may be up to 60% for some herds. Both agents induce suppurative lesions and reproductive system abscesses, including suppurative endometritis, salpingitis, and ovarian abscesses. Anterograde movement of bacteria just before parturition may result in placentitis and fetal death.

Treponema paraluiscuniculi (see Section 1.2) may decrease fertility in some animals but does not typically induce pyometra. Gross lesions are limited to perivulvar and perinasal crusting, ulceration, and hemorrhage.

Both **hypervitaminosis A** and **hypovitaminosis A** may induce similar fetal resorption, abortions, stillbirth, low neonatal survival, and hydrocephaly. Inadvertent errors in feed mixing are generally responsible for the problems noted in affected herds. Low dietary levels of **vitamin E** and **selenium** are also linked with abortions, stillbirth, infertility, and muscular dystrophy secondary to mineralization of the myocardium, tongue, and skeletal muscles in rabbits.

1.8.2.3 Female Reproductive Masses

Intact, adult does have a high incidence of uterine adenocarcinoma, which may approach 80% for some breeds, such as New Zealand white rabbits. The tumor is seen rarely in other breeds, such as Rex and Belgian. A bloody discharge associated with the tumor may be present and mistaken for hematuria. The uterus may be unilaterally or bilaterally enlarged, with a nodular appearance. Masses may be variably firm and contain multiloculated cysts filled with bloody material, as well as foci of necrosis (Figure 1.64). Histologic findings are characterized by endometrial gland anaplasia with proliferation and invasion of the myometrium. The stroma may have a myxomatous appearance and mitotic figures are variable. Areas of necrosis, superficial lumenal ulceration, and neutrophilic infiltrates may also be seen (Figure 1.65). Local seeding of abdominal tissues and pulmonary metastases occur late in the course of the disease. Mammary gland abnormalities (hyperplasia, dysplasia, and adenocarcinoma) are associated frequently with uterine adenocarcinomas in the rabbit, suggesting that these tumors are hormonally active.

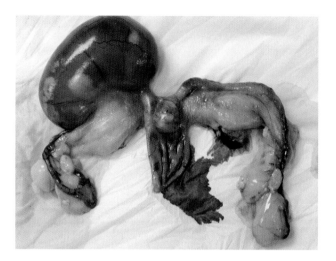

Figure 1.64 Uterine adenocarcinoma in a rabbit. *Source.* Courtesy of The Links Road Animal and Bird Clinic.

An important but uncommon differential diagnosis for uterine adenocarcinoma is choriocarcinoma. Choriocarcinoma is a rare and highly malignant tumor arising from trophoblasts within the placenta or ovary of does. A case was reported in a 3-year-old nongravid intact doe. The mass likely originated within the ovary and the animal presented with multiple uterine masses. The doe also had multiple metastases to the lungs and local seeding throughout the abdomen.

Leiomyomas are common in intact does and are usually detected during ovariohysterectomy of older animals or incidentally at necropsy. As for other species,

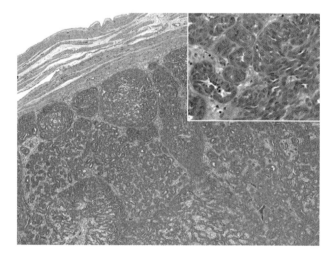

Figure 1.65 Photomicrograph of a uterus from a rabbit with adenocarcinoma. The tumor is composed of dense, variably-sized acini and tubules of neoplastic cells separated by a fine fibrovascular stroma invading the endometrium. Inset: Mitoses are frequent, up to 8/400x fields.

leiomyomas consist of benign, firm, pale masses that are composed of interlacing or palisading bundles of well differentiated spindle-shaped cells with indistinct cell borders. Mitoses are few in number, and positive cytoplasmic labeling of neoplastic cells can be seen with smooth muscle actin. Leiomyosarcoma occurs less commonly.

Uterine stromal polyps occur sporadically in does. Masses are generally pedunculated, project into the uterine lumen, and consist of spindle-shaped cells within a loose myxomatous stroma. In endometrial hemangiomatosis, the uterine horns are enlarged and turgid, and, on cross section, contain red-tinged watery fluid and a variable number of red-purple, firm, ovoid, pedunculated masses. The microscopic appearance of uterine hemangiomas includes congested and hemorrhagic polypoid nodules with laminated thrombi composed of layers of fibrin and red cells in the vascular spaces.

Granulosa cell tumors and ovarian carcinomas are uncommon tumors in does, with or without uterine adenocarcinoma. The gross and histologic appearances of both are similar to those seen in other domestic animal species. Cases of malignant mixed Mullerian tumor and a deciduosarcoma have also been reported in intact pet does. Ovarian teratomas are seen rarely in rabbits.

Ovarian cysts may be seen incidentally at post-mortem. Cysts are variably-sized and may be lined by ciliated epithelium (parovarian cysts), compressing the adjacent parenchyma into a thin surrounding rim. Cystic ovaries may be associated also with endometrial hyperplasia, in which proliferative changes of the endometrial glands are seen with formation of papillary or polypoid growths that project into the lumen (Figure 1.68B). Hyperplastic endometrial glands may also be cystic in appearance. Endometrial hyperplasia is commonly seen together with uterine adenocarcinoma, again, suggestive of a hormonal influence.

1.8.2.4 Male Reproductive Masses

Seminomas and interstitial cell tumors are reported sporadically in intact bucks, sometimes both tumors in the same animal. Seminomas may be uni- or bilateral and present as testicular enlargement. Tumors typically are firm and pale and are often well differentiated, although more invasive tumors have been reported. Neoplastic cells typically are round to polygonal with abundant pale granular basophilic cytoplasm and distinct cell borders, and a central round nucleus, set within a fine fibrovascular stroma. Masses may compress or replace adjacent normal parenchyma and mitoses are dependent upon the invasiveness. Small numbers of infiltrating lymphocytes may be present.

Interstitial cell tumors present as testicular enlargement with moderate firmness and a characteristic tan to orange appearance on cut section. Cells are round to polygonal with pale eosinophilic granular cytoplasm, indistinct cell borders, and a round nucleus. Intracytoplasmic crystals have been reported in one case. Surrounding seminiferous tubules are generally atrophied.

Other masses reported for intact bucks include testicular teratoma (in both cryptorchid and normal testes), testicular gonadoblastoma (Figure 1.66), granular cell tumor of the testes, and carcinoma *in situ* of the prostate gland.

Non-neoplastic differentials for testicular enlargement include trauma with associated swelling, abscessation, suppurative orchitis, cystic structures, scrotal hernia, and testicular torsion.

1.8.2.5 Pregnancy Toxemia

Pregnancy toxemia occurs in does within the final 2–3 weeks of gestation. Obesity and fasting are predisposing factors for ketosis in rabbits, and a similar metabolic syndrome with ketosis may be seen in obese buckss and does. Dutch, Polish, and English breeds have a predisposition to toxemia. Affected animals have a clinical history of acute anorexia, depression, and rapid death. Gross lesions include reduced gastric content, abundant body fat, dead and decomposed fetuses, uterine and placental hemorrhage, adrenal enlargement and hemorrhage, and a pale, greasy enlarged liver. Histologically, marked diffuse hepatic lipidosis with fatty degeneration of renal cortical tubular epithelium and the adrenal cortex is typical.

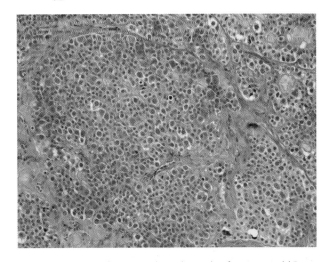

Figure 1.66 Tissue from an enlarged testicle of an 8 year-old Rex rabbit. The enlarged testicle is composed of lobules of tubules separated by fine fibrous stroma. Many of the tubules have central lumena containing pale eosinophilic fluid and contain Sertoli cells as well as variable numbers of large round cells resembling germ cells. Around the periphery of the testicle and also within the centre are nests and streams of neoplastic germ cells, consistent with a testicular gonadoblastoma.

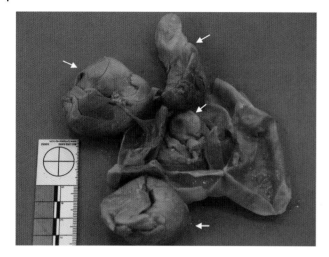

Figure 1.67 Large mass attached to the cecum of a doe opened to demonstrate three well-formed rabbit fetuses and a fourth undergoing maceration (arrows). The doe had given birth to eight live kits two days previously but was off feed. Another pendulous mass was attached to the stomach and contained a further three fetuses. This doe had been hand-mated twice and had no known risk factors for ectopic pregnancy.

1.8.2.6 Other Reproductive Conditions

Dystocia may occur in rabbits and may be related to fetal oversize or uterine inertia, secondary to calcium deficiency. Uterine prolapse also occurs and is typically managed clinically as an emergency condition.

Ectopic pregnancies occur sporadically in rabbits (Figure 1.67) and may be palpable as free masses within the abdomen. Often there are no associated clinical signs, although affected animals may be culled for perceived reproductive problems (that is, apparent failure to become pregnant). The condition is more common when artificial insemination techniques are used with inadvertent traumatic rupture of the uterine wall; however, spontaneous cases without uterine trauma are seen. In one case, a doe delivered eight kits without incident, retaining an additional seven kits intra-abdominally, in various stages of development and maceration. Abdominal masses containing developing fetuses may be free within the abdomen or attached to the omentum or parenchymatous organs by a long vascular placental stalk. Fetuses are typically necrotic at detection.

Endometrial venous varices may be seen sporadically in intact does (Figures 1.68 and 1.69). Affected vessels may rupture, leading to apparent hematuria or bloody vulvar discharge. Affected animals may be severely anemic and may die without surgical intervention (hysterectomy). On gross examination, aneurysms are visible as multifocal dark red dilatations bulging superficially from the endometrial surface. The etiopathogenesis is unknown.

Congenital lesions of the female rabbit reproductive tract are rare. **Uterine horn aplasia or partial agenesis** with cystic dilatation of remaining segments has been reported. Presumably, this arises from a developmental defect in fusion of the paramesonephric ducts with the urogenital sinus on one or both sides of the animal. **Cystic testes**, uni- or bilateral **undescended testes**, and **hypospadiasis** are congenital lesions reported in male rabbits. Similarly, congenital lesions of kits are highly uncommon. Endometrial fibrosis may be seen in aging does.

In rabbits fed **fumonisin B$_1$** contaminated food, mild to moderate testicular Sertoli cell degeneration was seen at levels equal to and exceeding 5 mg/kg (see Section 1.6.4.4).

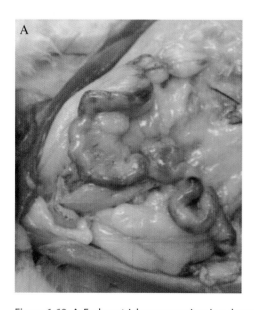

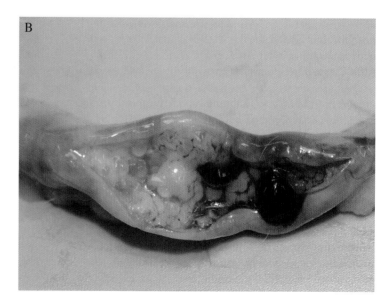

Figure 1.68 A: Endometrial venous varices in a doe with a chronic history of hematuria. B: Uterus opened to demonstrate the varices.

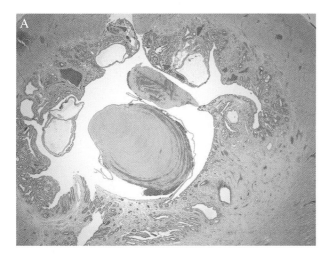 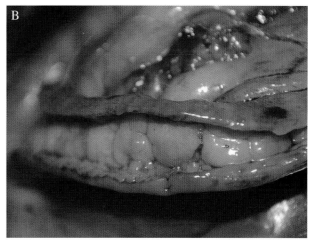

Figure 1.69 A: Cystic endometrial hyperplasia and venous varices in a mature doe. B: Uterus opened to demonstrate cystic endometrial hyperplasia.

A number of histologic alterations are seen in the testes in older aging bucks, including spermatid giant cells, cytoplasmic swelling of spermatogonia, hypospermatogenesis, and dilated seminiferous tubules.

1.9 Nervous System Conditions

Neurologic or apparent neurologic presenting signs are common in pet rabbits. As with musculoskeletal disorders, it is important to differentiate primary neurologic disease from other disorders that may produce neurologic signs. Causes of head tilt in rabbits may include conditions affecting the cerebellum and medulla oblongata; bacterial infection with resulting otitis media/interna or abscessation; viral infection including herpetic encephalitis or rabies virus infection; parasitic diseases such as toxoplasmosis, encephalitozoonosis, and larval migration; cerebrovascular accident (stroke); trauma; neurotoxicity; idiopathic central or peripheral vestibular disease; or neoplasia. Paresis and paralysis may be induced by vertebral fracture or luxation; intervertebral disk disease; osteoarthritis and spondylosis; abscess formation; parasitic diseases, such as toxoplasmosis, encephalitozoonosis, and larval migration; hypovitaminosis E; inappropriate flooring and overcrowding with acquired splayleg formation or other skeletal deformities; and neoplasia. Finally, the etiology of seizures in rabbits may include several bacterial, viral or parasitic diseases; abscesses; neurotoxicoses, pregnancy toxemia; end stage systemic disease; heat prostration; idiopathic epilepsy or neoplasia. The more common primary neurologic conditions are discussed below.

1.9.1 Encephalitozoonosis

Encephalitozoonosis remains an important cause of neurologic disease in rabbits (see Section 1.8.1.1). The disease is caused by the obligate intracellular microsporidial parasite, *Encephalitozoon cuniculi*, and it is considered enzootic in pet and commercial rabbit populations. In a recent retrospective study examining causes of neurologic disease in 118 pet rabbits over a 13-year period, almost 59% of the cases were attributed to infection by *E. cuniculi*. The parasite affects all breeds, ages, and both sexes of rabbits. Clinical disease is much more common in dwarf breeds. The life cycle is simple and direct, and spores are transmitted by ingestion or inhalation. Proliferative stages of merogeny and sporogony occur intracellularly and spores mature within a parasitophorous vacuole within the host cell cytoplasm. The vacuole enlarges until the host cell ruptures, releasing spores that infect adjacent cells. Spores are excreted from the kidneys in the urine of infected rabbits. Granulomatous lesions of the brain are not usually seen until at least 3–4 weeks post-infection.

Neurologic manifestations of encephalitozoonosis may range from subtle to overt, including vestibular disease (e.g., head tilt and ataxia), posterior paresis, behavioral changes, depression, seizures, and sudden death. Typically, there are no gross lesions associated with neurologic disease, although poor body condition and muscle mass may be seen in animals experiencing difficulty eating. Microscopic evaluation of the brain and spinal cord may demonstrate multifocal areas of nonsuppurative meningoencephalitis and astrogliosis within the neuropil with associated perivascular lymphoplasmacytic cuffing and, occasionally, vasculitis and mineraliza-

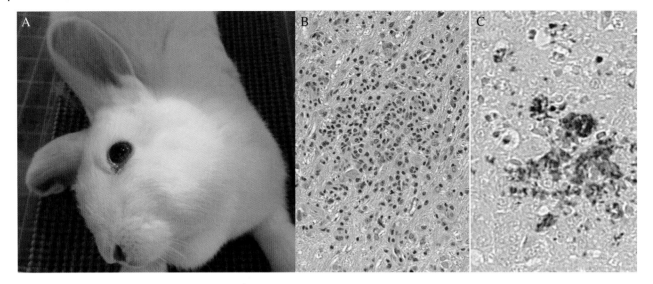

Figure 1.70 A: Torticollis in a young growing rabbit with *Encephalitozoon cuniculi* encephalitis. B: Microscopically, there are multifocal areas of nonsuppurative encephalitis and gliosis. C: Gram-positive microsporidial organisms can be seen in affected areas of the brain.

tion (Figure 1.70). Organisms are similar to coccobacilli in appearance, being approximately 1.5 x 2 μm, and are birefringent under polarized light. A modified Gram stain assists with visualization of parasitophorous vacuoles within lesions or in the parenchyma, unassociated with inflammation. Aggregations of the parasite are observed occasionally at necropsy in the brains of adult rabbits that have exhibited no clinical evidence of neurologic disease. Other organs with possible microsporidial lesions include the kidney (granulomatous nephritis) and eyes (cataracts and phacoclastic uveitis, see Section 1.8.1.1).

Experimentally infected animals typically shed spores in their urine between approximately 40–70 days post-infection. Spores (1.5 x 2.5 μm) persist for up to three months in the environment in moderate temperatures. The organism is zoonotic, and strict hand hygiene practices should be used following handling of rabbits. Similarly, rabbits may be infected with human strains of *Encephalitozoon*. Differential diagnoses for neurologic manifestations of encephalitozoonosis in rabbits include infections with *Pasteurella multocida* (Figure 1.71), *Listeria monocytogenes*, *Toxoplasma gondii* and *Baylisascaris* spp. larval migration.

1.9.2 Herpesvirus-1 Encephalitis

Human herpesvirus-1 (HHV-1; Herpes simplex 1) is an alphaherpesvirus with a seroprevalence of infection in the human population in North America estimated at

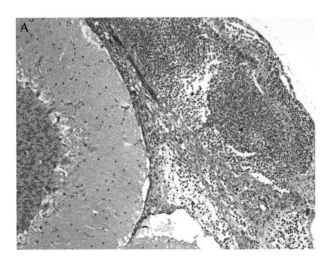

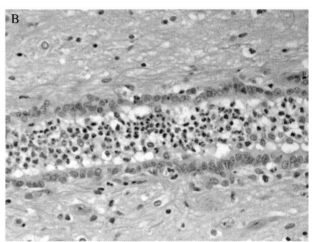

Figure 1.71 Marked fibrinosuppurative *Pasteurella*-associated meningitis (A) and myelitis (B) in a doe. The animal appeared "nervous" prior to clinical presentation for seizures.

over 80%. Rabbits are very sensitive to infection and because of this are used as an experimental animal model for HHV-1 infection. Although disease induced by HHV-1 in humans is frequently asymptomatic or mild, infection in rabbits may result in significant disease and death. Animals may shed live virus in their tears and other secretions prior to death.

1.9.2.1 Presenting Clinical Signs
A range of nonspecific signs may be seen ante mortem, including anorexia, bruxism, ataxia, inactivity, conjunctivitis, ptyalism, depression, and sudden death.

1.9.2.2 Pathology
No gross lesions are apparent in the brain or spinal cord; however, severe, diffuse nonsuppurative meningoencephalitis, primarily affecting the grey matter, may be seen, with lymphoplasmacytic perivascular cuffing. Glassy eosinophilic intranuclear inclusion bodies may be found in infected glia and neurons. Nonsuppurative keratitis and conjunctivitis are also reported with or without anterior uveitis.

1.9.2.3 Laboratory Diagnostics
A presumptive diagnosis may be made based on typical histopathologic findings, including characteristic eosinophilic intranuclear inclusion bodies in the brain or spinal cord. Definitive diagnosis is based on virus-specific PCR or immunohistochemical assay.

1.9.2.4 Differential Diagnoses
Other common neurologic conditions in rabbits with similar presenting signs to those of HHV-1 include *E. cuniculi* infection, *Baylisascaris* spp. larval migration, rabies virus infection, head trauma, brain abscess or bacterial meningitis, toxicity, and tumor. Conjunctivitis does not occur with any of the differential diagnoses listed, except for rabies virus infection, which is extremely uncommon in rabbits. When conjunctivitis is present, it may be an important diagnostic indicator of HHV-1 infection. Encephalitis has not been reported with leporid herpesvirus-4 infection in rabbits.

1.9.2.5 Group or Herd Management
Typical cases of HHV-1 encephalitis in rabbits are sporadic; however, infected animals may shed live virus that presents an infectious risk for other rabbits and is a zoonotic risk for humans.

1.9.3 Rabies

Rabies virus infection is caused by a rhabdovirus and is rarely reported in pet rabbits in North America. Some authors suggest the paucity of reports indicates a relative insensitivity of rabbits to the virus, however, rabbits were used for many years for rabies virus vaccine production, and they are a sensitive species. Rabies has been reported to occur in rabbits housed primarily outside or with exposure to potentially infected wildlife, such as raccoons, foxes, or skunks.

1.9.3.1 Presenting Clinical Signs
Rabbits typically develop the paralytic form of rabies and may present with sudden death or with nonspecific central nervous system signs of paresis, ataxia, conjunctivitis, head tilt, and anorexia, as well as bruxism. Clinical signs may occur up to one month post-exposure; however, death usually ensues within several days after clinical signs of infection appear.

1.9.3.2 Pathology
There are no gross lesions associated with the disease. Histopathology may demonstrate multifocal areas of lymphocytic infiltration with gliosis, perivascular lymphocytic cuffing, edema, and neurodegeneration. Negri bodies (eosinophilic intracytoplasmic inclusion bodies within affected neurons) may be seen in some infections.

1.9.3.3 Laboratory Diagnostics
Rabies virus infection is a reportable disease in Canada and the United States. Tissues or samples from suspect positive cases should be submitted according to the appropriate regulatory authorities. Direct fluorescence immunoassay on fresh or frozen brain is used by state and federal laboratories to confirm infection. Immunohistochemistry, RT-PCR, and virus isolation also may be used for viral detection.

1.9.3.4 Differential Diagnoses
Head trauma or other agents inducing central nervous system disease, such as *E. cuniculi*, HHV-1 infection, lead intoxication, brain abscess, neoplasia, and cerebrospinal parasitic larval migration are more common than rabies virus infection in rabbits. However, a history of exposure to feral or other potentially rabid animals or of outdoor housing may increase the diagnostic consideration of this disease.

1.9.3.5 Disease Management
No animal to human transmission of rabies virus has been reported from a domestic rabbit. Because there is no vaccine approved for rabies virus prophylaxis in pet rabbits in North America, clients who allow pet rabbits to graze outdoors or who house animals outside should be cautioned to protect them from feral animal exposures. Suspect cases should remain in a veterinary clinic

for close observation and the appropriate authorities contacted for advice.

1.9.4 Cerebrospinal Parasitic Larval Migration

Baylisascaris procyonis is a common nematode of raccoons and is a well-recognized agent of visceral and neural larval migrans in humans and various domestic animal species in North America; rabbits are a paratenic host. Eggs shed in the feces of raccoons require several weeks to become infective. After ingestion, larvae hatch and migrate within the body; approximately 8% going to the brain, where larvae continue to grow and migrate, inducing significant damage and marked inflammation.

1.9.4.1 Presenting Signs
Cerebrospinal larval migration (cerebral nematodiasis) presents as acute paresis or paralysis (spinal cord) or as head tilt with or without depression (Figure 1.72). As larvae continue to migrate, progressive signs of neurodegeneration occur, culminating in death.

1.9.4.2 Pathology
There are generally no gross lesions associated with larval migration in the brain; however, nodular larval granulomas may be seen occasionally on the epicardium, within the salivary gland and lung, and on the hepatic and renal capsules. Histologically, in the brain and spinal cord, there is marked neurodegeneration and necrosis with gliosis, marked eosinophilic and lymphocytic infiltrates, edema, focal hemorrhage, and spongiosis of affected areas. Although extensive tracts of necrosis and inflammation may be present, larvae are generally few in number and may not be readily apparent in tissue sections. Serial sec-

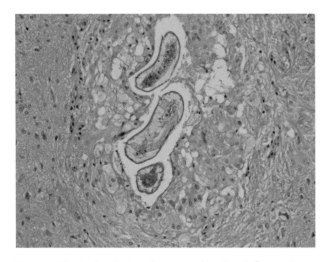

Figure 1.72 Focal malacia and pyogranulomatous inflammation in the brain of a rabbit surrounding several sections of nematode larvae, consistent in appearance with *Baylisascaris procyonis*. This rabbit presented with tetraparesis.

tioning of nervous tissue may be necessary to visualize the typical nematode larvae within the affected tissue.

In other tissues, eosinophilic myositis, interstitial nephritis, and eosinophilic interstitial pneumonia may be present and indicative of larval migration.

1.9.4.3 Laboratory Diagnostics
Microscopic visualization of nematode sections within tracts of neuronal inflammation and necrosis is generally diagnostic. No commercial serologic assay is available; however, PCR (tissue) assays are available from some human and primate diagnostic laboratories.

1.9.4.4 Differential Diagnoses
Trauma or infection with agents inducing myelitis or encephalitis, such as *E cuniculi*, HHV-1 infection, cerebrospinal abscess or neoplasia are potential differentials for *B. procyonis* larval migration. A history suggestive of exposure to raccoon feces may be helpful in the diagnosis.

Cerebral myiasis caused by unidentified fly larvae has also been reported in two Dutch rabbits that were housed outside.

1.9.4.5 Disease Management
Rabbits become intermediate hosts following exposure to environments contaminated by raccoon feces or following grooming of infective eggs on their hair coat. Exposure to contaminated bedding or food, or outdoor pasturing and housing may increase the risk of rabbit exposure in areas in which raccoons are common. Rabbits do not develop a patent infection and as such cannot transmit the disease; however, handling bedding or feed contaminated with raccoon feces poses similar concerns for humans, with risk of inadvertent ingestion or inhalation of infective eggs.

1.9.5 Neurotoxicoses

The most common neurotoxicant in rabbits is lead, generally following unsupervised access to furniture or building materials coated in lead paint. In addition to hematopoietic and renal signs (see Section 1.8.1.5, for a complete description), affected animals may present with tremors, blindness, seizures, and death. Basophilic stippling of erythrocytes may be seen on peripheral blood smears and blood lead levels in excess of 0.48 μmol/L are consistent with intoxication.

The mechanism by which lead-induced neurointoxication occurs is not clearly understood. Recent experimental studies in rats indicate that behavioral and locomotor changes induced by chronic lead consumption are linked to regional depletion of norepinephrine in the brain. Organolead compounds induce more direct nervous system damage, causing neuronal necrosis in the entorhinal complex, hippocampus, and amygdala, with neuronal chromatolysis, swelling, and cell death in the mid brain, brainstem, and spinal cord.

Organophosphate and permethrin toxicity have been reported in rabbits following dipping or spraying animals for cutaneous parasites. Animals presented with acute blindness, seizures, and rapid death.

1.9.6 Cerebrospinal Neoplasia

Multicentric lymphoma with focal or generalized meningeal or cerebral infiltration is the most commonly reported cerebrospinal tumor in rabbits.

Acidophil pituitary adenomas may occur in older New Zealand white rabbits and may secrete prolactin, resulting in associated mammary gland hyperplasia and dysplasia and endometrial gland hyperplasia. There is nodular or generalized enlargement of the anterior pituitary gland, formed by nests and cords of eosinophilic neoplastic cells contained within a fine fibrovascular stroma, which compress the adjacent parenchyma (see Sections 1.2.6.8 and 1.3.1).

Other cerebrospinal tumors are rare. Single cases of intracranial or intraspinal teratoma, ependymoma, and peripheral neurofibrosarcoma have been reported in rabbits.

1.9.7 Other Conditions of the Brain and Spinal Cord

Brain abscesses, and less commonly, suppurative meningitis, may occur in rabbits and are associated with systemic infection with *P. multocida* or *S. aureus*. **Cerebral ischemic lesions** have been reported in rabbits with severe myocardial degeneration and fibrosis. Idiopathic vestibular disease is described for rabbits, but no histologic lesions are reported. Random foci of mononuclear cell aggregates with intracellular accumulations of pigment (lipofuscin) can be seen within the neuropil of aging rabbits, but these foci may or may not be associated with clinical signs. The lesion is attributed to degenerative changes, as for other companion animal species.

Cerebellar cortical abiotrophy was reported in one litter of rabbits. Affected kits were normal at birth but displayed ataxia within four weeks. Microscopically, the molecular layer within the cerebellum of affected animals was thin with a decreased density of cells in granular layer. The pathogenesis of the condition was not determined.

Although exposure to *Toxoplasma gondii* in pet rabbits is presumed to be high, associated disease in rabbits is rare or subclinical and lesions are generally restricted to the liver, spleen, and heart (see Section 1.6.4.4).

Neuronal storage diseases are very rare in rabbits. In one case, a 1.5-year-old miniature pet lop rabbit present-ing with ataxia and rapidly progressive neurologic signs was euthanized. Microscopically, within the pyramidal neurons of the hippocampus, the perikarya were distended with fine granular to vacuolated material that stained deep purple with toluidine blue. Ultrastructural analysis and thin layer chromatography demonstrated the material to be consistent with lipid, specifically GM2 ganglioside, and biochemical analyses confirmed an absence of β-hexosaminidase A in the brain and liver of this animal. These findings are consistent with the lysosomal storage disease, **GM2 gangliosidosis** variant B1, as seen in children; affected individuals usually die before adolescence.

Self-mutilation of the hind limbs has been reported in rabbits receiving hind leg intramuscular injections of ketamine. Moderate mixed perineural and endoneural inflammation with edema and hemorrhage was seen in the sciatic and tibial nerves of affected animals, along with demyelination and myonecrosis. Ketamine is commercially available in North America as an injectable solution in 100 and 50 mg/mL formulations and has a low pH, which can be irritating. The lowest concentration (50 mg/mL) should always be used in small mammal pets to avoid tissue damage.

1.10 Hematopoietic and Lymphoid Conditions

Rabbits have no recognized blood groups and their erythrocytes have a relatively short lifespan of 50 days, thus nucleated red cells are seen commonly in peripheral smears in conditions inducing hemorrhage. Infections may not result in a leukocytosis, as in other species, and alterations in differential cell counts (i.e., predominantly lymphocytic to neutrophilic shifts) may be better indicators of the presence of an infection than the absolute total or differential white cell counts. Male rabbits have higher red blood cell counts and hemoglobin concentrations than do females. Traditionally, the rabbit neutrophil has been termed a heterophil because of the eosinophilic granules contained within the cytoplasm. The cell functions as a neutrophil; however, in all other respects, and differs considerably in appearance and function from heterophils found in avian and reptile species. Thus, the term "neutrophil" is used throughout the text when describing this cell. Differentiating the rabbit neutrophil from the eosinophil can occasionally be challenging in tissue sections, due to poor definition of eosinophilic granules. A Luna stain, which confers a rust-brown stain to eosinophil granules but not neutrophil granules, may be used to confirm the identity of eosinophils (Figure 1.73).

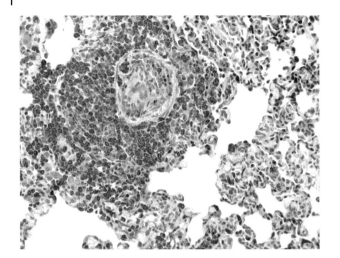

Figure 1.73 A Luna histochemical stain can be used to differentiate eosinophils from neutrophils in rabbits. Granules within eosinophils cuffing this pulmonary artery are stained brown, whereas neutrophils do not pick up the stain.

Causes of anemia in rabbits include lead or benzimidazole intoxication; chronic infectious diseases, such as pneumonia, dental disease, and renal disease; uterine adenocarcinoma; and endometrial venous aneurysms. Peracute anemia may be seen following infection with rabbit calicivirus, the agent of viral hemorrhagic disease.

1.10.1 Lymphoid and Hematopoietic Neoplasia

Lymphosarcoma is the most common tumor of rabbits and is seen frequently in young animals. Animals may present with lethargy, anorexia, depression, pallor, peripheral lymph node enlargement or cutaneous masses with overlying skin ulceration. Gross lesions include renal enlargement, often with multifocal firm pale nodules on the capsular surface, hepatosplenomegaly, nodules in the gastric fundus, and peripheral lymphadenopathy. Both thymic lymphoma with chylous effusion and cutaneous lymphosarcoma may be seen (see Section 1.2), but are less common presentations. Leukemia is rare, even in severely compromised animals, although white blood cell counts in excess of 30,000/μL have been reported. Histologically, masses are composed of dense infiltrates of neoplastic lymphoid cells. Cellular atypia and mitoses are variable. Neoplastic cells may be present throughout the bone marrow, spleen, lungs and hepatic sinusoids. Both B and T cell predominant patterns may be seen and definitive characterization requires immunohistochemical evaluation.

Thymomas are seen sporadically in older rabbits, and animals may present with dyspnea, exophthalmos, and radiographic evidence of a cranial mediastinal mass. Microscopically, neoplastic masses consist of mixed aggregations of large epithelial cells with clear cytoplasm and ovoid nuclei, and numerous small mature lymphocytes. Proliferating epithelial cells are positively immunolabeled for keratin and cytokeratin. Potential differential diagnoses include thymic hyperplasia, mediastinal abscess or hemorrhage, and thymic lymphoma. Bilateral exophthalmos may be seen as a sequela to vena caval compression by the mass, leading to decreased drainage of blood from the retroorbital sinuses. Exfoliative dermatoses may be seen in conjunction with thymomas in rabbits.

Other hematopoietic tumors are uncommon (Figure 1.74).

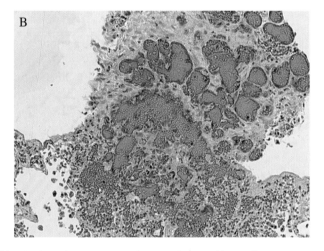

Figure 1.74 A: Pulmonary hemangiosarcoma in a 9-year-old male rabbit. B: The pulmonary parenchyma is disrupted by random, multifocal, well-demarcated, unencapsulated, expansile nodules of neoplastic cells that replace and efface approximately 40–50% of the parenchyma. Nodular aggregates are composed of polygonal to elongate plump cells arranged in nests or loose sheets supported by a highly vascular stroma. In occasional areas, the neoplastic cells are flattened and form variably sized irregular vascular channels supported by thin bands of collagenous stroma and channels containing variable numbers of erythrocytes. Mitoses are up to 8/400x field.

1.10.2 Lead Toxicosis

Lead intoxication remains an important cause of morbidity and death in rabbits. A history of chewing or licking lead painted surfaces is highly suggestive. Hematologic abnormalities include regenerative or nonregenerative anemia with basophilic stippling and nucleated red blood cells. Intravascular hemolysis may be seen with resultant renal tubular hemoglobin casts. For a complete discussion of lead intoxication, see Section 1.8.1.5.

1.10.3 Other Hematopoietic and Lymphoid Conditions

A rabbit-specific **parvovirus** has been identified. In experimental infections, rabbits demonstrated mild inappetence and moderate catarrhal enteritis.

Hemolytic anemia was reported as a sequela to iatrogenic valvular endocarditis in an experimental rabbit following inadvertent introduction of the Gram negative opportunistic bacterium, *Achromobacter xylosoxidans*, during surgery. Vegetative lesions may induce turbulence that results in intravascular hemolysis.

Benzimidazole intoxication has been reported in rabbits receiving high extralabel doses or prolonged courses of treatment with benzimidazoles, including albendazole and fenbendazole. Clinical signs noted in affected animals included sudden lethargy gastrointestinal stasis, pallor, petechiation, hemorrhage and sudden death. Bone marrow changes may range from severe anemia and erythroid precursor depletion to pancytopenia. Differential diagnoses for this toxicity include myelodysplasia or other drug hypersensitivity reactions. Because the drugs are metabolized by the liver, animals developing intoxications may have underlying hepatic disease and dysfunction.

1.11 Ophthalmic Conditions

Rabbits have large corneas and their eyes lack a lamina cribrosa, which creates a physiologic cup in the optic disk. They have a merangiotic vascular pattern to their retina and no tapetum lucidum. Binucleate cells are normally present in the retinal pigmented epithelium. The external jugular vein provides primary venous drainage of the head in the rabbit, with minimal collateral anastomoses with the internal jugular, such that prolonged occlusion of the external jugular vein leads to ocular swelling and protrusion. Rabbits have a large orbital venous sinus.

Ocular manifestations of respiratory and dental disease are relatively common in pet rabbits in that they have a single nasolacrimal puncta with a tortuous duct that readily becomes obstructed. Rabbits have a Harderian gland, larger in bucks than in does, which produces a milky product without porphyrins. It is important to examine oral, nasal, and ophthalmic structures in detail when evaluating ophthalmic disease, as secondary manifestations of disease are common.

1.11.1 Conditions of the Lacrimal Glands and Ducts

Epiphora is common in rabbits, resulting in an excessive milky secretion and periocular crusting. Epiphora may occur from excessive lacrimation following irritation to the eye, for example, from dusty food and bedding; or secondary to nasolacrimal duct obstruction from dental disease, infection, or impinging masses. The oral and nasal cavities should be closely evaluated in such cases. Bacterial rhinitis and associated dacryocystitis induce a purulent discharge with crusting and facial dermatitis, and *P. multocida* or *S. aureus* are commonly isolated from such cases.

Unilateral Harderian gland lymphoma with exophthalmos has been reported in a 2-year-old rabbit. The animal also had exposure keratitis and multicentric disease affecting the kidneys, spleen, and intestine, although no clinical signs were noted other than exophthalmos.

1.11.2 Conditions of the Eyelid and Conjunctiva

Suppurative conjunctivitis (Figure 1.75A) and blepharoconjunctivitis with or without periocular facial dermatitis and suppurative rhinitis are common manifestations of *P. multocida* infection (see Section 1.4.1 for more information). *S. aureus* or *P. aeruginosa* may also induce this condition. Blepharitis with erosion, ulceration, and crusting may also be indicative of *Chlamydia* sp. infection or spirochetosis (see Section 1.2 for more information) (Figure 1.75B). In cases of spirochetosis, biopsy of affected areas may reveal scant spirochetes (visualized by Warthin-Starry staining) and mixed inflammatory infiltrates. Lesions may be seen in juvenile animals as a result of early transmission from their dams. Perivulvar, anal, and nasal lesions may also be seen with this organism.

Uni- or bilateral prolapse of the deep gland of the third eyelid ("cherry eye") occurs in rabbits, usually secondary to infection, inflammation, or retrobulbar abscesses (Figure 1.76).

Aberrant conjunctival overgrowth, frequently termed pseudopterygium, although there is no associated inflammation as in humans, is a condition unique to rabbits (Figure 1.77). It appears as a progressive overgrowth of the cornea by a thin opaque double-layered fold of palpebral and bulbar elastic conjunctiva, and results in functional blindness if not corrected surgically.

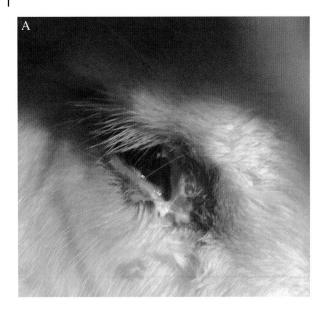

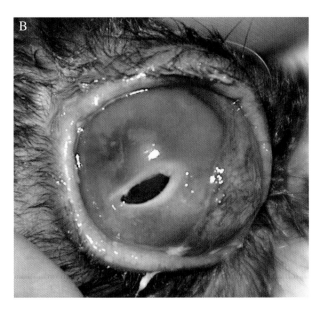

Figure 1.75 A: Suppurative conjunctivitis in a doe infected with *Pasteurella multocida*. B: Deep corneal ulcer secondary to irritation and self-trauma in a rabbit. *Source:* B: Courtesy of The Links Road Animal and Bird Clinic.

Self-trauma of the eyelids may result from exposure to irritants, including dust and ammonia, from ectropion or entropion, or may be indicative of underlying keratitis, and the entire eye should be examined closely. French rex rabbits are genetically predisposed to trichiasis and lid disorders.

Conjunctival papillomas may be seen following infection of rabbits with oral papilloma virus (ROPV, see Section 1.2.6.5). Masses may be single or multiple and are verrucoid with prominent folding of thickened epithelium. Intranuclear inclusion bodies may be visible and masses are usually self-limiting.

Squamous cell carcinoma of the eyelid occurs on occasion in rabbits and may induce a blepharitis if ulceration is present. Myxomatosis may also result in discrete or generalized subcutaneous swellings of the eyelid and face.

1.11.3 Conditions of the Cornea and Anterior Chamber

Trauma of the cornea with resulting ulceration occurs sporadically in rabbits and may be mechanical or secondary to inflammation from an orbital abscess or infection, particularly with *P. multocida*. Several cases of eosinophilic keratitis have been reported in middle-aged to older rabbits. Animals presented with blepharitis, con-

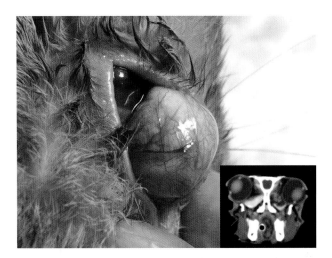

Figure 1.76 Manually extruded prolapsed third eyelid in a mature rabbit. Inset: CT scan of the same animal demonstrates an extensive mass ventrolateral to the medial canthus of the eye (red arrow) involving the third eyelid.

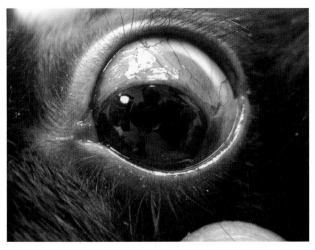

Figure 1.77 Pseudopterygium or aberrant conjunctival overgrowth. *Source:* Courtesy of The Links Road Animal and Bird Clinic.

junctivitis, ocular discharge and plaque formation, corneal neovascularization and cellular stromal infiltrates in which up to 95% of infiltrating cells were determined to be eosinophils. Corneal scrapings can be used to identify eosinophilic infiltrates, which can be further confirmed with Luna staining. The pathogenesis of the lesions is unknown, although in other species, eosinophilic keratitis has been attributed to an underlying Type I or IV hypersensitivity reaction. Corneal stromal abscessation may be seen secondary to ulceration. Exposure keratitis may occur following anesthesia thus lubricants should be applied during periods of anesthesia to minimize the likelihood of this condition. It is also hypothesized that direct exposure of rabbits to bright sunlight for periods of 30 minutes or more may induce photokeratitis.

Primary glaucoma with buphthalmos occurs in New Zealand white rabbits as an autosomal recessive trait with incomplete penetrance, and may result in keratitis and ulceration from exposure and self trauma (Figure 1.78). Most frequently, the onset is noted within the first six months of life in affected juvenile rabbits. The normal aqueous outflow tract, formed by iris pillars or pectinate ligaments (connective tissue strands lined by endothelium and inserted in the angle between Descemet's membrane and the iris) and a fine trabecular network is lacking in rabbits with buphthalmia, and the aqueous outflow tract is reduced to a narrow crescentic band with disorganized trabeculae. Glaucoma can also be acquired secondary to uveitis.

Corneal opacities are seen occasionally in rabbits and may be uni- or bilateral, focal or multifocal, and are likely secondary to previous injury or inflammation. Histologically, these appear as focal areas of subepithelial

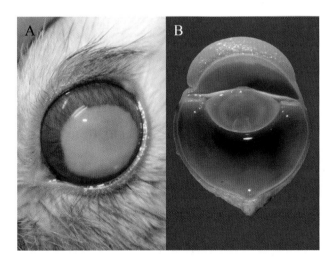

Figure 1.78 A: Glaucoma and marked corneal opacity in a mature rabbit with marked corneal opacity. B: Fixed and sectioned glaucomatous eye demonstrating severe corneal edema. *Source:* A: Courtesy of The Links Road Animal and Bird Clinic.

mineralization with stromal edema. Corneal lipidosis is a potential differential diagnosis. Experimentally, corneal lipidosis is associated with feeding an atherogenic diet to susceptible rabbit breeds, such as Watanabe. In these animals, foamy macrophages and cholesterol clefts are present within corneal stroma at the scleral junction and within the ciliary body and iris.

Shope fibroma virus-induced conjunctivitis and nonulcerative keratitis with perilimbal swelling has been reported in an aged rabbit. Microscopic evaluation of a biopsy of the affected conjunctiva indicated a mixture of bland polygonal and spindle-shaped cells within a myxocollagenous stroma. Intracytoplasmic eosinophilic viral inclusions were noted in the perilimbal mass.

Corneal epithelial dystrophy, similar clinically and microscopically to the condition noted in Boxer dogs, is reported rarely.

Corneal dermoid, a type of choristoma, is seen sporadically in rabbits. It is a rare congenital condition resulting in growth of normal skin in an abnormal location. Dermoids are composed of ectodermal and mesodermal tissues, and may elaborate hair follicles, sebaceous glands, adipose tissue, blood vessels, and cartilage. They often must be removed by superficial keratectomy because of ocular irritation from the long hairs that grow from them. Dermoids may also be found on the conjunctiva and palpebrae.

1.11.4 Uveal and Lenticular Conditions

Uveitis and cataracts in dwarf breeds of rabbits are most commonly manifestations of *E. cuniculi* infection. Lens infection with the organism likely represents in utero or early postnatal exposure, since the lens is largely avascular in older animals. Histologically, corneal neovascularization and scleral congestion may be seen with pyogranulomatous anterior uveitis and proteinaceous exudate within the anterior chamber. Degenerative lens fibers and multinucleated giant cells may also be present if lens rupture has occurred (phacoclastic uveitis) (Figure 1.79). Filtration angle collapse, anterior synechiae, and inflammatory cell infiltration into the posterior or anterior chambers may be present. *E. cuniculi* spores (1×2 um) are observed frequently within the lens epithelial cells and may also be identified by immunohistochemistry on fixed sections. Uveitis may also be seen secondary to systemic pasteurellosis or staphylococcosis.

Congenital cataracts are reported rarely in rabbits, but in a study of 946 cross-bred New Zealand white rabbits, an incidence of 4.3% was noted. Cataracts may also be seen secondary to *E. cuniculi* infection and following exposure to ionizing radiation and various heavy metals. Dutch rabbits are more sensitive to this effect than are

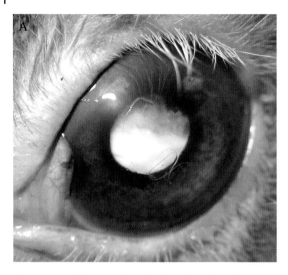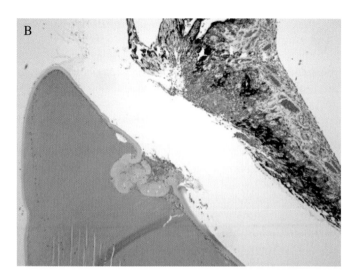

Figure 1.79 A: Cataract in a dwarf rabbit infected with *Encephalitozzon cuniculi*. B: Phacoclastic uveitis following lens rupture in a rabbit infected with *E. cuniculi. Source:* A: Courtesy of The Links Road Animal and Bird Clinic.

New Zealand white rabbits. Cataracts have also been reported following infection with Shope fibroma virus and are common in aging animals.

1.11.5 Fundic Conditions

Ocular colobomas are seen rarely in rabbits. Cupping of the optic disk may be seen in rabbits with glaucoma but must be distinguished from the normal background anatomy.

1.11.6 Exophthalmos

Exophthalmos may be induced by retrobulbar abscesses, generally secondary to dental disease; periorbital cellulitis, neoplasia, or salivary mucocele. It may also be seen secondary to any condition interfering with venous return from the head, such as thymoma or thymic lymphosarcoma. Unilateral exophthalmos was also reported in a young adult dwarf lop rabbit secondary to a coenurid cyst in the ventrolateral fornix. The cystic mass was surgically removed and contained numerous *Taenia serialis* immature scolices within dense fibrous tissue lined by macrophages, aggregates of lymphocytes, and abundant infiltrating eosinophils. The rabbit had been allowed to graze in the backyard and likely ingested eggs. Other sites of coenuri cysts reported for rabbits include the orbit, axilla, and facial muscles.

Bibliography

Introduction

Ekesbo, I. (2011) *Farm Animal Behaviour: Characteristics for Assessment of Health and Welfare.* CABI: Oxfordshire, UK.

FAO. (2012) *The Rabbit: Husbandry, Health and Production.* FAO Animal Production and Health Series, no. 21. http://www.fao.org/docrep/014/t1690e/t1690e.pdf (accessed: March 25).

Harkness, J.E., Turner, P.V., VandeWoude, S., and Wheler, C.L. (2010) *Harkness and Wagner's Biology and Medicine of Rabbits and Rodents,* 5th edn. Wiley-Blackwell: Ames, IA.

Maertens, L., and Coudert, P (eds.) (2006) *Recent Advances in Rabbit Sciences.* Institute for Agricultural and Fisheries Research: Melle, Belgium.

Alopecia

Allain, D. (2007) Fleece and fibre measurements in angora goats and angora rabbits. http://www.macaulay.ac.uk/europeanfibre/effnnew1da.htm

Beynen, A.C., Mulder, A., Nieuwenkamp, A.E., *et al.* (1992) Loose grass hay as a supplement to a pelleted diet reduces fur chewing in rabbits. *Journal of Animal Physiology Animal Nutrition,* **68**, 226–234.

Cox, A.B., Keng, P.C., Glass, N.L. and Lett, J.T. (1981) Effects of heavy ions on rabbit tissues: alopecia. *International Journal of Radiation Biology,* **40**(6), 645–657.

Fecteau, K.A., Deeb, B.J., Rickel, J.M., Kelch, W.J., and Oliver, J.W. (2007) Diagnostic endocrinology: Blood steroid concentrations in neutered male and female rabbits. *Journal of Exotic Pet Medicine,* **16**(4), 256–259.

Florizoone, K., Van der Luer, R., and Van den Ingh, T. (2007) Symmetrical alopecia, scaling and hepatitis in a rabbit. *Veterinary Dermatology,* **18**(3), 161–164.

Hoppman, E. and Wilson Barron, H. (2007) Ferret and rabbit dermatology. *Journal of Exotic Pet Medicine,* **16**(4), 225–237.

Hove, E.L. and Herndon, J.F. (1956) Vitamin B6 deficiency in rabbits. *Journal of Nutrition*, **61**(1), 127–136.

Iglauer, F., Beig, C., Dimigen, J., *et al.* (1995) Hereditary compulsive self-mutilating behaviour in laboratory rabbits. *Laboratory Animals (UK)*, **29**, 385–393.

Kanai, K., Nunoya, T., Yazawa, H., *et al.*. (2000) Congenital hypotrichosis in Japanese white strain (JW-NIBS) rabbits. *Journal of Toxicologic Pathology*, **13**, 21–27.

Oznurlu, Y., Celik, I., Sur, E., Telatae, T., and Ozparlak, H. (2009) Comparative skin histology of the white New Zealand and angora rabbits: Histometrical and Immunohistochemical evaluations. *Journal of Animal Veterinary Advances*, **8**(9), 1694–1701.

Paterson, S. (2006) *Skin Diseases of Exotic Pets*. Wiley-Blackwell: Ames, IA.

Powis, G. and Kooistra, K.L. (1987) Doxorubicin-induced hair loss in the Angora rabbit: a study of treatments to protect against hair loss. *Cancer Chemotherapy Pharmacology*, **20**, 291–296.

Sawin, P.B., Denenberg, V.H., Ross, S., Hafter, E., and Zarrow, M.X. (1960) Maternal behavior in the rabbit: hair loosening during gestation. *American Journal of Physiology*, **198**, 1099–1102.

Van Vleet, J.F. and Ferrans, V.J. (1980) Clinical and pathologic features of chronic adriamycin toxicosis in rabbits. *American Journal of Veterinary Research*, **41**(9), 1462–1469.

Whiteley, H.G. and Ghadially, F.N. (1958) Hair replacement in the domestic rabbit. *Journal of Anatomy*, **88**(1), 13–17.

Bacterial Dermatitis

Brash, M., Schutt, L., Draban, C., and Turner, P.V. (2009) Cutaneous spirochetosis due to *Treponema paraluiscuniculi* in a rabbit. *AHL Newsletter*, **13**(4), 30.

Cunliffe-Beamer, T.L., and Fox, R.R. (1981) Venereal spirochetosis of rabbits: epizootiology. *Laboratory Animal Science*, **4**, 372–378.

d'Ovidio, D. and Santoro, D. (2013) Orodental diseases and dermatological disorders are highly associated in pet rabbits: a case-control study. *Veterinary Dermatology*, **24**(5), 531–e125.

Garibaldi, B.A., Fox, J.G., and Musto, D.R. (1990) Atypical moist dermatitis in rabbits. *Laboratory Animal Science*, **40**(6), 652–653.

Hermans, K., De Herdta, P., Devriese, L.A., Hendrickx, W., Godard, C., and Haesebrouck, F. (1999) Colonization of rabbits with *Staphylococcus aureus* in flocks with and without chronic staphylococcosis. *Veterinary Microbiology*, **67**, 37–46.

Hermans, K., De Herdt, P., Devriese, L.A., Godard, C., and Haesebrouck, F. (2000) Colonisation of rabbits with *Staphylococcus aureus* after experimental infection with high and low virulence strains. *Veterinary Microbiology*, **72**, 277–284.

Hermans, K., Devriese, L.A., and Haesebrouck, F. (2003) Rabbit staphylococcosis: difficult solutions for serious problems. *Veterinary Microbiology*, **91**(1), 57–64.

Hoff, G.L., Bigler, W.J., and Hemmert, W. (1975) Tularemia in Florida: *Sylvilagus palustris* as a source of human infection. *Journal of Wildlife Diseases*, **11**, 560–561.

Kohler, R., Krause, G., Beutin, L., Stephan, R., and Zweifel, C. (2008) Shedding of food-borne pathogens and microbiological carcass contamination in rabbits at slaughter. *Veterinary Microbiology*, **132**, 149–157.

Leid, J.G., Willson, C.J., Shirtliff, M.E., Hassett, D.J., Parsek, M.R., and Jeffers, A.K. (2005) The exopolysaccharide alginate protects *Pseudomonas aeruginosa* biofilm bacteria from IFN-γ-mediated macrophage killing. *Journal of Immunology*. **175**, 7512–7518.

Lennox, A.M. (2010) Care of the geriatric rabbit. *Veterinary Clinics of North America: Exotic Animal Practice*, **13**, 123–133.

Lepitzki, D.A., Woolf, A., and Cooper, M. (1990) Serological prevalence of tularemia in cottontail rabbits of southern Illinois. *Journal of Wildlife Diseases*, **26**, 279–282.

Muller, M., Li, Z., and Mietz, P.K.M. (2009) *Pseudomonas* pyocyanin inhibits wound repair by inducing premature cellular senescence: Role for p38 mitogen-activated protein kinase. *Burn*, **35**(4), 500–508.

Narayanan, S.K., Nagaraja, T.G., Chengappa, M.M., and Stewart, G.C. (2001) Cloning, sequencing, and expression of the leukotoxin gene from *Fusobacterium necrophorum*. *Infection and Immunity*, **69**(9), 5447–5455.

Okerman, L., Devriese, L.A., Maertens, L., Okerman, F., and Godard, C. (1984) Cutaneous staphylococcosis in rabbits. *Veterinary Record*, **114**(13), 313–315.

Renquist, D. and Soave, O. (1969) Staphylococcal pneumonia in laboratory rabbit: An epidemiologic follow-up study. *Journal of the American Veterinary Medical Association* **155**, 1221–1223.

Saito, K. and Hasegawa, A. (2004) Clinical features of skin lesions in rabbit syphilis: A retrospective study of 63 cases (1999–2003). *Journal of Veterinary Medical Science*, **66**(10), 1247–9.

Saito, K., Tagawa, M., and Hasegawa, A. (2003) RPR test for serological survey of rabbit syphilis in companion rabbits. *Journal of Veterinary Medical Science*, **65**(7), 797–799.

Saito, K., Tagawa, M., and Hasegawa, A. (2003) Rabbit syphilis diagnosed clinically in household rabbits. *Journal of Veterinary Medical Science*, **65**(5), 637–639.

Segura, P., Martinez, J., Peris, B., *et al.* (2007) Staphylococcal infections in rabbit does on two industrial farms. *Veterinary Record*, **160**(25), 869–872.

Seps, S.L., Battles, A.H., Nguyen, L., Wardrip, C.L., and Li, X. (1999) Oropharyngeal necrobacillosis with septic thrombophlebitis and pulmonary embolic abscesses: Lemierre's syndrome in a New Zealand white rabbit. *Contemporary Topics in Laboratory Animal Science*, **38**(5), 44–46.

Tan, Z.L., Nagaraja, T.G., and Chengappa, M.M. (1996) *Fusobacterium necrophorum* infections: Virulence factors, pathogenic mechanism and control measures. *Veterinary Research Communications*, **20**, 113–140.

Tyrrell, K.L., Citron, D.M., Jenkins, J.R., Goldstein, E.J.C., and Veterinary Study Group. (2002) Periodontal bacteria in rabbit mandibular and maxillary abscesses. *Journal of Clinical Microbiology*, **40**(3), 1044–1047.

Vancraeynest, D., Hermans, K., Martel, A., Vaneechoutte, M., Devriese, L.A., and Haesebrouck, F. (2004) Antimicrobial resistance and resistance genes in *Staphylococcus aureus* strains from rabbits. *Veterinary Microbiology*, **101**, 245–251.

Viana, D., Selva, L., Segura, P., Penadés, J.R., and Corpa, J.M. (2007) Genotypic characterization of *Staphylococcus aureus* strains isolated from rabbit lesions. *Veterinary Microbiology*, **121**, 288–298.

Von Reyn, F.C., Barnes, A.M., Weber, N.S., and Hodgin, U.G. (1976) Bubonic plague from exposure to a rabbit: A documented case, and a review of rabbit-associated cases in the United States. *American Journal of Epidemiology.* **104**(1), 81–87.

Walther, B., Wieler, L.H., Friedrich, A.W., *et al.* (2008) Methicillin-resistant *Staphylococcus aureus* (MRSA) isolated from small and exotic animals at a university hospital during routine microbiological examinations. *Veterinary Microbiology*, **127**(1–2), 171–178.

Dermatophytoses

Cabanes, F.J., Vega, S., and Castella, G. (2011) *Malassezia cuniculi* sp. nov., a novel yeast species isolated from rabbit skin. *Medical Mycology*, **49**, 40–48.

Canny, C.J., and Gamble, C.S. (2003) Fungal diseases of rabbits. *Veterinary Clinics of North America: Exotic Animal Practice*, **6**, 429–433.

Chermette, R., Ferreiro, L., and Guillot, J. (2008) Dermatophytoses in animals. *Mycopathologia*, **166**, 385–405.

Hagen, K.W. (1969) Ringworm in domestic rabbits: Oral treatment with griseofulvin. *Laboratory Animal Care.* **19**(5), 635–638.

Kraemer, A., Mueller, R.S., Werckenthin, C., Straubinger, R.K., and Hein, J. (2012) Dermatophytes in pet Guinea pigs and rabbits. *Veterinary Microbiology*, **157**(1–2), 208–13.

Lane, R.F. (2003) Diagnostic testing for fungal diseases. *Veterinary Clinics of North America: Exotic Animal Practice*, **6**, 301–314.

Lopez-Martinez, R., Mier, T., and Quirarte, M. (1984) Dermatophytes isolated from laboratory animals. *Mycopathologia*, **88**, 111–113.

Radi, Z. (2004) Outbreak of sarcoptic mange and malasseziasis in rabbits (*Oryctolagus cuniculus*). *Comparative Medicine*, **54**, 434–437.

Rosen, L.B. (2011) Dermatologic manifestations of zoonotic diseases in exotic animals. *Journal of Exotic Pet Medicine*, **20**(1), 9–13.

Vangeel, I., Pasmans, F., Vanrobaeys, M., De Herdt, P., and Haesebrouck, F. (2000) Prevalence of dermatophytes in asymptomatic guinea pigs and rabbits. *Veterinary Record*, **146**(15), 440–441.

Van Rooij, P., Detandt, M., and Nolard, N. (2006) *Trichophyton mentagrophytes* of rabbit origin causing family incidence of kerion: an environmental study. *Mycoses.* **49**(5), 426–430.

Parasitic Dermatitis

Andersen, G.S., and Huitson, N.R. (2004) Myiasis in pet animals in British Columbia: The potential of forensic entomology for determining duration of possible neglect. *Canadian Veterinary Journal*, **45**, 993–998.

Baker, D.G. (2007) *Flynn's Parasites of Laboratory Animals*, 2nd edn. Wiley-Blackwell: Ames, IA.

Birke, L.L., Molina, P.E., Baker, D.G., *et al.* (2009) Comparison of selamectin and imidacloprid plus permethrin in eliminating *Leporacarus gibbus* infestation in laboratory rabbits (*Oryctolagus cuniculus*). *Journal of American Assoc Laboratory Animal Science*, **48**(6), 757–62.

Bisdorff, B., and Wall, R. (2006) Blowfly strike prevalence in domestic rabbits in southwest England and Wales. *Veterinary Parasitology*, **141**, 150–155.

Cutler, S.L. (1998) Ectopic *Psoroptes cuniculi* infestation in a pet rabbit. *Journal of Small Animal Practice*, **39**, 86–87.

Curtis, S.K. (1991) Diagnostic exercise: moist dermatitis on the hind quarters of a rabbit. *Laboratory Animal Science*, **41**(6), 623–4.

Dobrosavljevic, D.D., Popovic, N.D., and Radovanovic, S.S. (2007) Systemic manifestations of *Cheyletiella* infestation in man. *International Journal of Dermatology*, **46**, 397–399.

d'Ovidio, D., and Santoro, D. (2014) *Leporacarus gibbus* infestation in client-owned rabbits and their owner. *Veterinary Dermatology*, **25**(1), 46–e17.

Flatt, R.E., and Wiemers, J. (1976) A survey of fur mites in domestic rabbits. *Laboratory Animal Science*, **26**(5), 758–761.

Hallal-Calleros, C., Morales-Montor, J., Vázquez-Montiel, J.A.,*et al.* (2013) Hormonal and behavioral changes induced by acute and chronic experimental infestation with *Psoroptes cuniculi* in the domestic rabbit *Oryctolagus cuniculus. Parasite Vectors.* **6**(1), 361.

Harvey, R.G. (1990) *Demodex cuniculi* in dwarf rabbits (Oryctolagus cuniculi). *Journal of Small Animal Practice,* **31**, 204–207.

Jenkins, J.R. (2001) Skin disorders of the rabbit. *Veterinary Clinics of North America: Exotic Animal Practice,* **4**, 543–563.

Jones, J.M. (1984) Organophosphorus poisoning in two Rex rabbits. *New Zealand Veterinary Journal,* **32**(1–2), 9–10.

Kim, S.H., Jun, H.K., Song, K.H., Gram, D., and Kim, D.H. (2008) Prevalence of fur mites in pet rabbits in South Korea. *Veterinary Dermatology,* **19**(3), 189–190.

Kirwan, A.P., Middleton, B., and McGarry, J.W. (1998) Diagnosis and prevalence of *Leporacarus gibbus* in the fur of domestic rabbits in the UK. *Veterinary Record,* **3**, 20–21.

Loretti, A.P. and Lencewicz, C. (2010) Cerebral myiasis in a pet rabbit. 53rd *AAVLD Annual Conference Proceedings,* Minneapolis, MN.

Mellgren, M. and Bergvall, K. (2008) Treatment of rabbit cheyletiellosis with selamectin or ivermectin: a retrospective case study. *Acta Veterinaria Scand.* **50**, 1–6.

Niekrasz, M.A., Curl, J.L., and Curl, J.S. (1998) Rabbit fur mite (*Listrophorus gibbus*) infestation of New Zealand white rabbits. *Contemporary Topics in Laboratory Animal Science,* **37**(4), 73–75.

Patel, A., and Robinson, K.J.E. (1993) Dermatoses associated with *Listrophorus gibbus* in the Rabbit. *Journal of Small Animal Practice,* **34**, 409–411.

Pinter, L. (1999) *Leporacarus gibbus* and *Spilopsyllus cuniculi* infestation in a pet rabbit. *Journal of Small Animal Practice,* **40**(5), 220–221.

Radi, Z.A. (2004) Outbreak of sarcoptic mange and malasseziasis in rabbits (*Oryctolagus cuniculus*). *Comparative Medicine,* **54**(4), 434–437.

Sanders, A., Froggatt, P., Wall, R., and Smith, K.E. (2000) Life cycle stage morphology of *Psoroptes* mange mites. *Medical Veterinary Entomology,* **14**, 131–141.

Verocai, G.G., Fernandes, J.I., Ribeiro, F.A., *et al.* (2009) Furuncular myiasis caused by the human botfly, *Dermatobia hominis*, in the domestic rabbit: Case report. *Journal of Exotic Pet Medicine,* **18**(2), 153–155.

Mastitis

Blevins, S., Gardner, K., Wagner, A., *et al.* (2009) Mammary gland enlargement and discharge in an adult New Zealand white rabbit. *Laboratory Animals (NY).* **38**(8), 258–261.

Corpa, J.M., Hermans, K., and Haesebrouck, F. (2009) Main pathologies associated with *Staphylococcus aureus* infections in rabbits: A review. *World Rabbit Science,* **17**, 115–125.

Rosell, J.M., and de la Fuente, L.F. (2009) Culling and mortality in breeding rabbits. *Preventive Veterinary Medicine,* **88**(2), 120–127.

Segura, P., Martinez, J., Peris, B., Selva, L., Viana, D., Penades, J.R., and Corpa, J.M. (2007) Staphylococcal infections in rabbit does on two industrial farms. *Veterinary Record,* **160**, 869–872.

Viana, D., Selva, L., Callanan, J.J., Segura, P., and Corpa, J.M. (2008) The spectrum of pathology associated with natural chronic staphylococcal mastitis in rabbits. 9th World Rabbit Congress, Verona, IT, pp. 1107–1112.

Cutaneous Neoplasms and Masses

Benato, L. and Morrison, L.R. (2011) Apocrine gland hyperplasia in an 11-year-old rabbit (*Oryctolagus cuniculus*). *Journal of Exotic Pet Medicine,* **20**(1), 56–59.

Blevins, S., Gardner, K., Wagner, A., *et al.* (2009) Mammary gland enlargement and discharge in an adult New Zealand white rabbit. *Laboratory Animals (NY),* **38**(8), 258–261.

Brandão, J., Blair, R., Kelly, A., *et al.* (2015) Amelanotic melanoma in the rabbit: A case report with an overview of immunohistochemical characterization. *Journal of Exotic Pet Medicine,* **24**, 193–200.

Brash, M.L., Nagy, É., Pei, Y., *et al.* (2010) Acute hemorrhagic and necrotizing pneumonia, splenitis and dermatitis in a pet rabbit caused by a novel herpesvirus (leporid herpesvirus-4). *Canadian Veterinary Journal,* **51**(12), 1383–1386.

Budgeon, C., Mans, C., Chamberlin, T., *et al.* (2014) Diagnosis and surgical treatment of a malignant trichoepithelioma of the ear canal in a pet rabbit (*Oryctolagus cuniculus*). *Journal of American Veterinary Medical Association,* **245**(2), 227–231.

De Villiers, E-M., Fauquet, C., Broker, T.R., Bernard, H-U., and zur Hausen, H. (2004) Classification of papillomaviruses. *Virology.* **324**, 17–27.

Farsang, A., Makranszki, L., Dobos-Kovács, M., *et al.* (2009) *Giant cell sarcomas in pet rabbits.* AEMV Proceedings, Milwaukee, WI. pp. 85–86.

Hotchkiss, C.E., Norden, H., Collins, B.R., and Ginn, P.E. (1994) Malignant melanoma in two rabbits. *Laboratory Animal Science,* **44**(4), 377–385.

Hughes, J.E., Chapman, W.L., and Prasse, K.W. (1981) Cystic mammary disease in a rabbit. *Journal of the American Veterinary Medical Association,* **178**(2), 139–140.

Joiner, G.N., Jardine, J.H., and Gleiser, C.A. (1971) An epizootic of Shope fibromatosis in a commercial rabbitry. *Journal of the American Veterinary Medical Association,* **159**(11), 1583–1587.

Kanfer, S., and Reavill, D.R. (2013) Cutaneous neoplasia in ferrets, rabbits, and guinea pigs. *Veterinary Clinics of*

North America: Exotic Animal Practice, **16**(3), 579–598.

Krimer, P.M., Harvey, S.B., Blas-Machado, U., Lauderdale, J.D., and Moore, P.A. (2009) Reversible fibroadenomatous mammary hyperplasia in male and female New Zealand white rabbits associated with cyclosporine A administration. *Veterinary Pathology*, **46**(6), 1144–1148.

Krogstad, A.P., Simpson, J.E., and Korte, S.W. (2005) Viral diseases of rabbits. *Veterinary Clinics of North America: Exotic Animal Practice*, **8**, 123–138.

Kucsera, L., and Vetési, F. (2003) Occurrence of atypical myxomatosis in Central Europe: clinical and virological examinations. *Acta Veterinary Hungarica* **51**(4), 493–501.

Lipman, N.S., Zhao, Z.B., Andrutis, K.A., Hurley, R.J., Fox, J.G., and White, H.J. (1994) Prolactin-secreting pituitary adenomas with mammary dysplasia in New Zealand white rabbits. *Laboratory Animal Science*, **44**(2), 114–120.

Löhr, C.V., Hedge, Z.N., and Pool, R.R. (2012) Infiltrative myxoma of the stifle joint and thigh in a domestic rabbit (*Oryctolagus cuniculus*). *Journal of Comparative Pathology*, **147**(2–3), 218–222.

Mentre, V. and Bulliot, C. (2014) Idiopathic xanthoma in a pet rabbit. *Laboratory Animals (NY)*. **43**(8), 271–274.

Meredith, A.L. (2013) Viral skin diseases of rabbits. *Veterinary Clinics of North America: Exotic Animal Practice*, **16**, 705–714.

Mews, J.R., Ritchie, J.S.D., Romero-Mercado, C.H., and Scott, G.R. (1972) Detection of oral papillomatosis in a British rabbit colony. *Laboratory Animals (UK)*, **6**, 141–145.

Miwa, Y., Mochiduki, M., Nakayama, H., Shibuya, N., Ogawa, H., and Sasaki, N. (2006) Apocrine adenocarcinoma of possible sweat gland origin in a male rabbit. *Journal of Small Animal Practice*, **47**(9), 541–544.

Munday, J.S., Aberdein, D., Squires, R.A., Alfaras, A., and Wilson, A.M. (2007) Persistent conjunctival papilloma due to oral papillomavirus infection in a rabbit in New Zealand. *Journal of the American Association of Laboratory Animal Science*, **46**(5), 69–71.

Munday, J.S., and Kiupel. (2008) Papillomavirus-associated cutaneous neoplasia in mammals. *Veterinary Pathology*, **47**(2), 254–264.

Nicholls, P.K. and Stanley, M.A. (2000) The immunology of animal papillomaviruses. *Veterinary Immunology and Immunopathology*, **73**, 101–127.

Patton, N.M., and Holmes, H.T. (1977) Myxomatosis in domestic rabbits in Oregon. *Journal of the American Veterinary Medical Association*, **171**, 560–562.

Perkins, S.E., Murphy, J.C., and Alroy, J. (1996) Eosinophil granulocytic sarcoma in a New Zealand white rabbit. *Veterinary Pathology*, **33**(1), 89–91.

Petterino, C., Modesto, P., Strata, D., Vascellari, M., Mutinelli, F., Ferrari, A., and Ratto, A. (2009) A case of interscapular fibrosarcoma in a dwarf rabbit (*Oryctolagus cuniculus*). *Journal of Veterinary Diagnostic Investigation*, **21**, 900–905.

Reavill, D., and Schmidt, R. (2009) *Rabbit cutaneous basal cell tumors. AEMV Proceedings*, Milwaukee, WI, pp. 87.

Saito, K., Nakanishi, M., and Hasegawa, A. (2002) Uterine disorders diagnosed by ventrotomy in 49 rabbits. *Journal of Veterinary Medical Science*, **64**(6), 495–497.

Sawyer, D.R., Bunte, R.M., and Page, D.G. (1997) Basal cell adenoma in a rabbit. *Contemporary Topics in Laboratory Animal Science*, **36**(1), 90.

Schöniger, S., Horn, L.C., and Schoon, H.A. (2014) Tumors and tumor-like lesions in the mammary gland of 24 pet rabbits: a histomorphological and immunohistochemical characterization. *Veterinary Pathology*, **51**(3), 569–580.

Sikoski, P., Trybus, J., Cline, M., *et al.* (2008) Cystic mammary adenocarcinoma associated with a prolactin-secreting pituitary adenoma in a New Zealand white rabbit (*Oryctolagus cuniculus*). *Comparative Medicine*, **58**(3), 297–300.

Stanford, M.M., Werden, S.J., and McFadden, G. (2007) Myxoma virus in the European rabbit: Interactions between the virus and its susceptible host. *Veterinary Research*, **38**(2), 299–318.

Suckow, M.A., Rebelatto, M.C., Schulman, A.A., and HogenEsch, H. (2002) Sebaceous adenocarcinoma of the external auditory canal in a New Zealand white rabbit. *Journal of Comparative Pathology*, **127**(4), 301–303.

Summa, N.M., Eshar, D., Snyman, H.N., and Lillie, B.N. (2014) Metastatic anaplastic adenocarcinoma suspected to be of mammary origin in an intact male rabbit (*Oryctolagus cuniculus*). *Canadian Veterinary Journal*, **55**, 475–479.

Sundberg, J.P., Junge, R.E., and el Shazly, M.O. (1985) Oral papillomatosis in New Zealand white rabbits. *American Journal of Veterinary Research*, **46**(3), 664–668.

von Bomhard, W., Goldschmidt, M.H., Shofer, F.S., Perl, L., Rosenthal, K.L., and Mauldin, E.A. (2007) Cutaneous neoplasms in pet rabbits: A retrospective study. *Veterinary Pathology*, **44**, 579–588.

Walter, B., Poth, T., Böhmer, E., Braun, J., and Matis, U. (2010) Uterine disorders in 59 rabbits. *Veterinary Record*, **166**, 230–233.

White, S.D., Campbell, T., Logan, A., *et al.* (2000) Lymphoma with cutaneous involvement in three domestic rabbits (*Oryctolagus cuniculus*). *Veterinary Dermatology*, **11**(1), 61–67.

Zerfas, P.M., Brinster, L.R., Starost, M.F., Burkholder, T.H., Raffeld, M., and Eckhaus, M.A. (2010) Amelanotic melanoma in a New Zealand white rabbit (*Oryctolagus cuniculus*). *Veterinary Pathology*, **47**(5), 977–981.

Other

Banerjee, S.N., Banerjee, M., Fernando, K., Dong, M.Y., Smith, J.A, and Cook, D. (1995) Isolation of *Borrelia burdorferi*, the Lyme disease spirochete, from rabbit ticks, *Haemaphysalis leporispalustris* – Alberta. *Journal of Spirochete and Tick Diseases*, **2**, 23–24.

Blackmore, D.K., Schultze, W.H., and Absolon, G.C. (1986) Light intensity and fur-chewing rabbits. *New Zealand Veterinary Journal*, **34**(9), 158.

Blair, J. (2013) Bumblefoot: a comparison of clinical presentation and treatment of pododermatitis in rabbits, rodents, and birds. *Veterinary Clinics of North America: Exotic Animal Practice*, **16**(3), 715–735.

Florizoone, K., van der Luer, R., and van den Ingh, T. (2007) Symmetrical alopecia, scaling and hepatitis in a rabbit. *Veterinary Dermatology*, **18**(3), 161–164.

Florizoone, (2005) K. Thymoma-associated exfoliative dermatitis in a rabbit. *Veterinary Dermatology*, **16**(4), 28128–28124.

Kornblatt, A.N., Steere, A.C., and Brownstein, D.G. (1984) Experimental Lyme disease in rabbits: Spirochetes found in erythema migrans and blood. *Infection and Immunity*, **46**(1), 220–223.

Kovalik, M., Thoday, K.L., Eatwell, K., and van den Broek, A.H.M. (2012) Successful treatment of idiopathic sebaceous adenitis in a lionhead rabbit. *Journal of Exotic Pet Medicine*, **21**, 336–342.

Mancinelli, E., Keeble, E., Richardson, J., and Hedley, J. (2014) Husbandry risk factors associated with hock pododermatitis in UK pet rabbits (*Oryctolagus cuniculus*). *Veterinary Record*, **174**(17), 429.

Quinton, J-F., Prelaud, P., Poujade, A., and Faivre, N.C. (2015) A case of actinic keratosis in a rabbit. *Journal of Exotic Pet Medicine*, **23**, 283–286.

Sinke, J.D., van Dijk, J.E., and Willemse, T. (1997) A case of Ehlers-Danlos-like syndrome in a rabbit with a review of the disease in other species. *Veterinary Quarterly*, **19**(4), 182–185.

Snook, T.S., White, S.D., Hawkins, M.G., Tell, L.A., Wilson, L.S., Outerbridge, C.A., and Ihrke, P.J. (2013) Skin diseases in pet rabbits: a retrospective study of 334 cases seen at the University of California at Davis, USA (1984–2004). *Veterinary Dermatology*, **24**(6), 613–617, e148.

White, S.D., Linder, K., and Shultheiss, P. *et al.* (2000) Sebaceous adenitis in four domestic rabbits (*Oryctolagus cuniculus*). *Veterinary Dermatology*, **11**, 53–61.

General

Brewer, N.R. (2006) Biology of the rabbit. *Journal of the American Association of Laboratory Animal Science*, **45**(1), 8–24.

Harkness, J.E., Turner, P.V., VandeWoude, S., and Wheler, C.L. (2010) *Harkness and Wagner's Biology and Medicine of Rabbits and Rodents*, 5th edn. Wiley-Blackwell, Ames, IA.

Hoffman, K.L., Hernández Decasa, D.M., Beyer Ruiz, M.E., and González-Mariscal, G. (2010) Scent marking by the male domestic rabbit (*Oryctolagus cuniculus*) is stimulated by an object's novelty and its specific visual or tactile characteristics. *Behavioural Brain Research*, **207**(2), 360–367.

Kurosumi, K., Yanagishi, M., and Sekina, M. (1961) Mitochondrial deformation and apocrine secretory mechanism in the rabbit submandibular organ as revealed by electron microscopy. *Cell Tissue Research*, **55**, 297–312.

Van Praag, E., Maurer, A., and Saarony, T. (2010) *Skin Diseases of Rabbits*. MediRabbit.com:2010.

Other Endocrine Conditions

Cheeke, P.R. and Amberg, J.W. (1973) Comparative calcium excretion by rats and rabbits. *Journal of Animal Science*, **37**(2), 450–454.

Eckerman-Ross, C. (2008) Hormonal regulation and calcium metabolism in the rabbit. *Veterinary Clinics of North America: Exotic Animal Practice*, **11**, 139–152.

Fecteau, K.A., Deeb, B.J., Rickel, J.M., Kelch, W.J., and Oliver, J.W. (2007) Diagnostic endocrinology: Blood steroid concentrations in neutered male and female rabbits. *Journal of Exotic Pet Medicine*, **16**(4), 256–259.

Jekl, V., and Redrobe, S. (2013) Rabbit dental disease and calcium metabolism - the science behind divided opinions. *Journal of Small Animal Practice*, **54**(9), 481–490.

Lennox, A. and Chitty, J. (2006) Adrenal neoplasia and hyperplasia as a cause of hypertestosteronism in two rabbits. *Journal of Exotic Pet Medicine*, **15**(1), 56–58.

Lipman, N.S., Zhao, Z.B., and Andrutis, K.A., *et al.* (1994) Prolactin-secreting pituitary adenomas with mammary dysplasia in New Zealand white rabbits. *Laboratory Animal Science*, **44**(2), 114–120.

Roth, S.I. and Conaway, H.H. (1982) Spontaneous diabetes mellitus in the New Zealand white rabbit. *American Journal of Pathology*, **109**(3), 359–363.

Sikoski, P., Trybus, J., and Cline, J.M., *et al.* (2008) Cystic mammary adenocarcinoma associated with a prolactin-secreting pituitary adenoma in a New Zealand white rabbit (*Oryctolagus cuniculus*). *Comparative Medicine*, **58**(3), 297–300.

Pasteurellosis

Al-Haddawi, M.H., Jasni, S., Zamri-Saad, M., *et al.* (2000) *In vitro* study of *Pasteurella multocida* adhesion to trachea, lung and aorta of rabbits. *Veterinary Journal*, **179**, 274–281.

Chow, E.P., Bennett, R.A., and Dustin, L. (2009) Ventral bulla osteotomy for treatment of otitis media in a rabbit. *Journal of Exotic Pet Medicine*, **18**(4), 299–305.

de Matos, R., Ruby, J., Van Hatten, R.A., and Thompson, M. (2015) Computed tomographic features of clinical and subclinical middle ear disease in domestic rabbits (*Oryctolagus cuniculus*), 88 cases (2007–2014). *Journal of the American Veterinary Medical Association*, **246**(3), 336–343.

DiGiacomo, R.F., Garlinghouse, L.E. Jr, and Van Hoosier, G.L. Jr. (1983) Natural history of infection with *Pasteurella multocida* in rabbits. *Journal of the American Veterinary Medical Association*, **183**(11), 1172–1175.

DiGiacomo, R.F., Jones, C.D., and Wathes, C.M. (1987) Transmission of *Pasteurella multocida* in rabbits. *Laboratory Animal Science*, **37**(5), 621–623.

DiGiacomo, R.F., Deeb, B.J., Brodie, S.J., Zimmerman, T.E., Veltkamp, E.R., and Chrisp, C.E. (1993) Toxin production by *Pasteurella multocida* isolated from rabbits with atrophic rhinitis. *American Journal of Veterinary Research*, **54**(8), 1280–1286.

Dillehay, D.L., Paul, K.S., DiGiacomo, R.F., and Chengappa, M.M. (1991) Pathogenicity of *Pasteurella multocida* A:3 in Flemish giant and New Zealand white rabbits. *Laboratory Animals (UK)*, **25**(4), 337–341.

El Tayeb, A.B., Morishita, T.Y., and Angrick, E.J. (2004) Evaluation of *Pasteurella multocida* isolated from rabbits by capsular typing, somatic serotyping, and restriction endonuclease analysis. *Journal of Veterinary Diagnostic Investigation*, **16**, 121–125.

Ewers, C., Lubke-Becker, A., Bethe, A., *et al.* (2006) Virulence genotype of *Pasteurella multocida* strains isolated from different hosts with various disease status. *Veterinary Microbiology*, **114**, 304–317.

Jaglic, Z., Kucerova, Z., Nedbalcova1, K., Hlozek, P., and Bartos, M. (2004) Identification of Pasteurella multocida serogroup F isolates in rabbits. *Journal of Veterinary Medicine B*, **51**, 467–469.

Jaglic, Z., Kucerova, Z., Nedbalcova1, K., Kulich, P., and Alexa, P. (2006) Characterisation of *Pasteurella multocida* isolated from rabbits in the Czech Republic. *Veterinary Medicine*, **51**(5), 278–287.

Jaglic, Z., Jeklova, E., Leva, L., *et al.* (2008) Experimental study of pathogenicity of *Pasteurella multocida* serogroup F in rabbits. *Veterinary Microbiology*, **126**, 168–177.

Lax, A.J., Pullinger, G.D., Baldwin, M.R., *et al.* (2004) The *Pasteurella multocida* toxin interacts with signalling pathways to perturb cell growth and differentiation. *International Journal of Medical Microbiology*, **293**(7–8), 505–512.

Lennox, A.M. and Kelleher, S. (2009) Bacterial and parasitic diseases of rabbits. *Veterinary Clinics of North America: Exotic Animal Practice*, **12**, 519–530.

Marlier, D., Mainil, J., Linde, A., and Vindevogel, H. (2000) Infectious agents associated with rabbit pneumonia: isolation of amyxomatous myxoma virus strains. *Veterinary Journal*, **159**(2), 171–178.

Mercier, P., Rideaud, P., and Coudert, P. (1992) A study of the pathogenic influences of three strains of *Pasteurella multocida* on the rabbit–an experimental to control the effect by spiramycin. *Journal of Applied Rabbit Research*, **15**, 1401–1410.

Pathak, A.K., Boag, B., Poss, M., Harvill, E.T., and Cattadori, I.M. (2011) Seasonal breeding drives the incidence of a chronic bacterial infection in a free-living herbivore population. *Epidemiology Infection*, **139**(8), 1210–1219.

Per, H., Kumandaş, S., Gümüş, H., Oztürk, M.K., and Coşkun, A. (2010) Meningitis and subgaleal, subdural, epidural empyema due to *Pasteurella multocida*. *Journal of Emerging Medicine*, **39**(1), 35–38.

Rougier, S., Galland, D., Boucher, S., Boussarie, D., and Valle, M. (2006) Epidemiology and susceptibility of pathogenic bacteria responsible for upper respiratory tract infections in pet rabbits. *Veterinary Microbiology*, **115**, 192–198.

Snipes, K.P., Carpenter, T.E., Corn, J.L., Kasten, R.W., Hirsh, D.C., Hird, D.W., and McCapes, R.H. (1988) *Pasteurella multocida* in wild mammals and birds in California: Prevalence and virulence for turkeys. *Avian Diseases*, **32**(1), 9–15.

Stahel, A.B.J., Hoop, R.K., Kuhnert, P., and Korczak, B.M. (2009) Phenotypic and genetic characterization of *Pasteurella multocida* and related isolates from rabbits in Switzerland. *Journal of Veterinary Diagnostic Investigation*, **21**, 793–802.

Sterner-Kock, A., Lanske, B., Uberschär, S., and Atkinson, M.J. (1995) Effects of the *Pasteurella multocida* toxin on osteoblastic cells in vitro. *Veterinary Pathology*, **32**(3), 274–279.

Stieve-Caldwell, E.L., Morandi, F., Souza, M., and Adams, W.H. (2009) Veterinary Med Today: What's your diagnosis? *Journal of the American Veterinary Medical Association*, **235**(6), 665–666.

Suckow, M.A., Haab, R.W., Miloscio, L.J., and Guilloud, N.B. (2008) Field trial of a *Pasteurella multocida* extract vaccine in rabbits. *Journal of the American Association of Laboratory Animal Science*, **47**(1), 18–21.

Takashima, H., Sakai, H., Yanai, T., and Masegi, T. (2001) Detection of antibodies against *Pasteurella multocida* using immunohistochemical staining in an outbreak of rabbit pasteurellosis. *Journal of Veterinary Medical Science*, **63**(2), 171–174.

Other Bacterial Diseases

Boot, R., Bakker, R.H., Thuis, H., and Veenema, J.L. (1993) An enzyme-linked immunosorbent assay (ELISA) for monitoring guinea pigs and rabbits for *Bordetella bronchiseptica* antibodies. *Laboratory Animals (UK)*, **27**, 342–349.

Caniatti, M., Crippa, L., Giusti, M., Mattiello, S., Grilli, G., Orsenigo, R., and Scanziani, E. (1998) Cilia-associated respiratory (CAR) bacillus infection in conventionally reared rabbits. *Zentralblatt für Veterinärmedizin. Reihe B.* **45**(6), 363–371.

Cundiff, D.D., Besch-Williford, C.L., Hook, R.R. Jr, Franklin, C.L., and Riley, L.K. (1994) Characterization of cilia-associated respiratory bacillus isolates from rats and rabbits. *Laboratory Animal Science*, **44**, 305–312.

Cundiff, D.D., Besch-Williford, C.L., Hook, R.R. Jr, Franklin, C.L., and Riley, L.K. (1995) Characterization of cilia-associated respiratory bacillus in rabbits and analysis of the 16S rRNA gene sequence. *Laboratory Animal Science*, **45**(1), 22–26.

Deeb, B.J., DiGiacomo, R.F., Bernard, B.L., and Silbernagel, S.M. (1990) *Pasteurella multocida* and *Bordetella bronchiseptica* infections in rabbits. *Journal of Clinical Microbiology*, **28**(1), 70–75.

Glass, L.S., and Beasley, J.N. (1989) Infection with and antibody response to *Pasteurella multocida* and *Bordetella bronchiseptica* in immature rabbits. *Laboratory Animal Science*, **39**, 406–410.

Kurisu, K., Kyo, S., Shiomoto, Y., and Matsushita, S. (1990) Cilia-associated respiratory bacillus infection in rabbits. *Laboratory Animal Science*, **40**, 413–415.

Ludwig, E., Reischl, U., Janik, D., and Hermanns, W. (2009) Granulomatous pneumonia caused by *Mycobacterium genavense* in a dwarf rabbit (*Oryctolagus cuniculus*). *Veterinary Pathology*, **46**(5), 1000–1002.

Percy, D.H., Karrow, N., and Bhasin, J.L. (1988) Incidence of *Pasteurella* and *Bordetella* infections in fryer rabbits: an abattoir survey. *Journal of Applied Rabbit Research*, **11**, 245–246.

Ren, S.Y., Geng, Y., Wang, K.Y., Zhou, Z.Y., Liu, X.X., He, M., Peng, X., Wu, C.Y., and Lai, W.M. (2014) *Streptococcus agalactiae* infection in domestic rabbits, *Oryctolagus cuniculus*. *Transboundary Emerging Diseases*, **61**(6), e92–e95.

Rougier, S., Galland, D., Boucher, S., Boussarie, D., and Vallé, M. (2006) Epidemiology and susceptibility of pathogenic bacteria responsible for upper respiratory tract infections from pet rabbits. *Veterinary Microbiology*, **115**, 192–198.

Shoji-Darkye, Y., Itoh, T., and Kagiyama, N. (1991) Pathogenesis of CAR bacillus in rabbits, guinea pigs, Syrian hamsters, and mice. *Laboratory Animal Science*, **41**, 567–571.

Waggie, K.S., Spencer, T.H., and Allen, A.M. (1987) Cilia-associated respiratory (CAR) bacillus infection in New Zealand white rabbits. *Laboratory Animal Science*, **37**, 533.

Yokos, I.T. and Kagiyama, N. (1991) Pathogenesis of CAR bacillus in rabbits, guinea pigs Syrian hamsters, and mice. *Laboratory Animal Science*, **41**, 567–571.

Leporid herpesvirus-4

Brash, M.L., Nagy, É., Pei, Y., *et al.* (2010) Acute hemorrhagic and necrotizing pneumonia, splenitis and dermatitis in a pet rabbit caused by a novel herpesvirus (leporid herpesvirus-4). *Canadian Veterinary Journal*, **51**(12), 1383–1386.

Hesselton, R.M., Yang, W.C., Medveczky, P., and Sullivan, J.L. (1988) Pathogenesis of *Herpesvirus sylvilagus* infection in cottontail rabbits. *American Journal of Pathology*, **133**, 639–647.

Hinze, H.C. (1971) New member of the herpesvirus group isolated from wild cottontail rabbits. *Infection and Immunity*, **3**(2), 350–354.

Jin, L., Lohr, C.V., Vanarsdall, A.L., *et al.* (2008) Characterization of a novel alphaherpesvirus associated with fatal infections of domestic rabbits. *Virology*, **378**, 13–20.

Jin, L., Valentine, B.A., Baker, R.J., *et al.* (2008) An outbreak of fatal herpesvirus infection in domestic rabbits in Alaska. *Veterinary Pathology*, **45**, 369–374.

Onderka, D.K., Papp-Vid, G., and Perry, A.W. (1992) Fatal herpesvirus infection in commercial rabbits. *Canadian Veterinary Journal*, **33**, 539–543.

Schmidt, S.P., Bates, G.N., and Lewandoski, P.J. (1992) Probable herpesvirus infection in an eastern cottontail (*Sylvilagus floridanus*). *Journal of Wildlife Diseases*, **28**(4), 618–622.

Pneumocystosis

Aliouat-Denis, C.M., Chabé, M., Demanche, C., *et al.* (2008) Pneumocystis species, co-evolution and pathogenic power. *Infections, Genes, and Evolution*, **8**(5), 708–726.

Cere, N., Drouet-Viard, F., Dei-Cas, E., Chanteloup, N., and Coudert, P. (1997) In utero transmission of *Pneumocystis carinii* sp. f. *oryctolagi*. *Parasites*, **4**(4), 325–330.

Chabé, M., Aliouat-Denis, C.M., Delhaes, L., Aliouat, el M., Viscogliosi, E., and Dei-Cas, E. (2011) *Pneumocystis*: from a doubtful unique entity to a group of highly diversified fungal species. *FEMS Yeast Research*, **11**(1), 2–17.

Dei-Cas, E., Chabé, M., Moukhlis, M., *et al.* (2006) *Pneumocystis oryctolagi* sp. nov., an uncultured fungus causing pneumonia in rabbits at weaning: review of current knowledge, and description of a new taxon on genotypic, phylogenetic and phenotypic bases. *FEMS Microbiol Review*, **30**, 853–871.

Sanchez, C.A., Chabé, M., Aliouat, el M., *et al.* (2007) Exploring transplacental transmission of *Pneumocystis oryctolagi* in first-time pregnant and multiparous rabbit does. *Medical Mycology*, **45**(8), 701–707.

Swain, S.D., Han, S., Harmsen, A., Shampeny, K., and Harmsen, A.G. (2007) Pulmonary hypertension can be a sequela of prior *Pneumocystis* pneumonia. *American Journal of Pathology*, **171**(3), 790–799.

Viral Hemorrhagic Disease

Alexandrov, M., Peshev, R., Yanchev, I., Bozhkov, S., Doumanova, L., Dimitrov, T., and Zacharieva, S. (1992) Immunohistochemical localization of the rabbit haemorrhagic disease viral antigen. *Archives of Virology*, **127**, 355–363.

Bergin, I.L., Wise, A.G., Bolin, S.R., Mullaney, T.P., Kiupel, M., and Maes, R.K. (2009) Novel calicivirus identified in rabbits, Michigan, USA. *Emerging Infectious Diseases*, **15**(12), 1955–1962.

Bertagnoli, S., Gelfi, J., Le Gall, G., *et al.* (1996) Protection against myxomatosis and rabbit viral hemorrhagic disease with recombinant myxoma viruses expressing rabbit hemorrhagic disease virus capsid protein. *Journal of Virology*, **70**(8), 5061–5066.

Campagnolo, E.R., Ernst, M.J., Berninger, M.L., *et al.* (2003) Outbreak of rabbit hemorrhagic disease in domestic lagomorphs. *Journal of the American Veterinary Med Assoc.* **223**, 1151–1155, 1128.

Capucci, L., Fusi, P., Lavazza, A., Pacciarini, M.L., and Rossi, C. (1996) Detection and preliminary characterization of a new rabbit calicivirus related to rabbit hemorrhagic disease virus but nonpathogenic. *Journal of Virology*, **70**(12), 8614–8623.

Chasey, D. (1996) Rabbit hemorrhagic disease: The new scourge of *Oryctolagus cuniculus*. *Laboratory Animals (UK)*. **31**, 33–44.

Cooke, B.D. (2002) Rabbit haemorrhagic disease: field epidemiology and the management of wild rabbit populations. *Review Science Tech.* **21**(2), 347–358.

Duff, J.P., Chasey, D., Munro, R., and Wooldridge, M. (1994) European brown hare syndrome in England. *Veterinary Record*, **134**(26), 669–673.

Embury-Hyatt, C., Postey, R., *et al.* (2012) The first reported case of rabbit hemorrhagic disease in Canada. *Canadian Veterinary Journal*, **53**, 998–1002.

Gavier-Widen, D., and Momer, T. (1993) Descriptive epizootiological study of European brown hare syndrome in Sweden. *Journal of Wildlife Diseases*, **29**, 15–20.

Hukowska-Szematowicz, B., Tokarz-Deptuła, B., and Deptuła, W. (2012) Genetic variation and phylogenetic analysis of rabbit haemorrhagic disease virus (RHDV) strains. *Acta Biochimica Polonica*, **59**(4), 459–465.

Krogstad, A.P., Simpson, J.E., and Korte, S.W. (2005) Viral diseases of rabbits. *Veterinary Clinics of North America: Exotic Animal Practice*, **8**, 123–138.

Lawson, M. (1995) Rabbit virus threatens ecology after jumping the fence. *Nature*, **378**, 531.

Le Gall-Reculé, G., Lavazza, A., Marchandeau, S., *et al.* (2013) Emergence of a new lagovirus related to rabbit haemorrhagic disease virus. *Veterinary Research*, **44**, 81.

Liebermann, H., Bergmann, H., Lange, E., Schirrmeier, H., and Solisch, P. (1992) Some physicochemical properties of the virus of rabbit haemorrhagic disease. *Journal of Veterinary Medicine, Series B*, **39**(1–10), 317–326.

Meldrum, K.C. (1992) Viral haemorrhagic disease of rabbits. *Veterinary Record*, **130**, 407.

Ohlinger, V.F., Haas, B., Meyers, G., Weiland, F., and Thiel, H.J. (1990) Identification and characterization of the virus causing rabbit hemorrhagic disease. *Journal of Virology*, **64**(7), 3331–3336.

Nauwynck, H., Callebaut, P., Peeters, J., Ducatelle, R., and Uyttebroek, E. (1993) Susceptibility of hares and rabbits to a Belgian isolate of European brown hare syndrome virus. *Journal of Wildlife Diseases*, **29**(2), 203–208.

Pages Mante, A., and Artigas, C. (1992) Advisable vaccinal programme against myxomatosis and rabbit haemorrhagic disease viruses on wild rabbits. *Journal of Applied Rabbit Research*, **15**, 1448–1452.

Park, J.H., Ochiai, K., and Itakura, C. (1993) Aetiology of rabbit haemorrhagic disease in China. *Veterinary Record*, **133**, 67–69.

Parra, F., and Prieto, M. (1990) Purification and characterization of a calicivirus as the causative agent of a lethal hemorrhagic disease in rabbits. *Journal of Virology*, **64**, 4013–4015.

Puggioni, G., Cavadini, P., Maestrale, C., *et al.* (2013) The new French 2010 Rabbit Hemorrhagic Disease Virus causes an RHD-like disease in the Sardinian Cape hare (*Lepus capensis mediterraneus*). *Veterinary Research*, **44**, 96.

Smíd, B., Valícek, L., Rodák, L., Stěpánek, J., and Jurák, E. (1991) Rabbit haemorrhagic disease: an investigation of some properties of the virus and evaluation of an inactivated vaccine. *Veterinary Microbiology*, **26**(1–2), 77–85.

Other Respiratory Conditions

Bodon, L., Zsák, L., and Nagy, E. (1981) Detection of neutralizing antibodies to genuine rabbit adenovirus in rabbit antisera to human adenoviruses. *Acta Veterinaria Academiae Scientiarum Hungaricae*, **28**(4), 399–402.

Capello, V. (2014) Rhinostomy as surgical treatment of odontogenic rhinitis in three pet rabbits. *Journal of Exotic Pet Medicine*, **23**, 172–187.

Ludwig, E., Reischl, U., Janik, D., and Hermanns, W. (2009) Granulomatous pneumonia caused by Mycobacterium genavense in a dwarf rabbit (*Oryctolagus cuniculus*). *Veterinary Pathology*, **46**(5), 1000–1002.

Lennox, A.M., and Reavill, D. (2014) Nasal mucosal adenocarcinoma in a pet rabbit. *Journal of Exotic Pet Medicine*, **23**, 397–402.

Matsui, T., Taguchi-Ochi, S., Takano, M., *et al.* (1985) Pulmonary aspergillosis in apparently healthy young rabbits. *Veterinary Pathology*, **22**(3), 200–205.

Perpinan, D., Hernandez-Divers, S.J., Kelleher, S., Sanchez, S., and Shepherd, M. (2009) *Two cases of rabbit respiratory mycobacteriosis. AEMV Proceedings*, San Diego, CA, p. 97.

Phaneuf, L.R., Barker, S., Groleau, M.A., and Turner, P.V. (2006) Tracheal injury following endotracheal intubation and anesthesia in rabbits. *Journal of the American Association of Laboratory Animal Science*, **45**, 67–72.

Dysplastic and Degenerative Diseases

Baxter, J.S. (1975) Posterior paresis in the rabbit. *Journal of Small Animal Practice*, **16**, 267–271.

Green, P.W., Fox, R.R., and Sokoloff, L. (1984) Spontaneous degenerative spinal disease in the laboratory rabbit. *Journal of Orthopedic Research*, **2**(2), 161–168.

Joosten, H.F., Wirtz, P., Verbeek, H.O., and Hoekstra, A. (1981) Splayleg: a spontaneous limb defect in rabbits. Genetics, gross anatomy, and microscopy. *Teratology*, **24**(1), 87–104.

Lennox, A.M. (2010) Care of the geriatric rabbit. *Veterinary Clinics of North America: Exotic Animal Practice*, **13**, 123–133.

Owiny, J.R., Vandewoude, S., Painter, J.T., Norrdin, R.W., and Veeramachaneni, D.N.R. (2001) Hip dysplasia in rabbits: Association with nest box flooring. *Comparative Medicine*, **51**(1), 85–88.

Renberg, W.C. (2005) Pathophysiology and management of arthritis. *Veterinary Clinics of North America: Small Animal Practice*, **35**, 1073–1091.

Smith-Baxter, J. (1972) Posterior paralysis in a rabbit. *Journal of Small Animal Practice*, **16**, 267–271.

Nutritional Myopathy

Ringler, D.H. and Abrams, G.D. (1970) Nutritional muscular dystrophy and neonatal mortality in a rabbit breeding colony. *Journal of the American Veterinary Medical Association*, **157**(11), 1928–1934.

St Claire, M.B., Kennett, M.J., and Besch-Williford, C.L. (2004) Vitamin A toxicity and vitamin E deficiency in a rabbit colony. *Contemporary Topics in Laboratory Animal Science*, **43**(4), 26–30.

Stevenson, R.G. and Finley, G.G. (1976) Hypervitaminosis D in rabbits. *Canadian Veterinary Journal*, **17**, 54–57.

Yamini, B. and Stein, S. (1989) Abortion, stillbirth, neonatal death, and nutritional myodegeneration in a rabbit breeding colony. *Journal of the American Veterinary Medical Association*, **194**(4), 561–562.

Neoplasia

Amand, W.B., Riser, W.H., and Biery, D.N. (1973) Spontaneous osteosarcoma with widespread metastasis in a belted Dutch rabbit. *Journal of the American Animal Hospital Association*, **9**, 577–581.

Gibson, C.J., and Donnelly, T.M. (2011) What's your diagnosis: Lameness in a rabbit. *Laboratory Animals (NY)*, **40**(2), 39–40.

Haist, V., Hirschfeld, S.G., Mallig, C., Fehr, M., and Baumgärtner, W. (2010) Pathologic fracture of the femur due to endometrial adenocarcinoma metastasis in a female pet rabbit (*Oryctolagus cuniculus*). *Berliner und Münchener Tierärztliche Wochenschrift*, **123**(7–8), 346–351.

Higgins, S., Guzman, D.S-M., Sadar, M.J., *et al.* (2015) Coxofemoral amputation in a domestic rabbit (*Oryctolagus cuniculus*) with tibiofibular osteoblastic osteosarcoma. *Journal of Exotic Pet Medicine*, **24**, 455–463.

Hoover, J.P., Paulsen, D.B., Qualls, C.W., and Bahr, R.J. (1986) Osteogenic sarcoma with subcutaneous involvement in a rabbit. *Journal of the American Veterinary Medical Association*, **9**, 1156–1158.

Ishikawa, M., Kondo, H., Onuma, M., Shibuya, H., and Sato, T. (2012) Osteoblastic osteosarcoma in a rabbit. *Comparative Medicine*, **62**(2), 124–126.

Kondo, H., Ishikawa, M., Maeda, H., Onuma, M., Masuda, M., Shibuya, H., Koie, H., and Sato, T. (2007) Spontaneous osteosarcomas in a rabbit (*Oryctolagus cuniculus*). *Veterinary Pathology*, **44**, 691–694.

Mazzullo, G., Russo, M., Niutta, P.P., and De Vico, G. (2004) Osteosarcoma with multiple metastases and subcutaneous involvement in a rabbit (*Oryctolagus cuniculus*). *Veterinary Clinical Pathology*, **33**, 102–104.

Reed, S.D., Shaw, S., and Evans, D.E. (2009) Spinal lymphoma and pulmonary filariasis in a pet domestic rabbit (*Oryctolagus cuniculus domesticus*). *Journal of Veterinary Diagnostic Investigation*, **21**, 253–256.

Renfrew, H., Rest, R., and Holden, A.R. (2001) Extraskeletal fibroblastic osteosarcoma in a rabbit (*Oryctolagus cuniculus*). *Journal of Small Animal Practice*, **42**, 456–458.

Traumatic Injury

Jones, T., Lu, Y.S., Rehg, J., and Eckels, R. (1982) Diagnostic exercise: Fracture of the lumbar vertebrae. *Laboratory Animal Science*, **32**(5), 489–90.

Stiff, A.L., and Roe, F.J.C. (1962) Fracture-dislocation of lumbar spine occurring spontaneously in rabbits. *Journal of Animal Tech Association*, **12**(4), 1–3.

Villano, J.S., and Cooper, T.K. (2013) Mandibular fracture and necrotizing sialometaplasia in a rabbit. *Comparative Medicine*, **63**(1), 67–70.

Other Musculoskeletal Conditions

Bock, P., Peters, M., Bagó, Z., Wolf, P., Thiele, A., and Baumgärtner, W. (2007) Spontaneously occurring alimentary osteofluorosis associated with proliferative gastroduodenopathy in rabbits. *Veterinary Pathology*, **44**(5), 703–706.

Brewer, N.R. (2006) Biology of the rabbit. *Journal of the American Association of Laboratory Animal Science*, **45**(1), 8–24.

Delamaide Gasper, J.A., Rylander, H., Mans, C., Waller, K.R. 3rd, and Imai, D.M. (2014) Surgical management of vertebral synovial cysts in a rabbit (*Oryctolagus cuniculus*). *Journal of the American Veterinary Medical Association*, **244**(7), 830–834.

Gardner, D.G., Bunte, R.M., Sawyer, D.R., and Artwohl, J. (1997) Multicystic lesion of the jaw in a rabbit. *Contemporary Topics in Laboratory Animal Science*, **36**(3), 76–80.

Harcourt-Brown, F.M., and Baker, S.J. (2001) Parathyroid hormone, haematological and biochemical parameters in relation to dental disease and husbandry in rabbits. *Journal of Small Animal Practice*, **42**, 130–136.

Peixoto, P.V., Nogueira, V.A., Gonzaléz, A.P., Tokarnia, C.H., and França, T.N. (2009) Accidental and experimental salinomycin poisoning in rabbits. *Pesquisa Veterinária Brasileira*, **29**(9), 695–699.

Salles, M.S., Lombardo de Barros, C.S., and Barros, S.S. (1994) Ionophore antibiotic (narasin) poisoning in rabbits. *Veterinary and Human Toxicology*, **36**(5), 437–444.

Shientag, L.J., and Goad, M. (2011) Sudden hind limb injuries in two rabbits. *Laboratory Animals (NY)*, **40**(7), 212–216.

Oral Conditions

Bercier, M., Sanchez-Migallon Gullman, D., Stockman, J., *et al.* (2013) Salivary gland adenocarcinoma in a domestic rabbit (*Oryctolagus cuniculus*). *Journal of Exotic Pet Medicine*, **22**, 218–224.

Capello, V. (2008) Clinical technique: Treatment of periapical infections in pet rabbits and rodents. *Journal of Exotic Animal Practice*, **17**(2), 124–131.

Crossley, D.A. (2003) Oral biology and disorders of lagomorphs. *Veterinary Clinics of North America: Exotic Animal Practice*, **6**, 629–659.

Eckermann-Ross, C. (2008) Hormonal regulation and calcium metabolism in the rabbit. *Veterinary Clinics of North America: Exotic Animal Practice*, **11**, 139–152.

Harcourt-Brown, F.M. (1996) Calcium deficiency, diet and dental disease in pet rabbits. *Veterinary Record*, **139**, 567–571.

Harcourt-Brown, F.M., and Baker, S.J. (2001) Parathyroid hormone, haematological and biochemical parameters in relation to dental disease and husbandry in rabbits. *Journal of Small Animal Practice*, **42**, 130–136.

Harcourt-Brown, F.M. (2007) The progressive syndrome of acquired dental disease in rabbits. *Journal of Exotic Pet Medicine*, **16**(3), 146–157.

Harcourt-Brown, F.M. (2009) *Dental disease in pet rabbits 1.* Normal dentition, pathogenesis and aetiology. *In Practice*, **31**, 370–379.

Jekl, V., Hauptman, K., and Knotek, Z. (2008) Quantitative and qualitative assessments of intraoral lesions in 180 small herbivorous mammals. *Veterinary Record*, **162**(14), 442–9.

Joseph, C.E., Ashrafi, S.H., and Waterhouse, J.P. (1981) Structural changes in rabbit oral epithelium caused by zinc deficiency. *Journal of Nutrition*, **111**, 53–57.

Legendre, L.F.J. (2002) Malocclusions in guinea pigs, chinchillas and rabbits. *Canadian Veterinary Journal*, **43**, 385–390.

Lennox, A.M. (2008) Diagnosis and treatment of dental disease in pet rabbits. *Journal of Exotic Pet Medicine*, **17**(2), 107–113.

Mews, A.R., Ritchie, J.S.D., Romero-Mercado, H., and Scott, G.R. (1972) Detection of oral papillomatosis in a British rabbit colony. *Laboratory Animals (UK)*, **6**, 141–145.

Reiter, A.M. (2008) Pathophysiology of dental disease in the rabbit, guinea pig, and chinchilla. *Journal of Exotic Pet Medicine*, **17**(2), 70–77.

Tyrrell, K.L., Citron, D.M., Jenkins, J.R., Goldstein, E.J.C., and Veterinary Study Group. (2002) Periodontal bacteria in rabbit mandibular and maxillary abscesses. *Journal of Clinical Microbiology*, **40**(3), 1044–1047.

Villano, J.S. and Cooper, T.K. (2013) Mandibular fracture and necrotizing sialometaplasia in a rabbit. *Comparative Medicine*, **63**(1), 67–70.

Gastric Conditions

Harcourt-Brown, F.M. (2007) Gastric dilation and intestinal obstruction in 76 rabbits. *Veterinary Record*, **161**, 409–414.

Harcourt-Brown, T.R. (2007) Management of acute gastric dilation in rabbits. *Journal of Exotic Pet Medicine*, **16**(3), 168–174.

Hinton, M. (1980) Gastric ulceration in the rabbit. *Journal of Comparative Pathology*, **90**, 475–481.

Hood, S., Kelly, J., McBurney, S., and Burton, S. (1997) Lead toxicosis in two dwarf rabbits. *Canadian Veterinary Journal*, **38**, 721–722.

Johnson, M.S. Clinical toxicoses of domestic rabbits. *Veterinary Clinics of North America: Exotic Animal Practice*, **11**(2), 315–326.

Lichtenberger, M. and Lennox, A. (2010) Updates and advanced therapies for gastrointestinal stasis in rabbits. *Veterinary Clinics of North America: Exotic Animal Practice*, **13**, 525–541.

Mézes, M., and Balogh, K. (2009) Mycotoxins in rabbit feed: A review. *World Rabbit Science*, **17**, 53–62.

Pilny, A.A., and Hess, L. (2004) What is your diagnosis? Gastrointestinal stasis syndrome. *Journal of the American Veterinary Medical Association*, **225**, 681–682.

Van den Bulck, K., Baele, M., Hermans, K., *et al.* (2005) First report on the occurrence of '*Helicobacter heilmannii*' in the stomach of rabbits. *Veterinary Research Communications*, **29**, 271–279.

Van den Bulck, K., Decostere, A., Baele, M., *et al.* (2006) Low frequency of *Helicobacter* species in the stomachs of experimental rabbits. *Laboratory Animals (UK)*, **40**, 282–287.

Enteric Conditions

Bellier, R. and Gidenne, T. (1996) Consequences of reduced fibre intake on digestion, rate of passage and cecal microbial activity in the young rabbit. *British Journal of Nutrition*, **75**, 353–363.

Blanco, J.E., Blanco, M., Blanco, J., Rioja, L., and Ducha, J. (1994) Serotypes, toxins and antibiotic resistance of *Escherichia coli* strains isolated from diarrhoeic and healthy rabbits in Spain. *Veterinary Microbiology*, **38**, 193–201.

Camguilhem, R. and Milon, A. (1989) Biotypes and O serogroups of *Escherichia coli* involved in intenstinal infections of weaned rabbits: Clues to diagnosis of pathogenic strains. *Journal of Clinical Microbiology*, **27**(4), 743–747.

Caprioli, A., Morabito, S., Brugère, H., and Oswald, E. (2005) Enterohaemorrhagic *Escherichia coli*: emerging issues on virulence and modes of transmission. *Veterinary Research*, **36**(3), 289–311.

Carman, R.J. and Borriello, S.P. (1984) Infectious nature of *Clostridium spiroforme*-mediated rabbit enterotoxaemia. *Veterinary Microbiology*, **9**, 497–502.

Carman, R.J. and Evans, R.H. (1984) Experimental and spontaneous clostridial enteropathies of laboratory and free-living lagomorphs. *Laboratory Animal Science*, **34**(5), 443–452.

Catchpole, J. and Norton, C.C. (1979) The species of *Eimeria* in rabbits for meat production in Britain. *Parasitology*, **79**, 249–257.

Ciarlet, M., Gilger, M.A., Barone, C., McArthur, M., Estes, M.K., and Conner, M.E. (1998) Rotavirus disease, but not infection and development of intestinal histopathological lesions, is age restricted in rabbits. *Virology*, **251**(2), 343–360.

DeCubellis, J., and Graham, J. (2013) Gastrointestinal disease in guinea pigs and rabbits. *Veterinary Clinics of North America: Exotic Animal Practice*, **16**(2), 421–435.

DiGiacomo, R.F. and Thouless, M.E. (1986) Epidemiology of naturally occurring rotavirus infection in rabbits. *Laboratory Animal Science*, **36**(2), 153–156.

Duhamel, G.E., Klein, E.C., Elder, R.O., and Gebhart, C.J. (1998) Subclinical proliferative enteropathy in sentinel rabbits associated with *Lawsonia intracellularis*. *Veterinary Pathology*, **35**, 300–303.

Flatt, R.E. and Campbell, W.W. (1974) Cysticercosis in rabbits: Incidence and lesions of the naturally occurring disease in young domestic rabbits. *Laboratory Animal Science*, **24**(6), 914–918.

Ganaway, J.R., McReynolds, R.S., and Allen, A.M. (1976) Tyzzer's disease in free-living cottontail rabbits (*Sylvilagus floridanus*) in Maryland. *Journal of Wildlife Diseases*, **12**, 545–549.

Garcia, A., Marini, R.P., Feng, Y. *et al.* (2002) A naturally occurring rabbit model of enterohemorrhagic *Escherichia coli*-induced disease. *Journal of Infectious Diseases*, **186**, 1682–1686.

Garcia, A., and Fox, J.G. (2003) The rabbit as a new reservoir host of enterohemorrhagic *Escherichia coli*. *Emerging Infectious Diseases*, **9**(12), 1592–1597.

Garcia, A., Bosques, C.J., Wishnok, J.S., *et al.* (2006) Renal injury is a consistent finding in Dutch belted rabbits experimentally infected with enterohemorrhagic *Escherichia coli*. *Journal of Infectious Diseases*, **193**, 1125–1134.

Garmendia, J., Frankel, G., and Crepin, V.F. (2005) Enteropathogenic and enterohemorrhagic *Escherichia coli* infections: translocation, translocation, translocation. *Infection and Immunity*, **73**(5), 2573–2585.

Gidenne, T., Jehl, N., Lapanouse, A., and Segura, M. (2004) Inter-relationship of microbial activity, digestion and gut health in the rabbit: Effect of substituting fibre by starch in diets having a high proportion of rapidly fermentable polysaccharides. *British Journal of Nutrition*, **92**, 95–104.

Hahn, C.N., Whitwell, K.E., and Mayhew, I.G. (2001) Central nervous system pathology in cases of leporine dysautonomia. *Veterinary Record*, **149**(24), 745–746.

Hahn, C.N., Whitwell, K.E., and Mayhew, I.G. (2005) Neuropathological lesions resembling equine grass sickness in rabbits. *Veterinary Record*, **156**(24), 778–779.

Haligur, M., Ozmen, O., and Demir, N. (2009) Pathological and ultrastructural studies on mucoid enteropathy in New Zealand rabbits. *Journal of Exotic Pet Medicine*, **18**(3), 224–228.

Harris, I.E. and Portas, B.H. (1985) Enterotoxaemia in rabbits caused by *Clostridium spiroforme*. *Australian Veterinary Journal*, **62**(10), 342–343.

Harwood, D.G. (1989) *Salmonella typhimurium* infection in a commercial rabbitry. *Veterinary Record*, **125**, 554–555.

Horiuchi, N., Watarai, M., Kobayashi, Y., Omata, Y., and Furuoka, H. (2008) Proliferative enteropathy involving *Lawsonia intracellularis* infection in rabbits (*Oryctolagus cuniculus*). *Journal of Veterinary Medical Science*, **70**(4), 389–392.

Hotchkiss, C.E. and Collins, B.R. (1994) Imperforate anus with rectovaginal fistula in a dwarf rabbit. *Laboratory Animal Science*, **44**(2), 184–185.

Huybens, N., Houeix, J., Szalo, M., *et al.* (2008) Is epizootic rabbit enteropathy a bacterial disease? *9th World Rabbit Congress*, Verona, IT. pp 971–975.

Ishikawa, M., Maeda, H., Kondo, H., *et al.* (2007) A case of lymphoma developing in the rabbit cecum. *Journal of Veterinary Medical Science*, **69**(11), 1183–1185.

Kohler, R., Krause, G., Beutin, L., Stephan, R., and Zweifel, C. (2008) Shedding of food-borne pathogens and microbiological carcass contamination in rabbits at slaughter. *Veterinary Microbiology*, **132**, 149–157.

Lavazza, A., Cerioli, M., Martella, V., *et al.* (2008) Rotavirus in diarrheic rabbits: Prevalence and characterization of strains in Italian farms. 9th World Rabbit Congress, Verona, IT, pp. 993–997.

Macy, J.D., Weir, E.C., and Barthold, S.W. (1996) Colonic intussusception in a rabbit. *Contemporary Topics in Laboratory Animal Science*, **35**(6), 84–89.

Martella, V., Moschidou, P., Pinto, P., *et al.* (2011) Astroviruses in rabbits. *Emerging Infectious Diseases*, **17**(12), 2287–2293.

Német, Z., Szenci, O., Horváth, A., Makrai, L., Kis, T., Tóth, B., and Biksi, I. (2011) Outbreak of *Klebsiella oxytoca* enterocolitis on a rabbit farm in Hungary. *Veterinary Record*, **168**, 243b.

Ononiwu, J.C., and Julian, R.J. (1978) An outbreak of Tyzzer's disease in an Ontario rabbitry. *Canadian Veterinary Journal*, **19**, 107–109.

Pakandl, M., Hlásková, L., Poplstein, M., *et al.* (2008) Dependence of the immune response to coccidiosis on the age of rabbit suckling. *Parasitology Research*, **103**(6), 1265–1271.

Peddireddi, L., Myers, C., An, B., *et al.* (2010) *Providentia vermicola* septicemia resulting in acute death in a domestic rabbit (*Oryctolagus cuniculus*). *53rd AAVLD Conference Proceedings*, Minneapolis, MN, p. 62.

Peeters, J.E., Charlier, G., Antoine, O., and Mammerickx, M. (1984) Clinical and pathological changes after *Eimeria intestinalis* infection in rabbits. *Zentralblatt fuer Veterinaermedizin Reihe B.* **31**, 9–24.

Peeters, J.E., Pohl, P., Okerman, L., and Devriese, L.A. (1984) Pathogenic properties of *Escherichia coli* strains isolated from diarrheic commercial rabbits. *Journal of Clinical Microbiology*, **20**(1), 34–39.

Peeters, J.E., Charlier, G.J., and Raeymaekers, R. (1985) Scanning and transmission electron microscopy of attaching and effacing *Escherichia coli* in weanling rabbits. *Veterinary Pathology*, **22**, 54–59.

Peeters, J.E., Geeroms, R., Carman, R.J., and Wilkins, T.D. (1986) Significance of *Clostridium spiroforme* in the enteritis-complex of commercial rabbits. *Veterinary Microbiology*, **12**, 25–31.

Peeters, J.E., Geeroms, R., and Orskov, F. (1988) Biotype, serotype, and pathogenicity of attaching and effacing enteropathogenic *Escherichia coli* strains isolated from diarrheic commercial rabbits. *Infection and Immunity*, **56**(6), 1442–1448.

Percy, D.H., Muckle, C.A., Hampson, R.J., and Brash, M.L. (1993) The enteritis complex in domestic rabbits: A field study. *Canadian Veterinary Journal*, **34**, 95–102.

Pizzi, R., Hagen, R.U., and Meredith, A.L. (2007) Intermittent colic and intussusceptions due to a cecal polyp in a rabbit. *Journal of Exotic Pet Medicine*, **16**(2), 113–117.

Rehg, J.E., Lawton, G.W., and Pakes, S.P. (1979) *Cryptosporidium cuniculus* in the rabbit (*Oryctolagus cuniculus*). *Laboratory Animal Science*, **29**(5), 656–660.

Robins-Browne, R.M., Tokhl, A.M., *et al.* (1994) Adherence characteristics of attaching and effacing strains of *Escherichia coli* from rabbits. *Infection and Immunity*, **62**(5), 1584–1592.

Robinson, G., and Chalmers, R.M. (2010) The European rabbit (*Oryctolagus cuniculus*), a source of zoonotic cryptosporidiosis. *Zoonoses and Public Health.* **57**, e1–e13.

Sanchez-Migallon Guzman, D., Graham, J.E., Keller, K., Tong, N., and Morrisey, J.K. (2015) Colonic obstruction following ovariohysterectomy in rabbits: 3 cases. *Journal of Exotic Pet Medicine*, **24**, 112–119.

Schauer, D.B., McCathey, S.N., Daft, B.M., *et al.* (1988) Proliferative enterocolitis associated with dual infection with enteropathogenic *Escherichia coli* and *Lawsonia intracellularis* in rabbits. *Journal of Clinical Microbiology*, **36**(6), 1700–1703.

Schoeb, T.R., Casebolt, D.B., Walker, V.E., *et al.* (1986) Rotavirus-associated diarrhea in a commercial rabbitry. *Laboratory Animal Science*, **36**(2), 149–152.

Small, J.D., and Woods, R.D. (1987) Relatedness of rabbit coronavirus to other coronaviruses. *Advances in Experimental Medicine and Biology*, **218**, 521–527.

Spears, K.J., Roe, A.J., and Gally, D.L. (2006) A comparison of enteropathogenic and enterohaemorrhagic *Escherichia coli* pathogenesis. *FEMS Microbiology Letters*, **255**, 187–202.

Syverson, P.V., Juul, J., Rygg, M., Sletten, K., Husby, G., and Marhaug, G. (1993) The primary structure of rabbit serum amyloid A protein isolated from acute phase serum. *Scandinavian Journal of Immunology*, **37**, 447–451.

Tsalie, E., Kouzi, K., Poutahidis, T., *et al.* (2006) Effect of vitamin E nutritional supplementation on the pathological changes induced in the ileum of rabbits by experimental infection with enteropathogenic *Escherichia coli. Journal of Comparative Pathology*, **134**, 308–319.

Varga, I. (1982) Large-scale management systems and parasite populations: Coccidia in rabbits. *Veterinary Parasitology*, **11**, 69–84.

Wilkinson, M.J., Bell, S., McGoldrick, J., and Williams, A.E. (2001) Unexpected deaths in young New Zealand white rabbits (*Oryctolagus cuniculus*). *Contemporary Topics in Laboratory Animal Science*, **40**(4), 49–51.

Zanon, F., Siliotto, R., and Facchin, E. (1996) *Salmonella typhimurium* infection in a commercial rabbitry. *Proceedings of 6th World Rabbit Congress*, Toulouse, France. pp 131–133.

Hepatobiliary Conditions

Al-Mathal, E.M. (2008) Hepatic coccidiosis of the domestic rabbit *Oryctolagus cuniculus domesticus L.* in Saudi Arabia. *World Zoology Journal*, **3**(1), 30–35.

Birke, L., Cormier, S.A., You, D., *et al.* (2014) Hepatitis E antibodies in laboratory rabbits from 2 US vendors. *Emerging Infectious Diseases*, **20**(4), 693–696.

Diaolu, M., and Park, G. (2013) Acute torsion of the hepatic quadrate lobe in a mature pet rabbit. *AHL Newsletter*, **17**(2), 14.

Caruso, C., Modesto, P., Prato, R., *et al.* (2015) Hepatitis E virus: First description in a pet house rabbit. A new transmission route for humans? *Transboundary and Emerging Diseases*, **62**(3), 229–32.

Cossaboom, C.M., Córdoba, L., Dryman, B.A., and Meng, X.J. (2011) Hepatitis E virus in rabbits, Virginia, USA. *Emerging Infectious Diseases*, **17**(11), 2047–2049.

Cossaboom, C.M., Córdoba, L., Cao, D., Ni, Y.Y., and Meng, X.J. (2012) Complete genome sequence of hepatitis E virus from rabbits in the United States. *Journal of Virology*, **86**(23), 13124–13125.

DeCubellis, J., Kruse, A.M., McCarthy, R.J., *et al.* (2010) Biliary cystadenoma in a rabbit (*Oryctolagus cuniculus*). *Journal of Exotic Pet Medicine*, **19**(2), 177–192.

Dubey, J.P., Brown, C.A., Carpenter, J.L., and Moore, J.J. 3rd. (1992) Fatal toxoplasmosis in domestic rabbits in the USA. *Veterinary Parasitology*, **44**(3–4), 305–309.

Embury-Hyatt, C., Postey, R., Hisanaga, T., *et al.* (2012) The first reported case of rabbit hemorrhagic disease in Canada. *Canadian Veterinary Journal*, **53**(9), 998–1002.

Ewuola, E.O. (2009) Organ traits and histopathology of rabbits fed varied levels of dietary fumonisin B(1). *Journal of Animal Physiology and Animal Nutrition, (Berlin)*. **93**(6), 726–31.

Geng, J., Fu, H., Wang, L., *et al.* (2011) Phylogenetic analysis of the full genome of rabbit hepatitis E virus (rbHEV) and molecular biologic study on the possibility of cross species transmission of rbHEV. *Infection, Genetics and Evolution*, **11**(8), 2020–2025.

Geng, Y., Zhao, C., Song, A., *et al.* (2011) The serological prevalence and genetic diversity of hepatitis E virus in farmed rabbits in China. *Infection, Genetics and Evolution*, **11**(2), 476–482.

Graham, J., and Basseches, J. (2014) Liver lobe torsion in pet rabbits: clinical consequences, diagnosis, and treatment. *Veterinary Clinics of North America: Exotic Animal Practice*, **17**(2), 195–202.

Graham, J.E., Orcutt, C.J., Casale, S.A., Ewing, P.J., and Basseches, J. (2015) Liver lobe torsion in rabbits: 16 cases (2007 to 2012). *Journal of Exotic Pet Medicine*, **23**, 258–265.

Izopet, J., Dubois, M., Bertagnoli, S., *et al.* (2012) Hepatitis E virus strains in rabbits and evidence of a closely related strain in humans, France. *Emerging Infectious Diseases*, **18**(8), 1274–1281.

L'homme, S., Dubois, M., Abravanel, F., Top, S., Bertagnoli, S., Guerin, J.L., and Izopet, J. (2013) Risk of zoonotic transmission of HEV from rabbits. *Journal of Clinical Virology*, **58**(2), 357–362.

Liu, P., Bu, Q.N., Wang, L., *et al.* (2013) Transmission of hepatitis E virus from rabbits to cynomolgus macaques. *Emerging Infectious Diseases*, **19**(4), 559–565.

Meredith, A. and Rayment, L. (2000) Liver disease in rabbits. *Seminars in Avian and Exotic Veterinary Medicine*, **9**(3), 146–152.

Otto, P., Kohlmann, R., Müller, W., *et al.* (2015) Hare-to-human transmission of *Francisella tularensis* subsp. *holarctica*, Germany. *Emerging Infectious Diseases*, **21**(1), 153–155.

Park, J.H., Lee, Y.-S., and Itakura, C. (1995) Pathogenesis of acute necrotic hepatitis in rabbit hemorrhagic disease. *Laboratory Animal Science*, **45**(4), 445–449.

Ramirez, C.J., Kim, D.Y., Hanks, B.C., and Evans, T.J. (2013) Copper toxicosis in New Zealand white rabbits (*Oryctolagus cuniculus*). *Veterinary Pathology*, **50**(6), 1135–1138.

Taylor, H.R. and Staff, C.D. (2007) Clinical techniques: Successful management of liver lobe torsion in a domestic rabbit (*Oryctolagus cuniculus*) by surgical lobectomy. *Journal of Exotic Pet Medicine*, **16**(3), 175–178.

Wang, S., Dong, C., Dai, X., *et al.* (2013) Hepatitis E virus isolated from rabbits is genetically heterogeneous but with very similar antigenicity to human HEV. *Journal of Medical Virology*, **85**(4), 627–635.

Wenger, S., Barrett, E.L., Pearson, G.R., *et al.* (2009) Liver lobe torsion in three adult rabbits. *Journal of Small Animal Practice*, **50**, 301–305.

General Gastrointestinal Conditions

Bivolarski, B.L. and Vachkova, E.G. (2014) Morphological and functional events associated to weaning in rabbits. *Journal of Animal Physiology and Animal Nutrition (Berlin)*. **98**(1), 9–18.

Brewer, N.R. (2006) Biology of the rabbit. *Journal of the American Association of Laboratory Animal Science*, **45**(1), 8–24.

Combes, S., Gidenne, T., Cauquil, L., Bouchez, O., and Fortun-Lamothe, L. (2014) Coprophagous behavior of rabbit pups affects implantation of cecal microbiota and health status. *Journal of Animal Science*, **92**(2), 652–665.

Feinstein, R.E. and Nikkilä, T. (1988) Occurrence of multinucleated giant cells in the appendix of clinically healthy rabbits. *Journal of Comparative Pathology*, **99**(4), 439–447.

Harrenstein, L. (1999) Gastrointestinal disease of pet rabbits. *Seminars in Avian and Exotic Pet Medicine*, **8**(2), 83–89.

Heatley, J.J. and Smith, A.N. (2004) Spontaneous neoplasms of lagomorphs. *Veterinary Clinics of North America: Exotic Animal Practice*, **7**, 561–577.

Jekl, V. and Redrobe, S. (2013) Rabbit dental disease and calcium metabolism - the science behind divided opinions. *Journal of Small Animal Practice*, **54**(9), 481–490.

Kararli, T.T. (1995) Comparison of the gastrointestinal anatomy, physiology, and biochemistry of humans and commonly used laboratory animals. *Biopharmaceutics and Drug Disposition*, **16**(5), 351–380.

Kohles, M. (2014) Gastrointestinal anatomy and physiology of select exotic companion mammals. *Veterinary Clinics of North America: Exotic Animal Practice*, **17**(2), 165–178.

Krogstad, A.P., Simpson, J.E., and Korte, S.W. (2005) Viral diseases of rabbits. *Veterinary Clinics of North America: Exotic Animal Practice*, **8**, 123–138.

Lennox, A.M. and Kelleher, S. (2009) Bacterial and parasitic diseases of rabbits. *Veterinary Clinics of North America: Exotic Animal Practice*, **12**, 519–530.

Li, X., Fox, J.G., Erdman, S.E., and Lipman, N.S. (1996) Intestinal plasmacytosis in rabbits: a histologic and ultrastructural study. *Veterinary Pathology*, **33**(6), 721–724.

Rees Davies, R. and Rees Davies, J.A.E. (2003) Rabbit gastrointestinal physiology. *Veterinary Clinics of North America: Exotic Animal Practice*, **6**, 139–153.

Reusch, B. (2005) Rabbit gastroenterology. *Veterinary Clinics of North America: Exotic Animal Practice*, **8**, 351–375.

Cardiomyopathy

Bragdon, J.H. and Levine, H.D. (1949) Myocarditis in vitamin E-deficient rabbits. *American Journal of Pathology*, **25**(2), 265–271.

Downing, S.E. and Chen, V. (1985) Myocardial injury following endogenous catecholamine release in rabbits. *Journal of Molecular Cell Cardiology*, **17**(4), 377–387.

Hurley, R.J., Marini, R.P., Avison, D.L., *et al.* (1994) Evaluation of detomidine anesthetic combinations in the rabbit. *Laboratory Animal Science*, **44**(5), 472–478.

Lord, B., Devine, C., and Smith, S. (2011) Congestive heart failure in two pet rabbits. *Journal of Small Animal Practice*, **52**, 46–50.

Marini, R.P., Li, X., Harpster, N.K., and Dangler, C. (1999) Cardiovascular pathology possibly associated with ketamine/xylazine anesthesia in Dutch belted rabbits. *Laboratory Animal Science*, **49**(2), 153–160.

Pariault, R. (2009) Cardiovascular physiology and diseases of the rabbit. *Veterinary Clinics of North America: Exotic Animal Practice*, **12**, 135–144.

Rippy, M.K., Sandusky, G.E., and Pucak, G.J. (1994) Rabbit spontaneous cardiomyopathy. *Toxicologic Pathology*, **22**(6), 650–651.

Simons, M. and Downing, S.E. (1985) Coronary vasoconstriction and catecholamine cardiomyopathy. *American Heart Journal*, **109**(2), 297–304.

Myocarditis

Allison, S.O., Artwohl, J.E., Fortman, J.D., *et al.* (2007) Iatrogenic hemolytic anemia and endocarditis in New Zealand white rabbits secondary to *Achromobacter xylosoxidans* Infection. *Journal of the American Association of Laboratory Animal Science*, **46**(6), 58–62.

Cutlip, R.C., Amtower, W.C., Beall, C.W., and Matthews, P.J. (1971) An epizootic of Tyzzer's disease in rabbits. *Laboratory Animal Science*, **21**(3), 356–361.

Small, J.D., Aurelian, L., Squire, R.A., *et al.* (1979) Rabbit cardiomyopathy associated with a virus antigenically related to human coronavirus strain 229E. *American Journal of Pathology*, **95**(3), 709–729.

Myocardial Toxicity

Ali, M.A., Chanu, K.H.V., Singh, W.R., Shah, M.A.A., and Leishangthem, G.D. (2010) Biochemical and pathological changes associated with avocado leaves poisoning in rabbits - A case report. *International Journal of Research in Pharmaceutical Sciences*, **1**(3), 225–228.

Martino, P.E., Parrado, E., Sanguinetti, R., *et al.* (2009) Massive mortality in rabbits by maduramicin poisoning. *World Rabbit Science*, **17**, 45–48.

Oehme, F.W. and Pickrell, J.A. (1999) An analysis of the chronic oral toxicity of polyether ionophore antibiotics in animals. *Veterinary and Human Toxicology*, **41**(4), 251–257.

Singh, W.R., Rajkhowa, T.K., Chanu, K.H.V., *et al.* (2010) Histopathological changes caused by accidental avocado leaves toxicity in rabbits. *International Journal of Research in Pharmaceutical Science*, **1**(4), 517–520.

Other Cardiovascular Conditions

Crary, D.D. and Fox, R.R. (1975) Hereditary vestigial pulmonary arterial trunk and related defects in rabbits. *Journal of Heredity*, **66**(2), 50–55.

Fox, R.R., Schlager, G., and Laird, C.W. (1969) Blood pressure in thirteen strains of rabbits. *Journal of Heredity*, **60**(6), 312–314.

Guzman, R.E., Ehrhart, E.J., Wasson, K., and Andrews, J.J. (2000) Primary hepatic hemangiosarcoma with pulmonary metastases in a New Zealand white rabbit. *Journal of Veterinary Diagnostic Investigation*, **12**, 284–286.

Li, X., Murphy, J.C., and Lipman, N.S. (1995) Eisenmenger's syndrome in a New Zealand white rabbit. *Laboratory Animal Science*, **45**(5), 618–620.

Shell, L.G., and Saunders, G. (1989) Arteriosclerosis in a rabbit. *Journal of the American Veterinary Medical Association*, **194**(5), 679–680.

Zimmerman, T.E., Giddens, W.E. Jr, DiGiacomo, R.F., and Ladiges, W.C. (1990) Soft tissue mineralization in rabbits fed a diet containing excess vitamin D. *Laboratory Animal Science*, **40**(2), 212–215.

Encephalitozoonosis

Csokai, J., Joachim, A., Gruber, A., *et al.* (2009) Diagnostic markers for encephalitozoonosis in pet rabbits. *Veterinary Parasitology*, **163**, 18–26.

Flatt, R.E. and Jackson, S.J. (1970) Renal nosematosis in young rabbits. *Veterinary Pathology*, **7**, 492–497.

Harcourt-Brown, F.M. (2004) *Encephalitozoon cuniculi* infection in rabbits. *Seminars in Avian and Exotic Pet Medicine*, **13**(2), 86–93.

Hunt, R.D, King, N.W, and Foster, H.L. (1972) Encephalitozoonosis: Evidence for vertical transmission. *Journal of Infectious Diseases*, **126**, 212–214.

Keeble, E.J. and Shaw, D.J. (2006) Seroprevalence of antibodies to *Encephalitozoon cuniculi* in domestic rabbits in the United Kingdom. *Veterinary Record*, **158**, 539–544.

Künzel, F., Gruber, A., Tichy, A., *et al.* (2008) Clinical symptoms and diagnosis of encephalitozoonosis in pet rabbits. *Veterinary Parasitology*, **151**, 115–124.

Künzel, F. and Joachim, A. (2010) Encephalitozoonosis in rabbits. *Parasitology Research*, **106**, 299–309.

Ozkan, O., Ozkan, A.T, and Zafer, K. (2011) Encephalitozoonosis in New Zealand rabbits and potential transmission risk. *Veterinary Parasitology*, **179**(1–3), 234–237.

Chronic Renal Disease

Eckerman-Ross, C. (2008) Hormonal regulation and calcium metabolism in the rabbit. *Veterinary Clinics of North America: Exotic Animal Practice*, **11**, 139–152.

Garibaldi, B.A., Fox, J.G., Otto, G., Murphy, J.C. and Pecquet-Goad, M.E. (1987) Hematuria in rabbits. *Laboratory Animal Science*, **37**(6), 769–772.

Harcourt-Brown, F.M. (2013) Diagnosis of renal disease in rabbits. *Veterinary Clinics of North America: Exotic Animal Practice*, **16**(1), 145–174.

Hinton, M. (1981) Kidney disease in the rabbit: a histological survey. *Laboratory Animals (UK)*, **15**, 263–265.

Urolithiasis

Kamphues, J. (1991) Calcium metabolism of rabbits as an etiological factor for urolithiasis. *Journal of Nutrition*, **121**, S95–S96.

Lee, K.J., Johnson, W.D., Lang, C.M., and Hartshorn, R.D. (1978) Hydronephrosis caused by urinary urolithiasis in a New Zealand white rabbit. *Veterinary Pathology*, **15**, 676–678.

Renal Neoplasia

Atasever, A., Beyaz, L. and Deniz, K. (2007) A case of triphasic nephroblastoma with lung metastases in an angora rabbit. *Revue de médicine vétérinaire*, **158**(6), 303–308.

Durfee, W.J., Masters, W.G., Montgomery, C.A., *et al.* (1999) Spontaneous renal cell carcinoma in a New Zealand white rabbit. *Contemporary Topics in Laboratory Animal Science*, **38**(1), 89–91.

Gómez, L., Gázquez, A., Roncero, V., Sánchez, C., and Durán, M.E. (2002) Lymphoma in a rabbit: histopathological and immunohistochemical findings. *Journal of Small Animal Practice*, **43**(5), 224–226.

Lipman, N.S., Murphy, J.C., and Newcomer, C.E. (1985) Polycythemia in a New Zealand white rabbit with an embryonal nephroma. *Journal of American Veterinary Medical Association*, **187**(11), 1255–1256.

Lead Intoxication

Hood, S., Kelly, J., McBurney, S., and Burton, S. (1997) Lead toxicoses in two dwarf rabbits. *Canadian Veterinary Journal*, **38**, 721–722.

Johnston, M.S. (2008) Clinical toxicoses of domestic rabbits. *Veterinary Clinics of North America: Exotic Animal Practice*, **11**, 315–326.

Other Urinary Tract Conditions

Brammer, D.W., Doerning, B.J., Chrisp, C.E., and Rush, H.G. (1991) Anesthetic and nephrotoxic effects of Telazol in New Zealand white rabbits. *Laboratory Animal Science*, **41**(5), 432–435.

Crary, D.D., and Fox, R.R. (1980) Frequency of congenital abnormalities and of anatomical variations among JAX rabbits. *Teratology*, **21**, 113–121.

Evans, K.D., Dillehay, D.L., Huerkamp, M.J., and Webb, S.K. (1996) Diagnostic exercise: Azotemia in a rabbit (*Oryctolagus cuniculus*). *Laboratory Animal Science*, **46**(4), 442–443.

Grunkemeyer, V.L., Sura, P.A., Baron, M.L., and Souza, M.J. (2009) Inguinal herniation of the urinary bladder in a female rabbit. *AEMV Proceedings*, Milwaukee, WI, p. 79.

Maurer, K.J., Marini, R.P., Fox, J.G., and Rogers, A.B. (2004) Polycystic kidney syndrome in New Zealand white rabbits resembling human polycystic kidney disease. *Kidney International*, **65**, 482–489.

Metcalf, J.A., Lederman, M., Stout, E.R, and Bates R.C. (1989) Natural parvovirus infection of laboratory rabbits. *American Journal of Veterinary Research*, **50**(7), 1048–1051.

Nath, A.J., Juyal, R.C., Venkatesan, R., Kumar, M.J.M., and Nagarajan, P. (2006) Renal agenesis in a New Zealand white rabbit. *Scandinavian Journal of Laboratory Animal Science*, **33**(4), 197–200.

Petriz, Q.A., Guzman, D. S-M., Gandolfi, R.C., and Steffey, M.A. (2012) Inguinal-scrotal urinary bladder hernia in an intact male domestic rabbit (*Orytolagus cuniculus*). *Journal of Exotic Pet Medicine*, **21**(3), 248–254.

Sato, Y. (2005) A case of scrotal bladder hernia in a male rabbit. *Veterinary Medicine*, **58**, 992–994.

General Urinary Tract

Brewer, N.R. (2006) Biology of the rabbit. *Journal of American Association of Laboratory Animal Science*, **45**(1), 8–24.

Fisher, P.G. (2006a) Exotic mammal renal disease: causes and clinical presentation. *Veterinary Clinics of North America: Exotic Animal Practice*, **9**, 33–67.

Fisher PG. (2006b) Exotic mammal renal disease: diagnosis and treatment. *Veterinary Clinics of North America: Exotic Animal Practice*, **9**, 69–96.

Jenkins, J.R. (2010) Evaluation of the rabbit urinary tract. *Journal of Exotic Pet Medicine*, **19**(4), 271–279.

Listeriosis

Ayroud, M., Chirino-Trejo, M., and Kumor, L. (1991) Listeriosis in rabbits. *Canadian Veterinary Journal*, **32**, 44.

Iida, T., Kanzaki, M., Nakama, A., *et al.* (1998) Detection of *Listeria monocytogenes* in humans, animals and foods. *Journal of Veterinary Medical Science*, **160**(12), 1341–1343.

Watson, G.L., and Evans, M.G. (1985) Listeriosis in the rabbit. *Veterinary Pathology*, **22**, 191–193.

Other Causes of Pyometra and Abortion

DiGiacomo, R.F., Deeb, B.J., and Anderson, R.J. (1992) Hypervitaminosis A and reproductive disorders in rabbits. *Laboratory Animal Science*, **42**(3), 250–254.

Johnson, J.H. and Wolf, A.M. (1993) Ovarian abscesses and pyometra in a domestic rabbit. *Journal of the American Veterinary Medical Association*, **203**(5), 667–669.

Reproductive Neoplasia

Alexandre, N., Branco, S., Soares, T.F., and Soares, F. (2010) Bilateral testicular seminoma in a rabbit (*Oryctolagus cuniculus*). *Journal of Exotic Pet Medicine*, **19**(4), 304–308.

Brown, P.J., and Stafford, R.A. (1989) A testicular seminoma in a rabbit. *Journal of Comparative Pathology*, **100**, 353–355.

Cooper, T.K., Adelsohn, D., and Gilbertson, S.R. (2006) Spontaneous deciduosarcoma in a domestic rabbit (*Oryctolagus cuniculus*). *Veterinary Pathology*, **43**, 377–380.

Irizarry-Rovira, A.R., Lennox, A.M., and Ramos-Vara, J.A. (2008) Granular cell tumor in the testis of a rabbit: Cytologic, histologic, immunohistochemical, and electron microscopic characterization. *Veterinary Pathology*, **45**, 73–77.

Kaufmann-Bart, M. and Fischer, I. (2008) Choriocarcinoma with metastasis in a rabbit (*Oryctolagus cuniculus*). *Veterinary Pathology*, **45**(1), 77–79.

Kurotaki, T., Kokoshima, H., Kitamori, F., Kitamori, T., and Tsuchitani, M. (2007) A case of adenocarcinoma of the endometrium extending into the leiomyoma of the uterus in a rabbit. *Journal of Veterinary Medical Science*, **69**(9), 981–984.

Marino, F., Ferrara, G., Rapisarda, G., and Galofaro, V. (2003) Reinke's crystals in an interstitial cell tumour of a rabbit (*Oryctolagus cuniculus*). *Reproduction in Domestic Animals*, **38**(5), 421–422.

Meier, H., Myers, D.D., Fox, R.R., and Laird, C.W. (1970) Occurrence, pathological features, and propagation of gonadal teratomas in inbred mice and in rabbits. *Cancer Research*, **30**, 30–34.

Mutinelli, F., Carminato, A., Bozzato, E., *et al.* (2009) Retroperitoneal teratoma in a domestic rabbit (*Oryctolagus cuniculus*). *Journal of Veterinary Medical Science*, **71**(3), 367–370.

Roccabianca, P., Ghisleni, G., and Scanziani, E. (1999) Simultaneous seminoma and interstitial cell tumor in a rabbit with a previous cutaneous basal cell tumor. *Journal of Comparative Pathology*, **121**, 95–99.

Rosenbaum, M.D., Gardiner, D., and O'Rourke, D. (2013) Abdominal mass in a New Zealand white rabbit (*Oryctolagus cuniculus*). *Laboratory Animals (NY)*, **42**(1), 19–21.

Saito, K., Nakanishi, M., and Hasegawa, A. (2002) Uterine disorders diagnosed by ventrotomy in 47 rabbits. *Journal of Veterinary Medical Science*, **64**(6), 495–497.

Walter, B., Poth, T., Bohmer, E., Braun, J., and Matis, U. (2010) Uterine disorders in 59 rabbits. *Veterinary Record*, **166**, 230–233.

Zwicker, G.M., Killinger, J.M., and McConnel, R.F. (1985) Spontaneous vesicular and prostatic gland epithelial squamous metaplasia, hyperplasia, and keratinized nodule formation in rabbits. *Toxicologic Pathology*, **13**(3), 222–228.

Pregnancy Toxemia

Leland, S.E., Brownstein, D.G. and Weir, E.C. (1995) Pancreatitis and pregnancy toxemia in a New Zealand white rabbit. *Contemporary Topics in Laboratory Animal Science*, **34**(6), 84–85.

Other Reproductive Conditions

Bishop, C.R. (2002) Reproductive medicine of rabbits and rodents. *Veterinary Clinics of North America: Exotic Animal Practice*, **5**, 507–535.

Booth, J.L., Peng, X., Baccon, J., and Cooper, T.K. (2013) Multiple complex congenital malformations in a rabbit kit (*Oryctolagus cuniculus*). *Comparative Medicine*, **63**(4), 342–347.

Bray, M.V., Weir, E.C., Brownstein, D.G., and Delano, M.L. (1992) Endometrial venous aneurysms in three New Zealand white rabbits. *Laboratory Animal Science*, **42**(4), 360–362.

Brewer, N.R. (2006) Biology of the rabbit. *Journal of the American Association of Laboratory Animal Science*, **45**(1), 8–24.

Crary, D.D. and Fox, R.R. (1980) Frequency of congenital abnormalities and of anatomical variations among JAX rabbits. *Teratology* **21**, 113–121.

Corpa, J.C. (2006) Ectopic pregnancy in animals and humans. *Reproduction*, **131**, 631–640.

Dickie, E. (2011) Dystocia in a rabbit (*Oryctolagus cuniculus*). *Canadian Veterinary Journal*, **52**, 80–83.

Ewuola, E.O. (2009) Organ traits and histopathology of rabbits fed varied levels of dietary fumonisin B(1). *Journal of Animal Physiology and Animal Nutrition (Berlin)*, **93**(6), 726–731.

Harkness, J.E., Turner, P.V., VandeWoude, S., and Wheler, C.L. (2010) *Harkness and Wagner's Biology and Medicine of the Rabbits and Rodents*, 5th edn. Wiley-Blackwell, Ames, IA.

Gil, P.S., Palau, B.P., Martinez, J., Porcel, J.P., and Arena J.M.C. (2004) Abdominal pregnancies in farm rabbits. *Theriogenology*, **62**, 642–651.

Hill, W.A., and Brown, J.P. (2011) Zoonoses of rabbits and rodents. *Veterinary Clinics of North America: Exotic Animal Practice*, **14**(3), 519–531.

Johnston, M.S. (2009) Probable congenital uterine developmental abnormalities in two domestic rabbits. *Veterinary Record*, **164**, 242–244.

Matsuo, A. and Kast, A. (1995) Two decades of control Himalayan rabbit reproductive parameters and spontaneous abnormalities in Japan. *Laboratory Animals (UK)*, **29**, 78–82.

Morton, D., Weisbrode, S.E., Wyder, W.E., Maurer, J.K., and Capen, C.C. (1986) Spermatid giant cells, tubular hypospermatogenesis, spermatogonial swelling, cytoplasmic vacuoles, and tubular dilatation in the testes of normal rabbits. *Veterinary Pathology*, **23**(2), 176–183.

Sladakovic, I., Sanchez-Migallon Guczman, M., Petritz, O.A,, Mohr, F.C., and McGraw SN. (2015) Unilateral cervical and segmental uterine horn aplasia with endometrial hyperplasia, mucometra, and endometritis in a domestic rabbit (*Oryctolagus cuniculus*). *Journal of Exotic Pet Medicine*, **24**, 98–104.

Encephalitozoonosis

Harcourt-Brown, F.M. (2004) Encephalitozoon cuniculi infection in rabbits. *Seminars in Avian and Exotic Pet Medicine*, **13**(2), 86–93.

Hunt, R.D., King, N,W., and Foster, H.L. (1972) Encephalitozoonosis: Evidence for vertical transmission. *Journal of Infectious Diseases*, **126**, 212–214.

Künzel, F., Gruber, A., Tichy, A., *et al.* (2008) Clinical symptoms and diagnosis of encephalitozoonosis in pet rabbits. *Veterinary Parasitology*, **151**, 115–124.

Mathis, A., Michel, M., Kuster, H., *et al.* (1997) Two *Encephalitozoon cuniculi* strains of human origin are infectious to rabbits. *Parasitology*, **114** (Pt 1), 29–35.

Mathis, A., Weber, R., and Deplazes, P. (2005) Zoonotic potential of the microsporidia. *Clinical Microbiology Review*, **18**(3), 423–445.

Nast, R., Middleton, D.M., and Wheler, C.L. (1996) Generalized encephalitozoonosis in a Jersey wooly rabbit. *Canadian Veterinary Journal*, **37**, 303–305.

Valencakova, A., Balent, P., Petrovova, E., Novotny, F., and Luptakova, L. (2008) Encephalitozoonosis in household pet Netherland dwarf rabbits (*Oryctolagus cuniculus*). *Veterinary Parasitology*, **153**, 265–269.

Wasson, K. and Peper, R.L. (2000) Mammalian microsporidiosis. *Veterinary Pathology*, **37**, 113–128.

Human Herpes Virus-1 Encephalitis

Grest, P., Albicker, P., Hoelzle, L., Wild, P., and Pospischil, A. (2002) Herpes simplex encephalitis in a domestic rabbit (*Oryctolagus cuniculus*). *Journal of Comparative Pathology*, **126**, 308–311.

Müller, K., Fuchs, W., Heblinski, N, *et al.* (2009) Encephalitis in a rabbit caused by human herpesvirus-1. *Journal of the American Veterinary Medical Association*, **235**(1), 64–69.

Webre, J.M., Hill, J.M., Nolan, N.M., *et al.* Rabbit and mouse models of HSV-1 latency, reactivation, and recurrent eye diseases. *Journal of Biomedicine and Biotechnology*, **2012**, 612316.

Weissenböck, H., Hainfellner, J.A., Berger, J., Kasper, I., and Budka, H. (1997) Naturally occurring herpes simplex encephalitis in a domestic rabbit (*Oryctolagus cuniculus*). *Veterinary Pathology*, **34**, 44–47.

Rabies Virus Infections

Eidson, M., Matthews, S.D., Willsey, A.L., Cherry, B., Rudd, R.J., and Trimarchi, C.V. (2005) Rabies virus infection in a pet guinea pig and seven pet rabbits. *Journal of the American Veterinary Medical Association*, **227**, 932–935.

Fitzpatrick, J.L., Dyer, J.L., Blanton, J.D., Kuzmin, I.V., and Rupprecht, C.E. (2014) Rabies in rodents and lagomorphs in the United States, 1995–2010. *Journal of the American Veterinary Medical Association*, **245**(3), 333–337.

Karp, B.E., Ball, N.E., Scott, C.R., and Walcoff, J.B. (1999) Rabies in two privately owned domestic rabbits. *Journal of the American Veterinary Medical Association*, **215**, 1824–1827.

Krogstad, A.P., Simpson, J.E., and Korte, S.W. (2005) Viral diseases of rabbits. *Veterinary Clinics of North America: Exotic Animal Practice*, **8**, 123–138.

Lackay, S.N., Kuang, Y., and Fu, Z.F. (2008) Rabies in small animals. *Veterinary Clinics of North America: Small Animal Practice*, **38**(4), 851–860.

Cerebrospinal Parasitic Larval Migration

Deeb, B.J. and DiGiacomo, R.F. (1994) Cerebral larva migrans caused by *Baylisascaris* sp. in pet rabbits. *Journal of the American Veterinary Medical Association*, **205**(12), 1744–1747.

Gavin, P.J., Kazacos, K.R., and Shulman, S.T. (2005) Baylisascariasis. *Clinical Microbiology Review*, **18**(4), 703–718.

Kazacos, K.R., Reed, W.M., Kazacos, E.A., and Thacker, H.L. (1983) Fatal cerebrospinal disease caused by *Baylisascaris procyonis* in domestic rabbits. *Journal of the American Veterinary Medical Association*, **183**(9), 967–971.

Loretti, A.P. and Lencewicz, L. (2010) Cerebral myiasis in a pet rabbit. *Proceedings of the American Association of Veterinary Laboratory Diagnosticians*, Minneapolis, MN, p. 202.

Sato, H., Kamiya, H., and Furuoka, H. (2003) Epidemiological aspects of the first outbreak of *Baylisascaris procyonis* larva migrans in rabbits in Japan. *Journal of Veterinary Medical Science*, **65**(4), 453–457.

Cerebrospinal Neoplasia

Bishop, L. (1978) Intracranial teratoma in a domestic rabbit. *Veterinary Pathology*, **15**, 525–530.

Heatley, J.J. and Smith, A.N. (2004) Spontaneous neoplasms of lagomorphs. *Veterinary Clinics of North America: Exotic Animal Practice*, **7**, 561–577.

Lipman, N.S., Zhi-Bo, Z., Andrutis, K.A., *et al.* (1994) Prolactin-secreting pituitary adenomas with mammary dysplasia in New Zealand white rabbits. *Laboratory Animal Science*, **44**(2), 114–120.

Neurotoxicoses

Chang, L.W. (1990) The neurotoxicology and pathology of organomercury, organolead, and organotin. *Journal of Toxicologic Science*, **15** Suppl 4, 125–151.

Cox, A.B., Keng, P.C., Lee, A.C., and Lett, J.T. (1982) Effects of heavy ions on rabbit tissues: Damage to the forebrain. *International Journal of Radiation Biology*, **42**(4), 355–367.

DeCubellis, J. and Graham, J. (2013) Gastrointestinal disease in guinea pigs and rabbits. *Veterinary Clinics of North America: Exotic Animal Practice*, **16**(2), 421–435.

Johnston, M.S. (2008) Clinical toxicoses of domestic rabbits. *Veterinary Clinics of North America: Exotic Animal Practice*, **11**, 315–326.

Jones, J.M. (1984) Organophosphorus poisoning in two Rex rabbits. *New Zealand Veterinary Journal*, **32**, 9–10.

Sabbar, M., Delaville, C., De Deurwaerdère, P., Benazzouz, A., and Lakhdar-Ghazal, N. (2012) Lead intoxication induces noradrenaline depletion, motor nonmotor disabilities, and changes in the firing pattern of subthalamic nucleus neurons. *Neuroscience*, **210**, 375–383.

Other Neurologic Conditions

Dubey, J.P., Brown, C.A., Carpenter, J.L., and Moore, J.J. 3rd. (1992) Fatal toxoplasmosis in domestic rabbits in the USA. *Veterinary Parasitology*, **44**(3–4), 305–309.

Gruber, A., Pakozdy, A., Weissenböck, H., Csokai, J., and Kunzel, D.F. (2009) A retrospective study of neurological disease in 118 rabbits. *Journal of Comparative Pathology*, **140**, 31–37.

Harkness, JE., Turner, P.V., VandeWoude, S., and Wheler, C.L. (2010) *Harkness and Wagner's Biology and Medicine of Rabbits and Rodents*, 5th edn. Wiley-Blackwell, Ames, IA.

Keeble, E. (2006) Common neurological and musculoskeletal problems in rabbits. *In Practice*, **28**, 212–218.

Meredith, A.L. and Richardson, J. (2015) Neurological diseases of rabbits and rodents. *Journal of Exotic Pet Medicine*, **24**, 21–33.

Rickmeyer, T., Schöniger, S., Petermann, A., *et al.* (2013) GM2 gangliosidosis in an adult pet rabbit. *Journal of Comparative Parasitology*, **148**(2–3), 243–247.

Sato, J., Sasaki, S., Yamada, N., and Tsuchitani, M. (2012) Hereditary cerebellar degeneration disease (cerebellar cortical abiotrophy) in rabbits. *Veterinary Pathology*, **49**(4), 621–628.

Shientag, L.J., and Goad, M. (2011) Sudden hind limb injuries in two rabbits. *Laboratory Animals (NY)*, **40**(7), 212–216.

Hematopoietic and Lymphoid Neoplasia

Florizoone, K. (2005) Thymoma-associated exfoliative dermatitis in a rabbit. *Veterinary Dermatology*, **16**, 281–284.

Gomez, L., Gazquez, A., Roncero, V., Sanchez, C., and Duran, M.E. (2002) Lymphoma in a rabbit: Histopathological and immunohistochemical findings. *Journal of Small Animal Practice*, **43**, 224–226.

Heatley, J.J. and Smith, A.N. (2004) Spontaneous neoplasms of lagomorphs. *Veterinary Clinics of North America: Exotic Animal Practice*, **7**, 561–577.

Kostolich, M., and Panciera, R.J. (1992) Thymoma in a domestic rabbit. *Cornell Veterinarian*, **82**, 125–129.

Luna, L.G. (1968) *Histologic Staining Methods of the Armed Forces Institute of Pathology*. McGraw-Hill, New York.

Pignon, C. and Jardel, N. (2010) Bilateral exophthalmos in a rabbit. *Laboratory Animals (NY)*, **39**(9), 262–265.

Pilny, A.A., and Reaville, D. (2008) Chylothorax and thymic lymphoma in a pet rabbit (*Oryctolagus cuniculi*). *Journal of Exotic Pet Medicine*, **17**(4), 295–299.

Sanchez-Migallon, D.G., Mayer, J., Gould, J., and Azuma, C. (2006) Radiation therapy for the treatment of thymoma in rabbits (*Oryctolagus cuniculus*). *Journal of Exotic Pet Medicine*, **15**(2), 138–144.

Toth, L.A., Olson, G.A., Wilson, E., Rehg, J.E., and Classen, E. (1990) Lymphocytic leukemia and lymphosarcoma in a rabbit. *Journal of the American Veterinary Medical Association*, **197**(5), 627–629.

Vernau, K.M., Grahn, B.H., Clarke-Scott, H.A., and Sullivan, N. (1995) Thymoma in a geriatric rabbit with hypercalcemia and periodic exophthalmos. *Journal of the American Veterinary Medical Association*, **206**(6), 820–822.

Lead Toxicosis

Hood, S., Kelly, J., McBurney, S., and Burton, S. (1997) Lead toxicoses in two dwarf rabbits. *Canadian Veterinary Journal*, **38**, 721–722.

Johnston, M.S. (2008) Clinical toxicoses of domestic rabbits. *Veterinary Clinics of North America: Exotic Animal Practice*, **11**, 315–326.

Other Hematopoietic Conditions

Allison, S.O., Artwohl, J.E., Fortman, J.D., *et al.* (2007) Iatrogenic hemolytic anemia and endocarditis in New Zealand white rabbits secondary to *Achromobacter xylosoxidans* infection. *Journal of the American Association of Laboratory Animal Science*, **46**(6), 58–62.

Brewer, N.R. (2006) Biology of the rabbit. *Journal of the American Association of Laboratory Animal Science*, **45**(1), 8–24.

Graham, J.E., Garner, M.M., and Reavill, D.R. (2014) Benzimazole toxicosis in rabbits: 13 cases (2003 to 2011). *Journal of Exotic Pet Medicine*, **23**, 188–195.

Marshall, K.L. (2008) Rabbit hematology. *Veterinary Clinics of North America: Exotic Animal Practice*, **11**, 551–567.

Matsunaga, Y., Matsuno, S., and Mukoyama, J. (1977). Isolation and characterization of a parvovirus of rabbits. *Infection and Immunity*, **18**(2), 495–500.

Matsunaga, Y., and Chino, F. (2005) Experimental infection of young rabbits with rabbit parvovirus. *Archives of Virology*, **68**(3–4), 257–264.

Moore, D.M., Zimmerman, K., and Smith SA. (2015. Hematologic assessment in pet rabbits. *Veterinary Clinics of North America: Exotic Animal Practice*, **18**, 9–19.

Conditions of the Lacrimal Gland and Ducts

Florin, M., Rusanen, E., Haessig, M., Richter, M., and Spiess, B.M. (2009) Clinical presentation, treatment, and outcome of dacryocystitis in rabbits: A retrospective study of 28 cases (2003–2007). *Veterinary Ophthalmology*, **12**(6), 350–356.

Volopich, S., Gruber, A., Hassan, J., *et al.* (2005) Malignant B-cell lymphoma of the Harder's gland in a rabbit. *Veterinary Ophthalmology*, **8**(4), 259–263.

Conditions of the Eyelid and Conjunctiva

Allgoewer, I., Malho, P., Schulze, H., and Schaffer, E. (2008) Aberrant conjunctival stricture and overgrowth in the rabbit. *Veterinary Ophthalmology*, **11**(1), 18–22.

Munday JS, Aberdein D, Squires RA, Alfaras A, Wilson AM. (2007) Persistent conjunctival papilloma due to oral papillomavirus infection in a rabbit in New Zealand. *Journal of the American Association of Laboratory Animal Science*, **46**(5), 69–71.

Conditions of the Cornea and Anterior Chamber

Andrew, S.E. (2002) Corneal diseases of rabbits. (2002) *Veterinary Clinics of North America: Exotic Animal Practice*, **5**, 341–356.

Grinninger, P., Sanchez, R., Kraijer-Huver, I.M., *et al.* (2012) Eosinophilic keratoconjunctivitis in two rabbits. *Veterinary Ophthalmology*, **15**(1), 59–65.

Keller, R.L., Hendrix, D.V.H., and Greenacre, C. (2007) Shope fibroma virus keratitis and spontaneous cataracts in a domestic rabbit. *Veterinary Ophthalmology*, **10**(3), 190–195.

Knepper, P.A., McLone, D.G., Goossens, W., Vanden Hoek, T., and Higbee, R.G. (1991) Ultrastructural alterations in the aqueous outflow pathway of adult buphthalmic rabbits. *Experimental Eye Research*, **52**, 525–533.

Kouchi, M., Ueda, Y., Horie, H., and Tanaka, H. (2006) Ocular lesions in Watanabe heritable hyperlipidemic rabbits. *Veterinary Ophthalmology*, **9**(3), 145–148.

Styer, C.M., Ferrier, W.T., Labelle, P., Griffey, S.M., and Kendall, L.V. (2005) Limbic dermoid in a New Zealand white rabbit (*Oryctolagus cuniculus*). *Contemporary Topics in Laboratory Animal Science*, **44**(6), 44–48.

Watson, M.B. (2014) Vitamin D and ultraviolet B radiation considerations for exotic animal pets. *Journal of Exotic Pet Medicine*, **23**, 369–379.

Uveal and Lenticular Conditions

Ashton, N., Cook, C., and Clegg, F. (1976) Encephalitozoonosis (nosematosis) causing bilateral cataract in a rabbit. *British Journal of Ophthalmology*, **60**(9), 618–631.

Felchle, L..M, and Sigler, R,L. (2002) Phacoemulsification for the management of *Encephalitozoon cuniculi*-induced phacoclastic uveitis in a rabbit. *Veterinary Ophthalmology*, **5**(3), 211–215.

Giordano, C., Weigt, A., Vercelli, A., *et al.* (2005) Immunohistochemical identification of *Encephalitozoon cuniculi* in phacoclastic uveitis in four rabbits. *Veterinary Ophthalmology*, **8**(4), 271–275.

Keng, P.C., Lee, A,C., Cox, A.B., Bertgold, D.S., and Lett, J.T. (1982) Effects of heavy ions on rabbit tissues: cataractogenesis. *International Journal of Radiation Biology*, **41**(2), 127–137.

Munger, R.J., Langevin, N., and Podval, J. (2002) Spontaneous cataracts in laboratory rabbits. *Veterinary Ophthalmology*, **5**(3), 177–181.

Nastase, R. (1999) White Lesion in a dwarf rabbit's eye. *Laboratory Animals (NY)*, **28**(8), 21–23.

Ormerod, D., Koh, K., Juarez, R.S., *et al.* (1986) Anaerobic bacterial enophthalmitis in a rabbit. *Investigative Ophthalmology and Visual Science*, **27**, 115–118.

Exophthalmos

O'Reilly, A., McCowan, C., Hardman, C., and Stanley, R. (2002) *Taenia serialis* causing exopthalmos in a pet rabbit. *Veterinary Ophthalmology*, **5**(3), 227–230.

Pignon, C., and Jardel, N. (2010) Bilateral exophthalmos in a rabbit. *Laboratory Animals (NY)*, **39**(9), 262–265.

Vernau, K.M., Grahn, B.H., Clarke-Scott, H.A., and Sullivan, N. (1995) Thymoma in a geriatric rabbit with hypercalcemia and periodic exophthalmos. *Journal of the American Veterinary Medical Association*, **206**(6), 820–822.

Wagner, F., Beinecke, A., Fehr, M., *et al.* (2005) Recurrent bilateral exophthalmos associated with metastatic thymic carcinoma in a pet rabbit. *Journal of Small Animal Practice*, **46**, 393–397.

Ward, M.L. (2006) Diagnosis and management of a retrobulbar abscess of periapical origin in a domestic rabbit. *Veterinary Clinics of North America: Exotic Animal Practice*, **9**, 657–665.

General Ophthalmic Conditions

Donnelly, T.M. (2011) *Species differences in the anatomy of the eye. AEMV Proceedings*, Seattle, WA.

Kern, T.J. (1997) Rabbit and rodent ophthalmology. *Seminars in Avian and Exotic Pet Medicine*, **6**(3), 138–145.

Wagner, F. and Fehr, M. (2007) Common ophthalmic problems in pet rabbits. *Journal of Exotic Pet Medicine*, **16**(3), 158–167.

2

Ferrets

2.1 Introduction

The domestic ferret is descended from the European polecat, which is found in Europe and parts of Asia and Africa. Humans have used ferrets for hunting and as companion animals for over 2400 years and they are described in early Greek plays and writings in connection with rabbiting, because their long, tubular bodies and natural propensity for burrowing makes them well suited for flushing rabbits from their warrens. Ferrets were subsequently taken wherever rabbits were kept or released by various exploring nations, including to New Zealand in the mid-nineteenth century, where feral ferrets decimated terrestrial birds and other wildlife. Ferrets were initially promoted for pest control in North America in the early 1900s and subsequently became popular as pets. Ferrets are commonly used as an animal model for influenza virus research, as well as other disease conditions, such as *Helicobacter*-induced gastropathy.

Ferrets are crepuscular to nocturnal animals and belong to the Mustelidae, a family that includes weasels, badgers, mink, and otters. Most mustelids, including ferrets, are strict carnivores and have paired perianal scent glands that release strongly scented material for territorial marking. In North America, breeders extirpate these glands at 5–6 weeks of age. The word "ferret" means "thief," which aptly describes the behavior of many pet ferrets in stealing and hiding many small household items if they are left to roam unsupervised. Although solitary in the wild, domesticated ferrets are highly social, active, and curious animals.

Intact breeding ferrets display marked sexual dimorphism with male body weights being twice that of females, however, when neutered at an early age, this size difference is no longer apparent. Both sexes undergo marked seasonal variation in body weight of between 30–40% with deposition of body fat within the tail in the fall and loss of this body fat in the spring. The average lifespan in North America is approximately 6–7 years of age, but some animals can live to be 10 or more years old.

2.2 Integument Conditions

Ferrets have a dense hair coat composed of a soft, fine undercoat and long, coarse guard hairs. The guard hair color may become lighter as the animal ages. The coat is formed by compound hair follicles, which consist of one primary hair follicle surrounded by clusters of secondary follicles. The skin thickness varies depending upon the location in the body and may be very thick over the dorsum, with numerous sebaceous glands, occasional apocrine (sweat) glands, and accumulations of superficial yellow-red waxy secretions, particularly in intact males. The ferret pelage undergoes semi-annual hair growth cycles that are triggered by the external photoperiod, which induces neuroendocrine signaling largely via melatonin release. Skin, fiber density, and follicle number, are thickest and most abundant in winter and become thinner and sparser, respectively, in spring growth cycles, with a reduction in undercoat hairs. Ferrets have been bred to have a variety of coat colors, ranging from the natural sable color to albino.

Because of their highly territorial nature, ferrets use extensive environmental scent-marking, manifested by dragging or wiping their anal glands, body, and chin glands over various objects to release sulfur-containing secretions. These contribute to the general musky odor of ferrets, which is reduced in neutered and descented animals.

Ferrets require a diet that is high in animal protein and fat, and low in carbohydrates and fiber. Chronic feeding of an inappropriate diet may lead to a dry, dull hair coat. Tattoos (a single blue or green dot or a small numeral) may be present in the pinnae or on one or more footpads, depending upon the source of the animal. Breeders often use these to identify animals that have been descented and neutered. Areas of hair regrowth in dark-coated animals with previous alopecia or in ferrets that have been clipped for treatment or surgery may initially appear as bluish cutaneous discoloration until hair follicles erupt through the epidermis.

Pathology of Small Mammal Pets, First Edition. Patricia V. Turner, Marina L. Brash and Dale A. Smith.
© 2018 John Wiley & Sons, Inc. Published 2018 by John Wiley & Sons, Inc.

2.2.1 Alopecia

During the regular semi-annual molt, nonpruritic bilaterally symmetrical alopecia may be seen on the dorsal lumbosacral area of ferrets. This condition will resolve spontaneously if there is no other intercurrent disease. Pregnant jills will also lose hair around the teats and on their flanks and back up to two weeks prior to whelping.

The most common cause of pathologic alopecia in North American domestic ferrets results from adrenal gland-associated endocrinopathy (see Section 2.3.1). In this condition, hair loss may start at the tail and progress cranially with concurrent epidermal thinning, follicular atrophy such that only telogen hair follicles remain, mild orthokeratotic hyperkeratosis, and mild to moderate pruritus (Figure 2.1). Erythematous macules and linear bands of erythema and scaling (figurate erythema) associated with hyperplastic lymphohistiocytic perivascular dermatitis may be seen concurrently on the tail, inguinal, and lumbosacral areas.

Hyperestrogenism (estrogen toxicity) with associated alopecia is common in intact jills or in neutered jills with ovarian remnants. In both cases, elevated serum estrogen levels result in dermal follicular atrophy. This can be a life-threatening condition because of marked associated aplastic anemia or pancytopenia. The presence of an enlarged vulva and pale mucous membranes with petechiation or ecchymoses will also assist with the diagnosis of this condition.

2.2.1.1 Differential Diagnoses

Conditions to consider when presented with alopecia in ferrets include seasonal molt, adrenal gland disease (causing release of adrenal sex hormones), hyperestrogenism, ovarian remnants (incomplete spay), prostatic

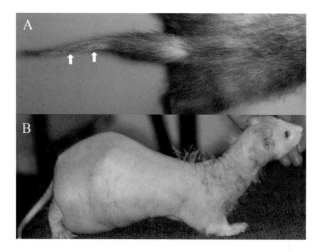

Figure 2.1 Alopecia in a ferret secondary to adrenal gland disease. A: Alopecia may start at the tail and progress cranially (arrows). B: Hair loss is almost complete in this animal. Bands of figurate erythema are seen on the side of the neck. *Source:* A and B: Courtesy of C. Wheler.

disease, hypothyroidism, iatrogenic Cushing's disease with corticosteroid use, flea or mite infestation (ear mites, demodicosis, sarcoptic mange), barbering or fur chewing, mechanical trauma from feeders or caging, and neoplasia. Investigations may include evaluation of crusts from lesions for parasites, skin scrapings, skin biopsy, clinical chemistry panels, and histopathology. Serum androgen hormone panels and abdominal ultrasound examination may be used to confirm ferret adrenal gland disease.

2.2.2 Bacterial Dermatitis and Abscesses

Bacterial skin diseases are uncommon in ferrets. Severe ulcerative dermatitis and superficial staphylococcal pyoderma were noted in the inguinal area of one ferret secondary to severe fire ant stings in the same area. Severe dermal necrosis in this case was attributed to a combination of staphylococcal exotoxins and alkaloids from the fire ant venom. There is a single historical report of dermatitis associated with *Actinomyces* sp. infection in a pet ferret. Abscesses may occur secondary to fighting, self-trauma, or playing and generally involve colonization by streptococcal or staphylococcal species. Perianal apocrine gland abscesses occur uncommonly in descented ferrets.

A definitive diagnosis may be made by culture of material aspirated from abscesses or of the lesion itself. In superficial infections, organisms are abundant and readily classified by Gram staining.

2.2.3 Dermatophytosis

Superficial cutaneous fungal infections are highly uncommon in ferrets and may be caused by either *Trichophyton mentagrophytes* or *Microsporum canis*. The clinical and microscopic appearances are similar to those seen in other small mammal species and most affected ferrets are not pruritic.

2.2.4 External Parasites

2.2.4.1 Ear Mites

Otodectes cynotis is a psoroptic mite that may superficially infest the ears of ferrets. These mites live on superficial secretions and sloughed cells within the ear canal and have a three-week life cycle. Many ferrets with otodectic mange are asymptomatic and mite infestation is more common in kits. In some animals, mild to moderate pruritus may be present with head shaking and scratching, and a dark brown, waxy aural exudate. Mites (0.3 x 0.5 mm) are readily visualized within the exudate and may be accompanied by hyperkeratosis, erosions, crusting, and secondary otitis externa (Figure 2.2). Mites may spread to other areas of the body. Otodectic mites

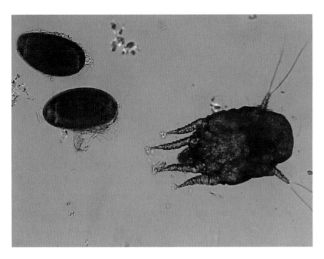

Figure 2.2 *Otodectes cynotis* ear mite and eggs in the aural exudate of a ferret. *Source:* Courtesy of K. Korber.

can transmit between ferrets and other companion animals, such as dogs and cats, by direct contact.

2.2.4.2 Other Mites

Sarcoptic mange, caused by *Sarcoptes scabiei*, occurs sporadically in ferrets as either a generalized or a local form of infestation. The localized form is limited to the feet (foot rot) and there is marked pruritus with swelling of the toes and feet, paronychia, and onychauxis. In the generalized form, there may be cutaneous thickening with crusting, erythema, and alopecia. Lesions can become secondarily infected with bacteria. Diagnosis of the burrowing mite occurs by deep skin scrapings or histopathology of affected skin. Acanthosis and orthokeratotic hyperkeratosis may be seen with erosions, crusting and ulceration of affected skin. Both mites (approximately 0.1–0.2 mm wide by 0.2–0.4 mm long) and eggs may be visible within tunnels within the stratum corneum. This condition is transmissible to other household pets and is zoonotic.

Low numbers of cigar-shaped *Demodex* spp. organisms, up to 200 μm in length, have been reported in the skin of normal, healthy ferrets of both sexes, without any associated clinical signs, and are seen in expanded hair follicles, and sebaceous and apocrine glands in the genital, perianal, and facial regions. Focal alopecia of the head and tail with erythema was described in a case of demodectic mange in a ferret with concurrent adrenal gland disease and lymphosarcoma. Demodectic mange was also reported in two ferrets with localized alopecia and pruritus being treated with a glucocorticoid-containing ointment for chronic ear mite infestations. In these animals, a mild, mixed superficial perivascular infiltrate was noted in the latter ferrets with mild, orthokeratotic hyperkeratosis was noted. Clinically apparent cases of demodectic mange in ferrets have also

been associated with conditions causing immunosuppression or following glucocorticoid therapy.

2.2.4.3 Fleas

There is no host-specific flea species of ferrets. Despite this, infestation with fleas is moderately common in ferret-exclusive households as well as in animals co-housed with infested cats or dogs (*Ctenocephalides felis* or *C. canis*, respectively). Very heavily infested animals may become anemic and may demonstrate intense pruritus with scratching and resultant alopecia around the head, neck, and thorax. Confirmation of infestation occurs by observation of fleas or flea dirt within the pelage. Differential diagnoses for flea infestations include sarcoptic or demodectic mange and dermatophytoses.

2.2.4.4 Lice

There are no louse species of domestic ferrets, although ferrets may become transiently infested with lice from other species, including humans.

2.2.4.5 Ticks

Ticks may be seen sporadically on ferrets used for hunting or with extensive exposure to the outdoors. They are unusual in pets.

2.2.4.6 Cutaneous Myiasis

Subcutaneous cysts containing *Cuterebra or Hypoderma* spp. larvae have rarely been reported in ferrets. Animals require access to the outdoors for transmission to occur. Cysts are composed of a thick fibrous capsule with a central pore and an encapsulated larva. A local granulomatous inflammatory reaction may be present.

Colony Management Because some ectoparasites may be transmitted to other companion animal pets or their human caregivers, it may be necessary to treat the environment extensively or determine whether other animals in the household require treatment when ectoparasites are identified.

2.2.5 Mastitis

Mastitis may occur in nursing jills and is characterized clinically by one or more erythematous, firm, swollen, and painful mammary glands on the ventrum. Microscopically, there may be marked neutrophilic infiltrates into the affected gland with local edema, hemorrhage, and necrosis of mammary gland alveoli and ducts. *E. coli* is the most common cause of mastitis in ferrets but the condition can also be caused by infection with *S. aureus*.

2.2.5.1 Differential Diagnoses

Mammary gland hyperplasia was reported in a 5-year-old castrated ferret with a concurrent adrenal gland carcinoma. In this case, two of six glands were enlarged and consisted of well-circumscribed, multilobular masses of proliferative ducts with scant stroma. Mammary gland tumors are very uncommon in ferrets, with a single report of a mammary papillary cystadenocarcinoma in a 12-year-old black-footed ferret (*Mustela nigripes*) being held at a wildlife center. The tumor had metastasized to iliac and mesenteric lymph nodes, as well as the liver and spleen.

2.2.6 Cutaneous Masses and Neoplasia

Cutaneous tumors or tumors with cutaneous manifestations are moderately common in ferrets of all ages, although most are benign or localized with low malignancy. The most common cutaneous masses reported in ferrets are basal cell tumors with sebaceous differentiation (sebaceous epithelioma or adenoma), mast cell tumors, and fibroma or fibrosarcoma (sometimes in association with vaccination) (Figure 2.3). Other neoplastic and nonneoplastic cutaneous masses that are seen occasionally include chordomas of the tail tip, lipomas and liposarcomas, piloleiomyomas and piloleiomyosarcomas, hemangiomas (Figure 2.10C), cutaneous lymphosarcomas, squamous cell carcinomas, papillomas, melanomas, and malignant histiocytic tumors.

Various cutaneous glandular hyperplastic and neoplastic are seen less commonly, including apocrine gland hyperplasia, adenoma, and adenocarcinoma of the head, neck, prepuce and vulva; mammary gland hyperplasia; perianal gland adenoma or adenocarcinoma; and aural ceruminous gland adenocarcinoma (Figures 2.4A and B). Some authors have reported rare cases of mesenchymal tumors with cutaneous manifestations, such as myxosarcoma, extraskeletal osteosarcoma, peripheral nerve sheath tumors, and hemangiosarcoma (Figures 2.4C and D).

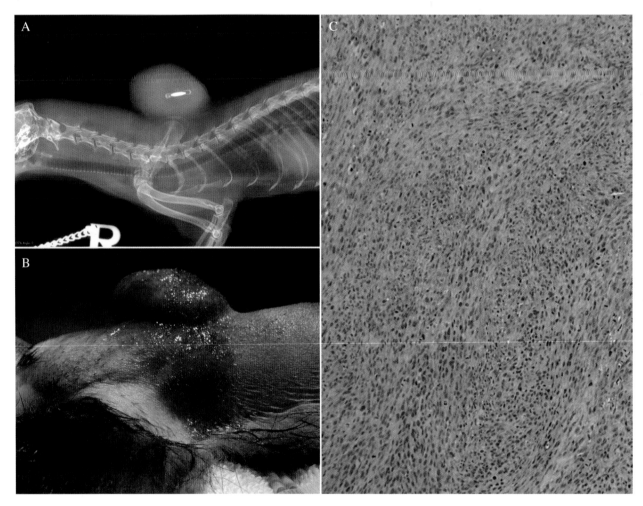

Figure 2.3 A: Radiograph of microchip-associated sarcoma in a ferret. B: Image of external mass prior to surgery. C: The mass is poorly circumscribed and composed of dense interlacing bands of spindle cells with a high mitotic rate. Vaccine-associated sarcomas are also seen sporadically in ferrets. *Source:* A and B: Courtesy of The Links Road Animal and Bird Clinic.

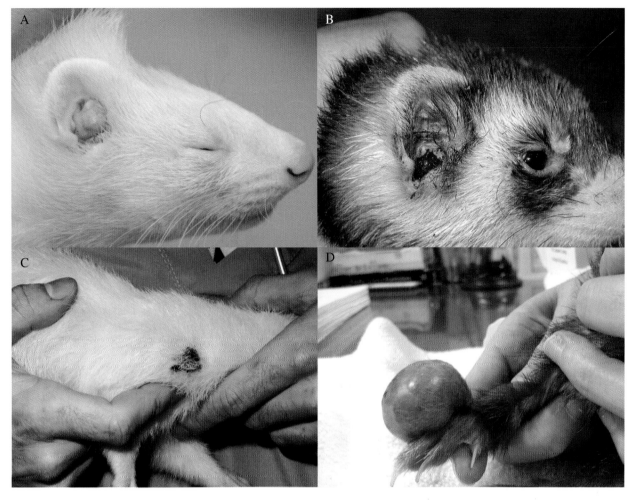

Figure 2.4 A: Aural ceruminous gland adenocarcinoma in a ferret. B: These tumors will ulcerate as a result of scratching and their presence may result in agitated behavior. C: Cutaneous hemangioma on the shoulder of a ferret. D: A slow-growing hemangiosarcoma on the forefoot of a ferret. Microscopically, within the dermis and invading the subcutis, the mass was comprised of a variably dense population of round to spindle-shaped cells arranged in short streams with dense hyaline collagen trabeculae and many irregularly-anastomosing blood-filled channels. Source: A and B: Courtesy of The Links Road Animal and Bird Clinic.

All tumor types have similar characteristics to those seen in other companion animal species and have similar prognoses, based on adequacy of resection of tumor margins, cellular atypia, necrosis, pleiomorphism, mitoses, and metastases. Masses that are more common or that are specific to ferrets are discussed in greater detail below.

2.2.6.1 Sebaceous Epithelioma
Basal cell tumors with sebaceous differentiation (sebaceous epithelioma) are the most common cutaneous tumors of ferrets and they are invariably benign. Masses may be found anywhere on the body, although they are more commonly found on the head and cervical areas, and are usually localized, nonencapsulated, solid or cystic, and plaque-like or exophytic. There may be hyperpigmentation of the mass and the surface may be ulcerated. On cut section, the masses are pale yellow to white and composed of irregular lobules. Microscopically,

the masses are composed of aggregates of basal cells arranged in nests surrounded by a fine fibrovascular stroma and forming a solid mass or fronds and papillary projections around narrow central stalks of mature connective tissue (Figure 2.5). Basal cells are commonly observed undergoing sebaceous and squamous differentiation, some with mild atypia. The mitotic rate is usually low and there may be mild, mixed leukocytic infiltrates within and around the tumor mass. The overlying epithelium may be variably hyperplastic and hyperkeratotic. Excisional biopsy is curative and the primary differential diagnosis is a mast cell tumor.

2.2.6.2 Mast Cell Tumors
Mast cell tumors are also very common in ferrets and may occur in animals as young as three years of age, with an average age of occurrence of 4.5 years. They appear as small, pigmented, flat plaque-like or nodular masses that

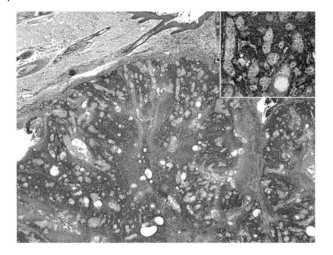

Figure 2.5 Sebaceous epitheliomas are common skin tumors in ferrets and are benign. They consist of nests of basal cells undergoing sebaceous differentiation (inset).

may be pruritic and erythematous (Figure 2.6). Masses are microscopically similar to those of domestic cats, and are composed of a nonencapsulated, densely packed, monomorphic, dermal population of round cells with fine, pale, metachromatic cytoplasmic granules, which are better visualized with toluidine blue staining. Anisocytosis and mitotic rates are usually low and there may be scattered eosinophils throughout the mass. Ulceration and crusting may occur if they are excoriated. Mast cell tumors are benign in ferrets and excision is curative.

2.2.6.3 Lymphosarcoma

As for other species, both epitheliotropic lymphosarcoma and multicentric lymphosarcoma with cutaneous manifestations occur in the ferret. In both cases, the overlying epithelium may be ulcerated, but the main microscopic distinction is whether neoplastic lymphocytes remain in the dermis or invade the epithelium (epitheliotropic

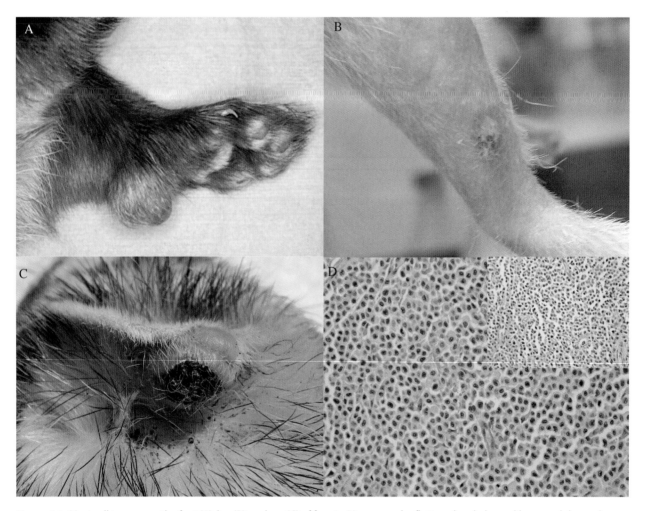

Figure 2.6 Mast cell tumors on the foot (A), leg (B), and ear (C) of ferrets. Masses can be flattened and plaque-like or nodular, and may be ulcerated. D: Mast cell tumors are generally benign and consist of well differentiated round cells with pale eosinophilic, granular cytoplasm. Cytoplasmic granules may or not be readily visualized with a toluidine blue stain (inset). *Source:* A, B, and C: Courtesy of The Links Road Animal and Bird Clinic.

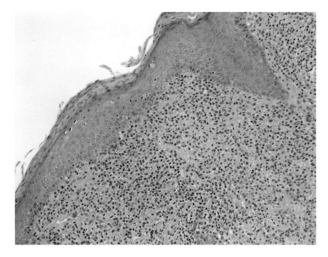

Figure 2.7 Cutaneous lymphosarcoma in a ferret. Neoplastic lymphocytes have not infiltrated the epithelium.

lymphoma) (Figure 2.7). Lymphosarcomas in ferrets may be initiated by retrovirus infection (see Section 2.10.4). Immunohistochemistry may be used to confirm the diagnosis.

2.2.6.4 Squamous Cell Carcinoma

Squamous cell carcinomas may appear as focal to multifocal cutaneous plaques with or without ulceration anywhere on the body, or as subcutaneous masses, particularly on the head and face, often extending to involve the oral cavity. Microscopically, the diagnosis of squamous cell carcinoma of the ferret is the same as for dogs and cats. Multicentric squamous cell carcinoma has been reported recently in a ferret associated with an uncharacterized papillomavirus, similar to squamous cell carcinoma *in situ* in cats. The prognosis depends on the site and completeness of excision. Tumors involving the face have a poor prognosis since they may be locally aggressive, invading the subtending bone of the face, mouth, and nasal cavity, as well as other soft tissue structures.

2.2.6.5 Chordoma

Chordomas are mesenchymal tumors that arise from embryonic notochord remnants and are most commonly found in association with the axial skeleton. They are unusual tumors in most mammals, but are moderately common in ferrets, typically occurring in animals 2 years of age or older. Clinically, they are often seen on the tail tip and present as a smooth, firm, poorly haired, and slow-growing mass (Figure 2.8). Focal and superficial ulceration of the mass with crusting may occur. On cut section, the mass is not associated with the terminal coccygeal vertebrae, although locally invasive chordomas may distort and compress subjacent vertebrae.

Chordomas have also been noted in association with cervical and thoracic vertebral bodies, with invasion of the spinal canal and impingement on the spinal cord. Tumors in these locations usually result in clinical presentations of ataxia, paresis, or ventral tracheal deviation, depending on the specific location and size of the mass. Diagnosis may be made by fine-needle aspiration or excisional biopsy and histopathology. Distinctive cytologic characteristics include scant clusters of large ovoid cells with multiple pale staining, granular, PAS-positive cytoplasmic vacuoles (physaliferous cells) and chondrocytes within a dense fibrillar metachromatic matrix. On histologic section, chordomas consist of clusters of large vacuolated cells (physaliferous cells) within a myxoid matrix, surrounding islands of cartilage and bone, with a variably lobulated pattern conferred by fine fibrovascular stroma. Chordomas are locally invasive and have a high rate of recurrence following surgical resection.

2.2.6.6 Piloleiomyoma

Piloleiomyomas (leiomyosarcomas) are rare tumors of the piloerector muscles in the skin. Masses are often found on the legs, tail, and trunk, and may be painful to the touch, although nonpruritic. There may be alopecia of the overlying skin. The tumors consist of an expansile, well demarcated but unencapsulated and not deeply invasive focal dermal masses of fusiform smooth muscle cells with closely packed vesicular nuclei, and that are oriented in whorls and bands, sometimes in parallel to the hair follicle (Figure 2.9). Strong immunopositive cytoplasmic labeling may be seen with smooth muscle actin, desmin, and vimentin. Depending on the site, these masses may be difficult to fully excise. Differential diagnoses for less well differentiated piloleiomyosarcomas include fibrosarcoma and malignant peripheral nerve sheath tumor.

2.2.6.7 Apocrine Gland Masses

Apocrine glands are found in highest concentrations on the head, neck, vulva, prepuce, and perineal areas, and cystic dilatations of the glands are common in ferrets. Cysts contain eosinophilic nonfibrillar proteinaceous material with variable numbers of mature and degenerate neutrophils, and the contents may be extruded with mild pressure. Excision of glands is curative (Figure 2.10). Glands may also become hyperplastic and less commonly, dysplastic, with development of an adenocarcinoma. Both intravascular metastases and local invasion of surrounding tissues may be seen in rare cases.

2.2.7 Other Skin Conditions

Pododermatitis (sore feet) occurs in ferrets kept in wet unsanitary conditions. One or more feet may be

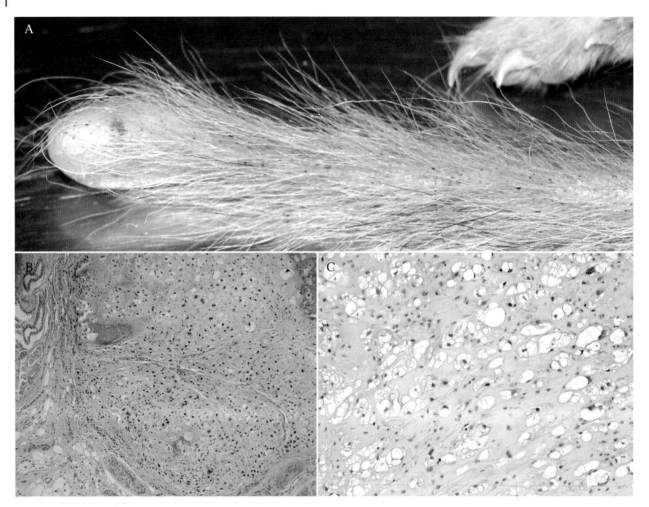

Figure 2.8 A: Tail chordoma in a ferret. B: The mass is composed of multiple expansile lobules in which bony spicules are interspersed. C: Vacuolated polygonal cells of varying size, so-called physaliferous cells, are a characteristic feature of chordomas. *Source:* A: Courtesy of J. Brandao.

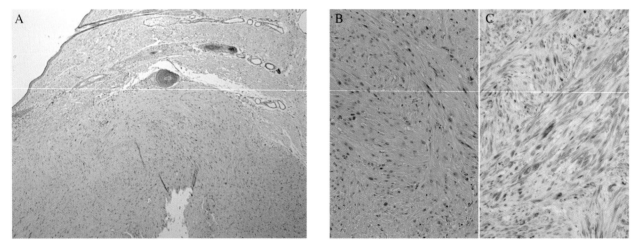

Figure 2.9 A: Piloleiomyosarcoma from a 2-year-old female ferret. B: The mass consists of interlacing spindle to strap-like cells with few mitotic figures, although spindle cells were infiltrating the dermis at the lateral margins of the mass. C: Strong positive cytoplasmic labeling is present for vimentin throughout the mass.

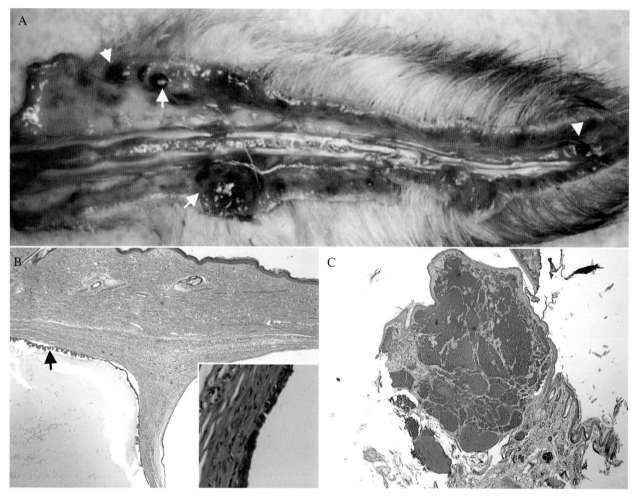

Figure 2.10 A: Apocrine gland carcinoma in the tail of a ferret. Multifocal pigmented masses are seen along the length of the tail (arrows). B: Cystic dilatation of a rapidly growing apocrine gland on the neck of a ferret. The cyst lining is occasionally thrown into papillary projections (arrow). Inset: The apical cytoplasm of the cyst contains golden-brown pigment with sporadic apical blebbing. C: Cutaneous hemangioma from a young ferret.

swollen, erythematous, crusted, and painful to touch. The tail tip may also be affected. *Staphylococcus aureus* is the most common infectious agent isolated.

An important differential diagnosis for cutaneous foot lesions in ferrets is canine distemper. Hyperkeratosis and erythema of the footpad ("hardpad disease") is a common finding in ferrets infected with canine distemper virus (see Section 2.9.3). The skin of the chin, lips, and face may also become quite thickened and erythematous in the early course of the disease. Atypical cutaneous lesions consisting of severe pruritus with generalized erythema and scaling of the feet have been reported in a vaccinated ferret that subsequently contracted canine distemper virus. In all cases of distemper, eosinophilic intranuclear and intracytoplasmic viral inclusion bodies are seen microscopically in affected skin sections. Immunohistochemistry may be used to confirm the presence of viral antigen.

Contact dermatitis and other forms of immune-mediated dermatitis have been reported anecdotally in ferrets, for example, after application of self-adhesive surgical drapes or certain types of bandaging. Clinical signs reported include moderate pruritus, erythema, and alopecia.

Erythema multiforme is an immune-mediated skin condition, in which keratinocytes are targeted for destruction by the host's immune system. The condition occurs acutely and affected animals present with erythematous macules and papules. Microscopically, there is patchy necrosis of keratinocytes, a marked interface dermatitis, and moderate hyperkeratosis and parakeratosis. A single case has been reported in a 5-year-old neutered male ferret. The inciting antigen was not determined and the animal was being treated concurrently for adrenal gland disease.

Preputial gland enlargement can occur in male ferrets, due to apocrine gland cyst formation, adenoma or adenocarcinoma (Figure 2.11).

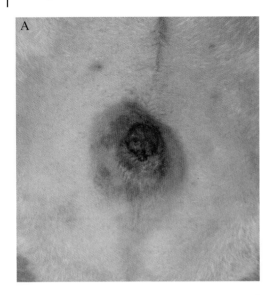
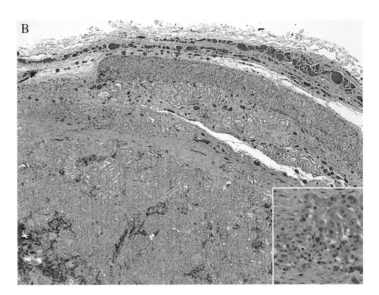

Figure 2.11 A: Preputial gland adenocarcinoma in a ferret. B: Microscopically, the mass is poorly circumscribed and consists of dermal nodules of glandular epithelium, arranged in tubules and acini, growing by expansion and compressing the adjacent hair follicles, sebaceous glands and aprocrine glands. Clusters of neoplastic cells are present multifocally outside the capsule at the base of the mass (inset), some invading blood vessels.

2.3 Endocrine Conditions

Endocrine diseases are very common in ferrets in both North America and Europe, and may affect both sexes and animals less than 3 years of age, although typically affected animals are older. Because of the pansystemic effects of hormonal signaling, it is not uncommon to find more than one endocrine condition in the same animal. The two primary conditions seen with almost equally high prevalence are adrenal gland disease and pancreatic islet cell tumor (insulinoma). Other endocrine disorders, such as pituitary tumors, Cushing's disease, and hypothyroidism are much less common in the ferret.

2.3.1 Adrenal Gland Disease

The structure of the adrenal gland is similar in ferrets to that of other companion animals. The right adrenal gland is more cranial and larger than the left gland, and is closely apposed to the vena cava. While the ferret adrenal gland synthesizes and secretes the same hormones as in other mammals, in animals with hyperadrenocorticism, sex steroidogenic cells resembling those found in the zona reticularis predominate. Thus, plasma levels of 17-hydroxyprogesterone, estradiol, dehydroepiandrosterone (DHEA, a sex steroid precursor), androstenedione may be elevated in ferrets with adrenal gland disease, rather than cortisol, as in dogs and humans with Cushing's disease. Both cortisol and DHEA are formed from cleavage of cholesterol via the activity of cytochrome P450 17a-hydroxylase/C17-C20 lyase. Cleavage activi-

ties of this enzyme and end product formation are differentially regulated, for example, increased expression of cytochrome b5 has been found to upregulate cleavage leading to DHEA formation. Cytochrome b5 is minimally expressed in normal ferret adrenocortical tissue (resulting in minimal sex steroid production by the adrenal glands), but expression is upregulated in ferrets with adrenocortical disease.

Despite being a commonly described condition for over 25 years, the etiopathogenesis of adrenal gland disease in ferrets is still elusive and is likely multifactorial. Age at neutering, diet, genetics, and indoor housing are all thought to play a role in disease susceptibility and onset. Some have postulated that early neutering alone may be responsible for initiating the condition, since North American pet ferrets are typically neutered at 6 weeks of age and have a high prevalence of adrenal gland disease. However, the condition is also seen with high prevalence in ferrets from the Netherlands, which are typically neutered later in life at the onset of sexual maturity. Ferrets are seasonal breeders and increasing day length triggers the release of gonadotropin-releasing hormone (GnRH) from the hypothalamus, which induces release of luteinizing hormone (LH) and follicle-stimulating hormone (FSH) from the pars distalis of the anterior pituitary gland. These hormones, in turn, induce the release of androgens, either estradiol from the ovaries or testosterone from the testes, both of which exert negative feedback on the hypothalamus and anterior pituitary gland, suppressing further secretion of GnRH, LH, and FSH. It is thought that in neutered ferrets, there is a loss of negative feedback inhibition resulting in continued secretion of GnRH, as well as LH and FSH, leading to continued stimulation of the adrenal cortex. This continuous hormonal stimulation may lead to the proliferation of and eventually transformation of sex steroidogenic cells within the adrenal cortex, leading to upregulation of cytochrome b5 expression and preferentially increased sex steroid synthesis. Other transcription factors, regulatory proteins, and hormones are likely to be involved in this condition.

2.3.1.1 Presenting Clinical Signs

Presenting signs include bilaterally symmetrical alopecia that initiates over the tail, head and flanks, a pot-bellied appearance, swollen vulva, petechiation, thinning of the skin, and dysuria in hobs from hypertrophy of prostatic ductular epithelium. Pruritus and increased aggression may also be noted.

2.3.1.2 Pathology

In the majority of cases, only the left adrenal gland is affected, but lesions may also be bilateral, and microscopic changes consistent with nodular hyperplasia, adenoma, or carcinoma may be seen. It is common to see the proliferation of the remaining adrenal gland following surgical removal of one adrenal gland and removal of both glands is incompatible with life (Figure 2.12). Adenomas are well demarcated and consist of well-differentiated cuboidal to polygonal cells with granular cytoplasm. In malignant tumors, cells may be less well differentiated with mildly increased mitotic rates, and the mass may demonstrate capsular invasion with areas of hemorrhage and necrosis. Production of myxoid material by neoplastic cells is associated with increased malignancy. Spindle cell proliferation may be present in some carcinomas, and may or not have prognostic significance. Caval invasion is common when the right adrenal gland is

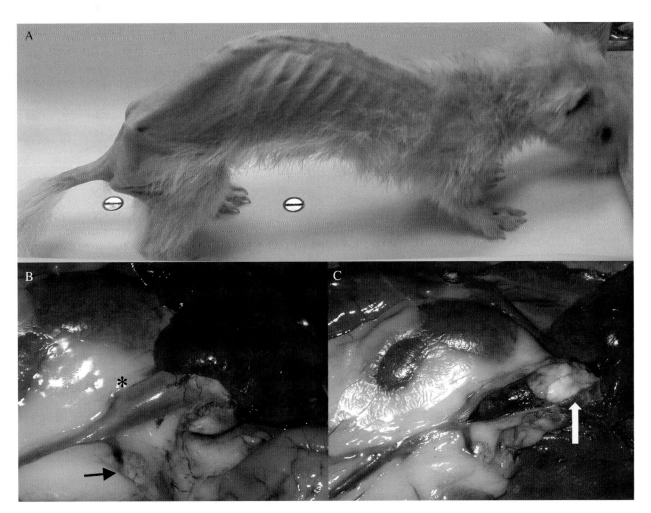

Figure 2.12 A: Severe muscle wasting in a ferret with chronic adrenal gland disease. B: Caval invasion can occur with malignant tumors of the right adrenal gland (*). The left adrenal gland (arrow) appears grossly normal. C: Vena cava opened to demonstrate invading adrenal gland adenocarcinoma (arrow). *Source:* A: Courtesy of The Links Road Animal and Bird Clinic.

affected. Metastases to the liver and lungs are uncommon. Carcinomas often demonstrate positive immunolabeling for inhibin and LH.

2.3.1.3 Laboratory Diagnostics

Increased serum levels of one or more sex hormones (17-hydroxyprogesterone, estradiol, dehydroepiandrosterone or androstenedione) are used to confirm a diagnosis of adrenal gland disease in ferrets, although these cannot be used to distinguish between benign or malignant conditions or an ovarian remnant (estradiol). Urinary corticoid: creatinine ratios are also commonly elevated in ferrets with adrenal gland disease. Traditional assays for detection and confirmation of Cushing's disease in dogs (e.g., ACTH plasma levels and dexamethasone suppression assays) are not appropriate for diagnosis of reproductive steroid-related endocrine disease in ferrets.

2.3.1.4 Differential Diagnoses

Adrenal gland disease is very common in ferrets and should be considered the primary differential diagnosis for enlarged adrenal glands, until proven otherwise. Primary hyperaldosteronism has been described in one ferret with an adrenal gland adenoma. Cushing's disease has also been reported in one ferret. In addition to having elevations in circulating levels of plasma estradiol, 17-hydroxyprogesterone, and androstenedione, this animal had significantly elevated levels of plasma aldosterone and glucocorticoids, which coincided with hypokalemia and persistent hypertension.

Pancreatic islet cell tumors are often present with adrenal gland tumors, although the etiopathogeneses for the two conditions has not been linked. Other occasional causes of adrenal gland enlargements include cysts, teratomas, and pheochromocytomas.

2.3.2 Pancreatic Islet Cell Tumors

The ferret pancreas is a pale pink, bilobed structure and has both exocrine and endocrine functions, as in other mammalian species. There are four primary cell types under neuroendocrine control within the islets of Langerhans: β cells, which form the bulk of the central portion of the islets and secrete insulin; α cells, which are located around the islet periphery and secrete glucagon; δ cells secrete somatostatin; and γ cells, which secrete pancreatic polypeptide.

Insulinomas or β cell proliferative lesions are very common in North American ferrets and are uncommon in the United Kingdom and Europe. This may be related to relatively limited genetic diversity within the North American population, as well as the frequent use of extruded diets, which are high in carbohydrates, compared with whole prey diets. Affected ferrets are usually at least three to five years of age, although the disease may occur rarely in younger animals. In humans and other animals, pancreatic islets cell tumors commonly occur in a subset of individuals with mutations in the MEN-1 gene, leading to a syndrome of multiple endocrine neoplasias. It is unknown whether this gene is mutated in ferrets with insulinomas.

2.3.2.1 Presenting Clinical Signs

The clinical signs in cases of insulinoma are related to the inappropriate and episodic secretion of insulin. This eventually results in hypoglycemia, with related adrenergic and neurologic symptoms of ptyalism, paresis, ataxia, seizures, and collapse. Severe untreated cases may progress to coma and death. The onset of clinical signs may be slow and insidious. Most nodules are too small to be detected with current imaging techniques although they may be readily palpated at laparotomy. Both nodulectomy and partial pancreatectomy may eliminate clinical signs and extend the lifespan of animals with pancreatic islet cell tumors.

2.3.2.2 Pathology

Pancreatic islet cell tumors appear as raised red discrete nodules grossly and may vary from a few mm to over one cm in diameter (Figure 2.13). Multiple nodules are common and masses appear as expansile well circumscribed islet cell hyperplasias or adenomas, microscopically. Carcinomas occur much less commonly and local seeding of tumor or metastasis to regional lymph nodes and the liver are unusual. The typical histologic appearance

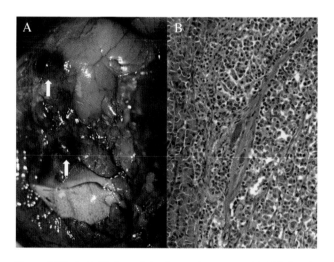

Figure 2.13 A: Multiple nodules (arrows) are present in this ferret and diagnosed as pancreatic islet cell tumors. B: Microscopically, the nodules of neoplastic islet cells grow by expansion compressing the adjacent exocrine pancreas (left side of image). The neoplastic cells are arranged in packets enclosed in a fine fibrovascular stroma and have up to two-fold anisokaryosis with infrequent mitotic figures.

of a mass is that of a homogeneous population of round to polygonal cells packeted into ribbons and nests by a delicate fibrovascular stroma. Cells have indistinct cell borders, abundant pale eosinophilic, finely granular cytoplasm, a central round nucleus with finely stippled chromatin, and often a prominent nucleolus. Anisokaryosis and anisocytosis may be up to three-fold with occasional binucleate cells. Mitoses range from 0–5 per high power field. An encircling fibrous capsule may be present. Immunohistochemistry for insulin demonstrates strong positive cytoplasmic labeling within a suspect populations of cells.

2.3.2.3 Laboratory Diagnostics

Both insulin and glucose blood levels may be measured in suspected cases, although insulin levels may be within normal reference intervals because of the episodic nature of the secretion. Fasting blood glucose levels less than 3.3 mmol/L are consistent with a diagnosis of insulinoma.

2.3.2.4 Differential Diagnoses

Neoplasms of other islet cell types are very rare in the ferret. Hyperplasia of exocrine pancreatic acinar cells may produce a nodular appearance. Adrenal gland disease is often present in ferrets with pancreatic islet cell tumors.

2.3.3 Diabetes Mellitus

Diabetes mellitus is seen sporadically in ferrets and may occur alone or in combination with other endocrine disorders. Animals with this disease may present with alopecia, muscle wasting, polyuria and polydipsia, and poor body condition. Vacuolar degeneration of pancreatic islet cells is reported in uncomplicated cases. Secondary diabetes mellitus with severe ketoacidosis has been described in a ferret with hyperadrenocorticism, pancreatitis, and corticosteroid administration.

2.3.4 Thyroid Gland Carcinomas

Thyroid gland tumors are very uncommon in ferrets. A C-cell thyroid carcinoma has been reported in a 4-year-old castrated male ferret with concurrent adrenocortical adenoma, pheochromocytoma, and insulinoma. In this animal, the thyroid tumor consisted of lobules and cords of neoplastic neuroendocrine cells separated by thin branching fibrovascular stroma. Stroma was positive for amyloid, which is also deposited in human and canine C-cell carcinomas.

A thyroid follicular carcinoma was diagnosed in a 5-year-old neutered male pet ferret presenting with dyspnea, alopecia, poor body condition, and a rapidly growing ventral cervical mass. The mass consisted of large cuboidal neoplastic cells arranged in cords around lakes of colloid, and neoplastic cells were strongly positive for thyroglobulin immunostaining.

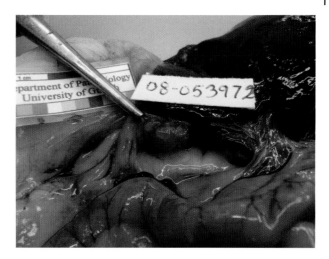

Figure 2.14 Adrenal gland cysts in a ferret. In this animal 50% of the adrenal cortex was replaced by cysts up to 3 mm in diameter, which were filled with eosinophilic amorphous material.

2.3.5 Other Endocrine Conditions

Adrenal gland cysts (Figure 2.14) and **pheochromocytomas** are occasionally seen in ferrets.

Adrenal-hepatic fusion without intervening capsule is seen commonly in ferrets, often in association with adrenal gland cysts at the tissue junction. The right adrenal gland is generally involved and this is interpreted as an incidental finding.

Hypothyroidism has been reported anecdotally in pet ferrets. Affected animals present with vague signs of lethargy, obesity, hind end weakness, and increased sleeping activity and may have concurrent pancreatic islet cell tumors and/or adrenal gland disease. Suspect cases should be evaluated for serum T3/T4 levels. In general, the etiopathogenesis of hypothyroidism in ferrets is unknown; No further pathology information is available, but hypothyroidism may represent an emerging potential differential diagnosis for both insulinoma and adrenal gland disease in older ferrets.

Mineralized debris can be seen occasionally in thyroid follicles of aging animals.

Extramedullary hematopoiesis can be seen at times within and surrounding the pancreas, and thyroid and adrenal glands.

2.4 Respiratory Conditions

Ferrets have a large cone-shaped thorax with a more caudally located heart than is seen in other companion animal species. They have a large pulmonary capacity for their size and can breathe through both their nose and mouth, similar to other carnivores. The left lung is divided into cranial and caudal lobes, while the right lung has four

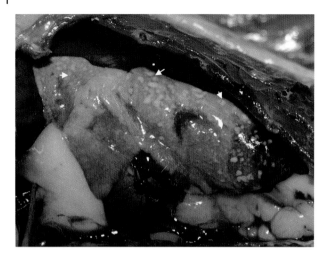

Figure 2.15 Alveolar histiocytosis in a ferret, characterized by multifocal, raised, white subpleural plaques (arrows). Microscopically, areas are filled with macrophages containing foamy cytoplasm. These are considered a common incidental finding in aging ferrets.

lobes: cranial, middle, caudal, and accessory. Alveolar histiocytosis can be seen as an incidental lesion in aging animals (Figure 2.15). While pneumonia is generally uncommonly seen in ferrets, there are several respiratory conditions that are important in this species.

2.4.1 Influenza

Influenza infections are caused by negative sense, single-stranded RNA viruses in the Orthomyxoviridae family. Ferrets are very susceptible to human influenza viruses (both type A, which is more common, and type B) and this represents an important anthropozoonosis with similar upper respiratory clinical signs evinced by both species. Avian, swine, and equine influenza viruses are also known to infect ferrets. Influenza virus subtypes are further classified based on surface antigens for hemagglutinin (H) and neuraminidase (N), e.g., H5N1. While infection with most subtypes results in rapid replication of the virus within the upper respiratory, more virulent subtypes may induce viral replication in both the upper and lower respiratory system, with more significant clinical signs and related pathology. Antigenic drift and antigenic shift account for the highly mutable nature of the influenza virus, such that antibodies produced from prior infection with one virus strain are rarely cross-protective against others.

2.4.1.1 Presenting Clinical Signs

In ferrets that are otherwise healthy, viral infection usually results in transient pyrexia with catarrhal nasal discharge and perinasal crusting, sneezing, exaggerated swallowing attempts, coughing, anorexia, and lethargy. Exudative conjunctivitis with periocular crusting and photophobia may also be seen. Persistent severe dyspnea and death may occur, especially in neonatal or juvenile animals or in ferrets that are already debilitated from intercurrent disease.

2.4.1.2 Pathology

In uncomplicated disease, gross lesions are limited to nasal mucosal and tracheal congestion, and periocular and perinasal serous crusting, sometimes with conjunctivitis. With infection by more virulent strains, a severe acute bronchopneumonia may be present. Secondary bacterial infections may result in more complicated pneumonias. In experimental infections, intestinal infection has been reported with mild resultant enteritis.

Microscopically, in mild cases, nasal changes consist of generalized mucosal congestion with mixed, predominantly lymphocytic infiltrates and mild, focal ulceration. Ulceration and hemorrhage with loss of cilia may be more severe in some cases, with cell debris admixed with serosanguinous exudate within the sinus. Bronchointerstitial pneumonia with alveolar septal thickening by mixed leukocytic infiltrates, marked alveolar edema, and patchy necrosis has been reported in young ferrets during a colony-wide outbreak of H1N1 influenza virus.

2.4.1.3 Laboratory Diagnostics

Transient lymphopenia and increased circulating neutrophils may be seen in the early course of an infection. There are no consistent changes in serum biochemistry parameters. Human ELISA assays for type A influenza viruses have been used to verify suspected viral infections in ferrets. PCR assays, virus isolation, and immunohistochemistry may be used when confirmation of virus is critical.

2.4.1.4 Differential Diagnoses

The most important differential diagnosis in the early course of influenza infection is canine distemper virus infection, as both viruses may initially cause pyrexia and oculonasal discharge. Influenza infection is much more common and self-limiting, whereas infection with canine distemper virus has a rapid disease course, frequently results in clinical signs not seen with influenza virus infection, such as facial dermatitis and footpad hyperkeratosis, and is invariably fatal in affected ferrets. Influenza infection may predispose ferrets to secondary bacterial invaders, such as *Streptococcus pneumoniae* infection. Other causes of nasal discharge and sneezing in ferrets include intranasal foreign bodies, less common mycotic nasal infections, seasonal or environmental hypersensitivities, and tooth root abscessation. Heartworm infections in ferrets may induce coughing and dyspnea. Pneumonia, otherwise uncommon in ferrets, can also be caused by systemic coronavirus infection, bacterial and mycotic infections and aspiration. Endogenous lipid pneumonia has also been described.

2.4.1.5 Colony Management

Influenza viruses are readily transmitted by aerosol or from oculonasal secretions from humans or other species to ferrets. Signs of infection generally occur within 1–2 days following exposure, with clinical signs resolving 7–10 days after onset in uncomplicated cases. Human caregivers with viral respiratory disease should avoid handling ferrets and minimize any contact with jills and kits until their clinical signs resolve. If caregiver tasks cannot be delegated, owners should wash their hands carefully before feeding, watering, or performing other routine husbandry duties. Similarly, ferrets with clinical signs of influenza disease should be isolated from other ferrets, and handling should be minimized. Vaccination of ferrets against influenza virus is generally not recommended, because disease is generally mild and self-limiting in ferrets, and because virus mutations quickly render vaccines ineffective.

2.4.2 Canine Distemper

Canine distemper virus (CDV) is caused by a single stranded, negative sense RNA virus of the genus Morbillivirus, which belongs to the Paramyxoviridae family. It is a highly contagious pathogen that is transmitted by aerosol, fomites or direct contact. There is no treatment for this disease in ferrets and unvaccinated animals are highly susceptible to infection and subsequent death. The virus typically enters the host through the upper respiratory tract, replicating locally, as well as in oropharyngeal lymphoid tissues, with a secondary viremia after 4–5 days, resulting in pansystemic infection and disease. CDV is shed by infected ferrets in all body secretions and excreta as early as 2 days post-infection.

2.4.2.1 Presenting Clinical Signs

The initial presenting signs in the ferret occur approximately 1 week after infection and include pyrexia, anorexia, and mucopurulent oculonasal discharge with periocular swelling and crusting. Conjunctivitis, corneal ulceration and photophobia, cheilitis, and a pruritic, papular dermatitis of the chin are common sequelae (Figure 2.16). Later, more variable clinical signs include hyperkeratosis of the footpads, which gives rise to the common term, hardpad disease, and nasal planum, melena, and bronchopneumonia. Neurologic signs may also be present, including severe depression, convulsions, blindness, and coma. Viral infection induces profound immunosuppression and secondary bacterial infections are common.

2.4.2.2 Pathology

Gross pathology lesions in ferrets infected with CDV correlate with the clinical signs. Microscopically, there is

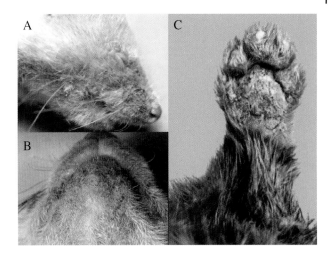

Figure 2.16 Variable skin changes are seen in ferrets presenting with canine distemper virus infections, including hyperkeratosis of the nasal planum, ear tips (A), and feet (C), as well as papular dermatitis of the chin (B).

a suppurative rhinitis and tracheitis, in addition to a necrosuppurative bronchopneumonia in animals with more severe respiratory signs (Figure 2.17). Dermal lesions consist of regional parakeratotic hyperkeratosis and acanthosis with occasional loss of keratinocytes. Nonsuppurative encephalitis, erythroid depletion of the bone marrow, and multifocal lymphoid necrosis may also be apparent. Eosinophilic intracytoplasmic and intranuclear viral inclusion bodies may be found in epithelial and other cells, in addition to virus-induced multinucleate syncytia; these are useful features for confirming the diagnosis. Secondary bacterial, parasitic, and mycotic infections are common in animals surviving the initial viral infection, leading to further debilitation and death. Potential underlying viral disease, such as that caused by canine distemper virus, should be investigated in ferrets dying of opportunistic infections.

2.4.2.3 Laboratory Diagnostics

CDV infection induces a profound leukopenia in infected animals. A mild, nonregenerative anemia may also be present in the early course of infection. Serum chemistry parameters are often within reference ranges. In live animals, direct immunofluorescence assay of the buffy coat may be used to confirm infection. Immunohistochemistry and PCR assays may be useful for biopsy or post mortem specimens.

2.4.2.4 Differential Diagnoses

Rare cases of CDV infection lacking the typical ocular and respiratory signs have been reported in ferrets. In these cases, dermal lesions have been misinterpreted as arising from environmental allergies. While initial pyrexia and respiratory signs may be suggestive of influenza, distemper

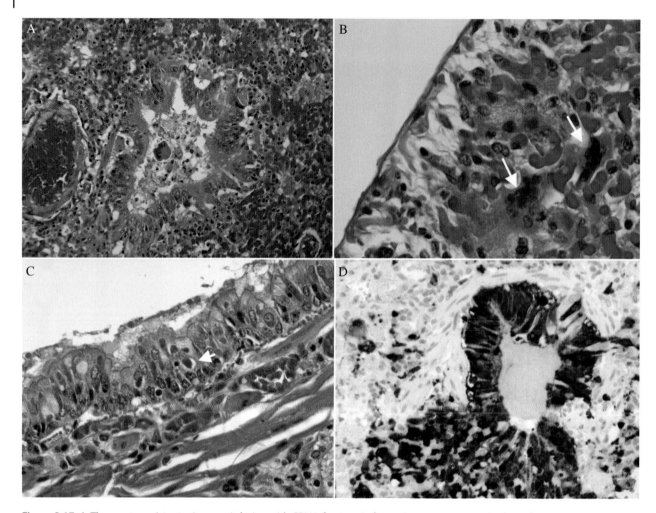

Figure 2.17 A: The most consistent microscopic lesion with CDV infections in ferrets is a necrosuppurative bronchopneumonia. B: Multinucleated syncytial cells (arrows) are often present. C: Eosinophilic intracytoplasmic viral inclusion bodies (arrow) are present within the bronchiolar epithelial cells. D: Immunohistochemistry for CDV antigen demonstrating strong positive nuclear and cytoplasmic immunolabeling (brown staining), counterstained with Mayer's hematoxylin.

progresses to include dermal and other lesions, and is almost always fatal.

2.4.2.5 Colony Management
Regular immunization of animals with CDV vaccines specifically approved for ferrets is helpful for preventing disease, however, reports exist of vaccinated ferrets contracting distemper following exposure to infected and sick animals. Healthy animals should be immediately isolated from ferrets with clinical signs of distemper and a rigid quarantine imposed. Ferrets should not be exposed to dogs of unknown CDV vaccination status.

2.4.3 Mycobacterial Respiratory Diseases

Mycobacterial infections are uncommon in pet ferrets, however, *M. bovis*, *M. avium* or other atypical mycobacterial species have been cultured from lymph nodes of 2% of feral ferrets in New Zealand (representing approximately 480 positive cultures out of a sample size of 21,500 ferrets). It is unknown whether these infected animals serve as a reservoir for domestic cattle and other wildlife or whether ferrets are being infected from domestic animals.

2.4.3.1 Presenting Clinical Signs
Sporadic cases of *Mycobacterium* spp. infection are reported in pet ferrets, including several case reports of ferrets infected with *M. celatum*. Ferrets infected with mycobacteria may present with a chronic history of weight loss, lethargy, depression, coughing or dyspnea, and diarrhea with scattered radiodense foci visible in survey radiographs.

2.4.3.2 Pathology
Upon post-mortem examination, multifocal gray, firm nodules may be present throughout the lungs and mediastinal tissue with marked regional to generalized

enlargement of lymph nodes. Alternatively, nodular lesions may be localized to the gut, spleen, or liver, without involving the respiratory tree or the disease may be disseminated, affecting multiple tissues and skin. Microscopically, nodules consist of predominantly granulomatous inflammation with scattered neutrophils, lymphocytes, and plasma cells, epithelioid and multinucleated giant cells, and necrotic debris. Numerous slender, sometimes branching, intracellular acid-fast bacilli may be found in nodules and enlarged lymph nodes.

2.4.3.3 Laboratory Diagnostics
Bacterial culture with PCR follow-up and molecular species typing by 16S rDNA sequencing is required for definitive identification of mycobacterial species.

2.4.3.4 Differential Diagnoses
Differential diagnoses include other bacterial infections; such as those caused by *Pseudomonas* spp., as well as systemic coronavirus infection. Concurrent infection with influenza or other diseases leading to debilitation, such as lymphosarcoma, may enhance ferret susceptibility to infection. Mycobacterial infections are zoonotic but may also be transmitted to pet ferrets from their owners.

2.4.4 Other Bacterial Respiratory Diseases

Infection of young, adult ferrets with *Pseudomonas luteola* has been reported to result in a pyogranulomatous pleuropneumonia and mediastinitis. In all cases, animals presented with acute depression, anorexia, and dyspnea. Pure cultures of yellow colonies of encapsulated Gram negative bacteria were isolated from affected animals. *P. luteola* is considered an opportunistic pathogen found in water that infects humans with prosthetic heart valves or immunocompromised individuals, however, no intercurrent disease was reported in any of the affected animals. Other differentials for mediastinal masses include lymphosarcoma, mycobacteriosis, and systemic coronavirus infections.

An outbreak of a novel, unspeciated *Mycoplasma*-associated respiratory disease has been recently described in ferrets from a single large breeding colony. Affected animals had clinical signs largely consisting of mild coughing and dyspnea and although very high colony morbidity was noted, the disease was typically subclinical to mild, with almost no mortality. Tissues from animals exhibiting clinical signs showed mild, multifocal, pale tan-gray nodules centered on airways correlating microscopically to mild to moderate bronchointerstitial pneumonia with marked peribronchiolar lymphoid aggregates. In this report, novel *Mycoplasma* organisms were identified by electron microscopy and PCR analyses.

Primary bacterial respiratory infections are otherwise uncommon in pet ferrets. Potential underlying viral disease, e.g., CDV or influenza, should be investigated in ferrets dying of opportunistic respiratory infections.

2.4.5 Other Respiratory Conditions

Aspiration pneumonia may occur in ferrets secondary to oral medication, megaesophagus, light anesthesia, or as a terminal event prior to death. As for other small animal species, grossly, there is patchy congestion and consolidation of lung lobes, sometimes with obvious lines of demarcation and necrosis. Depending on the material aspirated, the lesion may range from suppurative or granulomatous inflammation to coagulation necrosis and are usually localized around small airways. Food particles may be refractile.

Nasal and pulmonary mycoses are uncommon in ferrets but case reports exist for rare infections with *Coccidoides*, *Blastomyces*, and *Cryptococcus* spp. In one case, pulmonary blastomycosis caused by *B. dermatitidis* was diagnosed in a ferret housed strictly indoors. The most likely source of exposure was potting soil from houseplants. Nodular pyogranulomatous inflammation with multinucleated giant cells and characteristic 10–20 cm round broad-based budding yeast with refractile thick walls was noted microscopically.

Naturally occurring ***Sarcocystis neurona*** rhinitis has been reported in a young male ferret purchased from a pet store and vaccinated with a modified live CDV vaccine. The animal developed respiratory disease and hind end paresis and was euthanized. *S. neurona* merozoites were found throughout the lung, brain, heart, skeletal muscle, adrenal glands, liver, spleen, lymph nodes, and kidneys and schizonts were present within the nasal turbinates. Imunohistochemistry was used to confirm that the organisms were *S. neurona*. Tissues from this ferret were also PCR-positive for canine distemper virus and it is speculated that the resulting immunosuppression and lymphopenia predisposed this animal to *S. neurona* infection.

Endogenous lipid pneumonia or subpleural histiocytosis is a common incidental finding in adult ferrets and may appear grossly as pale plaques on the parenchymal surface (Figure 2.15). The microscopic appearance consists of subpleural aggregates of lipid-laden, foamy alveolar macrophages with scant inflammatory cells and occasional cholesterol clefts.

Systemic coronavirus infection and disease may result in dyspnea in affected animals. Pyogranulomatous pulmonary nodules and bronchiolar lymphadenopathy may be present, however, pyogranulomatous abdominal lesions and marked mesenteric lymphadenopathy are the major lesions in affected animals (see Section 2.6.5.1).

Primary pulmonary neoplasms are very rare in ferrets. In contrast, local tumor seeding and metastases can commonly be seen with **intrathoracic lymphosarcomas**. A single report exists for **adenosquamous tracheal carcinoma** in a 4-year-old neutered male ferret. This neoplasm is typically an aggressive malignant tumor that is associated with chronic cigarette smoke exposure in humans and other animals, however, there was no known exposure to cigarette smoke in the affected ferret.

Dental disease, including tooth root abscesses should be explored in ferrets presenting with chronic suppurative nasal discharge. Various **environmental particulates** and **foreign bodies** may become lodged within the nasal cavities, resulting in rhinitis, sneezing and purulent discharge.

Dyspnea, coughing, and pleural effusion may occur secondary to **congestive heart failure**, **intrathoracic neoplasia**, and **heartworm infection** in ferrets. **Hypoglycemia**, secondary to insulinoma, **acidosis** from any cause, and **adverse vaccine reactions** to immunization against distemper or rabies viruses may result in tachypnea. The latter condition may be associated with sudden death in rare cases.

2.5 Musculoskeletal Conditions

Ferrets in appropriate body condition have long, lean tubular bodies with large vertebrae and a flexible spinal column. Their musculature and skeletal systems are similar to those of dogs except ferrets have two sesamoid bones associated with their first digit and their clavicle is quite rudimentary. Primary musculoskeletal disease is uncommon in ferrets. Congenital skeletal malformations are also rare. Weakness, particularly of the hind end, can be seen relatively frequently in ferrets and is a non-specific sign related to the presence of underlying cardiovascular disease or endocrine disturbances, such as occurs with pancreatic islet cell tumors, adrenal gland disease, and anemia secondary to estrogen toxicity in intact jills. These conditions should always be considered unless there is obvious soft tissue or bony trauma, or neoplasia of the affected part.

2.5.1 Disseminated Idiopathic Myofasciitis

Disseminated idiopathic myofasciitis is a recently recognized systemic inflammatory disease of ferrets that affects skeletal, smooth, and cardiac muscles, adipose tissue, and associated fascia. It occurs in juvenile through to adult animals and affected ferrets may appear depressed and be pyrexic, painful, and reluctant to move, and have difficulty eating and swallowing. Serous oculonasal discharge, bruxism, panting, and abnormal stools may also be present. The clinical course of the condition may be days to weeks and animals may become anemic with a moderate mature neutrophilia and increased white blood cell count.

Grossly, muscle atrophy may be observed on the trunk, legs, and diaphragm, the esophagus may become markedly edematous and erythematous, and there may be splenic pallor and enlargement secondary to marked myelopoiesis. Microscopically, there is multifocal pyogranulomatous fasciitis surrounding muscle bundles and extending along fascial planes and affecting adipose tissue, with associated myofibre degeneration and atrophy. Esophageal changes result from circumferential inflammation within fascia and adventitia along the length of the esophagus. Mild neutrophilic inflammation may be seen in other tissues, such as the brain and liver. The pathogenesis of this condition is unknown but is possibly related to one or more of viral infections, genetic predisposition, and vaccine-induced inflammation resulting in activation of autoimmune responses in predisposed ferrets. The disease is not transmissible between animals.

2.5.2 Intervertebral Disc Disease

Several clinical cases of intervertebral disc disease resulting from disc protrusion have been reported in ferrets ranging in age from 7 months to 6 years and in normoweight to obese animals. Animals have presented with hind limb paresis to tetraparesis, depending upon the area of spinal cord impingement. No consistent cause has been identified, although trauma and discospondylitis were each suspected in single cases.

2.5.3 Musculoskeletal Neoplasia

There are no published reports of osteosarcoma in ferrets and rare reports of chondroma and chondrosarcomas, both of which may interfere with the animal's ability to ambulate. Osteomas are seen on occasion and present as slow-growing, firm, irregular protrusions involving the flat bones of the face, calvarium, ribs, and vertebrae, which, in the latter location, may impinge on the spinal cord, inducing paresis or paralysis. Microscopically, the masses consist of bony spicules and trabeculae lined by well differentiated osteoblasts separated by connective tissue and mineralized matrix.

An intramedullary lumbosacral teratoma has also been reported in an 18-month-old spayed female ferret, which led to clinical signs of paresis because of subtotal effacement of the spinal cord.

Other neoplasms of ferrets that may induce paresis include plasma cell myeloma (see Section 2.10), chordoma (see Section 2.2), fibrosarcoma, and lymphosarcoma (see Section 2.10).

2.5.4 Trauma

Fractures of the pelvis and long bones and soft tissue wounds may result from inadvertent crushing injuries or attacks by other animal species. Pet ferrets will burrow into furniture and cushions and may be injured inadvertently in these locations by an unsuspecting human. This emphasizes the importance of close supervision of this species when they are allowed to roam freely.

2.5.5 Other Musculoskeletal Conditions

Myasthenia gravis has been reported in a 7-month-old neutered male ferret. Acquired myasthenia gravis was suspected in this animal based on presenting signs of flaccid tetraparesis, elevated serum acetylcholine receptor antibodies (0.35 nmol/L compared with an average value of <0.06 nmol/L obtained from clinically normal ferrets), and complete remission of signs when treated with oral pyridostigmine bromide.

Rupture of the posterior cruciate ligament has been reported in a ferret, although the etiopathogenesis was not determined.

Osteoarthritis is reported anecdotally in pet ferrets but has not been described in the literature. Posterior cruciate ligament rupture is also described in a 4-year-old neutered female ferret.

Weakness, ataxia, and recumbency have been seen in ferrets after accidental ingestion of **ibuprofen**, with signs occurring within 4–8 hours after ingestion. Renal papillary necrosis and gastrointestinal hemorrhage were commonly present in these animals. **Botulism** will also result in flaccid paralysis and potentially death in ferrets, and may be due to ingestion of *Clostridium botulinum* toxin in poorly preserved or contaminated feed.

Congenital skeletal malformations are reported sporadically in ferrets. A case of **occipitoatlantoaxial malformation** has been noted in a 3-month-old ferret with progressive tetraparesis.

2.6 Gastrointestinal Conditions

Ferrets are true carnivores and have a simple stomach and short gastrointestinal tract, which empties within 2–4 hours after eating a meal. Ferrets have five paired salivary glands, including the zygomatic, parotid, submandibular, sublingual, and molar glands. The intestine is composed of a duodenum and a jejunoileum, which empties directly into the colon and discharges through the rectum. Ferrets do not have a cecum or a grossly obvious ileocolic junction but do have a gall bladder. The paired apocrine anal glands are usually removed at a young age in pet ferrets to reduce their musky odor.

Gastrointestinal conditions are moderately common in ferrets and often arise from bacterial or viral infections, as well as foreign body ingestion. Recent large-scale viral molecular screening of ferret rectal swabs has suggested that pet, laboratory, and commercially-reared ferrets within Europe may be subclinically infected with a range of novel, previously unidentified viruses, including picornaviruses, astrovirus, and hepatitis E virus. Whether and how these agents contribute to enteric disease of ferrets as co-pathogens or opportunistic agents remains to be determined.

2.6.1 Oral Conditions

Ferrets have 28–30 deciduous teeth, as the second mandibular molars may be congenitally absent in some animals. Supernumerary teeth may also be found on occasion between the first and second maxillary incisors.

2.6.1.1 Dental Disease

Dental disease is common in ferrets and includes malocclusion, gingivitis, periodontal disease, dental calculus, extrusion of canine teeth, and canine tooth fractures with or without dental pulp exposure. Periapical abscesses may also be present in incisors or other teeth, sometimes with foul-smelling fistulous tracts that exit onto the face or within the nasal cavity.

2.6.1.2 Oral Neoplasia

Oral tumors are seen infrequently in ferrets. Sporadic cases of squamous cell carcinoma are seen in young adult animals of both sexes (Figure 2.18). Tumors appear as ulcerated plaques or masses on the lips, palate or surrounding teeth, and microscopic characteristics are similar to oral squamous cell carcinomas seen in cats. Neoplasms may be very invasive with late metastases to cervical lymph nodes or other tissues.

2.6.1.3 Other Oral Conditions

Idiopathic oral ulcers and oral foreign bodies occur periodically in ferrets. Both may present with a history of hyperptyalism and pawing at the mouth. The latter sign may also be seen in ferrets with any gastrointestinal or systemic condition that induces nausea. Most commonly, foreign bodies become lodged across the roof of the mouth, between the upper dental arcades. Material may also become impacted between or around teeth.

2.6.2 Salivary Gland Conditions

Salivary gland microliths may be seen in the parotid glands of ferrets and are not usually associated with inflammation or ductal obstruction, although focal acinar cell degeneration may be present. Microliths in ferrets are

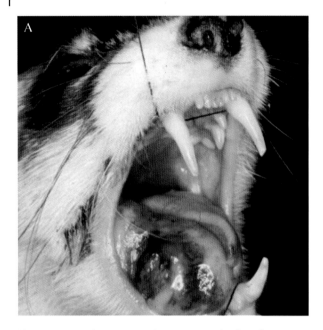
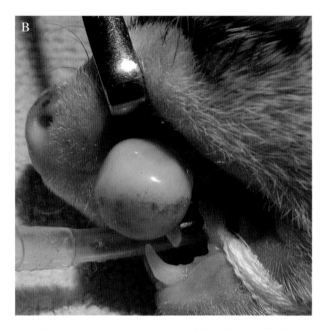

Figure 2.18 Oral tumors may be seen sporadically in ferrets. A: Squamous cell carcinoma in a ferret with loss of the right mandibular canine. Radiographs demonstrated significant lysis of mandibular bone. B: Acanthomatous ameloblastoma in a ferret. *Source:* B: Courtesy of The Links Road Animal and Bird Clinic.

less calcified compared with those occurring in cats or humans and may induce less local irritation because of this.

Mucoceles are rarely reported and are thought to occur secondary to trauma. They may result in concurrent periorbital swelling, exophthalmos, and prolapse of the third eyelid or soft, fluctuant cervical swellings, depending upon which gland is involved.

2.6.3 Megaesophagus

Megaesophagus refers to intracervical and intrathoracic esophageal dilatation and the condition may be congenital or acquired (Figure 2.19). Animals with this condition may have a clinical history of regurgitation and dysphagia, which should be distinguished from vomiting. Congenital megaesophagus is highly uncommon in most domestic animal species. More common causes of acquired megaesophagus include myasthenia gravis, intrathoracic esophageal or mediastinal obstruction (e.g., thymoma, mediastinal lymphosarcoma, esophageal foreign body), lead intoxication, tetanus, botulism, and hypoadrenocorticism, although the etiopathogenesis of most cases of megaesophagus in ferrets is unknown. Stasis of ingesta within the dilated esophagus may induce a mild suppurative esophagitis with focal erosions or ulcerations along the length of the esophagus, and secondary aspiration may occur resulting in a necrosuppurative bronchopneumonia of varying severity. Myasthenia gravis has been documented in a young adult pet ferret presenting with flaccid tetraparesis and mild

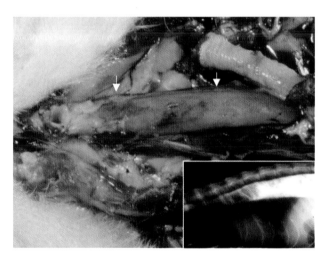

Figure 2.19 Megaesophagus (arrows) in a 6-year-old neutered male ferret with a chronic history of regurgitation. Inset: This condition was diagnosed ante-mortem following barium contrast imaging.

megaesophagus. The diagnosis was confirmed by the presence of antibodies to acetylcholine receptors.

2.6.4 Gastric Conditions

Vomiting is a relatively uncommon sign in ferrets and may occur sporadically or have a sudden and regular onset with or without diarrhea and anorexia. Common causes for vomiting include *Helicobacter mustelae* infection, gastric ulceration from other causes, such as adverse stress or nonsteroidal anti-inflammatory drug administration, foreign body ingestion, gastric tumors, hepatic disease, or various enteric conditions, including enteric or systemic coronavirus infection and inflammatory bowel disease.

2.6.4.1 *Helicobacter mustelae* Infection

Helicobacter mustelae was identified in ferrets over 25 years ago and is now known to be a very common opportunistic bacterium, which may be present in pet ferrets from the age of 6 weeks and older. The bacterium is a Gram-negative, microaerophilic and argyrophilic, urease-positive, spiral rod that has multiple sheathed flagellae at both ends. Ferrets are infected around weaning by fecal-oral bacterial transmission and infections are lifelong without treatment. Hypersecretion of gastrin can occur in infected animals, likely a response to chronic gastric inflammation, and this may contribute to duodenal ulceration.

2.6.4.2 Presenting Clinical Signs

Infection with *H. mustelae* is often asymptomatic, despite the high prevalence estimated in North American ferrets. Clinical signs may include bruxism, vomiting, melena, pallor, inappetence, abdominal tenderness, and weight loss. Infections may be longstanding but remain undetected until comorbidities, adverse stress, tumors, treatment with ulcerogenic therapeutics, or other conditions induce overt disease.

2.6.4.3 Pathology

The pathology associated with *Helicobacter* infection is variable and dependent on the chronicity of infection, including gastroesophageal reflux, chronic gastritis, gastric and duodenal erosion and ulceration with or without perforation, gastric adenocarcinoma, and gastric mucosa-associated lymphosarcoma (MALT lymphosarcoma). Bacteria colonize cells of the antrum and pylorus by means of adhesion pedestals, inducing a moderate, localized lymphoplasmacytic infiltrate with glandular atrophy and regeneration. Gastric MALT may be markedly expanded in chronic cases and there may be concurrent hyperplasia and reactivity of the gastric lymph node. Pinpoint to focal to multifocal erosions and ulcers may be present on gross examination of the gastric mucosa (Figure 2.20) and scant bacteria are visible microscopically around the crater edges or in gastric mucosa peripheral to leukocytic infiltrates. Visualization of bacteria within the gastric glands or superficial mucus can be enhanced with a Warthin-Starry stain.

Low-grade gastric adenocarcinomas can occur in ferrets chronically infected with *H. mustelae*. The pylorus is the most common site and masses are characterized by nests of proliferating but well differentiated glandular epithelial cells with mild atypia and few mitoses, and

marked dissecting fibrosis within a background of chronic lymphoplasmacytic inflammation. Tumors may extend into the underlying submucosa and bacteria may be present within areas of inflammation.

As in humans infected with *H. pylori*, chronic infection with *H. mustelae* may result in B-cell lymphosarcomas of the gastric MALT, characterized by clonal expansion of neoplastic lymphocytes within the mucosa and submucosa with marked thickening and replacement of glandular cells and disruption of normal architecture.

2.6.4.4 Laboratory Diagnostics

Helicobacter mustelae can be diagnosed ante-mortem by PCR conducted on feces or gastric mucosal scrapings or biopsies, or by microscopic examination of pyloric biopsies. Fecal culture and serologic tests are available but less commonly used. Microscopic identification of short argyrophilic rods within gastric pits associated with antral or pyloric lymphoplasmacytic inflammation is highly consistent with *H. mustelae* infection.

2.6.4.5 Differential Diagnoses

Vomiting may be induced by a number of infectious and noninfectious conditions, including incidental cases of dietary indiscretion and nonspecific stress. The age of the animal, frequency and temporal occurrence of vomition, and nature of the content are important considerations for determining the cause of vomiting. The presence of digested blood within the vomitus may increase the clinical index of suspicion for gastric ulceration caused or exacerbated by an underlying *H. mustelae* infection. Clinicians often use a response to therapy to diagnose potential cases of *Helicobacter*-induced gastritis. Other considerations for melena in ferrets include viral or bacterial enterocolitis, gastroenteric foreign body or enteric neoplasia.

2.6.4.6 Disease/Herd Management

While ferrets can be cured of *H. mustelae* infection, they may become reinfected if exposed to *Helicobacter*-positive animals. This is particularly true for younger animals. Hence, all animals in a group-housed setting should be treated at the same time to completely eradicate the agent. New ferrets should be quarantined, tested for *Helicobacter* infection, and treated, if positive, prior to direct contact with a stable *Helicobacter*-negative group or colony.

2.6.4.7 Gastrointestinal Foreign Bodies

Ferrets are notorious chewers and esophageal, gastric, and enteric foreign bodies are a common occurrence (Figure 2.21). A clinical history of anorexia, vomiting, or abdominal distension may be reported and the condition may occur in ferrets of any age. Undiagnosed foreign

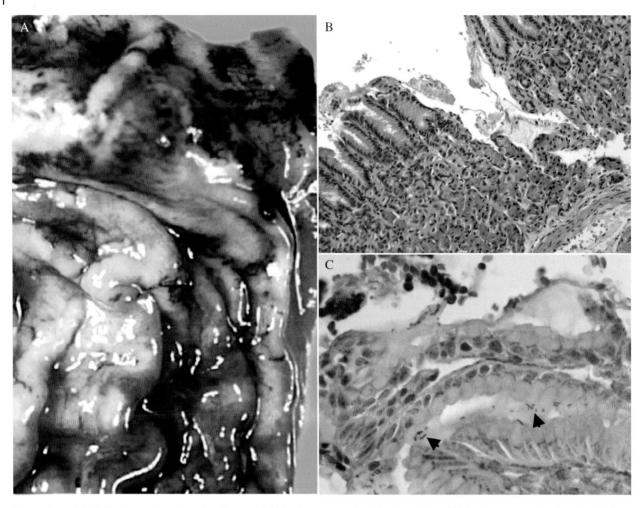

Figure 2.20 A: Multifocal gastric erosions in a ferret with *Helicobacter mustelae* infection. B: Focal *Helicobacter*-associated erosion in the gastric mucosa. C: Small, agyrophilic, curved, rod-shaped bacteria, consistent with *Helicobacter* sp. (arrows), are associated with the mucosal defect.

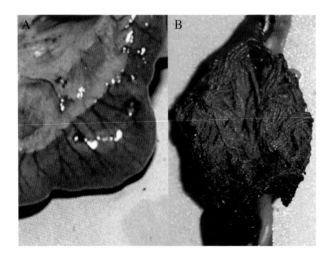

Figure 2.21 A: Intestinal foreign bodies with obstruction are common in ferrets. B: Mass of green string obstructing the small intestine of a ferret. *Source:* A and B: Courtesy of C. Wheler.

bodies may eventually induce ischemic necrosis and rupture. Gastric foreign bodies, including trichobezoars, may also be seen as incidental findings at post-mortem.

2.6.4.8 Gastric Neoplasia

Gastric adenocarcinoma unassociated with *Helicobacter* infection can be seen infrequently in older ferrets. Microscopic characteristics are as described above, but do not include chronic lymphoplasmacytic inflammation. Osseous metaplasia may occur within some masses.

2.6.4.9 Other Gastric Conditions

Gastric bloat with sudden death has been reported in black-footed ferrets in zoo settings. The condition is correlated with overeating resulting in secondary *Clostridium perfringens* type A overgrowth, elaboration of α toxin, and fatal enterotoxemia. Animals presented with marked gastric distension and dyspnea and died peracutely. Microscopic examination of gastric sections indicated acute mucosal erosion of the stomach and proximal small intestine with abundant Gram-positive bacilli blanketing the necrotic epithelium.

Gastric polyps have been reported anecdotally in pet ferrets.

Gastric ulcers are also commonly found in ferrets negative for *Helicobacter mustelae* infection. Ulcers may occur spontaneously in animals experiencing stress secondary to systemic disease, management changes, or other factors.

2.6.5 Enteric Conditions

The feces of healthy ferrets may be soft because of the short gastrointestinal transit time, and sporadic diarrhea may occur for both infectious and noninfectious causes, including nonspecific stress, dietary indiscretion or dietary change, foreign body ingestion, neoplasia, or heat stress. As for cases of vomiting in ferrets, it is important to consider animal age, comorbidities, duration of illness, and character of feces in cases of suspect enteritis. Infectious enteropathies are less common in mature ferrets, particularly in closed colonies.

2.6.5.1 Coronaviral Enteritis

Coronaviruses are large, enveloped, positive-stranded RNA viruses, divided into three groups based on sequence homology. Group 1 coronaviruses include porcine transmissible gastroenteritis virus, feline coronavirus, ferret enteric coronavirus (FRECV), and ferret systemic coronavirus (FRSCV), a closely related variant.

Epizootic catarrhal enteritis (ECE) (green slime disease) was first described in 1993 in the United States and the etiologic agent was later confirmed to be a ferret enteric coronavirus. In 2004, a syndrome resembling the granulomatous or dry form of feline infectious peritonitis (FIP) was reported in ferrets from Spain, and subsequently has been seen in the United States, Europe, and Canada. Similar to coronaviral disease in cats, FRECV causes self-limiting enteric disease in ferrets while pathogenic FRECV variant, FRSCV, may be associated with a progressive, fatal, systemic pyogranulomatous peritonitis and perivasculitis in ferrets. This FIP-like syndrome is now recognized as ferret systemic coronavirus-associated disease after positive identification by immunohistochemical labeling of intralesional macrophages for coronaviral particles and sequence analysis of the isolated

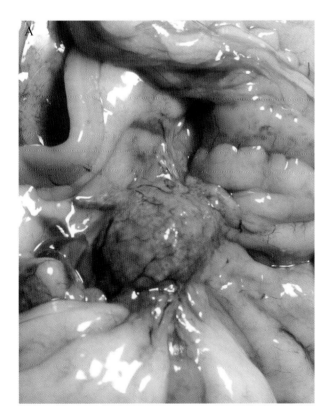
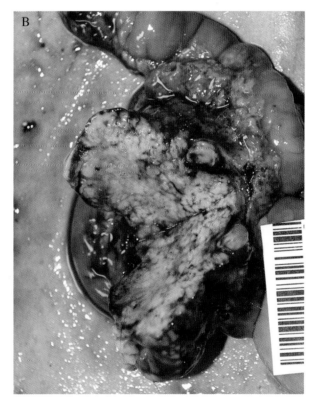

Figure 2.22 A: Systemic FIP-like coronavirus enteritis in a young ferret. The mesenteric lymph node is enlarged and firm. Segmentally, the small intestine is thickened with serosal reddening. B: Mesenteric lymph node from a different ferret with systemic FIP-like coronavirus disease sectioned to demonstrate marked pyogranulomatous inflammation. The primary differential diagnosis for mesenteric lymphadenopathy in a ferret is lymphosarcoma.

virus. FRSCV-associated disease is typically seen in young adult ferrets and is almost invariably fatal.

There are several prevailing theories regarding the pathogenesis of FIP-like disease in ferrets. The current hypothesis is that the condition arises from spontaneous internal mutation from less virulent FRECV variants to highly pathogenic FRSCV variants. Despite this theory, FIP-like disease has been noted in ferrets infected only with FRECV variants, indicating that further work is needed to understand the etiopathogenesis of the disease. It is likely that enteric coronaviruses are enzootic in pet and colony ferrets. One study from Japan examining the prevalence of virus using PCR analysis of fecal samples from 79 pet ferrets determined that 56% of samples were positive.

2.6.5.2 Presenting Clinical Signs
ECE is characterized by a foul-smelling, bright green, mucoid diarrhea in association with lethargy, dehydration, and anorexia. ECE infection induces almost 100% morbidity but very low mortality. Clinical signs in juveniles are subclinical to mild, while adults are more severely affected. Despite this, the disease is often self-limiting with supportive care. Chronic malabsorptive clinical signs may persist or develop later in life in rare cases.

Ferrets with FIP-like disease may also present with similar signs of watery green diarrhea that progress to weight loss, severe anorexia and dehydration, depression, and eventually death, despite efforts at supportive care. Large, discrete abdominal masses and splenomegaly may be palpated in affected animals. The clinical course of disease is generally 5 days to 2 weeks but can be longer if animals are given supportive care.

2.6.5.3 Pathology
In cases of ECE, affected animals may have dilated, erythematous loops of small intestine with watery content. Histology of affected sections demonstrates moderate to marked lymphoplasmacytic infiltrates within the lamina propria of affected segments with marked vacuolar degeneration of enterocytes on the villus tips with resulting villus blunting and fusion.

On post-mortem examination, animals with FIP-like disease may have abundant serous pleural and peritoneal effusion. Generalized petechiation may be present on the intestinal serosa, as well as the hepatic capsule and body wall. Multifocal, miliary to 2 cm diameter nodules are seen on the serosa of the gastrointestinal tract, the capsules of other abdominal organs, within the mesentery in association with vasculature, as well as on the pleural surface of the lungs and diaphragm. Depending on the chronicity of infection, marked fibrinous to fibrous adhesions may be present between loops of bowel, hepatic lobes, and mesenteric lymph nodes. The

spleen and mesenteric lymph nodes are often markedly enlarged, firm, and pale on cut section (Figure 2.22).

Microscopically, FIP-like lesions consist of pyogranulomatous lymphadenitis, enteritis, pneumonia, and peritonitis. The architecture of enlarged mesenteric lymph nodes is effaced by foamy histiocytic infiltrates with lesser numbers of neutrophils, lymphocytes, and plasma cells. Affected small intestinal sections are diffusely thickened with nodular to coalescing areas of foamy histiocytic and lymphoplasmacytic infiltrates effacing the muscularis, submucosa, and sometimes, the mucosa. Variable fibrosis and scattered multinucleated giant cells may be seen within lesions from animals surviving for longer periods. Within parenchymatous tissues, inflammation is often localized around small vessels and occasionally associated with necrosis and fibrin deposition within the tunica media. Mild to moderate segmental villus atrophy and fusion with associated enterocyte vacuolar degeneration and mixed leukocytic infiltrates may also be present within the lamina propria of less affected segments of small intestine (Figure 2.23).

2.6.5.4 Laboratory Diagnostics
Hematologic changes may include nonregenerative anemia, hypergammaglobulinemia, hypoalbuminemia, and thrombocytopenia.

Coronavirus antigens can be detected within affected macrophages by immunohistochemistry. RT-PCR assay for specific virus spike proteins is used to differentiate between FRECV and FRSCV variants. Coronaviral particles may also be visualized in feces or affected tissue of infected ferrets by transmission electron microscopy.

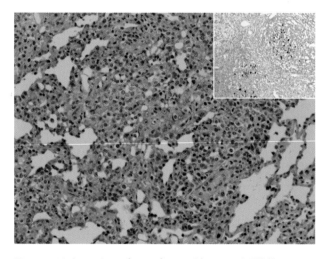

Figure 2.23 Lung tissue from a ferret with systemic FIP-like coronavirus disease. There are marked histiocytic infiltrates. Inset: immunohistochemistry against FIP antigens in a ferret with systemic coronavirus disease demonstrating marked cytoplasmic immunolabeling (brown staining) of affected cells. Counter stain: Mayer's hematoxylin.

2.6.5.5 Differential Diagnoses

Differential diagnoses for hypergammaglobulinemia and/or abdominal masses include Aleutian disease, lymphosarcoma, chronic infection (e.g., proliferative colitis, helicobacteriosis), idiopathic splenomegaly, multiple myeloma, other neoplasms, and inflammatory bowel disease. Other causes of lymphadenopathy include lymphosarcoma and mycobacterial infection.

Counter-immunoelectrophoresis for anti-Aleutian disease parvovirus antibodies can be conducted to exclude Aleutian disease.

2.6.5.6 Disease/Group Management

While occurrences of severe ECE are rare, serology and fecal PCR screening of ferret colonies indicate that FRECV is widely distributed in large ferret breeding operations in the United States. Ferret coronaviruses are highly contagious and animals with diarrhea should be isolated from other animals. There is no specific treatment for this condition and affected animals may be provided with supportive nursing care.

2.6.5.7 Rotaviral Diarrhea

Rotaviruses are double-stranded, nonenveloped RNA viruses in the family Reoviridae and a significant cause of viral enteritis in infant or juvenile animals of many species, including ferrets. There are seven serogroups of rotavirus (A–G) but only Group C rotavirus has been definitively diagnosed in juvenile ferrets, in association with an outbreak of enteritis in juvenile animals. Affected kits were a week old and were thin and dehydrated, with distended abdomens. Sections of small intestine were grossly dilated and filled with fluid and gas. Microscopically, degeneration, necrosis, and sloughing of terminal villus enterocytes are seen with subsequent villus blunting. Definitive diagnosis requires identification of characteristic viral particles by electron microscopy or by specific PCR assay (VP6 consensus sequence from porcine, human, and bovine viral DNA alignment). The virus is transmitted by fecal-oral contamination and it is resistant to environmental decontamination. Differential diagnoses for rotavirus enteritis of young kits include colibacillosis and coccidiosis.

2.6.5.8 Inflammatory Bowel Disease

Idiopathic inflammatory bowel disease occurs in ferrets and likely has a multifactorial etiology, possibly involving dietary or environmental allergens. Affected animals are generally 4 months of age or older and they present with vomiting, diarrhea, anorexia, and weight loss or may be asymptomatic. Biopsies or tissue sections from the stomach, duodenum, and jejunum of affected animals often demonstrate moderate to marked lymphoplasmacytic infiltrates within the lamina propria with scant eosinophils and other inflammatory cells, similar to inflammatory bowel disease lesions in dogs and cats. Villi may be blunted or fused and crypts may be hyperplastic with sporadic abscessation. Mesenteric lymph nodes in affected animals are often moderately enlarged and appear reactive, microscopically. Differential diagnoses include eosinophilic gastroenteritis, helicobacteriosis, coronaviral enteritis, and Aleutian disease. The diagnosis of inflammatory bowel disease is one of exclusion. The disease requires lifelong immunomodulatory therapy and the etiology is unknown.

2.6.5.9 Eosinophilic Gastroenteritis

Eosinophilic gastroenteritis is a distinct idiopathic inflammatory condition of young adult ferrets. Affected animals may present with vomiting, diarrhea, and lethargy, and a marked eosinophilia may be noted during routine hematologic evaluation. Lesions may consist of segmental erythema and thickening of the gastric and intestinal walls, and other tissues may be affected, included mesenteric lymph nodes, liver, and lung. Histologic examination of surgical biopsies demonstrates marked eosinophilic and histiocytic infiltrates into the lamina propria of affected gut segments with dilated lymphatics and occasional eosinophilic vasculitis. Splendore-Hoeppli material may be present in areas of eosinophilic inflammation within affected lymph nodes. Differential diagnoses are similar to those for inflammatory bowel disease and treatment involves lifelong immunomodulatory therapy.

2.6.5.10 Proliferative Colitis

Proliferative colitis is a sporadic condition affecting juvenile and young adult ferrets. Animals with this condition are afebrile and generally maintain normal activity and eating patterns but have a persistent mucoid diarrhea. These ferrets may become dehydrated and lose body condition with time, and repeated tenesmus during defecation may result in rectal prolapse. Upon gross examination, the colon is turgid and thickened with a cobblestone appearance to the mucosa and mesenteric lymph nodes may be enlarged (Figure 2.24). Full thickness colonic biopsies or tissue sections demonstrate marked mucosal epithelial hyperplasia with extension of convoluted mucosal glands into the submucosa, and a moderate, mixed, predominantly lymphoplasmacytic mucosal and submucosal infiltrate. Abundant short, slightly curved bacterial rods may be seen within the apical epithelial cytoplasm of affected colonic segments and visualization is enhanced with Warthin-Starry staining. Mesenteric lymph nodes are reactive, containing confluent lymphoid follicles and prominent germinal centers. The 16S ribosomal DNA sequence of the bacteria is consistent with *Lawsonia intracellularis*, which also induces

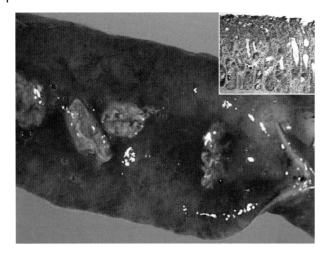

Figure 2.24 Proliferative colitis in a young ferret with chronic diarrhea, wasting, and rectal prolapse. Inset: Microscopically, there is marked colonic mucosal hyperplasia. *Lawsonia intracellularis* infection was presumed based on positive Warthin-Starry staining of superficial bacteria within the colonic mucosa.

proliferative enteropathy in hamsters, rabbits, and pigs. *Lawsonia* sp. do not appear to be highly contagious, such that only one or a few ferrets in a group or colony may be infected, and other co-factors may be required for infection to occur. The bacterium can only be grown on cell culture under specific conditions and gross and histologic findings are generally sufficient for a diagnosis. Some commercial porcine fecal PCR assays for *Lawsonia intracellularis* are cross-reactive for infected ferret tissues or feces, affording a definitive diagnosis.

2.6.5.11 Granulomatous Enteritis

Mycobacterial disease, including granulomatous enteritis with or without splenitis, hepatitis, and disseminated mycobacteriosis, has been reported in ferrets. Infections are rare and chronic, usually involving older adult animals. Animals may present with intermittent anorexia, vomition, mild diarrhea, weight loss, and palpably enlarged mesenteric lymph nodes. During exploratory surgery or post-mortem evaluation, intestinal constrictions, mesenteric lymphadenopathy, and hepatosplenomegaly with or without miliary gray-white nodules may be seen. Nodular lesions generally consist of pyogranulomatous inflammation and local fibrosis with abundant intracellular acid-fast bacilli. Ferrets are susceptible to infection with a variety of mycobacterial species, including *M. bovis, M. avium, M. celatum, M. chelonae, M. genavense,* and other disease syndromes, such as respiratory disease, may be seen following infection. Infected animals may also be asymptomatic, carrying the organism in their oral cavity, and represent a zoonotic risk for human caregivers, veterinarians, and other personnel if bitten. Identification of the bacterial species requires culture or 16S ribosomal RNA

sequencing. Differential diagnoses for the clinical syndrome include lymphosarcoma, intestinal foreign body, eosinophilic gastroenteritis, inflammatory bowel disease, and proliferative enteropathy.

2.6.5.12 Enteric Coccidiosis

Intestinal coccidiosis can occur in infant, juvenile, and adult ferrets, and is most commonly caused by infection with *Eimeria furonis* and *Isospora (Cystoisospora) laidlawi*, although several different coccidial species have been identified in ferrets, including *E. ictidea*. Infected animals may be asymptomatic depending on their overall health and immune status or may be inappetent, thin, and dehydrated with pasty to mucoid to black tarry feces. Gross lesions are usually confined to the small intestine, which appears reddened and dilated. Initial microscopic lesions include enterocyte proliferation with numerous coccidial schizonts, oocysts, and gametocytes present within enterocytes and a moderate, mixed neutrophilic and lymphoplasmacytic infiltrate within the lamina propria. Infected enterocytes rupture and are shed, resulting in villus atrophy, blunting, and fusion.

Two reports exist of *E. furonis*-induced biliary coccidiosis in which the affected adult ferrets presented with lethargy, jaundice and abdominal distension. One of these animals was receiving prednisolone, cyclosporine, and azathioprine to treat a severe, chronic nonregenerative anemia and presented with serum biochemistry results consistent with cholestasis (increased bilirubin, alkaline phosphatase, and gamma glutamyl transferase) 80 days after initiation of this therapy. Grossly, icterus of internal connective and adipose tissues, hepatomegaly, thickening of the gall bladder wall by mucosal proliferation and transmural neutrophilic and lymphoplasmacytic infiltrates, and dilatation and hyperplasia of bile ductules with peribiliary fibrosis were seen in these animals with marked numbers of *E. furonis* oocysts, micro- and macrogametocytes, and merozoites.

Transmission is direct and outbreaks of coccidiosis with high morbidity and moderate mortality can be seen in animal shelters or under conditions of intensive ferret housing. These can be challenging to manage without effective quarantine and isolation practices. Differential diagnoses include infection with rotavirus, coronavirus, and various bacteria. Definitive coccidial typing requires sequence analysis, although this is usually not required for effective treatment of animals.

2.6.5.13 Enteric Neoplasia

Lymphosarcoma may occur anywhere along the gastrointestinal tract, as well as within mesenteric lymph nodes, and the resultant masses are often palpable clinically (see Section 2.10.4). Ferrets with enteric lymphosarcoma may present with lethargy, anorexia, weight loss, abdominal distension, and diarrhea. Other forms of intestinal neoplasia are uncommon in ferrets. Intestinal and rectal adenocarcinomas have been identified in rare cases, as well as leiomyosarcomas of the large intestine and rectum. Perirectal/perineal hemangiosarcoma has been reported in a 4-year-old ferret. This animal had numerous cutaneous metastases as well as neoplastic masses in the omentum and sacral lymph node. Colonic polyps have also been described.

2.6.5.14 Other Conditions

Infection with *Campylobacter jejuni*, a slender, curved, argyrophilic and Gram-negative bacterial rod, may produce self-limiting mucoid or blood-tinged diarrhea in young ferrets. Animals may be persistently infected with lifelong episodic bouts of diarrhea occurring under conditions of stress or with intercurrent disease. Non-specific lesions of epithelial loss and neutrophilic and lymphocytic mucosal infiltrates may be found in the small and large intestines of affected animals, and a diagnosis may be confirmed with darkfield identification of characteristic motile rods from fresh feces or from culture of feces or tissue under selective conditions or by using 16S ribosomal DNA analysis for the bacteria. Ferrets may act as reservoirs for human *Campylobacter* infections. Because bacterial transmission occurs by fecal-oral exposure, human caregivers should always wash their hands carefully after handling ferrets with diarrhea.

Salmonella Typhimurium has been reported historically in ferrets that were fed raw meat diets that were improperly handled and should be considered a potential differential diagnosis of bloody diarrhea in febrile ferrets, particularly those fed raw diets. Microscopic findings include a necrohemorrhagic enteritis with mixed leukocytic mucosal and submucosal infiltrates and multifocal hepatic and splenic necrosis.

Cryptosporidium parvum infection can occur in young ferrets but is generally asymptomatic and self-limiting. Transmission occurs by direct consumption of sporulated oocysts and confirmation of infection is made by identifying of characteristic trophozoites within the brush border of enterocytes in tissue sections or within feces.

Giardia intestinalis has rarely been reported as a cause of diarrhea in debilitated ferrets and may be found incidentally in clinically normal animals. Dogs or cats may act as potential reservoirs for ferrets.

Some variants of **canine distemper virus** can induce diarrhea, in addition to other systemic signs of disease, in unvaccinated ferrets.

Systemic candidiasis presenting as vomiting and persistent hemorrhagic enteritis has been reported in a young ferret following infection with *Candida tropicalis*. The affected animal had enlarged mesenteric lymph nodes, and blastospores, pseudomycelia, and mycelia were identified in several tissues, including kidney and heart.

Rectal prolapse may occur in ferrets with diarrhea and is a nonspecific indication of tenesmus.

Other types of gastrointestinal parasites, including various nematodes, are rare in ferrets.

2.6.6 Hepatobiliary Conditions

There are generally six lobes to the ferret liver (left and right medial and lateral lobes, caudate, and quadrate) and the relative liver to body weight ratio of 0.43 for adult ferrets is high compared with other small mammal pets and companion animals. Liver inflammation or disease is relatively common in sick ferrets and may be secondary to other conditions. Hepatic lipidosis, with characteristic hepatocellular macrovesiculation, is common in obese adult pet ferrets. Clinical signs of hepatic disease are nonspecific and include lethargy, anorexia, and intermittent vomiting, and diarrhea with or without pyrexia. Because of skin and eye pigmentation, icterus may only be visible within the oral cavity, on the nose plenum or deep within the external ear or nares.

2.6.6.1 Infectious Hepatic Conditions

Multifocal hepatic necrosis, in addition to cholangiohepatitis, can be seen with almost any bacterial agent inducing septicemia in ferrets, including *Salmonella* spp., *Pseudomonas* sp., *Mycobacterium* spp., *Escherichia coli*, and *Aeromonas* sp. *Helicobacter cholecystus* has been isolated as an agent of hepatitis in a ferret colony but infection with this agent is otherwise uncommon. Hepatic coccidiosis and toxoplasmosis are seen sporadically in ferrets. Similarly, systemic viral disease caused by infection with canine distemper virus, influenza virus, Aleutian disease (a parvovirus infection), and coronavirus may induce foci of hepatic necrosis and inflammation. In all cases, further diagnostic tests are required to determine the causative agent. Although a novel hepatitis E virus has been isolated by PCR from the feces of pet, breeding, and laboratory ferrets in the United States, the Netherlands, and Japan, virus infection has not been correlated with hepatic disease to date. Furthermore, the ferret virus was not transmissible to either rats or monkeys, suggesting that it is unlikely to be zoonotic.

Nonspecific lymphoplasmacytic hepatitis may be seen with moderate regularity in surgical biopsies or tissue sections from adult ferrets as an extension of gastrointestinal inflammatory conditions.

2.6.6.2 Copper Toxicoses

Chronic hepatopathy, with periportal mononuclear leukocytic infiltrates, generalized fibrosis, scattered hepatocyte necrosis, and hepatic cord atrophy, was reported in two adult female ferrets from the same litter. Copper deposition was noted within hepatocytes and macrophages in both animals and one ferret additionally had hemoglobinuric nephrosis, likely secondary to intravascular hemolysis from copper intoxication. The mean liver copper levels in the two affected ferrets were ≥ 200 ppm (normal reference range 7–66 ppm). A genetic mutation in hepatic copper transport or storage mechanisms was considered the most likely underlying etiology.

2.6.6.3 Hepatic and Biliary Neoplasia

Hepatic neoplasia, both primary and metastatic, is moderately common in pet ferrets and includes nodular hyperplasia, hepatic adenomas, and hepatocellular carcinomas (Figure 2.25). In one animal, peliosis hepatis was noted in conjunction with hepatocellular carcinoma. Hepatic cysts are common in domestic ferrets while biliary cysts and cystadenomas are common in black-footed ferrets. Cystic mucinous hyperplasia of the gall bladder with consequent hepatomegaly and icterus have been reported in an 8-year-old ferret. Primary hepatic hemangiosarcoma is seen infrequently in adult ferrets whereas lymphosarcoma with hepatic involvement is common.

2.6.6.4 Other Hepatic and Biliary Conditions

Rare cases of **hepatic torsion** are seen in pet ferrets with resulting hepatocellular ischemia and necrosis.

Adrenohepatic fusion is seen commonly as an incidental finding in ferrets. No changes in hepatic or adrenal gland function are associated with the condition.

Acetaminophen intoxication with resulting hepatic necrosis and death of the animal has been reported anecdotally in a pet ferret. Glucuronidation of acetaminophen is slow in ferrets, similar to cats, which may contribute to increased susceptibility to intoxication.

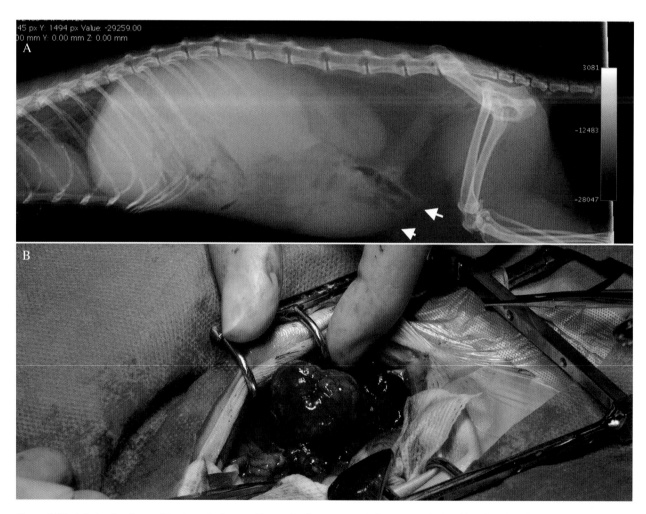

Figure 2.25 A: Lateral radiographic view of a ferret with massive hepatomegaly (arrows mark distal border of the liver) that was later determined to be due to hepatocellular carcinoma. B: Surgical resection of the mass. Histopathology was consistent with a hepatocellular carcinoma.

Other intoxications are reported sporadically in ferrets. Most veterinary insecticides and flea treatments have a wide therapeutic margin and do not cause intoxications when used at label doses.

A **ruptured gall bladder** was reported in a 6-year-old ferret presenting acutely for a painful abdomen. A cholecystectomy was conducted and a marked chronic lymphocytic cholehepatitis was diagnosed from surgical biopsies of the liver and resected gall bladder. *Pseudomonas aeruginosa* was isolated from both tissues.

Intra- and extrahepatic cholelithiasis due to an accumulation of bile sediment with resultant cholestasis were also seen sporadically in pet ferrets.

2.6.7 Conditions of the Exocrine Pancreas

Pancreatitis may be diagnosed in obese adult ferrets and may also occur secondary to diabetes mellitus. Exocrine pancreatic carcinoma and adenocarcinoma are sporadic, aggressive tumors in ferrets and local seeding of the liver, gastrointestinal tract, or peritoneal cavity as well as pulmonary metastases often results. Animals can present with abdominal effusions as a sequela to carcinomatosis. In several cases, adult ferrets presented with clinical chemistry changes consistent with biliary obstruction (increased total bilirubin and alkaline phosphatase) because of involvement and obstruction of the bile duct papilla in the duodenum. Neoplastic cells contain apical zymogen and may form rosettes.

Mesotheliomas arise from the relatively undifferentiated mesothelial cells that line various body cavities, including the peritoneum, pleura, and pericardium. These tumors are rare in ferrets and present grossly as generalized, small to miliary, soft white nodules scattered throughout the mesentery as well as lining the parietal surface of the coelomic wall (Figure 2.26).

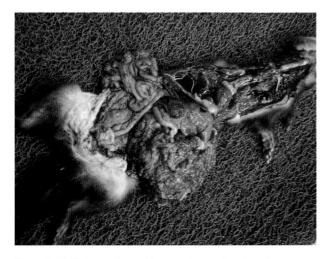

Figure 2.26 Peritoneal mesothelioma in a mature ferret.

2.7 Cardiovascular Conditions

Cardiac disease is relatively common in pet ferrets and may be asymptomatic or present as lethargy, inactivity, hypothermia, coughing, exercise intolerance, and hind end weakness or generalized weakness. Except for infant ferrets with congenital heart lesions, most cases are diagnosed in middle-aged, adult animals. Ascites and hepatic or splenic enlargement may also be present.

2.7.1 Cardiomyopathy

Dilated, hypertrophic, and restrictive forms of cardiomyopathy are all seen in ferrets. In most cases, no underlying cause is ever determined, although historically, taurine deficiency in poor quality diets was suspected as an underlying etiology. Dilated cardiomyopathy is the most common form and untreated chronic disease frequently progresses to congestive heart failure. Grossly, the heart is enlarged and flabby with dilatation of both the atria and ventricles and thinning of the ventricular free walls (Figure 2.27). Microscopically, myocyte degeneration, and myofibre loss and necrosis are present with replacement by fibrous connective tissue and scattered mononuclear cell infiltrates. Hydrothorax, and, to a lesser extent, ascites and hepatomegaly may be present. Centrilobular necrosis, edema, and fibrosis may be present in the liver of chronically affected animals.

Hypertrophic cardiomyopathy is less common and is characterized by abnormal thickening of the interventricular septum and left ventricular free wall. Myofiber hypertrophy and fibrosis may be seen in tissue sections. Thromboembolic disease secondary to cardiomyopathy has not been reported in ferrets.

In restrictive cardiomyopathy, the overall heart size may be normal or slightly enlarged but there is widespread replacement of myofibers with fibrous connective tissue. Either or both ventricles may be affected.

2.7.2 Heartworm Disease

Ferrets are highly susceptible to natural infection with *Dirofilaria immitis* and because of their small heart size, only one or two adult worms are sufficient to induce sudden fatal cardiac insufficiency, particularly if they are located within the pulmonary artery or right ventricle. Right atrial or ventricular enlargement may occur with chronic infections, as well as ascites and pleural effusions. Microfilaria may be seen microscopically within pulmonary capillaries, in addition to pulmonary endarteritis, calcified adult worms, and generalized pulmonary edema.

2.7.3 Myocarditis

Toxoplasmosis, sarcocystosis and Aleutian disease (see Section 2.10.1) may result in nonsuppurative myocardi-

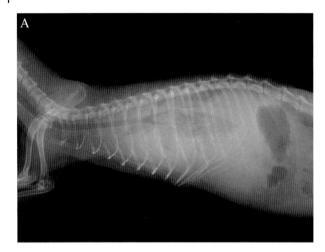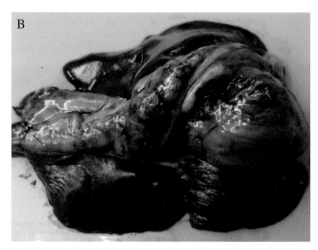

Figure 2.27 A: Radiographic appearance of the thorax in a ferret with congestive heart failure. Severe pleural effusion obscures the heart. B: At post-mortem, the heart was markedly enlarged and flabby, and the lungs were atelectic, wet and heavy. Together with ventricular dilatation, these findings were consistent with dilated cardiomyopathy.

tis with myofiber degeneration, necrosis and localized myocardial necrosis. Characteristic *Toxoplasma* or *Sarcocystis* cysts may be found within myofibers of infected animals.

Idiopathic polymyositis and myofasciitis have been described in ferrets with involvement of cardiac muscle, in addition to skeletal and smooth muscle (see Section 2.5.1). Affected animals present with lethargy, weakness, pain, and fever, and patchy white streaking is seen on the heart and within other muscle tissues at post-mortem. Moderate to severe pyogranulomatous myocarditis can be seen with loss of cross-striations and eventual fibrosis. There is no known cause or treatment and the condition is invariably fatal.

2.7.4 Other Cardiovascular Conditions

Mitral or **aortic valvular** endocardiosis is common in ferrets and presents clinically as valvular regurgitation with echocardiography. Nodular thickening of valve leaflets is seen at post-mortem in addition to atrial dilatation. **Nonbacterial thrombotic endocarditis** has been reported in one 4-year-old ferret with aortic valvular endocardiosis.

Although rare in ferrets, congenital heart lesions have been described and include **atrial** and **ventricular septal defects**, **patent ductus arteriosus**, and **tetralogy of Fallot** (characterized by nonrestrictive ventricular septal defect, overriding aorta, pulmonic stenosis, and secondary right ventricular hypertrophy). Abnormalities may be subclinical and go undetected for a year or more until animals present for surgery or other medical procedures. Common presenting signs include abdominal distension from ascites and muscle wasting.

Primary cardiac tumors are not reported in ferrets, although **thoracic lymphosarcoma** is common. Affected animals may be dyspneic and present with pleural effusion.

2.8 Genitourinary Conditions

Ferrets have multipapillate kidneys that sit just under the sublumbar muscles in the retroperitoneal space. The wall of the urinary bladder is usually quite thin and the bladder does not normally accommodate more than about 10 mL of urine in healthy animals. Unlike some other small mammal species, the urethral orifice of female ferrets exits just cranial to the clitoral fossa within the vaginal vestibule, such that there is a single external orifice. The uterine body is very short in the jill, with long horns. Males have an os penis that lies dorsal to the urethra and the distal end is J-shaped, curving dorsally. The only accessory sex gland in male ferrets is the prostate gland, which is inconspicuous in neutered ferrets. Ferrets use both anal gland secretions and urine marking for recognition of individual animals and differentiation between males and females.

Ferrets with renal disease often exhibit elevated blood urea nitrogen (BUN). Serum creatinine is considered a less sensitive parameter for evaluating renal function in ferrets, compared with cats and dogs, and may show only mild elevations or remain within normal reference values in ferrets with kidney problems.

2.8.1 Urinary Tract Conditions

Urinary tract and renal diseases are moderately common in aging ferrets as in other small mammal pet species.

2.8.1.1 Cystic Renal Disease

Congenital renal tubular cysts, either singular or multiple, occur in 10–5% of ferrets, and are often incidental in nature, being identified during ultrasound or routine post mortem examination. Cortical cysts may be up to 1 cm in diameter and clinically palpable. They are generally thin-walled, fluid-filled, and bulge from the capsular surface (Figure 2.28A). Microscopically, cysts are lined by simple flattened to cuboidal epithelium, and are usually found within the cortex. Pericyst fibrosis is variable, ranging from none to moderate interstitial fibrosis with nonsuppurative inflammation and scattered tubular degeneration.

2.8.1.2 Cystitis

Primary cystitis and pyelonephritis are less common in neutered pet ferrets compared with rabbits and rodents. Jills are more susceptible to bacterial cystitis because of their shorter urethra. In sporadic cases, *Escherichia coli*, *Staphylococcus aureus*, *Pseudomonas* sp., or *Proteus* sp. may be cultured from urine or affected tissue of an animal with cystitis. Bacterial cystitis may also occur secondary to urolithiasis.

2.8.1.3 Urolithiasis

Uroliths occur sporadically and are more common in adult animals chronically fed poor quality diets. Male ferrets are 2.5 times more likely to develop uroliths than females because of their J-shaped os penis, which leads to narrowing of the distal urethra. Ferrets fed a high-quality, high-protein diet will generally have a urine pH of 6.0–6.5. Feeding ferrets low protein diets will make the urine pH alkaline, increasing their susceptibility to struvite (magnesium ammonium phosphate) crystal precipitation. Calcium oxalate and cystine uroliths can also occur, although they are much less common and the etiopathogenesis for these types of crystals is less clear. Cystine precipitates in acidic urine, and as in humans and dogs, cystine urolithiasis is often familial. It has been speculated that a familial disorder may predispose ferrets to this cysteine urolithiasis, however, this requires further investigation.

Clinically, animals may present with vocalization during urination, stranguria, urine dribbling and scalding, genital overgrooming, and hematuria. Bladder rupture may occur in cases of complete urethral obstruction. Single or multiple variably-sized calculi can occur anywhere along the urogenital tract, although less commonly in the ureters.

2.8.1.4 Chronic Renal Disease

Chronic renal disease is common in middle-aged to aging ferrets. Kidneys may be pitted with capsular adhesions (see Figure 2.28B). In some cases, membranoproliferative glomerulonephropathy is seen, consisting of thickening of Bowman's capsule and the mesangial tufts as well as hyalinization of glomerular capillary walls, scattered pyknosis of mesangial cell nuclei, and glomerular sclerosis. Mild lymphoplasmacytic interstitial inflammation and fibrosis with patchy tubular degeneration and regeneration may also be present, and may be accompanied by widespread tubular dilatation with attenuation of the epithelial lining and sloughing of pyknotic renal tubular epithelial cells. Eosinophilic proteinaceous material may be present within tubules, as well as mineralized debris. In other cases, the lesions are predominantly interstitial with mild to moderate lymphoplasmacytic infiltrates and fibrosis.

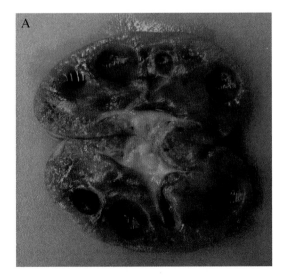 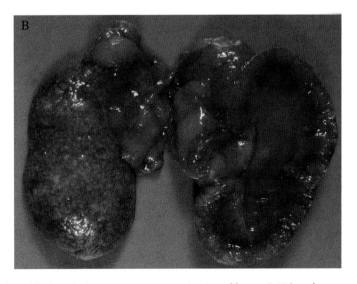

Figure 2.28 A: Multifocal cortical renal cysts are often an incidental finding during post-mortem examination of ferrets. B: Kidney from an aging ferret. The capsular surface is pitted and undulating. Pallor due to cortical fibrosis is evident on cut section.

Infection with Aleutian disease virus (see Section 2.10.1) can result in multi-organ immune complex deposition and chronic membranous glomerulonephropathy. Parvovirus infection should be considered as a potential differential diagnosis for chronic renal disease in adult ferrets. A definitive diagnosis can be made using counter-immunoelectrophoresis to detect viral antibodies or PCR assays of tissues or fecal swabs.

2.8.1.5 Renal Neoplasia

Primary renal neoplasms are rare in pet ferrets, with only sporadic reports of renal carcinoma and transitional cell tumors of the urinary bladder. Renal lymphosarcoma is not uncommon, however, and hemangiosarcoma has also been reported in the kidney. Renal tubular cell neoplasms, often with central osseous metaplasia, have been reported as a familial condition in captive black-footed ferrets.

2.8.1.6 Other Renal Conditions

Hydronephrosis and **hydroureter** are sporadic entities that may occur secondary to urethral obstruction, prostatic hypertrophy, paraurethral cysts or obstructive urolithiasis.

Large, single or multiple thin-walled *cysts* filled with clear fluid and adherent to the serosal surface of the urinary bladder and ureters have been found in both male and female adult ferrets. The cysts were palpable clinically as caudal abdominal masses and several animals presented with dysuria and hematuria. Cysts were lined with nonkeratinized flattened to cuboidal epithelium and epithelial erosions, ulceration and nonsuppurative inflammation were noted in the adjacent urinary bladder mucosa of several animals. The cysts were likely congenital and may have arisen from mesonephric or paramesonephric duct remnants.

Ectopic ureter with urinary incontinence was seen in a 6-month-old female spayed ferret. In this animal, the ureter entered the urinary bladder caudal to the urethral sphincter, resulting in constant urine dribbling.

Ureteral rupture can be seen in cases of motor vehicle or blunt force trauma to the abdomen.

2.8.2 Reproductive Tract Conditions

Female ferrets become sexually mature around 7 months of age, whereas males are mature at 8 months of age or older. Ferrets are long day seasonal breeders and jills are induced ovulators. Plasma estrogen levels become elevated in jills in estrus resulting in swelling and erythema of the vulva (Figure 2.29). Failure to ovulate, either by natural mating or mechanical stimulation of the cervix, can result in estrogen-induced bone marrow suppression (see: Section 2.10.2).

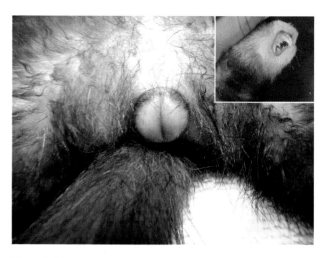

Figure 2.29 Hyperestrogenemia and vulvar swelling in an intact jill. Inset: Many jills will remain in estrus if not bred, resulting in estrogen-related bone marrow depression, anemia (inset), and death, if untreated. *Source:* Courtesy of C. Wheler.

Ferret embryos implant approximately 12 days after successful mating and ovulation and the gestation period lasts for about 42 days. Progesterone from corpora lutea is required for the duration of pregnancy. Corpora lutea are maintained by prolactin released from the anterior pituitary gland. Any conditions affecting either formation of corpora lutea or release of prolactin may result in pregnancy failure.

2.8.2.1 Congenital Malformations and Neonatal Mortality

Ferret litter sizes can range up to 15–18 kits but the average size is about 8 kits. Preweaning mortality may be as high as 20%, although it is usually less than 7% in well-managed colonies. Congenital malformations are found in <1% of kits that die before weaning, primarily consisting of cranioschisis, palatoschisis, kinked tail, short tail, open eyes, and splay leg.

Kits are altricial and require constant maternal care in their early life. Causes of neonatal mortality include agalactia, poor mothering, cannibalism (if the jill is disturbed), diarrhea (induced by bacteria or rotavirus), and umbilical cord entangling. Parturition normally lasts only a few hours and any delays, for example, due to dystocia from fetal-maternal size mismatch or malpresentation, may result in stillborn kits.

2.8.2.2 Uterine Conditions

Pyometra can occur in older, intact pseudopregnant jills and is characterized clinically by a foul-smelling red-brown discharge, lethargy, depression, anorexia, and pyrexia. Grossly, the uterus is markedly enlarged, hyperemic, and filled with purulent exudate. Microscopically, endometrial glands are dilated and cystic, with sloughing of epithelial cells and moderate to marked neutrophilic infiltrates. Bacterial isolates from affected animals include *Escherichia coli*, *Staphylococcus* sp., *Streptococcus* sp. and *Corynebacterium* sp. Cystic endometrial hyperplasia and stump pyometras can occur in neutered jills if ovarian remnants are present. These animals are also at risk for developing estrogen-associated bone marrow suppression (see Section 2.10.2).

Hydrometra is common in jills in parts of Europe in which animals undergo ovariectomy at sexual maturity but the uterus is left intact. The condition is thought to arise from ovarian remnants, estrogen signaling from ovarian-related neoplasms, or hormonal signaling from adrenal gland disease. Animals may present with alopecia and marked abdominal enlargement.

Metritis may occur after fetal abortion or if placentas are retained postpartum. Histologic characteristics are as for other small animals.

2.8.2.3 Ovarian Remnants

Ovarian remnants occur sporadically in North American ferrets, likely because of the technique used for ovariectomy in 6-week-old ferrets. Ovaries in very young animals may be freed during surgery by tearing the ovarian pedicles instead of clamping, ligating, and sectioning the pedicles, as is done in older animals. The former method may result in small pieces of ovarian tissue remaining in the animal. Ovarian remnants should be considered as a differential diagnosis for vulvar swelling, alopecia, and estrogen-induced bone marrow toxicity in jills, along with adrenal gland disease. In general, signs of estrus and estrogen-related side effects occur earlier in jills with ovarian remnants (less than 2 years of age) than in jills with adrenal gland disease (more than 2 years of age). Various neoplasms may also arise from the ovarian remnants (see below).

2.8.2.4 Pregnancy Toxemia and Postparturient Hypocalcemia

Pregnancy toxemia can occur during the last quarter of gestation, more frequently in primiparous jills, and is initiated by a period of anorexia due to stress, poor nutritional management, dietary changes, or intercurrent illness. Animals are often in shock when diagnosed, presenting comatose or with severe lethargy and depression, hypothermia, and dehydration. They may also die peracutely. The prognosis for the jill and kits is very poor, even with treatment for acidosis and caesarian section removal of the kits. The pathogenesis of the condition is the same as for ruminants or rabbits, with acidosis and accumulation of ketone bodies secondary to massive fatty acid mobilization. Grossly, the liver may be enlarged,

pale, and greasy with marked macrovesiculation of hepatocytes noted microscopically.

Post-parturient hypocalcemia (milk fever) can occur in jills within 3–4 weeks after parturition. The condition is initiated by poor nutrition and animals may present with hind end paresis or convulsions. No gross or microscopic lesions may be present.

2.8.2.5 Prostatic Conditions

Adrenal gland disease and the resulting chronic increase in circulating sex steroid hormone levels may stimulate proliferation and hypertrophy of prostatic tissue in male ferrets, leading to accumulation of secretions, squamous metaplasia of the gland lining, and keratin production, eventually leading to cyst formation (Figure 2.30). Sludging of proteinaceous material within cysts can also lead to ascending bacterial infections, prostatitis, abscessation, chronic suppurative inflammation, and stromal fibrosis. As the prostate surrounds the neck of the urinary bladder and proximal urethra in the ferret, prostatic hyperplasia, with or without the development of prostatic cysts, may result in partial or complete urethral obstruction and dysuria or anuria. This is the leading cause of urethral obstruction in North American male ferrets. Affected animals may present with stranguria, urine dribbling, tenesmus, inappropriate genital grooming, and abdominal swelling. Cystic prostatic enlargement can also cause obstipation.

2.8.2.6 Female Reproductive Masses

Ovarian tumors are seen sporadically in spayed jill, likely due to ovarian remnants. In addition to presenting with an abdominal mass, animals may have other signs related

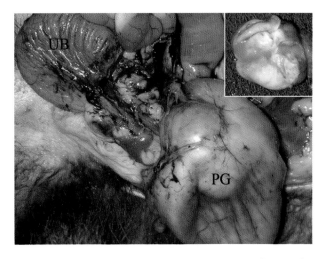

Figure 2.30 Multiloculated prostatic cysts in an aging ferret with adrenal gland adenocarcinoma. (UB = urinary bladder, PG = cysts in prostate gland). Inset: Large prostatic cyst opened to reveal suppurative content and connecting channels between cysts.

to estrogen production, such as alopecia and vulvar swelling. Tumors reported include thecoma, leiomyoma, teratoma, and granulosa cell tumor. Uterine leiomyoma and teratoma have also been reported.

2.8.2.7 Male Reproductive Masses

Testicular tumors are very uncommon, may involve a cryptorchid testicle, and include Sertoli and interstitial cell tumors, as well as seminomas. Tumors are grossly and microscopically similar to those seen in dogs and cats. An intratesticular peripheral nerve sheath tumor has also been noted in a 6-year-old male ferret kept at a zoo.

2.8.2.8 Other Reproductive Conditions

Ferret testes normally descend into the scrotum during fetal development, but if not, they should descend by no later than 6 months of age. Occasionally, one testicle may not have descended in a male kit by 6 weeks of age, the time that these kits are usually neutered in North America, and only one testicle will be removed during the surgery. Owners may notice a scrotal "swelling" as these animals become sexually mature, which will usually turn out to be a normal testicle. Sexually intact male ferrets will have a thicker neck and heavier coat than males that are castrated at six weeks of age. True **cryptorchidism** is uncommon in male ferrets and reported to be seen in <0.75% of males.

Penile trauma with hematoma formation is seen occasionally in male ferrets.

A **cloaca-like congenital malformation** was reported in a 2-month-old female ferret that was lacking external genitalia and a tail. Following euthanasia, a post-mortem examination demonstrated an intrapelvic structure into which the distal colon, uterus and urethra emptied. The right kidney was also misshapen.

2.9 Nervous System Conditions

Although ferrets commonly present for ataxia, weakness, and seizures, primary neurologic disease is uncommon. There are many potential causes of apparent neurologic disease in the ferret including systemic infection, hypoglycemia from a pancreatic islet cell tumor, toxin ingestion (e.g., lead or ibuprofen), hepatic or renal failure, cardiac disease and related hypoxia, anemia, trauma or primary or secondary neoplasia with impingement of the brain or spinal cord.

2.9.1 Congenital Malformations or Defects

Compared to a cat, the ferret brain is slightly smaller and narrower, although sulci and gyri are present. Congenital malformations of the neural tube, including inencephaly, which consists of a defect in the back of the skull, a spinal column fissure and cervical retroflexion, have been reported in two litters of ferret kits. Kits had other congenital malformations, including anencephaly. The two litters were sired by the same male to different dams, suggesting a genetic defect in the male.

Congenital peripheral vestibular syndrome was reported in a 3 month-old male ferret with a 2-month history of ataxia. The animal presented with a marked head tilt and was noted to have mild, bilateral asymmetry of the inner ear labyrinth and cochlea, based on MRI evaluation, as well as unilateral deafness. The animal was treated supportively and no pathology work-up was undertaken.

Coat color-linked bilateral or unilateral congenital sensorineural deafness is reported in pet ferrets at a prevalence of up to 29%. Similar to other species, the condition is usually associated with a white or white-marked coat color (examples of the latter include panda, silver, blaze, and mitt), and prevalence is particularly high in animals with premature graying, although albino animals are usually unaffected. The condition is linked to dysfunction of or failure of neural crest melanocytes to migrate within the stria vascularis of the cochlea and can be tested for under general anesthesia via a brainstem auditory evoked response test. Albino animals are generally unaffected because they have melanocytes in the inner ear but the melanocytes are homozygous negative for the tyrosinase gene. This enzyme catalyzes several important steps needed for melanin synthesis, resulting in albinism. Because albinism is dominant over other coat colors, it can mask underlying white or white-marked coat colors resulting in deafness in sporadic albino ferrets.

2.9.2 Rabies

Rabies virus infection is caused by a Rhabdovirus and is rarely reported in pet ferrets in North America, although they are susceptible to virus infection and natural cases of rabies have occurred in ferrets. Some experimentally infected ferrets have recovered from rabies virus infection. Following inoculation with rabies virus, a subset of ferrets survived infection but had lasting paresis.

2.9.2.1 Presenting Clinical Signs

Clinical signs of rabies in ferrets include ascending paralysis, ataxia, cachexia, bladder atony, pyrexia, hyperactivity, tremors, and paresthesia. Clinical signs occur within one month post-exposure, however, death usually ensues within four to five days after clinical signs of infection appear.

2.9.2.2 Pathology

There are no gross lesions associated with the disease. Histopathology may demonstrate multifocal areas of lymphocytic infiltrates with gliosis, perivascular lymphocytic cuffing, edema, and neurodegeneration. Negri bodies (eosinophilic intracytoplasmic inclusion bodies within affected neurons) can sometimes be seen in infected ferrets.

2.9.2.3 Laboratory Diagnostics

Rabies virus infection is a reportable disease in Canada and the United States. Tissues or samples from suspect positive cases should be submitted to the appropriate regulatory authorities. Direct fluorescence immunoassay on fresh or frozen brain is used by state and federal laboratories to confirm infection. Immunohistochemistry, RT-PCR, and virus isolation also may be used for viral detection.

2.9.2.4 Differential Diagnoses

Head trauma or other agents inducing central nervous system disease, such as canine distemper virus infection, Aleutian disease, lead intoxication, brain abscess, neoplasia, and cryptococcosis are more common than rabies virus infection in ferrets. However, a history of exposure to feral or other potentially rabid animals or outdoor housing may increase the diagnostic consideration of this disease.

2.9.2.5 Disease Management

In North America, ferret vaccination against rabies virus is required in many jurisdictions using a product specifically licensed for ferrets. Because ferrets often nip other ferrets or their owners during play, suspect cases should remain in a veterinary clinic for close observation. Anaphylactic reactions to vaccination occur in <1% of ferrets receiving rabies vaccine, either alone or in combination with canine distemper virus vaccine.

2.9.3 Canine Distemper Virus

Infection with canine distemper virus (see Section 2.4.2 for a fuller discussion) may result in severe neurologic disease in ferrets. Central nervous system signs occur later in the course of infection, and include myoclonus, paresis, muscular tremors, hyperexcitability, convulsions, and coma. Viral inclusions bodies may be seen within neurons and glial cells, as well as within a variety of epithelial tissues.

2.9.4 Aleutian Disease

Infection with Aleutian disease virus (see Section 2.10.1), a parvovirus, may result in tremors, ataxia, paresis, and convulsions. Affected ferrets may also demonstrate generalized lymphadenopathy, chronic wasting, and hyper-gammaglobulinemia. Brain and spinal cord lesions in infected ferrets are nonspecific and include lymphoplasmacytic meningitis, perivascular lymphoplasmacytic cuffing, and focal cerebral malacia.

2.9.5 Cryptococcosis

Lethargy, depression, and anorexia have been reported in ferrets infected systemically with *Cryptococcus* spp. Splenomegaly, lymphadenopathy and miliary multi-organ nodules are seen in affected animals. The nodules consist of granulomatous to pyogranulomatous inflammation surrounding numerous thick-walled, narrow-based, budding yeast organisms. DNA typing is required for definitive speciation.

2.9.6 Cerebrospinal Neoplasia

Tumors of the brain and spinal cord are very rare in ferrets with single reports of meningioma, astrocytoma, and glioma (Figure 2.31).

Pituitary adenomas may be found occasionally in adult ferrets with adrenal gland disease and hyperadrenocorticism. Neoplastic cells from pituitary masses are negative for prolactin, ACTH, TSH, GH, LH, and FSH markers, immunologically, suggesting that they are not gonadotroph adenomas and that adrenal tumors in ferrets form independent of pituitary tumor stimulation. Masses are unencapsulated and expansile and may induce ischemic necrosis in surrounding tissue as they grow.

A large, white, expansile and compressive forebrain mass was noted in a ferret euthanized for seizures that were refractory to treatment. Histologically, the mass was composed of sheets of polygonal cells within a fine fibrovascular stroma and the center of the mass was necrotic. Neoplastic cells were large with a pale, finely granular cytoplasm and had eccentric small nuclei and mitoses were scant. A granular cell tumor was diagnosed based on the histopathology.

A 6-year-old ferret presenting with a short history of progressive head tilt and ataxia was diagnosed with an obstructive choroid plexus papilloma arising from the fourth ventricle, which resulted in development of hydrocephalus. Microscopically, the mass consisted of well-differentiated neoplastic epithelial cells arranged in papillary fingers within a fine fibrovascular stroma.

Many other nonneuronal neoplasias, including lymphosarcoma, chordoma of the vertebrae, plasma cell myeloma with vertebral erosion, osteoma, teratoma, and fibrosarcoma, may occur within the brain or spinal cord or within the skull or vertebrae of the ferret, resulting in impingement upon and necrosis of neural tissue. Clinical signs will depend upon the location of the neoplastic mass.

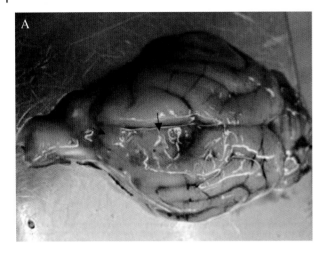
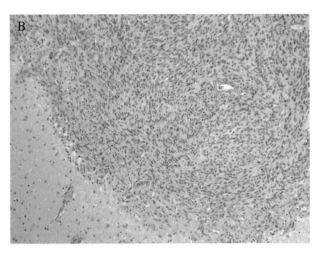

Figure 2.31 A: A unilateral, locally extensive area of widened gyri with flattening (arrows), consistent with cerebral edema and a cerebral mass, in a 2-year-old neutered female ferret presenting with an acute onset of weakness and seizures. B: A fibrous meningioma was diagnosed, based on the spindle-shaped cells embedded in an abundant collagenous matrix. The tumor is both compressing the subtending parenchyma and beginning to invade along vascular pathways.

2.9.7 Other Conditions of the Brain and Spinal Cord

Thoracolumbar **intervertebral disk herniation** is seen sporadically in adult ferrets and causes acute paresis to paralysis. The pathogenesis of the condition is variable and includes trauma, discospondylitis, and degeneration of disk material.

***Clostridium botulinum* type C endotoxin** may induce profound ataxia, paresis, and salivation within 8–12 hours of ingestion, which can progress to flaccid paralysis and death. The cause is related to improper storage and handling of fresh meat diets leading to bacterial reproduction and toxin production and accumulation. There are no characteristic gross or microscopic signs in affected animals.

Subclinical nonsuppurative encephalitis, lymphoplasmacytic perivascular cuffing, and focal cerebral hemorrhages have been reported in asymptomatic ferrets after experimental inoculation with H5N1 **influenza virus** variants.

Idiopathic neuronal vacuolation has been reported in a 5-year-old ferret presenting with acute ataxia and convulsions. No infectious agent was isolated from the brain of this animal.

2.10 Hematopoietic and Lymphoid Conditions

Ferrets have no recognized blood groups and do not require cross-matching for transfusion therapy. The red blood cell count, hematocrit, hemoglobin levels, and reticulocyte count are higher in ferrets than in cats and dogs and the lifespan of an erythrocyte is shorter, giving rise to polychromasia in blood smears of normal animals. White blood cell counts are normally low and neutrophils are the predominant white blood cell type. Cytoplasmic granules in ferret neutrophils are paler than those found within neutrophils of cats and dogs. Caution should be used when interpreting the ferret hemogram as ferrets do not always display a left shift in white blood cell counts in response to acute infections. There are both sex- and age-related differences in the ferret hemogram and specific reference ranges should be consulted when interpreting hematology results. In addition, isoflurane inhalant anesthesia has been demonstrated to induce splenic sequestration of erythrocytes in ferrets, significantly altering apparent values for red blood cell count, hematocrit, and hemoglobin levels. It has a lesser effect on circulating white blood cell counts. It is important for the pathologist to remember that extramedullary hematopoiesis is common in ferrets.

2.10.1 Aleutian Disease

Aleutian disease (AD) virus is a parvovirus of mustelids and is a commercially important disease of farmed mink. Several mutations have occurred within the mink virus genome and ferret-specific mutants cause disease in ferrets. The prevalence of AD virus infection in pet ferret populations in North America is unknown. A serologic survey of ferrets in a club of ferret enthusiasts in the UK indicated 8.5% of animals were seropositive for AD antibodies. The severity of the disease in ferrets depends on the strain of virus, age of animal, and presence of intercurrent disease. The disease may be more acute and severe in younger animals. In some ferrets, the virus persists for years while in others the infection is acute and self-limiting.

2.10.1.1 Presenting Clinical Signs

AD virus infections in ferrets may be asymptomatic but animals may also show signs of lethargy, depression, anorexia, melena, and chronic weight loss that progress in severity over time. Depending on the body systems affected, posterior paresis with urine soiling, tremors, and convulsions may also be seen. Animals initially mount an ineffective humoral response to the virus and may demonstrate hypergammaglobulinemia.

2.10.1.2 Pathology

Gross findings in ferrets with Aleutian disease are nonspecific and include splenomegaly, hepatomegaly, and generalized lymphadenopathy. Multi-organ lymphoplasmacytic or plasmacytic infiltrates may be seen microscopically, including within the renal interstitium and splenic red pulp, surrounding portal triads in the liver, within the medulla of lymph nodes, and in the bone marrow. Within the brain and spinal cord there may be perivascular lymphoplasmacytic cuffing, focal to locally extensive malacia and astrocytosis, and mild nonsuppurative meningitis. Deposition of immune complexes within tissues can result in membranous glomerulonephropathy and multi-organ vasculitis.

2.10.1.3 Laboratory Diagnostics

Counter-immunoelectrophoresis is a simple and rapid assay commonly used in suspect cases of AD to determine ferret antibody levels. PCR assays also exist to directly detect viral nucleic acids, however, the routine availability of these assays in diagnostic laboratories is limited.

2.10.1.4 Differential Diagnoses

There are many other conditions of ferrets that can cause signs of ataxia, anorexia, and incoordination, as well as chronic wasting disease, including gastrointestinal ulcers, proliferative enteritis, cardiomyopathy, bacterial enteritis, lymphosarcoma, multiple myeloma, anemia of any cause, ferret coronavirus infection, and eosinophilic gastroenteritis. Canine distemper virus also results in fatal nonsuppurative encephalitis, however, the disease time course is shorter than typically seen for AD. Posterior paresis with urine soiling may occur with intervertebral disk disease, vertebral fractures, and tumors of the vertebral column or spinal cord.

2.10.1.5 Disease/Group Management

AD virus is shed in the saliva, urine, and feces and transmission occurs directly by respiratory droplets. Asymptomatic infected ferrets can shed virus into the environment for many months. There is no treatment or preventative for AD in ferrets. Introducing ferrets of unknown health status from shelters into multiferret households can be risky. Best practices would include quarantining animals prior to introductions or after returning from shows or trials in which animals are in contact with other ferrets, and testing new introductions for AD antibodies.

2.10.2 Anemia

Anemia is a very common clinical finding in pet ferrets and has many potential etiologies, including lymphosarcoma, adrenal gland tumors, hyperestrogenism, pancreatic islet cell tumors, gastric ulcers, chronic systemic inflammation or infection, or hepatic or renal disease. Gross and microscopic examinations should help to direct investigations as to the root cause of the condition.

Hyperestrogenism or estrogen-induced bone marrow toxicity is an important cause of pancytopenia in intact jills that experience prolonged estrus, neutered jills with ovarian remnants, and male and female ferrets with adrenal gland disease. Nonregenerative anemia occurs in these animals because of severe estrogen-induced bone marrow suppression and increased blood loss from thrombocytopenia. Untreated animals may die from hemorrhage. Clinically, ferrets with hyperestrogenism may present with a swollen and erythematous vulva, pallor, alopecia, petechiation, hematuria, and melena. Bone marrow evaluation will demonstrate severe depletion of all cell types.

Pure red cell aplasia has been reported in ferrets and should be considered as a potential differential diagnosis for aplastic anemia, when more common causes have been ruled out. The condition is likely acquired and is thought to be due to antibody-mediated targeting of erythrocytes or their precursors or erythropoietin. To date, animals with this condition have tested negative for Aleutian disease virus and canine distemper virus antibodies.

2.10.3 Splenomegaly

Splenic enlargement is a very common and nonspecific finding in adult ferrets, although it can occasionally be seen in animals less than a year of age. The ferret spleen is normally quite large for the size of the animal, but when enlarged and engorged, it can hamper movement of animals and can readily be seen and palpated as a longitudinal ventral abdominal mass up to 10 cm in length (Figure 2.32). The potential causes of splenomegaly are multiple and include extramedullary hematopoiesis, lymphosarcoma and other neoplasias such as hemangiosarcoma, chronic infections, and cardiomyopathy.

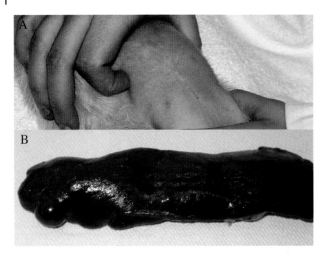

Figure 2.32 A: Idiopathic splenomegaly in a ferret. The spleen can be readily visualized as well as palpated through the abdominal wall. B: The spleen in this animal was surgically resected and was markedly enlarged. The red pulp was expanded, however, there was no evidence of neoplasia.

In the vast majority of cases, splenic enlargement is caused by increased extramedullary hematopoiesis, which results in diffuse enlargement of the spleen and marked expansion of the red pulp, with high mitotic rates and proliferation of all cell types, including erythroid, myeloid, and platelet precursors. There are no accompanying changes in peripheral blood cell counts. Nodular splenic enlargement can occur with chronic mycotic infections and neoplasias, and other lymph nodes may be enlarged with these conditions.

Enlarged spleens are friable and prone to rupture, and rarely, torsion. Affected animals may present with hemoabdomen and microscopically, multifocal areas of coagulation necrosis surrounded by neutrophilic infiltrates and granulation tissue may be present in the spleen.

2.10.4 Lymphosarcoma

Lymphosarcoma is the most common neoplasm seen in ferrets of any age and accounts for up to 15% of all neoplasms seen in ferrets. Traditionally, lymphoid tumors have been supposed to arise spontaneously in ferrets, however, clusters of lymphosarcoma in multiferret households and experimental horizontal transmission of lymphosarcoma in ferrets have suggested that an infectious agent, possibly a type C retrovirus, may be responsible for tumor initiation.

Clinical signs of lymphosarcoma include anorexia, chronic weight loss, splenomegaly, and internal and peripheral lymphadenopathy. A marked lymphocytosis may be seen on the complete blood count and differential, and anemia and thrombocytopenia may also be present. Elevated serum calcium levels can be seen in some ferrets with lymphosarcoma, similar to hypercalcemia of malignancy seen in other species.

Classically, two primary presentations of lymphosarcoma are seen in ferrets, based on age of animal and anatomic location. The juvenile form of the disease has an acute onset and is rapidly progressive with a mean survival time of less than two months. It is multicentric and lymphoblastic in nature, and may involve the kidneys, spleen, liver, lung, and thymus, leading to dyspnea and pleural effusion, which may be misdiagnosed as respiratory or cardiac disease. In rare cases, only the spleen may be involved. Microscopically, there is effacement of the normal architecture of affected tissues by a monomorphic population of large lymphocytes with both cleaved and noncleaved nuclei. Nuclei are round to oval, cytoplasmic borders are distinct and the mitotic rate is high (>6–8/high power field). Smaller numbers of well differentiated lymphocytes may be present within infiltrates. Immunophenotyping with anti-human CD3 polyclonal antibodies indicates that the majority of these tumors are of T cell origin. Animals in terminal stages of the disease may have a lymphocytic leukemia.

The adult form is usually chronic in nature, affecting animals older than 3 years of age and clinical signs may wax and wane over the course of months. These animals often are lymphopenic and anemic, and present with peripheral lymphadenopathy with later spread to visceral organs (Figure 2.33). Involvement of vertebral bone marrow may result in paresis following bony fracture and extension into the vertebral canal. Microscopically, infiltrates consist of well-differentiated neoplastic lymphocytes with noncleaved nuclei and modest mitotic rates.

Epitheliotropic lymphoma, retroorbital lymphoma, and immunoblastic polymorphous lymphoma are also seen in ferrets. In the latter disease, animals older than 2 years of age are affected and small to large polymorphic lymphocytes are present, many with bizarre nuclei. Epitheliotropic lymphoma is of T cell origin and presents as single or multiple, sometimes hairless, pruritic cutaneous plaques anywhere on the body, including the prepuce and toes. Retroorbital lymphoma may present in adult ferrets as exophthalmos and exposure keratitis in addition to the presence of peripheral lymphadenopathy. Rare cases of gastric MALT lymphosarcoma have been correlated with chronic *Helicobacter mustelae* infection in ferrets. In these animals, only the gastric wall and one or two local lymph nodes are involved (Figure 2.34).

Consistent with trends in veterinary pathology to more accurately develop tumor classification schemes and to assist with prognostication for clinicians and owners, a standard approach to description of lymphosarcomas in ferrets has been proposed that would include the clinical

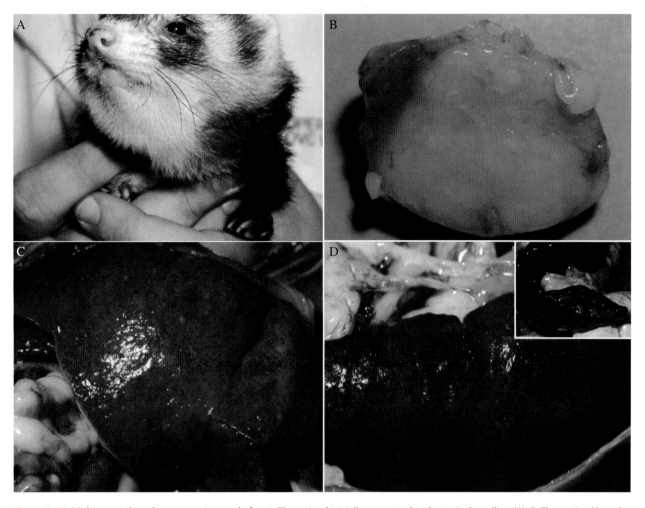

Figure 2.33 Multicentric lymphosarcoma in a male ferret. The animal initially presented with cervical swelling (A). B: The excised lymph node was enlarged, firm, and white on cut section and was microscopically consistent with a B cell lymphosarcoma. C: The disease progressed, resulting in eventual euthanasia. At post-mortem, the liver was markedly enlarged. D: Splenomegaly was also noted in this ferret at post-mortem, and neoplastic tissue bulged from the cut surface (inset).

stage of the disease based on anatomic site and lesion distribution, histologic description of the tumor, and immunophenotyping to determine the primary cell of origin (i.e., B or T lymphocyte). Anti-human antibodies for CD3 (T cell) and CD79 (B cell) generally show good cross-reactivity in ferret tumors. There is poor correlation between classification of lymphosarcomas diagnosed by fine needle aspirate versus histopathology, and surgical biopsy is the preferred diagnostic method.

2.10.5 Other Hematopoietic Neoplasms

Hemangiomas and **hemangiosarcomas** are diagnosed occasionally in the liver, spleen or skin of ferrets and microscopic characteristics are the same as for dogs (Figure 2.35).

Thymomas are rare tumors in ferrets and affected animals may present with dyspnea, coughing, reduced exercise tolerance, and episodic vomiting, and a radiographically visible mediastinal mass may be present. Grossly, a large tan tumor is present in the cranial mediastinum, which consists, microscopically, of an expansile and infiltrative dense mass of neoplastic epithelial cells admixed with normal lymphocytes arranged in solid and glandular patterns within a fine fibrovascular stroma. Neoplastic cells have a round to ovoid nucleus with abundant heterochromatin and a single nucleolus and may have vacuolated cytoplasm, and mitoses are generally scant. The primary and more common differential diagnosis for a cranial mediastinal mass is lymphosarcoma.

Splenic myelolipoma has been reported in a 5-year-old pet ferret. Myelolipomas are rare, benign masses consisting of an admixture of adipose and hematopoietic tissues. Grossly there was marked splenic enlargement in this animal and multifocal yellow nodules up to 0.4 cm diameter were present on the surface of the spleen and throughout the parenchyma. Similar nodules were present on the kid-

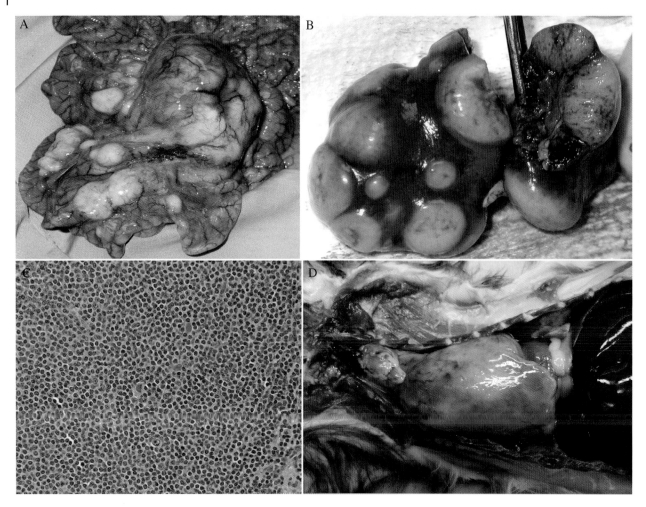

Figure 2.34 A: Adult form of lymphosarcoma with multifocally enlarged mesenteric lymph nodes. B: Multiple firm renal nodules were found in the same animal. C: The histologic appearance consists of dense, monomorphic sheets of round cells with variable mitotic rates. D: Thymic lymphosarcoma also occurs in ferrets but much less commonly. *Source:* A and B: Courtesy of The Links Road Animal and Bird Clinic.

ney and pancreas. Histologically, the masses were nonencapsulated and compressive and composed of clusters of adipocytes and hematopoietic cells of all lineages. The etiopathogenesis of this condition is unknown.

2.10.6 Other Hematopoietic and Lymphoid Conditions

***Cryptococcus* spp.** is a dimorphic fungus found in the environment, more commonly in hot, arid climates, and infection of humans and animals is typically acquired through inhalation of yeast-like forms. Both *C. gattii* and *C. neoformans* have been associated with chronic lymphadenopathy and multi-organ granulomas in pet ferrets. Cryptococcosis is a zoonotic condition and asymptomatically infected human caregivers and other pet ferrets have been identified within the same household as infected animals with clinical signs of disease. Granulomatous lesions within the spleen and lymph node may demonstrate numerous macrophages and multinucleated giant cells, and lesser numbers of neutrophils, lymphocytes and plasma cells. Within the granulomas, numerous fungal organisms (5 to 10 um in diameter) are present with a PAS-positive thick capsule that appears as a clear halo around the organism in hematoxylin and eosin-stained tissue sections. A latex cryptococcal antigen agglutination assay can be used to detect polysaccharide capsular antigen.

Mycobacterium celatum has been diagnosed as a cause of chronic splenitis in several pet ferrets presenting with chronic weight loss and malaise. Numerous Ziehl-Neelsen-positive bacilli were visualized within macrophages and granulomatous lesions within the spleen. Definitive diagnosis requires 16S rDNA sequence analysis. The source of mycobacterial exposure remained obscure in all cases. This agent is zoonotic to humans and has been diagnosed in people with overt immunosuppression.

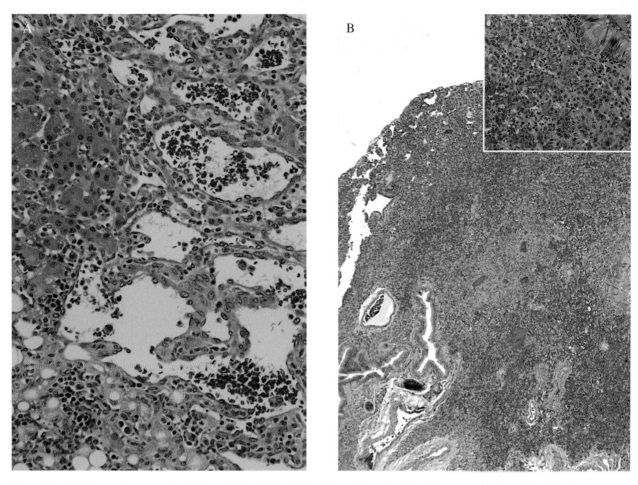

Figure 2.35 A: Hemangiosarcoma in the liver of a ferret. Blood-filled channels are lined by plump, neoplastic endothelial cells. B: Hemangiosarcoma in the lung of a ferret. Alveolar spaces are filled with hemosiderin-laden macrophages (inset).

Benzocaine-induced methemoglobinemia occurred in ferrets treated topically within the oral cavity to facilitate endotracheal intubation. P-aminobenzoic acid, a benzocaine metabolite, induces the oxidation of hemoglobin to methemoglobin. If methemoglobin is present in significant concentrations, the oxygen-carrying capacity of erythrocytes is reduced. Lidocaine is not associated with methemoglobinemia in clinically relevant doses.

Splenosis, the presence of heterotypic splenic tissue, and the presence of an **accessory spleen** are rarely seen in ferrets. Splenosis is an acquired condition in which splenic tissue embeds within the abdominal cavity, using following splenic rupture. It is often asymptomatic but in one case, presented as a large torsed abdominal mass in a young adult ferret with acute abdominal pain and ambulatory weakness. Accessory spleens are congenital lesions arising from incomplete fusion of the splenic anlage during embryogenesis. These may be found on the tail of the pancreas, splenic hilum, and within the mesentery.

2.11   Ophthalmic Conditions

Ferrets have a holangiotic retinal vascular pattern and a well-developed retrobulbar venous plexus, which can bleed extensively during enucleation surgery. They also have a third eyelid and two lacrimal glands, one located dorsolaterally and the other within the nictitating membrane. *Staphylococcus* sp. and *Corynebacterium* sp. have been isolated from the lid margins and conjunctival sacs of healthy ferrets and may be part of the normal eye flora. Albino ferrets lack tyrosinase, which is critical for melanin synthesis in the retinal pigmented epithelium. Lack of melanin within the retina leads to alterations in fetal retinal development and function with the end result being that these ferrets have motion detection defects compared with pigmented ferrets, and may also have hearing deficits.

Other than cataracts and corneal ulcers, ocular lesions are not commonly reported in ferrets.

2.11.1 Conditions of the Eyelid and Conjunctiva

Neonatal conjunctivitis can be seen in kits up to three weeks of age. Kits present with an accumulation of purulent material within the conjunctival sac, which presents as bulging eyelids, since the eyes are still closed at that time. Several different bacterial agents have been cultured from affected kits, including *E. coli* originating from a dam with mastitis. The etiopathogenesis of this condition is unknown but thought to be due to environmental exposure and contamination.

Conjunctivitis in older ferrets can be caused by a number of different infectious agents, including canine distemper virus, influenza virus, *Mycobacterium* spp., and *Salmonella* spp. Other systemic signs of disease and accompanying pathology should be used to assist with the diagnosis in these cases.

A single report exists for squamous cell carcinoma of the eyelid in a ferret.

2.11.2 Conditions of the Cornea and Anterior Chamber

Congenital corneal dermoid is seen sporadically in young ferrets and is microscopically similar to the same condition in dogs.

Ferrets kept on dusty bedding may have corneal irritation and tearing, which can be exacerbated by self-trauma.

Pyogranulomatous panophthalmitis has been reported in a young adult ferret with a systemic coronavirus infection (see Section 2.6.5.1). In addition to depression and behavioral changes, a unilateral corneal opacity was detected at presentation, which was later correlated to marked infiltrates of macrophages, neutrophils, lymphocytes, and plasma cells within the ciliary body and cornea. Virus presence was confirmed with immunohistochemistry.

2.11.3 Uveal and Lenticular Conditions

Persistent hyperplastic primary vitreous (persistent fetal ocular circulation) occurs sporadically in ferrets and results from retention of hyaloid vessels, proliferation of fibrovascular tissue within the posterior chamber, and eventual formation of cataracts. Osseous metaplasia can be seen at times as well as retinal detachment. This condition has been determined to be due to an autosomal dominant genetic mutation and is also associated with microphthalmia and progressive retinal degeneration.

Acquired cataracts are very common in pet ferrets, although the etiopathogenesis is usually undetermined. Ferrets with diabetes mellitus may be at higher risk for developing cataracts. Primary and secondary glaucoma are unusual in ferrets.

2.11.4 Retinal Conditions

Uveitis and chorioretinitis can occur in ferrets systemically infected with *Cryptococcus* sp. (see Section 2.10.6).

2.11.5 Exophthalmos

Exophthalmos with exposure keratitis is a common presenting sign in ferrets with lymphosarcoma. It can also occur with other retrobulbar tumors as well as a zygomatic salivary gland mucocele.

Bibliography

Introduction

Bell, J.A. (1999) Ferret nutrition. *Veterinary Clinics of North America: Exotic Animal Practice.* **2**(1), 169–192.

Clapperton, B.K. (1989) Scent-marking behaviour of the ferret (*Mustela furo* L.). *Animal Behaviour*, **38**(3), 436–446.

Kondo, K. (2000) The diversity of mammalian pelage. *Journal of Faculty of Agriculture, Hokkaido University*, **70**(1), 9–17.

Lewington, J.H. (2007) *Ferret Husbandry, Medicine and Surgery*, 2nd edn. Saunders, Philadelphia, PA.

Quesenberry, K.E. and Carpenter, J.W. (eds.) (2012) *Ferrets, Rabbits, and Rodents, 3rd edn.* Elsevier, Saunders, St Louis, MO.

Thomson, A.P.D. (1951) A history of the ferret. *Journal of the History of Medicine and Allied Sciences*, **VI** (Autumn), 471–480.

Alopecia

Kelleher, S.A. (2002) Skin diseases of ferrets. *Seminars in Avian and Exotic Pet Medicine*, **11**(3), 136–140.

Patterson, M.M., Rogers, A.B., Schrenzel, M.D., Marini, R.P., and Fox, J.G. (2003) Alopecia attributed to neoplastic ovarian tissue in two ferrets. *Comparative Medicine*, **53**(2), 213–217.

Scott, D.W., Gould, W.J., Cayatte, S.M., Lawrence, H.J., and Miller, Jr W.M. (1994) Figurate erythema resembling erythema annulare centrifugum in a ferret with adrenocortical adenocarcinoma-associated alopecia. *Veterinary Dermatology*, **5**(3), 111–115.

Wheler, C.L., and Kamieniecki, C.L. (1998) Ferret adrenal-associated endocrinopathy. *Canadian Veterinary Journal*, **39**(3), 175–176.

Bacterial Dermatitis

King, W.W., Lemarie, S.L., Veazey, R.S., and Hodgin E.C. (1996) Superficial spreading pyoderma and ulcerative dermatitis in a ferret. *Veterinary Dermatology*, **7**, 43–47.

Skukski, G. and Symmers, W.S. (1954) Actinomycosis and torulosis in the ferret (*Mustela furo* L). *Journal of Comparative Pathology*, **64**(4), 306–311.

Dermatophytoses

Donnelly, T.M., Rush, E.M., and Lackner, P.A. (2000) Ringworm in small exotic pets. *Seminars in Avian and Exotic Pet Medicine*, **9**(2), 82–93.

Greenacre, C.B. (2003) Fungal diseases of ferrets. *Veterinary Clinics of North America: Exotic Animal Practice*, **6**, 435–448.

Hoppmann, E., and Wilson Barron, H. (2007) Ferret and rabbit dermatology. *Journal of Exotic Pet Medicine*, **16**(4), 225–237.

Parasitic Dermatitis

Beaufrere, H., Neta, M., Smith, D.A., and Taylor, W.M. (2009) Demodectic mange associated with lymphoma in a ferret. *Journal of Exotic Pet Medicine*, **18**(1), 57–61.

Erdman, S.E., Brown, S.A., and Kawasaki, T.A., *et al.* (1996) Clinical and pathologic findings in ferrets with lymphoma: 60 cases (1982–1994). *Journal of the American Veterinary Medical Association*, **208**, 1285–1289.

Hoppmann, E., and Wilson Barron, H. (2007) Ferret and rabbit dermatology. *Journal of Exotic Pet Medicine*, **16**(4), 225–237.

Kelleher, S.A. (2002) Skin diseases of ferrets. *Seminars in Avian and Exotic Pet Medicine*, **11**(3), 136–140.

Lohse, J., Rinder, H., Gothe, R., and Zahler, M. (2002) Validity of species status of the parasitic mite *Otodectes cynotis*. *Medical and Veterinary Entomology*, **16**(2), 133–138.

Morrisey, J.K. (1996) Parasites of ferrets, rabbits, and rodents. *Seminars in Avian and Exotic Pet Medicine*, **5**(2), 106–114.

Noli, C., van der Horst, H.H., and Willemse, T. (1996) Demodicosis in ferrets (*Mustela putorius furo*). *Veterinary Quarterly*, **18**(1), 28–31.

Patterson, M.M., and Kirchain, S.M. (1999) Comparison of three treatments for control of ear mites in ferrets. *Laboratory Animal Science*, **49**(6), 655–657.

Phillips, P.H., O'Callaghan, M.G., Moore, E., and Baird, R.M. (1987) Pedal *Sarcoptes scabiei* infestation in ferrets (*Mustela putorius* furo). *Australian Veterinary Journal*, **64**(9), 289–290.

Cutaneous Neoplasms and Masses

Beach, J.E., and Greenwood, B. (1993) Spontaneous neoplasia in the ferret (*Mustela putorius furo*). *Journal of Comparative Pathology*, **108**(2), 133–147.

Berrocal, A. (2007) Dermal and subcutaneous extraskeletal osteosarcomas in eight dogs, two cats, and one ferret. *Veterinary Dermatology*. **15**, 61.

Bonel-Raposo, J., Silveira, M.F., Gamba, C.D.O., *et al.* (2008) Sebaceous epithelioma in a ferret (*Mustela putorius furo*). *Brazilian Journal of Veterinary Pathology*, **1**(2), 70–72.

Camus, M.S., Rech, R.R., Choy, F.S., Fiorello, C.V., and Howerth, E.W. (2009) Pathology in practice: Chordoma on the tip of the tail of a ferret. *Journal of the American Veterinary Medical Association*, **235**(8), 949–951.

Carpenter, J.W., Davidson, J.P., Novilla, M.N., and Huang, J.C. (1980) Metastatic, papillary cystadenocarcinoma of the mammary gland in a black-footed ferret. *Journal of Wildlife Diseases*, **16**(4), 587–592.

Dillberger, J.E., and Altman, N.H. (1989) Neoplasia in ferrets: eleven cases with a review. *Journal of Comparative Pathology*, **100**(2), 161–176.

D'Ovidio, D., Rossi, G., Melidone, R., Menna, F., and Fioretti, A. (2012) Subcutaneous liposarcoma in a ferret (*Mustela putorius furo*). *Journal of Exotic Pet Medicine*, **21**, 230–242.

Dunn, D.G., Harris, R.K., Meis, J.M., and Sweet, D.E. (1991) A histomorphologic and immunohistochemical study of chordoma in twenty ferrets (*Mustela putorius furo*). *Veterinary Pathology*, **28**(6), 467–473.

Fox-Alvarez, W., Morena, A.R., and Bush, J. (2015) Diagnosis and successful surgical removal of an aural ceruminous gland adenocarcinoma in a domestic ferret (*Mustela putorius furo*). *Journal of Exotic Pet Medicine*, **24**, 350–355.

Garner, M.M., and Powers, L. (2010) Diseases of domestic ferrets. *AEMV Proceedings*, San Diego, CA, pp. 209–219.

Graham, J., Fidel, J., and Mison, M. (2006) Rostral maxillectomy and radiation therapy to manage squamous cell carcinoma in a ferret. *Veterinary Clinics of North America: Exotic Animal Practice*, **9**(3), 701–706.

Hamilton, T., and Morrison, W. (1991) Bleomycin chemotherapy for metastatic squamous cell carcinoma in a ferret. *Journal of the American Veterinary Medical Association*, **198**(1), 107–108.

Kanfer, S., and Reavill, Dr. (2013) Cutaneous neoplasia in ferrets, rabbits and guinea pigs. *Journal of Exotic Pet Medicine*, **16**, 579–598.

Li, X., Fox, J.G., Erdman, S.E., and Aspros, D.G. (1995) Cutaneous lymphoma in a ferret (*Mustela putorius furo*). *Veterinary Pathology*, **32**, 55–56.

Mialot, M., Prata, D., Girard-Luc, A., Rakotovao, F., Cuveillier, J.F., and Bernex, F. (2011) Multiple progressive piloleiomyomas in a ferret (*Mustela putorius furo*), a case report. *Veterinary Dermatology*, **22**(1), 100–103.

Mikaelian, I., and Garner, M.M. (2002) Solitary dermal leiomyosarcomas in 12 ferrets. *Journal of Veterinary Diagnostic Investigation*, **14**(3), 262–265.

Munday, J.S., Brown, C.A., and Richey, L.J. (2004) Suspected metastatic coccygeal chordoma in a ferret (*Mustela putorius furo*). *Journal of Veterinary Diagnostic Investigation*, **16**(5), 454–458.

Olsen, G.H., Turk, M.A., and Foil, C.S. (1985) Disseminated cutaneous squamous cell carcinoma in a ferret. *Journal of the American Veterinary Medical Association*, **186**(7), 702–703.

Parker, G.A., and Picut, C.A. (1993) Histopathologic features and post-surgical sequelae of 57 cutaneous neoplasms in ferrets (*Mustela putorius furo* L.). *Veterinary Pathology*, **30**(6), 499–504.

Pye, G.W., Bennett, R.A., Roberts, G.D., and Terrell, S.P. (2000) Thoracic vertebral chordoma in a domestic ferret (*Mustela putorius furo*). *Journal of Zoo and Wildlife Medicine*, **31**(1), 107–111.

Rickman, B.H., Craig, L.E., and Goldschmidt, M.H. (2001) Piloleiomyosarcoma in seven ferrets. *Veterinary Pathology*, **38**(6), 710–711.

Rodrigues, A., Gates, L., Payne, H.R., Kiupel, M., and Mansell, J. (2010) Multicentric squamous cell carcinoma in situ associated with papillomavirus in a ferret. *Veterinary Pathology*, **47**(5), 964–968.

Rosenbaum, M.R., Affolter, V.K., Usborne, A.L., and Beeber, N.L. (1996) Cutaneous epitheliotropic lymphoma in a ferret. *Journal of the American Veterinary Medical Association*, **209**(8), 1441–1444.

Roth, L., and Takata, I. (1992) Cytological diagnosis of chordoma of the tail in a ferret. *Veterinary Clinical Pathology*, **21**(4), 119–121.

Rudmann, D.G., White, M.R., and Murphey, J.B. (1994) Complex ceruminous gland adenocarcinoma in a brown-footed ferret (*Mustela putorius furo*). *Laboratory Animal Science*, **44**(6), 637–638.

Schultheiss, P.C. (2004) A retrospective study of visceral and nonvisceral hemangiosarcoma and hemangiomas in domestic animals. *Journal of Veterinary Diagnostic Investigation*, **16**(6), 522–526.

Smith, S.H., Goldschmidt, M.H., and McManus, P.M. (2002) A comparative review of melanocytic neoplasms. *Veterinary Pathology*, **39**(6), 651–678.

Tunev, S.S., and Wells, M.G. (2002) Cutaneous melanoma in a ferret (*Mustela putorius furo*). *Veterinary Pathology*, **39**(1), 141–143.

Vannevel, J. (1999) Unusual presentation of hemangiosarcoma in a ferret. *Canadian Veterinary Journal*, **40**(11), 808.

Williams, B.H., Eighmy, J.J., Berbert, M.H., and Dunn, D.G. (1993) Cervical chordoma in two ferrets (*Mustela putorius furo*). *Veterinary Pathology*, **30**(2), 204–206.

Zwicker, G.M., and Carlton, W.W. (1974) Spontaneous squamous cell carcinoma in a ferret. *Journal of Wildlife Diseases*, **10**(3), 213–216.

Other Integumentary Conditions

Carpenter, J.W., Davidson, J.P., Novilla, M.N., and Huang, J.C. (1980) Metastatic, papillary cystadenocarcinoma of the mammary gland in a black-footed ferret. *Journal of Wildlife Diseases*, **16**(4), 587–92.

Fisher, P.G. (2013) Erythema multiforme in a ferret (*Mustela putorius furo*). *Journal of Exotic Pet Medicine*, **16**, 599–609.

Mor, N., Qualls, C.W. Jr, and Hoover, J.P. (1992) Concurrent mammary gland hyperplasia and adrenocortical carcinoma in a domestic ferret. *Journal of the American Veterinary Medical Association*, **201**(12), 1911–2.

Zehnder, A.M., Hawkins, M.G., Koski, M.A., Luff, J.A., Benak, J., Lowenstine, L.J., and White, S.D. (2008) An unusual presentation of canine distemper virus infection in a domestic ferret (*Mustela putorius furo*). *Veterinary Dermatology*, **19**(4), 232–238.

General Information

Clapperton, B.K. (1989) Scent-marking behaviour of the ferret (*Mustela furo* L.). *Animal Behaviour*, **38**(3), 436–446.

Crump, D.R. (1980) Anal gland secretion of the ferret (*Mustela putorius* forma *furo*). *Journal of Chemistry and Ecology*, **6**, 837–844.

Kelleher, S.A. (2002) Skin diseases of ferrets. *Seminars in Avian Exotic Pet Medicine*, **11**(3), 136–140.

Kondo, K. (2000) The diversity of mammalian pelage. *Journal of Faculty of Agriculture, Hokkaido University*, **70**(1), 9–17.

Lewington, J.H. (2007) *Ferret Husbandry, Medicine and Surgery*, 2nd edn, Saunders, Philadelphia, PA.

Martin, A.L., Irizarry-Rovira, A.R., Bevier, D.E., Glickman, L.G., Glickman, N.W., and Hullinger, R.L. (2007) Histology of ferret skin: preweaning to adulthood. *Veterinary Dermatology*, **18**(6), 401–411.

Nixon, A.J., Ashby, M.G., Saywell, D.P., and Pearson, A.J. (1995) Seasonal fiber growth cycles of ferrets (*Mustela putorius furo*) and long-term effects of melatonin treatment. *Journal of Experimental Zoology*, **272**(6), 435–445.

Adrenal Gland Disease

Bielinska, M., Kiiveri, S., Parviainen, H., Mannisto, S., Heikinheimo, M., and Wilson, D.B. (2006) Gonadectomy-induced adrenocortical neoplasia in the domestic ferret (*Mustela putorius furo*) and laboratory mouse. *Veterinary Pathology*, **43**(2), 97–117.

Desmarchelier, M., Lair, S., Dunn, M., and Langlois, I. (2008) Primary hyperaldosteronism in a domestic ferret with an adrenocortical adenoma. *Journal of the American Veterinary Medical Association*, **233**(8), 1297–1301.

Garner, M.M., and Powers, L. (2010) *Diseases of domestic ferrets. AEMV Proceedings*, San Diego, CA, pp. 209–219.

Gould, W.J., Reimers, T.J., Bell, J.A., Lawrence, H.J., Randolph, J.F., Rowland, P.H., and Scarlett, J.M. (1995) Evaluation of urinary cortisol:creatinine ratios for the diagnosis of hyperadrenocorticism associated with adrenal gland tumors in ferrets. *Journal of the American Veterinary Medical Association*, **206**(1), 42–46.

Neuwith, L., Isaza, R., Bellah, J., Ackerman, N., and Collins, B. (1993) Adrenal neoplasia in seven ferrets. *Veterinary Radiology and Ultrasound*, **34**(5), 340–346.

Peterson, R.A. 2nd, Kiupel, M., and Capen, C.C. (2003) Adrenal cortical carcinomas with myxoid differentiation in the domestic ferret (*Mustela putorius furo*). *Veterinary Pathology*, **40**(2), 136–142.

Schoemaker, N.J. (2009) Ferrets: endocrine and neoplastic diseases, in E. Keeble, and A. Meredith (eds) *BSAVA Manual of Rodents and Ferrets*, BSAVA, Gloucester, pp. 320–329.

Schoemaker, N.J., Teerds, K.J., Mol, J.A., *et al.* (2002) The role of luteinizing hormone in the pathogenesis of hyperadrenocorticism in neutered ferrets. *Molecular and Cellular Endocrinology*, **197**(1–2), 117–125.

Schoemaker, N.J., van der Hage, M.H., Flik, G., Lumeij, J.T., and Rijnberk, A. (2004) Morphology of the pituitary gland in ferrets (*Mustela putorius furo*) with hyperadrenocorticism. *Journal of Comparative Pathology*, **130**(4), 255–265.

Schoemaker, N.J., Wolfswinkel, J., Mol, J.A., Voorhout, G., Kik, M.J., Lumeij, J.T., and Rijnberk, A. (2004) Urinary glucocorticoid excretion in the diagnosis of hyperadrenocorticism in ferrets. *Domestic Animal Endocrinology*, **27**(1), 13–24.

Simone-Freilicher, E. (2008) Adrenal gland disease in ferrets. *Veterinary Clinics of North America; Exotic Animal Practice*, **11**(1), 125–137.

Wagner, S., Kiupel, M., Peterson, R.A. 2nd, Heikinheimo, M., and Wilson, D.B. (2008) Cytochrome b5 expression in gonadectomy-induced adrenocortical neoplasms of the domestic ferret (*Mustela putorius furo*). *Veterinary Pathology*, **45**(4), 439–442.

Weiss, C.A., and Scott, M.V. (1997) Clinical aspects and surgical treatment of hyperadrenocorticism in the domestic ferret: 94 cases (1994–1996). *Journal of the American Animal Hospital Assoiattion*, **33**(6), 487–493.

Wheler, C.L., and Kamieniecki, C.L. (1998) Ferret adrenal-associated endocrinopathy. *Canadian Veterinary Journal*, **39**(3), 175–176.

Pancreatic Islet Cell Tumors

Buchanan, K.C., and Belote, D.A. (2003) Pancreatic islet cell tumor in a domestic ferret. *Contemporary Topics in Laboratory Animal Science*, **42**(6), 46–48.

Caplan, E.R., Peterson, M.E., Mullen, H.S., *et al.* (1996) Diagnosis and treatment of insulin-secreting pancreatic islet cell tumors in ferrets: 57 cases (1986–1994). *Journal of the American Veterinary Medical Association*, **209**(10), 1741–1745.

Chen, S. (2008) Pancreatic endocrinopathies in ferrets. *Veterinary Clinics of North America: Exotic Animal Practice*, **11**(1), 107–123.

Eatwell, K. (2004) Two unusual tumours in a ferret (*Mustela putorius furo*). *Journal of Small Animal Practice.* **45**(9), 454–459.

Ehrhart, N., Withrow, S.J., Ehrhart, E.J., and Wimsatt, J.H. (1996) Pancreatic beta cell tumor in ferrets: 20 cases (1986–1994). *Journal of the American Veterinary Medical Association*, **209**(10), 1737–1740.

Garner, M.M., and Powers, L. (2010) Diseases of domestic ferrets. *AEMV Proceedings*, San Diego, CA, pp. 209–219.

Johnson-Delaney, C.A. (2009) Ferret neoplasia. *AEMV Proceedings*, Milwaukee, WI.

Shin, J.J., Gorden, P., and Libutti, S.K. (2010) Insulinoma: pathophysiology, localization and management. *Future Oncology*, **6**(2), 229–237.

Weiss, C.A., Williams, B.H., and Scott, M.V. (1998) Insulinoma in the ferret: clinical findings and treatment comparison of 66 cases. *Journal of the American Animal Hospital Association*, **34**(6), 471–475.

Other Endocrine Disorders

Benoit-Biancamano, M.O., Morin, M., and Langlois, I. (2005) Histopathologic lesions of diabetes mellitus in a domestic ferret. *Canadian Veterinary Journal*, **46**(10), 895–897.

Boari, A., Papa, V., Di Silverio, F., Aste, G., Olivero, D., and Rocconi, F. (2010) Type 1 diabetes mellitus and hyperadrenocorticism in a ferret. *Veterinary Research Communications*, **34**(Suppl. 1), S107–S110.

Fox, J.G., Dangler, C.A., Snyder, S.B., Richard, M.J., and Thilsted, J.P. (2000) C-cell carcinoma (medullary thyroid carcinoma) associated with multiple endocrine neoplasms in a ferret (*Mustela putorius*). *Veterinary Pathology*, **37**(3), 278–282.

Lennox, A.M. (2009) Hypothyroidism in an obese pet ferret. *AEMV Proceedings*, Milwaukee, WI.

Li, X., Fox, J.G., and Padrid, P.A. (1998) Neoplastic diseases in ferrets: 584 cases (1968–1998). *Journal of the American Veterinary Medical Association*, **212**, 1402–1406.

Phair, K.A., Carpenter, J.W., Schermerhorn, T., Ganta, C.K., and DeBey, B.M. (2011) Diabetic ketoacidosis with concurrent pancreatitis, pancreatic β islet cell tumor, and adrenal disease in an obese ferret (*Mustela putorius furo*). *Journal of the American Association of Laboratory Animal Science*, **50**(4), 531–535.

Quesada-Canales, O., Suárez-Bonnet, A., Ramírez, G.A., *et al.* (2013) Adrenohepatic fusion in domestic ferrets

(*Mustela putorius furo*). *Journal of Comparative Pathology*,

Williams, B.H., Yantis, L.D., Craig, S.L., Geske, R.S., Li, X., and Nye, R. (2001) Adrenal teratoma in four domestic ferrets (*Mustela putorius furo*). *Veterinary Pathology*, **38**(3), 328–331.

Wills, T.B., Bohn, A.A., Finch, N.P., Harris, S.P., and Caplazi, P. (2005) Thyroid follicular adenocarcinoma in a ferret. *Veterinary Clinical Pathology*, **34**(4), 405–408.

Wyre, N.R., Michels, D., and Chen, S. (2013) Selected emerging diseases in ferrets. *Veterinary Clinics of North America: Exotic Animal Practice*, **16**(2), 469–493.

Mycobacterial Disease

Butler, W.R., O'Connor, S.P., Yakrus, M.A., *et al.* (1993) *Mycobacterium celatum* sp. nov. *International Journal of Systemic Bacteriology*, **43**(3), 539–548.

de Lisle, G.W., Kawakami, R.P., Yates, G.F., and Collins, D.M. (2008) Isolation of *Mycobacterium bovis* and other mycobacterial species from ferrets and stoats. *Veterinary Microbiology*, **132**(3–4), 402–407.

Ludwig, E., Reischl, U., Holzmann, T., Melzl, H., Janik, D., Gilch, C., and Hermanns, W. (2011) Risk for *Mycobacterium celatum* infection from ferret. *Emerging Infectious Diseases*, **17**(3), 553–555.

Piseddu, E., Trotta, M., Tortoli, E., Avanzi, M., Tasca, S., and Solano-Gallego, L. (2011) Detection and molecular characterization of *Mycobacterium celatum* as a cause of splenitis in a domestic ferret (*Mustela putorius furo*). *Journal of Comparative Pathology*, **144**(2–3), 214–218.

Pollock, C. (2012) Mycobacterial infection in the ferret. *Veterinary Clinics of North America: Exotic Animal Practice*, **15**(1), 121–129.

Ragg, J.R., Walderup, K.A., and Moller, H. (1995) The distribution of gross lesions of tuberculosis caused by *Mycobacterium bovis* in feral ferrets (*Mustela furo*) from Otago, New Zealand. *New Zealand Veterinary Journal*, **43**, 338–341.

Saunders, G.K., and Thomsen, B.V. (2006) Lymphoma and *Mycobacterium avium* infection in a ferret (*Mustela putorius furo*). *Journal of Veterinary Diagnostic Investigation*, **18**(5), 513–515.

Valheim, M., Djønne, B., Heiene, R., and Caugant, D.A. (2001) Disseminated *Mycobacterium celatum* (type 3) infection in a domestic ferret (*Mustela putorius furo*). *Veterinary Pathology*, **38**(4), 460–463.

Other Bacterial Diseases

Casalta, J.P., Fournier, P.E., Habib, G., Riberi, A., and Raoult, D. (2005) Prosthetic valve endocarditis caused by *Pseudomonas luteola*. *BMC Infectious Diseases*, **5**, 82.

Kiupel, M., Desjardins, D.R., *et al.* (2012) Mycoplasmosis in ferrets. *Emerging Infectious Diseases*, **18**(11), 1763–1770.

Martínez, J., Martorell, J., Abarca, M.L., *et al.* (2012) Pyogranulomatous pleuropneumonia and mediastinitis in ferrets (*Mustela putorius furo*) associated with *Pseudomonas luteola* infection. *Journal of Comparative Pathology*, **146**(1), 4–10.

Mentre, V., and Bulliot, C. (2015) A retrospective study of 17 cases of mycobacteriosis in domestic ferrets (*Mustela putorius furo*) between 2005 and 2013. *Journal of Exotic Pet Medicine*, **24**, 340–349.

Canine Distemper Virus

Beineke, A., Puff, C., Seehusen, F., and Baumgärtner, W. (2009) Pathogenesis and immunopathology of systemic and nervous canine distemper. *Veterinary Immunology and Immunopathology*, **127**(1–2), 1–18.

Langlois, I. (2005) Viral diseases of ferrets. *Veterinary Clinics of North America: Exotic Animal Practice*, **8**(1), 139–160.

Perpiñán, D., Ramis, A., Tomás, A., Carpintero, E., and Bargalló, F. (2008) Outbreak of canine distemper in domestic ferrets (*Mustela putorius furo*). *Veterinary Record*. **163**(8), 246–250.

Thomas, S. (2012) Canine distemper outbreak in ferrets in the UK. *Veterinary Record*, **170**, 27.

Zehnder, A.M., Hawkins, M.G., Koski, M.A., Luff, J.A., Benak, J., Lowenstine, L.J., and White, S.D. (2008) An unusual presentation of canine distemper virus infection in a domestic ferret (*Mustela putorius furo*). *Veterinary Dermatology*, **19**(4), 232–238.

Influenza

Campagnolo, E.R., Moll, M.E., Tuhacek, K., *et al.* (2013) Concurrent 2009 pandemic influenza A (H1N1) virus infection in ferrets and in a community in Pennsylvania. *Zoonoses and Public Health*, **60**(2), 117–124.

Langlois, I. (2005) Viral diseases of ferrets. *Veterinary Clinics of North America: Exotic Animal Practice*, **8**(1), 139–160.

Patterson, A.R., Cooper, V.L., Yoon, K.J., Janke, B.H., and Gauger, P.C. (2009) Naturally occurring influenza infection in a ferret (*Mustela putorius furo*) colony. *Journal of Veterinary Diagnostic Investigation*, **21**(4), 527–530.

Pignon, C., and Mayer, J. (2011) Zoonoses of ferrets, hedgehogs, and sugar gliders. *Veterinary Clinics of North America: Exotic Animal Practice*, **14**(3), 533–549.

Sanford, B.A., and Ramsay, M.A. (1989) In vivo localization of *Staphylococcus aureus* in nasal tissues of healthy and influenza A virus-infected ferrets. *Proceedings of the Society of Experimental Biology and Medicine*, **191**(2), 163–169.

Souza, M.J. (2011) Influenza. *Journal of Exotic Pet Medicine*, **20**(1), 4–8.

Smith, J.H., Nagy, T., Driskell, E., Brooks, P., Tompkins, S.M., and Tripp, R.A. (2011) Comparative pathology in ferrets infected with H1N1 influenza A viruses isolated from different hosts. *Journal of Virology*, **85**(15), 7572–7581.

Swenson, S.L., Koster, L.G., Jenkins-Moore, M., *et al.* (2010) Natural cases of 2009 pandemic H1N1 influenza A virus in pet ferrets. *Journal of Veterinary Diagnostic Investigation*, **22**(5), 784–788.

van den Brand, J., Stittelaar, K., van Amerongen, G., *et al.* (2013) Comparison of temporal and spatial dynamics of seasonal H3N2, pandemic H1N1 and highly pathogenic avian influenza H5N1 virus infections in ferrets. *ESVP/ECVP Proceedings*, **148**, 1.

Wyre, N.R., Michels, D., and Chen, S. (2013) Selected emerging diseases in ferrets. *Veterinary Clinics of North America: Exotic Animal Practice*, **16**(2), 469–493.

Other Respiratory Conditions

Britten, A.P., Dubey, J.P., and Rosenthal, B.M. (2010) Rhinitis and disseminated disease in a ferret (*Mustela putorius furo*) naturally infected with *Sarcocystis neurona. Veterinary Parasitology*, **169**, 226–231.

Darrow, B.G., Mans, C., Drees, R., Pinkerton, M.E., and Sladky, K.K. (2014) Pulmonary blastomycosis in a domestic ferret (*Mustela putorius furo*). *Journal of Exotic Pet Medicine*, **23**, 158–164.

Duval-Hudelson, K.A. (1990) Coccidiomycosis in three European ferrets. *Journal of Zoo and Wildlife Medicine*, **21**(3), 353–357.

Eshar, D., Mayer, J., Parry, N.M., Williams-Fritze, M.J., and Bradway, D.S. (2010) Disseminated, histologically confirmed *Cryptococcus* sp. infection in a domestic ferret. *Journal of the American Veterinary Medical Association*, **236**(7), 770–774.

Garner, M.M., Ramsell, K., Morera, N., *et al.* (2008) Clinicopathologic features of a systemic coronavirus-associated disease resembling feline infectious peritonitis in the domestic ferret (*Mustela putorius*). *Veterinary Pathology*, **45**(2), 236–246.

Greenacre, C.B. (2003) Incidence of adverse events in ferrets vaccinated with distemper or rabies vaccine: 143 cases (1995–2001). *Journal of the American Veterinary Medical Association*, **223**(5), 663–665.

Greenacre, C.B. (2003) Fungal diseases of ferrets. *Veterinary Clinics of North America: Exotic Animal Practice*, **6**, 435–448.

Lenhard, A. (1985) Blastomycosis in a ferret. *Journal of the American Veterinary Medical Association*, **186**(1), 70–72.

Malik, R., Martin, P., McGill, J., Martin, A., and Love, D.N. (2000) Successful treatment of invasive nasal cryptococcosis in a ferret. *Australian Veterinary Journal*, **78**(3), 158–159.

Perpinan, D., and Ramas, A. (2011) Endogenous lipid pneumonia in a ferret (*Mustela putorius furo*). *Journal of Exotic Pet Medicine*, **20**(1), 51–55.

Petritz, O.A., Antinoff, N., Pfent, C., Corapi, W., Pool, R.R., Fabiani, M., and Chen, S. (2013) Adenosquamous carcinoma of the trachea in a domestic ferret (*Mustela putorius furo*). *Journal of Exotic Pet Medicine*, **22**, 287–292.

General Respiratory Conditions

Johnson-Delaney, C.A., and Orosz, S.E. (2011) Ferret respiratory system: clinical anatomy, physiology, and disease. *Veterinary Clinics of North America: Exotic Animal Practice.* **14**(2), 357–367.

Disseminated Idiopathic Myofasciitis

Garner, M., and Ramsell, K. (2006) Myofasciitis: an emerging fatal disease of the domestic ferret. *Exotic DVM*, **8**(3), 23–25.

Garner, M.M., Ramsell, K., Schoemaker, N.J., *et al.* (2007) Myofasciitis in the domestic ferret. *Veterinary Pathology* **44**(1), 25–38.

Ramsell, K.D., and Garner, M.M. (2010) Disseminated idiopathic myofasciitis in ferrets. *Veterinary Clinics of North America: Exotic Animal Practice*, **13**(3), 561–575.

Neoplasia

Dillberger, J.E., and Altman, N.H. (1989) Neoplasia in ferrets: eleven cases with a review. *Journal of Comparative Pathology*, **100**(2), 161–176.

Huynh, M., Guillaumot, and Boussarie, D. (2009) Osteoma of the zygomatic arch in a ferret. *AEMV Proceedings*, Milwaukee, WI. p. 95.

Johnson, J.G., Brandao, J., Fowlkes, N., Rich, G., Rademacher, N., and Tully, Jr T.N. (2014) Calvarial osteoma with cranial vault invasion in the skull of a ferret (*Mustela putorius furo*). *Journal of Exotic Pet Medicine*, **23**, 266–269.

Keller, D.L., Schneider, L.K., Chamberlin, T., Ellison, M., and Steinberg, H. (2012) Intramedullary lumbosacral teratoma in a domestic ferret (*Mustela putorius furo*). *Journal of Veterinary Diagnostic Investigation*, **24**(3), 621–624.

Li, X., Fox, J.G., and Padrid, P. (1998) Neoplastic diseases in ferrets: 574 cases (1968–1997). *Journal of the American Veterinary Medical Association*, **212**, 1402–1406.

Maguire, R., Maguire, P., and Jenkins, J.R. (2014) Chondrosarcoma associated with the appendicular skeleton of 2 domestic ferrets. *Journal of Exotic Pet Medicine*, **23**, 165–171.

Perpiñán, D., Bargalló, F., Ramis, A., and Grífols, J. (2008) Thoracic vertebral osteoma in a domestic ferret (*Mustela putorious furo*). *Journal of Exotic Pet Medicine*, **17**(2), 144–147.

Other Musculoskeletal Conditions

De Castro, N., and Espino, L. (2014) What is your diagnosis. Congenital malformation in a pet ferret. *Journal of the American Veterinary Medical Association*, **245**(6), 631–633.

Huynh, M., Cauzinille, L., and Shelton, G.D. (2009) Autoimmune myasthenia gravis in a ferret. *AEMV Proceedings*, Milwaukee, WI. p. 93.

Lu, D., Lamb, C.R., Patterson-Kane, J.C., and Cappello, R. (2004) Treatment of a prolapsed lumbar intervertebral disc in a ferret. *Journal of Small Animal Practice*, **45**(10), 501–503.

Morera, N., Valls, X., and Mascort, J. (2006) Intervertebral disk prolapse in a ferret. *Veterinary Clinics of North America: Exotic Animal Practice*, **9**(3), 667–671.

Pignon, C., and Jardel, N. (2011) Rupture of a posterior cruciate ligament in a ferret. *AEMV Proceedings*, Seattle, WA, p. 347.

Richardson, J.A., and Balabuszko, R.A. (2001). Ibuprofen ingestion in ferrets: 43 cases (January 1996–March 2000). *Journal of Veterinary Emergency Critical Care* **11**(1), 53–59.

Ritzman, T.K., and Knapp, D. (2002) Ferret orthopedics. *Veterinary Clinics of North America: Exotic Animal Practice*, **5**(1), 129–155, vii.

Coccidiosis

Abe, N., Tanoue, T., Ohta, G., and Iseki, M. (2008) First record of *Eimeria furonis* infection in a ferret, Japan, with notes on the usefulness of partial small subunit ribosomal RNA gene sequencing analysis for discriminating among *Eimeria* species. *Parasitology Research*, **103**, 967–970.

Blankenship-Paris, T.L., Chang, J., and Bagnell, C.R. (1993) Enteric coccidiosis in a ferret. *Laboratory Animal Science*, **43**(4), 361–363.

Sledge, D.G., Bolin, S.R., Lim, A., Kaloustian, L.L., Heller, R.L., Carmona, F.M., and Kiupel, M. (2011) Outbreaks of severe enteric disease associated with *Eimeria furonis* infection in ferrets (*Mustela putorius furo*) of 3 densely populated groups. *Journal of the American Veterinary Medical Association*, **239**(12), 1584–1588.

Coronavirus Enteritis

Autieri, C.R., Miller, C.L., Scott, K.E., *et al.* (2015) Systemic coronaviral disease in 5 ferrets. *Comparative Medicine*, **65**(6), 508–516.

Garner, M.M., Ramsell, K., Morera, N., *et al.* (2008) Clinicopathologic features of a systemic coronavirus-associated disease resembling feline infectious peritonitis in the domestic ferret (*Mustela putorius*). *Veterinary Pathology*, **45**(2), 236–246.

Martinez, J., Ramis, A.J., Reinacher, M., and Perpinan, D. (2006) Detection of feline infectious peritonitis virus-like antigen in ferrets. *Veterinary Record*, **158**(15), 523.

Martinez, J., Reinacher, M., Perpinan, D., and Ramis, A. (2008) Identification of group 1 coronavirus antigen in multisystemic granulomatous lesions in ferrets (*Mustela putorius furo*). *Journal of Comparative Pathology*, **138**, 54–58.

Michimae, Y., Mikami, S., Okimoto, K., Toyosawa, K., Matsumoto, I., Kouchi, M., Koujitani, T., Inoue, T., and Seki, T. (2010) The first case of feline infectious peritonitis-like pyogranuloma in a ferret infected by coronavirus in Japan. *Journal of Toxicologic Pathology*, **23**, 99–101.

Murray, J., Kiupel, M., and Maes, R. (2010) Ferret coronavirus-associated diseases. *Veterinary Clinics of North America: Exotic Animal Practice*, **13**(3), 543–560.

Perpinan, D., and Lopez, C. (2008) Clinical aspects of systemic granulomatous inflammatory syndrome in ferrets (*Mustela putorius furo*). *Veterinary Record*, **162**(6), 180–184.

Provacia, L.B., Smits, S.L., Martina, B.L., *et al.* (2011) Enteric coronavirus in ferrets, The Netherlands. *Emerging Infectious Diseases*, **17**(8), 1570–1571.

Shigemoto, J., Muroaka, Y., Wise, A.G., Kiupel, M., Maes, R.K., and Torisu, S. (2014) Two cases of systemic coronavirus associated disease resembling feline infectious peritonitis in domestic ferrets in Japan. *Journal of Exotic Pet Medicine*, **23**, 196–200.

Terada, Y., Minami, S., Noguchi, K., *et al.* (2014) Genetic characterization of coronaviruses from domestic ferrets, Japan. *Emerging Infectious Diseases*, **20**(2), 284–287.

Williams, B., Kiupel, M., West, K., Raymond, J.T., Grant, C., and Glickman, L. (2000) Coronavirus associated epizootic catarrhal enteritis in ferrets. *Journal of the American Veterinary Medical Association*, **217**(4), 526–530.

Wise, A., Kiupel, M., and Maes, R. (2006) Molecular characterization of a novel coronavirus associated with epizootic catarrhal enteritis (ECE) in ferrets. *Virology*, **349**, 169–174.

Wise, A., Kiupel, M., Garner, M., Clark, A., and Maes, R. (2010) Comparative sequence analysis of the distal one-third of the genomes of a systemic and an enteric ferret coronavirus. *Virus Research*, **149**(1), 42–50.

Enteric Conditions

Burgess, M., and Garner, M.M. (2002) Clinical aspects of inflammatory bowel disease in ferrets. *Exotic DVM*, **4**, 29–34.

Carmel, B. (2006) Eosinophilic gastroenteritis in three ferrets. *Veterinary Clinics of North America: Exotic Animal Practice*, **9**, 707–712.

Castillo-Alcala, F., Mans, C., Bos, A.S., Taylor, W.M., and Smith, D.A. (2010) Clinical and pathologic features of an adenomatous polyp of the colon in a domestic ferret (*Mustela putorius furo*). *Canadian Veterinary Journal*, **51**(11), 1261–1264.

Dixon, R.J. (1984) Systemic candidosis in a fitch. *New Zealand Veterinary Journal*, **32**, 132–133.

Fox, J.G. (1991) Campylobacter infections and salmonellosis. *Seminars in Veterinary Medicine and Surgery (Small Animal)*, **6**(3), 212–218.

Fox, J.G., Ackerman, J.I., and Newcomer, C.E. (1983) Ferret as a potential reservoir for human campylobacteriosis. *American Journal of Veterinary Research*, **44**(6), 1049–1052.

Fox, J.G., Ackerman, J.I., Taylor, N., Claps, M., and Murphy, J.C. (1987) *Campylobacter jejuni* infection in the ferret: an animal model of human campylobacteriosis. *American Journal of Veterinary Research*, **18**(1), 85–90.

Gomez-Villamandos, J.C., Carrasco, L., Mozos, E., and Hervas, J. (1995) Fatal cryptosporidiosis in ferrets (*Mustela putorius furo*), A morphopathological study. *Journal of Zoo and Wildlife Medicine*, **26**(4), 539–544.

Iyengar, K.P., Nadkarni, J.B., Gupta, R., Beeching, N.J., Ullah, I., and Loh, W.Y. (2013) *Mycobacterium chelonae* hand infection following ferret bite. *Infection*, **41**(1), 237–241.

Johnson-Delaney, C.A. (2010) Emerging ferret diseases. *Journal of Exotic Pet Medicine*, **19**(3), 207–215.

Kaye, S.W., Ossiboff, R.J., Noonan, B., *et al.* (2015) Biliary coccidiosis associated with immunosuppressive treatment of pure red cell aplasia in an adult ferret (*Mustela putorius furo*). *Journal of Exotic Pet Medicine*, **24**, 215–222.

Ludwig, E., Reischl, U., Holzmann, T., Melzl, H., Janik, D., Gilch, C., and Hermanns, W. (2011) Risk for *Mycobacterium celatum* infection from ferret. *Emerging Infectious Diseases*, **17**(3), 553–555.

Mentre, V., and Bulliot, C. (2015) A retrospective study of 17 cases of mycobacteriosis in domestic ferrets (*Mustela putorius furo*) between 2005–2013. *Journal of Exotic Pet Medicine*, **24**, 340–349.

Nemelka, K.W., Brown, A.W., Wallace, S.M., *et al.* (2009) Immune response to and histopathology of Campylobacter jejuni infection in ferrets (*Mustela putorius furo*). *Comparative Medicine*, **59**(4), 363–371.

Piseddu, E., Trotta, M., Tortoli, E., Avanzi, M., Tasca, S., and Solano-Gallego, L. (2011) Detection and molecular characterization of Mycobacterium celatum as a cause of splenitis in a domestic ferret (*Mustela putorius furo*). *Journal of Comparative Pathology*, **144**(2–3), 214–218.

Pollock, C. (2012) Mycobacterial infection in the ferret. *Veterinary Clinics of North America: Exotic Animal Practice*, **15**(1), 121–129.

Powers, L.V. (2009) Bacterial and parasitic diseases of ferrets. *Veterinary Clinics of North America: Exotic Animal Practice*, **12**, 531–561.

Rehg, J.E., Gigliotti, F., and Stokes, D.C. (1988) Cryptosporidiosis in ferrets. *Laboratory Animal Science*, **38**(2), 155–158.

Saunders, G.K., and Thomsen, B.V. (2006) Lymphoma and *Mycobacterium avium* infection in a ferret (*Mustela putorius furo*). *Journal of Veterinary Diagnostic Investigation*, **18**(5), 513–515.

Schultheiss, P.C., and Dolginow, S.Z. (1994) Granulomatous enteritis caused by Mycobacterium avium in a ferret. *Journal of the American Veterinary Medical Association*, **204**(8), 1217–1218.

Torres-Medina, A. (1987) Isolation of an atypical rotavirus causing diarrhea in neonatal ferrets. *Laboratory Animal Science*, **37**(2), 167–171.

Valheim, M., Djønne, B., Heiene, R., and Caugant, D.A. (2001) Disseminated *Mycobacterium celatum* (type 3) infection in a domestic ferret (*Mustela putorius furo*). *Veterinary Pathology*, **38**(4), 460–463.

Vannevel, J. (1999) Unusual presentation of hemangiosarcoma in a ferret. *Canadian Veterinary Journal*, **40**(11), 808.

Wise, A.G., Smedley, R.C., Kiupel, M., and Maes, R.K. (2009) Detection of group C rotavirus in juvenile ferrets (*Mustela putorius furo*) with diarrhea by reverse transcription polymerase chain reaction: sequencing and analysis of the complete coding region of the VP6 gene. *Veterinary Pathology*, **46**(5), 985–991.

Wyre, N.R., Michels, D., and Chen, S. (2013) Selected emerging diseases in ferrets. *Veterinary Clinics of North America: Exotic Animal Practice*, **16**(2), 469–493.

Exocrine Pancreas Conditions

Hoefer, H.L., Patnaik, A.K., and Lewis, A.D. (1992) Pancreatic adenocarcinoma with metastasis in two ferrets. *Journal of the American Veterinary Medical Association*, **201**(3), 466–467.

Kornegay, R.W., Morris, J.M., Cho, D., and Lozano-Alarcon, F. (1991) Pancreatic adenocarcinoma with osseous metaplasia in a ferret. *Journal of Comparative Pathology*, **105**(1), 117–121.

Li, X., Fox, J.G., and Padrid, P.A. (1998) Neoplastic diseases in ferrets: 574 cases (1968–1997). *Journal of the American Veterinary Medical Association*, **212**(9), 1402–1406.

Phair, K.A., Carpenter, J.W., Schermerhorn, T., Ganta, C.K., and DeBey, B.M. (2011) Diabetic ketoacidosis with concurrent pancreatitis, pancreatic β islet cell tumor, and adrenal disease in an obese ferret (*Mustela putorius furo*). *Journal of the American Association Lab Animal Science*, **50**(4), 531–535.

Rhody, J.L., and Williams, B.H. (2013) Exocrine pancreatic adenocarcinoma and associated extrahepatic biliary obstruction in a ferret. *Journal of Exotic Pet Medicine*, **22**, 206–211.

Whittington, J.K., Emerson, J.A., Satkus, T.M., Tyagi, G., Barger, A., and Pinkerton, M.E. (2006) Exocrine pancreatic carcinoma and carcinomatosis with abdominal effusion containing mast cells in a ferret (*Mustela putorius furo*). *Veterinary Clinics of North America: Exotic Animal Practice*, **9**(3), 643–650.

Gastric Conditions

Beach, J.E., and Greenwood, B. (1993) Spontaneous neoplasia in the ferret (*Mustela putorius furo*). *Journal of Comparative Pathology*, **108**(2), 133–147.

Nakanishi, M., Kuwamura, M., Yamate, J., Fujita, D., and Sasai, H. (2005) Gastric adenocarcinoma with ossification in a ferret (*Mustela putorius furo*). *Journal of Veterinary Medical Science*, **67**(9), 939–941.

Rice, L.E., Stahl, S.J., and McLeod, C.G. Jr. (1992) Pyloric adenocarcinoma in a ferret. *Journal of the American Veterinary Medical Association*, **200**(8), 1117–1118.

Saunders, G.K., and Thomsen, B.V. (2006) Lymphoma and *Mycobacterium avium* infection in a ferret (*Mustela putorius furo*). *Journal of Veterinary Diagnostic Investigation*, **18**(5), 513–515.

Schulman, F.Y., Montali, R.J., and Hauer, P.J. (1993) Gastroenteritis associated with *Clostridium perfringens* type A in black-footed ferrets (*Mustela nigripes*). *Veterinary Pathology*, **30**(3), 308–310.

Sleeman, J.M., Clyde, V.L., Jones, M.P., and Mason, G.L. (1995) Two cases of pyloric adenocarcinoma in the ferret (*Mustela putorius furo*). *Veterinary Record*, **137**(11), 272–273.

Helicobacteriosis

Erdman, S.E., Correa, P., Coleman, L.A., *et al.* (1997) *Helicobacter mustelae*-associated gastric MALT lymphoma in ferrets. *American Journal of Pathology*, **151**(1), 273–280.

Forester, N.T., Parton, K., Lumsden, J.S., and O'Toole, P.W. (2000) Isolation of *Helicobacter mustelae* from ferrets in New Zealand. *New Zealand Veterinary Journal*, **48**(3), 65–69.

Fox, J.G., Dangler, C.A., Sager, W., Borkowski, R., and Gliatto, J.M. (1997) *Helicobacter mustelae*-associated gastric adenocarcinoma in ferrets (*Mustela putorius furo*). *Veterinary Pathology*, **34**(3), 225–229.

Fox, J.G., and Marini, R.P. (2001) *Helicobacter mustelae* infection in ferrets: Pathogenesis, epizootiology, diagnosis and treatment. *Seminars in Avian and Exotic Pet Medicine*, **110**(1), 36–44.

Fox, J.G., Otto, G., Taylor, N.S., Rosenblad, W., and Murphy, J.C. (1991) *Helicobacter mustelae*-induced gastritis and elevated gastric pH in the ferret (*Mustela putorius furo*). *Infection and Immunity*, **59**(6), 1875–1880.

Johnson-Delaney, C.A. (2005) The ferret gastrointestinal tract and *Helicobacter mustelae* infection. *Veterinary Clinics of North America: Exotic Animal Practice*, **8**, 197–212.

O'Toole, P.W., Snelling, W.J., Canchaya, C., *et al.* (2010) Comparative genomics and proteomics of *Helicobacter mustelae*, an ulcerogenic and carcinogenic gastric pathogen. *BMC Genomics.* **11**, 164.

Perkins, S.E., Fox, J.G., and Walsh, J.H. (1996) *Helicobacter mustelae*-associated hypergastrinemia in ferrets (*Mustela putorius furo*). *American Journal of Veterinary Research*, **57**(2), 147–150.

Hepatobiliary Conditions

Batchelder, M.A., Bell, J.A., Erdman, S.E., Marini, R.P., Murphy, J.C., and Fox, J.G. (1999) Pregnancy toxemia in the European ferret (*Mustela putorius furo*). *Laboratory Animal Science*, **49**(4), 372–379.

Beach, J.E., and Greenwood, B. (1993) Spontaneous neoplasia in the ferret (*Mustela putorius furo*). *Journal of Comparative Pathology*, **108**(2), 133–147.

Bradley, G.A., Orr, K., and Reggiardo, C., *et al.* (2001) Enterotoxigenic *Escherichia coli* infection in captive black-footed ferrets. *Journal of Wildlife Diseases*, **37**, 617–620.

Court, M.H. (2001) Acetaminophen UDP-glucuronosyltransferase in ferrets: species and gender differences, and sequence analysis of ferret UGT1A6. *Journal of Veterinary Pharmacologic Therapy*, **24**(6), 415–422.

Cross, B.M. (1987) Hepatic vascular neoplasms in a colony of ferrets. *Veterinary Pathology*, **24**(1), 94–96.

Dalrymple, E.F. (2004) Pregnancy toxemia in a ferret. *Canadian Veterinary Journal*, **45**(2), 150–152.

Darby, C., and Ntavlourou, V. (2006) Hepatic hemangiosarcoma in two ferrets (*Mustela putorius furo*). *Veterinary Clinics of North America: Exotic Animal Practice*, **9**(3), 689–694.

Dunayer, E. (2008) Toxicology of ferrets. *Veterinary Clinics of North America: Exotic Animal Practice*, **11**(2), 301–314.

Fox, J.G., Zeman, D.H., and Mortimer, J.D. (1994) Copper toxicosis in sibling ferrets. *Journal of the American Veterinary Medical Association*, **205**(8), 1154–1156.

García, A., Erdman, S.E., Xu, S., Feng, Y., Rogers, A.B., Schrenzel, M.D., Murphy, J.C., and Fox, J.G. (2002) Hepatobiliary inflammation, neoplasia, and argyrophilic bacteria in a ferret colony. *Veterinary Pathology*, **39**(2), 173–179.

Hall, B.A., and Ketz-Riley, C.J. (2011) Cholestasis and cholelithiasis in a domestic ferret (*Mustela putorius furo*). *Journal of Veterinary Diagnostic Investigation*, **23**(4), 836–839.

Hauptman, K., Jekl, V., and Knotek, Z. (2011) Extrahepatic biliary tract obstruction in two ferrets (*Mustela putorius furo*). *Journal of Small Animal Practice*, **52**(7), 371–375.

Hiruma, M., Ike, K., and Kume, T. (1986) Focal heaptic necrosis in young ferrets infected with *Aeromonas* species. *Japanese Journal of Veterinary Science*, **48**, 159–162.

Huynh, M., Guillamot, P., and Boussarie, D. (2011) Ruptured gall bladder in a ferret. *AEMV Proceedings*, Seattle, WA, p. 361.

Huynh, M., Huynh, M., and Laloi, F. (2013) Diagnosis of liver disease in domestic ferrets (*Mustela putorius*). *Veterinary Clinics of North America: Exotic Animal Practice*, **16**(1), 121–144.

Jones, Y., Wise, A., Maes, R., and Kiupel, M. (2006) Peliod hepatocellular carcinoma in a domesticated ferret (*Mustela putorius furo*). *Journal of Veterinary Diagnostic Investigation*, **18**(2), 228–231.

Lair, S., Barker, I.K., Mehren, K.G., and Williams, E.S. (2002) Epidemiology of neoplasia in captive black-footed ferrets (*Mustela nigripes*), 1986–1996. *Journal of Zoo and Wildlife Medicine*, **33**(3), 204–213.

Li, T.C., Yang, T., Ami, Y., *et al.* (2014) Complete genome of hepatitis E virus from laboratory ferrets. *Emerging Infectious Diseases*, **20**, 709–712.

Li, T.C., Yonemitsu, K., Terada, Y., Takeda, N., Takaji, W., and Maeda, K. (2015) Ferret hepatitis E virus infection in Japan. *Japanese Journal of Infectious Diseases*, **68**(1), 60–62.

Li, T.C., Yoshizaki, S., Ami, Y., *et al.* (2015) Monkeys and rats are not susceptible to ferret hepatitis E virus infection. *Intervirology*, **58**(3), 139–142.

Overman, M.C. (2015) A review of ferret toxicosis. *Journal of Exotic Pet Medicine*, **24**, 398–402.

Quesada-Canales, O., Suárez-Bonnet, A., *et al.* (2013) Adrenohepatic fusion in domestic ferrets (*Mustela putorius furo*). *Journal of Comparative Pathology*, **149**(2–3), 314–317.

Raj, V.S., Smits, S.L., Pas, S.D., Provacia, L.B., Moorman-Roest, H., Osterhaus, A.D., and Haagmans, B.L. (2012) Novel hepatitis E virus in ferrets, the Netherlands. *Emerging Infectious Diseases*, **18**(8), 1369–1370.

Reindel, J.F., and Evans, M.G. (1987) Cystic mucinous hyperplasia in the gallbladder of a ferret. *Journal of Comparative Pathology*, **97**(5), 601–604.

Williams, B.H., Chimes, M.J., and Gardiner, C.H. (1996) Biliary coccidiosis in a ferret (*Mustela putorius furo*). *Veterinary Pathology*, **33**(4), 437–439.

Megaesophagus

Blanco, M.C., Fox, J.G., Rosenthal, K., Hillyer, E.V., Quesenberry, K.E., and Murphy, J.C. (1994) Megaesophagus in nine ferrets. *Journal of the American Veterinary Medical Association*, **205**(3), 444–447.

Caligiuri, R., Bellah, J.R., Collins, B.R., and Ackerman, N. (1989) Medical and surgical management of esophageal foreign body in a ferret. *Journal of the American Veterinary Medical Association*, **195**(7), 969–971.

Couturier, J., Huynh, M., Boussarie, D., Cauzinille, L., and Shelton, G.D. (2009) Autoimmune myasthenia gravis in a ferret. *Journal of the American Veterinary Medical Association*, **235**(12), 1462–1466.

Harms, C.A., and Andrews, G.A. (1993) Megaesophagus in a domestic ferret. *Laboratory Animal Science*, **43**(5), 506–508.

Oral Conditions

Berkovitz, B.K. Supernumerary deciduous incisors and the order of eruption of the incisor teeth in the albino ferret. *Journal of Zoology*, **155**, 445.

Eroshin, V.V., Reiter, A.M., Rosenthal, K., Fordham, M., Latney, L., Brown, S., and Lewis, J.R. (2011) Oral examination results in rescued ferrets: clinical findings. *Journal of Veterinary Dentistry*, **28**(1), 8–15.

Graham, J., Fidel, J., and Mison, M. (2006) Rostral maxillectomy and radiation therapy to manage squamous cell carcinoma in a ferret. *Veterinary Clinics of North America: Exotic Animal Practice.* **9**(3), 701–706.

Hamilton, T.A., and Morrison, W.B. (1991) Bleomycin chemotherapy for metastatic squamous cell carcinoma in a ferret. *Journal of the American Veterinary Medical Association*, **198**(1), 107–108.

Johnson-Delaney. C.A. (2008) Diagnosis and treatment of dental disease in ferrets. *Journal of Exotic Pet Medicine*, **17**(2), 132–137.

Thas, I., and Cohen-Solal, N.A. (2014) Acquired oronasal fistula in a domestic ferret (*Mustela putorius furo*). *Journal of Exotic Pet Medicine*, **23**, 409–414.

Zwicker, G.M., and Carlton, W.W. (1974) Spontaneous squamous cell carcinoma in a ferret. *Journal of Wildlife Diseases*, **10**, 213–216.

Proliferative Colitis

Fox, J.G., Curry, C., and Leathers, C.W. (1986) Proliferative colitis in a pet ferret. *Journal of the American Veterinary Medical Association*, **189**(11), 1475–1476.

Fox, J.G., and Lawson, G.H. (1988) Campylobacter-like omega intracellular antigen in proliferative colitis of ferrets. *Laboratory Animal Science*, **38**(1), 34–36.

Fox, J.G., Murphy, J.C., Ackerman, J.I., Prostak, K.S., Gallagher, C.A., and Rambow, V.J. (1982) Proliferative colitis in ferrets. *American Journal of Veterinary Research*, **43**(5), 858–864.

Fox, J.G., Murphy, J.C., Otto, G., Pecquet-Goad, M.E., Lawson, G.H., and Scott, J.A. (1989) Proliferative colitis in ferrets: epithelial dysplasia and translocation. *Veterinary Pathology*, **26**(6), 515–517.

Garner, M.M., and Powers, L. (2010) Diseases of domestic ferrets *(Mustela putorius)*. *AEMV Proceedings*, San Diego, CA.

Li, X., Pang, J., and Fox, J.G. (1996) Coinfection with intracellular *Desulfovibrio* species and coccidia in ferrets with proliferative bowel disease. *Laboratory Animal Science*, **46**(5), 569–571.

Salivary Gland Conditions

Miller, P.E., and Pickett, J.P. (1989) Zygomatic salivary gland mucocele in a ferret. *Journal of the American Veterinary Medical Association*, **1194**(10), 1477–1479.

Triantafyllou, A., Fletcher, D., and Scott, J. (2006) Histological and histochemical observations on salivary microliths in ferret. *Archives of Oral Biology*, **51**(3), 198–205.

Triantafyllou, A., Harrison, J.D., and Garrett, J.R. (2009) Microliths in the parotid of ferret investigated by electron microscopy and microanalysis. *International Journal of Experimental Pathology*, **90**(4), 439–447.

General Gastrointestinal Conditions

Johnson-Delaney, C. (2009) The gastrointestinal system: Exotic companion animals. *AEMV Proceedings*, Madison, WI.

Lennox, A.M. (2005) Gastrointestinal diseases of the ferret. *Veterinary Clinics of North America: Exotic Animal Practice.* **8**, 213–225.

Schwarz, L.A., Solano, M., Manning, A., Marini, R.P., and Fox, J.G. (2003) The normal upper gastrointestinal examination in the ferret. *Veterinary Radiology and Ultrasound*, **44**(2), 165–172.

Smits, S.L., Raj, V.S., Oduber, M.D., *et al.* (2013) Metagenomic analysis of the ferret fecal viral flora. *PLoS ONE*, **8**(8), e71595.

Cardiomyopathy

Atkinson, R.M. (1992) Case reports on cardiomyopathy in the domestic ferret. *Mustela putorius furo. Journal of Small Exotic Animal Medicine*, **2**(2), 75–78.

Ensley, P.K., and Van Winkle, T. (1982) Treatment of congestive heart failure in a ferret. *Journal of Zoo Animal Medicine*, **13**, 23–25.

Greenlee, P.G., and Stephens, E. (1984) Meningeal cryptococcosis and congestive cardiomyopathy in a ferret. *Journal of the American Veterinary Medical Association*, **184**(7), 840–841.

Lipman, N.S., Murphy, J.C., and Fox, J.G. (1987) Clinical, functional and pathologic changes associated with a case of dilatative cardiomyopathy in a ferret. *Laboratory Animal Science*, **37**(2), 210–212.

Myocarditis

Garner, M.M., Ramsell, K., Schoemaker, N.J., *et al.* (2007) Myofasciitis in the domestic ferret. *Veterinary Pathology*, **44**(1), 25–38.

Powers, L.V. (2009) Bacterial and parasitic diseases of ferrets. *Veterinary Clinics of North America: Exotic Animal Practice*, **12**, 531–561.

Heartworm Disease

Bradbury, C., Saunders, A.B., Heatley, J.J., *et al.* (2010) Transvenous heartworm extraction in a ferret with caval syndrome. *Journal of the American Animal Hospital Association*, **46**(1), 31–35.

Moreland, A.F., Battles, A.H., and Nease, J.H. (1986) Dirofilariasis in a ferret. *Journal of the American Veterinary Medical Association*, **188**(8), 864.

Parrott, T.Y., Greiner, E.C., and Parrott, J.D. (1984) *Dirofilaria immitis* infection in three ferrets. *Journal of the American Veterinary Medical Association*, **184**(5), 582–583.

Powers, L.V. (2009) Bacterial and parasitic diseases of ferrets. *Veterinary Clinics of North America: Exotic Animal Practice.* **12**(3), 531–561.

Other Cardiovascular Conditions

Di Girolamo, N., Critelli, M., Zeyen, U., and Selleri, P. (2012) Ventricular septal defect in a ferret (*Mustela putorius furo*). *Journal of Small Animal Practice*, **53**(9), 549–553.

Kottwitz, J.J., Luis-Fuentes, V., and Micheal, B. (2006) Nonbacterial thrombotic endocarditis in a ferret (*Mustela putorius furo*). *Journal of Zoo and Wildlife Medicine*, **37**(2), 197–201.

Laniesse, D., Hebert, J., Larrat, S., Helie, P., Pouleur-Larrat, B., and Belanger, M.C. (2014) Tetralogy of Fallot in a 6-year old albino ferret (*Mustela putorius furo*). *Canadian Veterinary Journal*, **55**, 456–461.

Malakoff RL, Laste NJ, and Orcutt CJ. (2012. Echocardiographic and electrocardiographic findings in client-owned ferrets: 95 cases (1994–2009). *Journal of the American Veterinary Medical Association*, **241**(11), 1484–1489.

Stamoulis, M.E. (1995) Cardiac disease in ferrets. *Seminars in Avian and Exotic Pet Medicine*, **4**(1), 43–48.

Truex, R.C., Belej, R., Ginsberg, L.M., and Hartman, R.L. (1974) Anatomy of the ferret heart: an animal model for cardiac research. *Anatomical Record*, **179**(4), 411–422.

Van Schaik-Gerritsen, K.M., Shoemaker, N.J., Kik, M.J.L., and Beijerink, N.J. (2013) Atrial septal defect in a ferret (*Mustela putorius furo*). *Journal of Exotic Pet Medicine*, **22**, 70–75.

Wagner, R.A. (2009) Ferret cardiology. *Veterinary Clinics of North America: Exotic Animal Practice*, **12**(1), 115–134.

Williams, J.G., Graham, J.E., Laste, N.J., and Malakoff, R.L. (2011) Tetralogy of Fallot in a young ferret. *Journal of Exotic Pet Medicine*, **20**(3), 232–236.

Chronic Renal Disease

Antinoff, N. (1998) Urinary disorders in ferrets. *Seminars in Avian and Exotic Pet Medicine*, **7**(2), 89–92.

Garner, M.M., Raymond, J.T., O'Brien, T.D., Nordhausen, R.W., and Russell, W.C. (2007) Amyloidosis in the black-footed ferret (*Mustela nigripes*). *Journal of Zoo and Wildlife Medicine*, **38**(1), 32–41.

Cystic Urogenital Disease

Dillberger, J.E. (1985) Polycystic kidneys in a ferret. *Journal of the American Veterinary Medical Association*, **186**(1), 74–75.

Jackson, C.N., Rogers, A.B., Maurer, K.J., Lofgren, J.L., Fox, J.G., and Marini, R.P. (2008) Cystic renal disease in the domestic ferret. *Comparative Medicine*, **58**(2), 161–167.

Urolithiasis

Del Angel-Caraza, J., Chávez-Moreno, O., García-Navarro, S., and Pérez-García, C. (2008) Mixed urolith (struvite and calcium oxalate) in a ferret (*Mustela putorius furo*). *Journal of Veterinary Diagnostic Investigation*, **20**(5), 682–683.

Nguyen, H.T., Moreland, A.F., and Shields, R.P. (1979) Urolithiasis in ferrets (*Mustela putorius*). *Laboratory Animal Science*, **29**(2), 243–245.

Nwaokorie, E.E., Osborne, C.A., Lulich, J.P., and Albasan, H. (2013) Epidemiological evaluation of cystine urolithiasis in domestic ferrets (*Mustela putorius furo*), 70 cases (1992–2009). *Journal of the American Veterinary Medical Association*, **242**(8), 1099–1103.

Nwaokorie, E.E., Osborne, C.A., Lulich, J.P., Albasan, H., and Lekcharoensuk, C. (2011) Epidemiology of struvite uroliths in ferrets: 272 cases (1981–2007). *Journal of the American Veterinary Medical Association*, **239**(10), 1319–1324.

Palmore, W.P., and Bartos, K.D. (1987) Food intake and struvite crystalluria in ferrets. *Veterinary Research Communications*, **11**(6), 519–526.

Renal Neoplasia

Bell, R.C., and Moeller, R.B. (1990) Transitional cell carcinoma of the renal pelvis in a ferret. *Laboratory Animal Science*, **40**(5), 537–538.

Kawaguchi, H., Miyoshi, N., Souda, M., *et al.* (2006) Renal adenocarcinoma in a ferret. *Veterinary Pathology*, **43**(3), 353–356.

Lair, S., Barker, I.K., Mehren, K.G., and Williams, E.S. (2006) Renal tubular-cell neoplasms in black-footed ferrets (*Mustela nigripes*) - 38 cases. *Veterinary Pathology*, **43**(3), 276–280.

Other Urinary Tract Conditions

Langlois, I. (2005) Viral diseases of ferrets. *Veterinary Clinics of North America: Exotic Animal Practice*, **8**(1), 139–160.

Li, X., Fox, J.G., Erdman, S.E., Lipman, N.S., and Murphy, J.C. (1996) Cystic urogenital anomalies in ferrets (*Mustela putorius furo*). *Veterinary Pathology*, **33**(2), 150–158.

MacNab, T.A., Newcomb, B.T., Ketz-Riley, C., Pechman, R.D., and Rochat, M.C. (2010) Extramural ectopic ureter in a domestic ferret (*Mustela putorius furo*). *Journal of Exotic Pet Medicine*, **19**(4), 313–316.

Pennick, K.E., Stevenson, M.A., Latimer, K.S., Ritchie, B.W., and Gregory, C.R. (2005) Persistent viral shedding during asymptomatic Aleutian mink disease parvoviral infection in a ferret. *Journal of Veterinary Diagnostic Investigation*, **17**(6), 594–597.

Porter, H.G., Porter, D.D., and Larsen, A.E. (1982) Aleutian disease in ferrets. *Infection and Immunity*, **36**(1), 379–386.

Une, Y., Wakimoto, Y., Nakano, Y., Konishi, M., and Nomura, Y. (2000) Spontaneous Aleutian disease in a ferret. *Journal of Veterinary Medical Science*, **62**(5), 553–555.

Weisse, C., Aronson, L.R., and Drobatz, K. (2002) Traumatic rupture of the ureter: 10 cases. *Journal of the American Animal Hospital Association*, **38**(2), 188–192.

Welchman, D de B., Oxenham, M., and Done, S.H. (1993) Aleutian disease in domestic ferrets: diagnostic findings and survey results. *Veterinary Record*, **132**(19), 479–484.

General Urinary Tract Conditions

Fisher, P.G. (2006) Exotic mammal renal disease: diagnosis and treatment. *Veterinary Clinics of North America: Exotic Animal Practice*, **9**(1), 69–96.

Orcutt, C.J. (2003) Ferret urogenital diseases. *Veterinary Clinics of North America: Exotic Animal Practice*, **6**(1), 113–138.

Zhang, J.X., Soini, H.A., Bruce, K.E., *et al.* (2005) Putative chemosignals of the ferret (*Mustela putorius furo*) associated with individual and gender recognition. *Chemistry and Senses*, **30**(9), 727–737.

Reproductive Neoplasia

Batista-Arteaga, M., Suárez-Bonnet, A., Santana, M., *et al.* (2011) Testicular neoplasms (interstitial and Sertoli cell tumours) in a domestic ferret (*Mustela putorius furo*). *Reproduction of Domestic Animals*, **46**(1), 177–180.

Cotchin, E. (1980) Smooth-muscle hyperplasia and neoplasia in the ovaries of domestic ferrets (*Mustela putorius furo*). *Journal of Pathology*, **130**(3), 169–171.

Dillberger, J.E., and Altman, N.H. (1989) Neoplasia in ferrets: eleven cases with a review. *Journal of Comparative Pathology*, **100**(2), 161–176.

Hohšteter, M., Smolec, O., Gudan Kurilj, A., *et al.* (2012) Intratesticular benign peripheral nerve sheath tumour in a ferret (*Mustela putorius furo*). *Journal of Small Animal Practice*, **53**(1), 63–66.

Li, X., Fox, J.G., and Padrid, P.A. (1998) Neoplastic diseases in ferrets: 574 cases (1968–1997). *Journal of the American Veterinary Medical Association*, **212**(9), 1402–1406.

Martinez, A., Martinez, J., Burballa, A., and Martorell, J. (2011) Spontaneous thecoma in a spayed pet ferret (*Mustela putorius furo*) with alopecia and swollen vulva. *Journal of Exotic Pet Medicine*, **20**(4), 308–312.

Patterson, M.M., Rogers, A.B., Schrenzel, M.D., Marini, R.P., and Fox, J.G. (2003) Alopecia attributed to neoplastic ovarian tissue in two ferrets. *Comparative Medicine*, **53**(2), 213–217.

Pinches, M.D., Liebenberg, G., and Stidworthy, M.F. (2008) What is your diagnosis? Preputial mass in a ferret. *Veterinary Clinical Pathology*, **37**(4), 443–446.

Pregnancy Toxemia

Batchelder, M.A., Bell, J.A., Erdman, S.E., Marini, R.P., Murphy, J.C., and Fox, J.G. (1999) Pregnancy toxemia in the European ferret (*Mustela putorius furo*). *Laboratory Animal Science*, **49**(4), 372–379.

Dalrymple, E.F. (2004) Pregnancy toxemia in a ferret. *Canadian Veterinary Journal*, **45**(2), 150–152.

Other Reproductive Conditions

Batista-Arteaga, M., Alamo, D., Herráez, P., *et al.* (2007) Segmental atresia of the uterus associated with hydrometra in a ferret. *Veterinary Record*, **161**(22), 759–760.

Bodri, M.S. (2000) Theriogenology question of the month. Cryptorchid testis. *Journal of the American Veterinary Medical Association*, **217**(10), 1465–1466.

Coleman, G.D., Chavez, M.A., and Williams, B.H. (1998) Cystic prostatic disease associated with adrenocortical lesions in the ferret (*Mustela putorius furo*). *Veterinary Pathology*, **35**(6), 547–549.

D'Ovidio, D., Melidone, R., Rossi, G., Albarella, S., Noviello, E., and Meomartino, L. (2015) Multiple congenital malformations in a ferret (*Mustela putorius furo*). *Journal of Exotic Pet Medicine*, **24**, 92–97.

Jekl, V., Hauptman, K., Jeklová, E., Dorrestein, G.M., and Knotek, Z. (2006) Hydrometra in a ferret-case report. *Veterinary Clinics of North America: Exotic Animal Practice*, **9**(3), 695–700.

Huang, J.L., Powell, M., and Mead, R.A. (1993) Luteal protein secretion during preimplantation in the ferret. *Biology of Reproduction*, **48**(3), 647–654.

Lindeberg, H. (2008) Reproduction of the female ferret (*Mustela putorius furo*). *Reproduction of Domestic Animals*, **43**(Suppl 2), 150–156.

Martinez-Jiminez, D., Chary, P., Barron, H.W., Hernandez-Divers, S.J., and Basseches, J. (2009) Cystic endometrial hyperplasia-pyometra complex in two female ferrets (*Mustela putorius furo*). *Journal of Exotic Pet Medicine*, **18**(1), 62–70.

McLain, D.E., Harper, S.M., Roe, D.A., Babish, J.G., and Wilkinson, C.F. (1985) Congenital malformations and variations in reproductive performance in the ferret: effects of maternal age, color and parity. *Laboratory Animal Science*, **35**(3), 251–255.

Murphy, B.D. (1979) The role of prolactin in implantation and luteal maintenance in the ferret. *Biology and Reproduction*, **21**(2), 517–521.

Powers, L.V., Winler, K., Garner, M.M., Reavill, D., and LeGrange, S.M. (2007) Omentalization of prostatic abscesses and large cysts in ferrets (*Mustela putorius furo*). *Journal of Exotic Animal Practice*, **16**(3), 186–194.

Aleutian Disease

Palley, L.S., Corning, B.F., Fox, J.G., Murphy, J.C., and Gould, D.H. (1992) Parvovirus-associated syndrome (Aleutian disease) in two ferrets. *Journal of the American Veterinary Medical Association*, **201**(1), 100–106.

Pennick, K.E., Stevenson, M.A., Latimer, K.S., Ritchie, B.W., and Gregory, C.R. (2005) Persistent viral shedding during asymptomatic Aleutian mink disease parvoviral infection in a ferret. *Journal of Veterinary Diagnostic Investigation*, **17**(6), 594–597.

Porter, H.G., Porter, D.D., and Larsen, A.E. (1982) Aleutian disease in ferrets. *Infection and Immunity*, **36**(1), 379–386.

Rozengurt, N., Stewart, D., and Sanchez, S. (1995) Diagnostic exercise: ataxia and incoordination in ferrets. *Laboratory Animal Science*,. **45**(4), 432–434.

Une, Y., Wakimoto, Y., Nakano, Y., Konishi, M., and Nomura, Y. (2000) Spontaneous Aleutian disease in a ferret. *Journal of Veterinary Medical Science*, **62**(5), 553–555.

Welchman Dde, B., Oxenham, M., and Done, S.H. (1993) Aleutian disease in domestic ferrets: diagnostic findings and survey results. *Veterinary Record*, **132**(19), 479–484.

Cryptococcosis

Eshar, D., Mayer, J., Parry, N.M., Williams-Fritze, M.J., and Bradway, D.S. (2010) Disseminated, histologically confirmed *Cryptococcus* spp. infection in a domestic ferret. *Journal of the American Veterinary Medical Association*, **236**(7), 770–774.

Lester, S.J., Kowalewich, N.J., Bartlett, K.H., Krockenberger, M.B., Fairfax, T.M., and Malik, R. (2004) Clinicopathologic features of an unusual outbreak of cryptococcosis in dogs, cats, ferrets, and a bird: 38 cases (January to July 2003). *Journal of the American Veterinary Medical Association*, **225**(11), 1716–1722.

Morera, N., Juan-Sallés, C., Torres, J.M., Andreu, M., Sánchez, M., Zamora, M.Á., and Colom, M.F. (2011) *Cryptococcus gattii* infection in a Spanish pet ferret (*Mustela putorius furo*) and asymptomatic carriage in ferrets and humans from its environment. *Medical Mycology*, **49**(7), 779–784.

Cerebrospinal Neoplasia

Hanley, C.S., Wilson, G.H., Frank, P., *et al.* (2004) T cell lymphoma in the lumbar spine of a domestic ferret (*Mustela putorius furo*). *Veterinary Record*, **155**(11), 329–332.

Ingrao, J.C., Eshar, D., Vince, A., *et al.* (2014) Focal thoracolumbar spinal cord lymphosarcoma in a ferret (*Mustela putorius furo*). *Canadian Veterinary Journal*, **55**(7), 667–671.

Keller, D.L., Schneider, L.K., Chamberlin, T., Ellison, M., and Steinberg, H. (2012) Intramedullary lumbosacral teratoma in a domestic ferret (*Mustela putorius furo*). *Journal of Veterinary Diagnostic Investigation*, **24**(3), 621–624.

Schoemaker, N.J., van der Hage, M.H., Flik, G., Lumeij, J.T., and Rijnberk, A. (2004) Morphology of the pituitary gland in ferrets (*Mustela putorius furo*) with hyperadrenocorticism. *Journal of Comparative Pathology*, **130**(4), 255–265.

Sleeman, J.M., Clyde, V.L., and Brenneman, K.A. (1996) Granular cell tumour in the central nervous system of a ferret (*Mustela putorius furo*). *Veterinary Record*, **138**(3), 65–66.

Suran, J.N., and Wyre, N.R. (2013) Imaging findings in 14 domestic ferrets (*Mustela putorius furo*) with lymphoma. *Veterinary Radiology and Ultrasound*, **54**(5), 522–531.

van Zeeland, Y., Schoemaker, N., Passon-Vastenburg, M., and Kik, M. (2009) Vestibular syndrome due to a choroid plexus papilloma in a ferret. *Journal of the American Animal Hospital Association*, **45**(2), 97–101.

Rabies

Hamir, A.N., Niezgoda, M., and Rupprecht, C.E. (2011) Recovery from and clearance of rabies virus in a domestic ferret. *Journal of the American Association Laboratory Animal Science*, **50**(2), 248–251.

Moore, G.E., Glickman, N.W., Ward, M.P., Engler, K.S., Lewis, H.B., and Glickman, L.T. (2005) Incidence of and risk factors for adverse events associated with distemper and rabies vaccine administration in ferrets. *Journal of the American Veterinary Medical Association*, **226**(6), 909–912.

Niezgoda, M., Briggs, D.J., Shaddock, J., Dreesen, D.W., and Rupprecht, C.E. (1997) Pathogenesis of experimentally induced rabies in domestic ferrets. *American Journal of Veterinary Research*, **58**(11), 1327–1331.

Niezgoda, M., Briggs, D.J., Shaddock, J., and Rupprecht, C.E. (1998) Viral excretion in domestic ferrets (*Mustela putorius furo*) inoculated with a raccoon rabies isolate. *American Journal of Veterinary Research*, **59**(12), 1629–1632.

Other Neurologic Conditions

Diaz-Figueroa, O., and Smith, M.O. (2007) Clinical neurology of ferrets. *Veterinary Clinics of North America: Exotic Animal Practice*, **10**(3), 759–773.

Hamir, A.N., Miller, J.M., and Yaeger, M.J. (2007) Neuronal vacuolation in an adult ferret. *Canadian Veterinary Journal*, **48**(4), 389–391.

Harrison, S.G., and Borland, E.D. (1973) Deaths in ferrets (*Mustela putorius*) due to *Clostridium botulinum* type C. *Veterinary Record*, **93**(22), 576–577.

Langlois, I. (2005) Viral diseases of ferrets. *Veterinary Clinics of North America: Exotic Animal Practice*, **8**(1), 139–160.

Lockard, B.I. (1985) The forebrain of the ferret. *Laboratory Animal Science*, **35**(3), 216–228.

Lu, D., Lamb, C.R., Patterson-Kane, J.C., and Cappello, R. (2004) Treatment of a prolapsed lumbar intervertebral disc in a ferret. *Journal of Small Animal Practice*, **45**(10), 501–503.

McLain, D., Harper, S.M., Roe, D.A., Babish, J.G., and Wilkinson, C.F. (1985) Congenital malformations and variations in reproductive performance in the ferret: effects of maternal age, color and parity. *Laboratory Animal Science*, **35**, 251–255.

Morera, N., Valls, X., and Mascort, J. (2006) Intervertebral disk prolapse in a ferret. *Veterinary Clinics of North America: Exotic Animal Practice*, **9**(3), 667–671.

Moya, A., Martorell, J., Gallinato, M.J., and Rcio, A. (2014) Congenital peripheral vestibular syndrome in a domestic ferret (*Mustela putorius furo*). *Journal of Exotic Pet Medicine*, **23**, 287–293.

Piazza, S., Abitbol, M., Gnirs, K., Huynh, M., and Cauzinille, L. (2014) Prevalence of deafness and association with coat variations in client-owned ferrets.

Journal of the American Veterinary Medical Association, **244**(9), 1047–1052.

Steel, K.P., and Barkway, C. (1989) Another role for melanocytes: their importance for normal stria vascularis development in the mammalian inner ear. *Development*, **107**(3), 453–463.

Williams, B.H., Popek, E.J., Hart, R.A., and Harris, R.K. (1994) Iniencephaly and other neural tube defects in a litter of ferrets (*Mustela putorius furo*). *Veterinary Pathology*, **31**(2), 260–262.

Aleutian Disease

Chitty, J. (2009) Aleutian disease in ferrets: diagnostics and controversies. *AEMV Proceedings*, Milwaukee, WI, pp. 75–78.

Langlois, I. (2005) Viral diseases of ferrets. *Veterinary Clinics of North America: Exotic Animal Practice*, **8**(1), 139–160.

Palley, L.S., Corning, B.F., Fox, J.G., Murphy, J.C., and Gould, D.H. (1992) Parvovirus-associated syndrome (Aleutian disease) in two ferrets. *Journal of the American Veterinary Medical Association*, **201**(1), 100–106.

Pennick, K.E., Stevenson, M.A., Latimer, K.S., Ritchie, B.W., and Gregory, C.R. (2005) Persistent viral shedding during asymptomatic Aleutian mink disease parvoviral infection in a ferret. *Journal of Veterinary Diagnostic Investigation*, **17**(6), 594–597.

Porter, H.G., Porter, D.D., and Larsen, A.E. (1982) Aleutian disease in ferrets. *Infection and Immunity*, **36**(1), 379–386.

Rozengurt, N., Stewart, D., and Sanchez, S. (1995) Diagnostic exercise: ataxia and incoordination in ferrets. *Laboratory Animal Science*, **45**(4), 432–434.

Une, Y., Wakimoto, Y., Nakano, Y., Konishi, M., and Nomura, Y. (2000) Spontaneous Aleutian disease in a ferret. *Journal of Veterinary Medical Science*, **62**(5), 553–555.

Welchman Dde, B., Oxenham, M., and Done, S.H. (1993) Aleutian disease in domestic ferrets: diagnostic findings and survey results. *Veterinary Record*, **132**(19), 479–484.

Anemia

Lennox, A.M., and Powers, L. (2009) Aplastic myeloid anemia in ferrets. *AEMV Proceedings*, Milwaukee, MI, p. 63.

Lymphosarcoma

Batchelder, M.A., Erdman, S.E., Li, X., and Fox, J.G. (1996) A cluster of cases of juvenile mediastinal lymphoma in a ferret colony. *Lab Animal Science*, **46**(3), 271–274.

Coleman, L.A., Erdman, S.E., Schrenzel, M.D., and Fox, J.G. (1998) Immunophenotypic characterization of lymphomas

from the mediastinum of young ferrets. *American Journal of Veterinary Research*, **59**(10), 1281–1286.

Erdman, S.E., Brown, S.A., Kawasaki, T.A., Moore, F.M., Li, X., and Fox, J.G. (1996) Clinical and pathologic findings in ferrets with lymphoma: 60 cases (1982–1994). *Journal of the American Veterinary Medical Association*, **208**(8), 1285–1289.

Erdman, S.E., Kanki, P.J., Moore, F.M., Brown, S.A., Kawasaki, T.A., Mikule, K.W., Travers, K.U., Badylak, S.F., and Fox, J.G. (1996) Clusters of lymphoma in ferrets. *Cancer Investigation*, **14**(3), 225–230.

Erdman, S.E., Reimann, K.A., Moore, F.M., Kanki, P.J., Yu, Q.C., and Fox, J.G. (1995) Transmission of a chronic lymphoproliferative syndrome in ferrets. *Laboratory Investigations*, **72**(5), 539–546.

Hammond, D.L. (1990) Splenic lymphosarcoma in a ferret. *Journal of the American Animal Hospital Association*, **26**, 101–103.

Hess, L. (2005) Ferret lymphoma: The old and the new. *Seminars in Avian and Exotic Pet Medicine*, **14**(3), 199–204.

Mayer, J., and Burgess, K. (2012) An update on ferret lymphoma: A proposal for standardized classification of ferret lymphoma. *Journal of Exotic Pet Medicine*, **21**, 343–346.

Onuma, M., Kondo, H., Ono, S., Shibuya, H., and Sato, T. (2008) Cytomorphological and immunohistochemical features of lymphoma in ferrets. *Journal of Veterinary Medical Science*, **70**(9), 893–898.

Saunders, G.K., and Thomsen, B.V. (2006) Lymphoma and Mycobacterium avium infection in a ferret (*Mustela putorius furo*). *Journal of Veterinary Diagnostic Investigation*, **18**(5), 513–515.

Other Hematopoietic and Lymphoid Neoplasia

Altman, N.H., and Lamborn, P.B. Jr. (1984) Lymphocytic leukemia in a ferret (*Mustela furo*). *Veterinary Pathology*, **21**(3), 361–362.

Dillberger, J.E., and Altman, N.H. (1989) Neoplasia in ferrets: eleven cases with a review. *Journal of Comparative Pathology*, **100**(2), 161–76.

Li, X., Fox, J.G., and Erdman, S.E. (1996) Multiple splenic myelolipomas in a ferret (*Mustela putorius furo*). *Laboratory Animal Science*, **46**(1), 101–103.

Li, X., Fox, J.G., and Padrid, P.A. (1998) Neoplastic diseases in ferrets: 574 cases (1968–1997). *Journal of the American Veterinary Medical Association*, **212**(9), 1402–1406.

Taylor, T.G., and Carpenter, J.L. (1995) Thymoma in two ferrets. *Laboratory Animal Science*, **45**(4), 363–365.

Other Hematopoietic Conditions

Davis, J.A., Greenfield, R.E., and Brewer, T.G. (1993) Benzocaine-induced methemoglobinemia attributed to topical application of the anesthetic in several laboratory animal species. *American Journal of Veterinary Research*, **54**(8), 1322–1326.

Ferguson, D.C. (1985) Idiopathic hypersplenism in a ferret. *Journal of the American Veterinary Medical Association*, **186**(7), 693–695.

Greenacre, C.B. (2003) Fungal diseases of ferrets. *Veterinary Clinics of North America: Exotic Animal Practice.* **6**, 435–448.

Hanley, C.S., MacWilliams, P., Giles, S., and Paré, J. (2006) Diagnosis and successful treatment of *Cryptococcus neoformans* variety *grubii* in a domestic ferret. *Canadian Veterinary Journal*, **47**(10), 1015–1017.

Ludwig, E., Reischl, U., Holzmann, T., Melzl, H., Janik, D., Gilch, C., and Hermanns, W. (2011) Risk for *Mycobacterium celatum* infection from ferret. *Emerging Infectious Diseases*, **17**(3), 553–555.

Malka, S., Hawkins, M.G., Zabolotzky, S.M., Mitchell, E.B., and Owens, S.D. (2010) Immune-mediated pure red cell aplasia in a domestic ferret. *Journal of the American Veterinary Medical Association*, **237**(6), 695–700.

Marini, R.P., Callahan, R.J., Jackson, L.R., Jyawook, S., Esteves, M.I., Fox, J.G., Wilkinson, R.A., and Strauss, H.W. (1997) Distribution of technetium 99m-labeled red blood cells during isoflurane anesthesia in ferrets. *American Journal of Veterinary Research*, **58**(7), 781–785.

Martorell, J., Vrabelova, D., Reberte, L., and Ramis, A. (2011) Diagnosis of an abdominal splenosis in a case of ambulatory paraparesis of the hind limbs in a ferret (*Mustela putorius furo*). *Journal of Exotic Pet Medicine*, **20**(3), 227–231.

Morera, N., Juan-Sallés, C., Torres, J.M., Andreu, M., Sánchez, M., Zamora, M.Á., and Colom, M.F. (2011) *Cryptococcus gattii* infection in a Spanish pet ferret (*Mustela putorius furo*) and asymptomatic carriage in ferrets and humans from its environment. *Medical Mycology*, **49**(7), 779–784.

Piseddu, E., Trotta, M., Tortoli, E., Avanzi, M., Tasca, S., and Solano-Gallego, L. (2011) Detection and molecular characterization of *Mycobacterium celatum* as a cause of splenitis in a domestic ferret (*Mustela putorius furo*). *Journal of Comparative Pathology*, **144**(2–3), 214–218.

Schultheiss, P.C. (2004) A retrospective study of visceral and nonvisceral hemangiosarcoma and hemangiomas in domestic animals. *Journal of Veterinary Diagnostic Investigation*, **16**(6), 522–526.

Siperstein, L.J. (2008) Ferret hematology and related disorders. *Veterinary Clinics of North America: Exotic Animal Practice.* **11**(3), 535–550.

Smith, S.A., Zimmerman, K., and Moore, D.M. (2015) Hematology of the domestic ferret (*Mustela putorius furo*). *Journal of Exotic Pet Medicine*, **18**, 1–8.

Stephen, C. (2002) Multi-species outbreak of cryptococcosis on southern Vancouver Island, British Columbia. *Canadian Veterinary Journal*, **43**, 792–794.

Valheim, M., Djønne, B., Heiene, R., and Caugant, D.A. (2001) Disseminated *Mycobacterium celatum* (type 3) infection in a domestic ferret (*Mustela putorius furo*). *Veterinary Pathology*, **38**(4), 460–463.

Wyre, N.R., Michels, D., and Chen, S. (2013) Selected emerging diseases in ferrets. *Veterinary Clinics of North America: Exotic Animal Practice*, **16**(2), 469–493.

Conditions of the Cornea and Anterior Chamber

Lindemann, D.M., Eshar, D., Schumacher, L.L., Almes, K.M., and Rankin, A.J. (2016) Pyogranulomatous panophthalmitis with systemic coronavirus disease in a domestic ferret (*Mustela putorius furo*). *Veterinary Ophthalmology*, **19**(2), 167–171.

Ringle, M.J., Lindley, D.M., and Krohne, S.G. (1993) Lymphoplasmacytic keratitis in a ferret with lymphoma. *Journal of the American Veterinary Medical Association*, **203**(5), 670–672.

Uveal and Lenticular Conditions

Lipsitz, L., Ramsey, D.T., Render, J.A., Bursian, S.J., and Auelrich, R.J. (2001) Persistent fetal intraocular vasculature in the European ferret (*Mustela putorius*), clinical and histological aspects. *Veterinary Ophthalmology*, **4**(1), 29–33.

Miller, P.E., Marlar, A.B., and Dubielzig, R.R. (1993) Cataracts in a laboratory colony of ferrets. *Laboratory Animal Science*, **43**(6), 562–568.

Retinal Conditions

Morera, N., Juan-Sallés, C., Torres, J.M., Andreu, M., Sánchez, M., Zamora, M.Á., and Colom, M.F. (2011) *Cryptococcus gattii* infection in a Spanish pet ferret (*Mustela putorius furo*) and asymptomatic carriage in ferrets and humans from its environment. *Medical Mycology*, **49**(7), 779–784.

Ropstad, E.O., Leiva, M., Peña, T., Morera, N., and Martorell, J. (2011) *Cryptococcus gattii* chorioretinitis in a ferret. *Veterinary Ophthalmology*, **14**(4), 262–366.

General Ophthalmic Conditions

Donnelly, T.M. (2011) Species differences in the anatomy of the eye. *AEMV Proceedings*, Seattle, WA.

Good, K.L. (2002) Ocular disorders of pet ferrets. *Veterinary Clinics of North America: Exotic Animal Practice*, **5**(2), 325–339.

Hess, L. (2005) Ferret lymphoma: The old and the new. *Seminars in Avian Exotic Pet Medicine*, **14**(3), 199–204.

Hupfeld, D., Distler, C., and Hoffmann, K.P. (2006)
Motion perception deficits in albino ferrets
(*Mustela putorius furo*). *Vision Research*, **46**(18),
2941–2948.

McBride, M., Mosunic, C.B., Barron, G.H., *et al.* (2009)
Successful treatment of a retrobulbar adenocarcinoma
in a ferret (*Mustela putorius furo*). *Veterinary Record*,
165(7), 206–208.

Miller, P.E. (1996) Ferret ophthalmology. *Seminars in Avian
and Exotic Pet Medicine*, **6**(3), 146–151.

Montiani-Ferreira, F., Mattos, B.C., and Russ, H.H. (2006)
Reference values for selected ophthalmic diagnostic tests
of the ferret (*Mustela putorius furo*). *Veterinary
Ophthalmology*, **9**(4), 209–213.

3

Guinea Pigs

3.1 Introduction

Guinea pigs (*Cavia porcellus*), also known as cavies, are popular and gentle companion animals that were domesticated from a wild cavid species (*C. aperea*) originating in the mountainous regions of the Andes between 3000 and 6000 years ago. They belong to the class of hystricomorph rodents, and were traditionally raised for food and medicinal use by different indigenous populations in South America. Guinea pigs continue to be bred today in large numbers for domestic consumption in Peru, Ecuador, and Bolivia, and have been raised as microlivestock species in parts of Asia and Africa in recent years. The cultural importance of guinea pigs in the rituals of Andean society are demonstrated in several Peruvian paintings of the Last Supper made in 1670, approximately 130 years after Spanish conquest of the region, in which Jesus is portrayed surrounded by his disciples with a plate of cooked guinea pig (*cuy*) on the table. The conquistadors brought guinea pigs back to Europe in the mid-sixteenth century, where they were bred and kept as curiosities, and later, as pets. Guinea pigs are bred primarily as companions or for research use in North America and Western Europe today, although limited commercial breeding for reptile feeding also occurs. Most breeds of guinea pigs have a lifespan of five to seven years when housed conventionally. Guinea pigs readily adapt to a range of environments, are inquisitive and friendly, and easy to handle.

3.2 Integument Conditions

Different guinea pig breeds and strains come with a wide variety of hair coat lengths, colors, and patterns, ranging from the classic short-haired, smooth-coated English breeds and strains, such as Dunkin-Hartley, to short, wavy coats (rex), to coarse coats with rosettes (Abyssinian), to long-haired coats (Peruvian). Thirteen different breeds are recognized by the American Rabbit Breeders Association, which sets breed standards for cavies in North America.

Hairless or relatively nonhaired breeds (e.g., Skinny, Baldwin) have emerged in recent years, arising from hairless strains originally bred for research. These should not be confused with other specific hairless and athymic strains, which are immunodeficient.

3.2.1 Alopecia

Guinea pigs shed small quantities of hair all year round, as each hair follicle has an individual growth cycle, similar to hair follicles in human skin. Sparsely haired or hairless patches may normally be present behind the ears of guinea pigs. These areas are also devoid of sebaceous glands and are often heavily pigmented in pigmented breeds. Juvenile animals may appear to be sparsely haired as their adult coat and guard hairs are growing in. Hairless breeds may be born with variable amounts of hair on their heads or bodies, which is lost as the animal matures.

3.2.1.1 Presenting Clinical Signs

Alopecia may occur anywhere on the body. Pregnant sows may develop bilaterally symmetrical alopecia on their backs or flanks, which is more obvious in multiparous sows; however, the condition resolves spontaneously post partum. In group-housed animals, hair loss secondary to fighting may be accompanied by lacerations or abscesses.

3.2.1.2 Pathology

Alopecia accompanied by pruritus, moist dermatitis, localized swellings, discharge, or skin scaling and flaking is highly suggestive of an underlying disease or an infectious process induced by bacterial, fungal or parasitic agents, and additional diagnostic work is warranted. Hypovitaminosis C is an important condition of guinea pigs, and must be considered when animals present with poor hair coat and other nonspecific signs (Figures 3.1A and B).

3.2.1.3 Laboratory Diagnostics

Skin scrapings, biopsies, histopathology, special histologic staining, and fungal or microbiologic culturing are

Pathology of Small Mammal Pets, First Edition. Patricia V. Turner, Marina L. Brash and Dale A. Smith.
© 2018 John Wiley & Sons, Inc. Published 2018 by John Wiley & Sons, Inc.

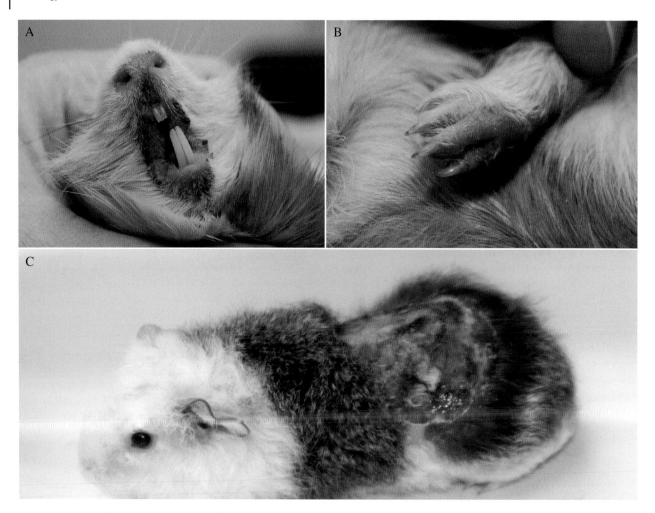

Figure 3.1 A: Cheilitis and perinasal dermatitis in a young guinea pig with hypovitaminosis C. B: The feet on this same animal were erythematous and swollen with a mild scaling dermatitis. C: Severe ulcerative dermatitis over the dorsum of a guinea pig. Lesions may be initiated by fighting, particularly in group-housed males, with secondary bacterial contamination. *Source:* A, B, and C: Courtesy of The Links Road Animal and Bird Clinic.

all suitable ancillary techniques for further determining an etiologic basis for suspected infectious causes of alopecia in guinea pigs. Serum ascorbate levels are infrequently used to evaluate hypovitaminosis C in guinea pigs, as it may be difficult to find a diagnostic laboratory that routinely assesses this nutrient. Response to supplementation is frequently used as an alternative and indirect means of confirming the condition.

3.2.1.4 Differential Diagnoses

Nonpruritic alopecia may arise from mechanical abrasions from cages or feeders, chronic ingestion of low protein diets, or nutritional deficiencies, such as parakeratotic hyperkeratosis and alopecia seen with chronic zinc deficiency, and poor hair coat, alopecia, scaling, and seborrhea due to hypovitaminosis C (see Section 3.5.1). Other causes of uncomplicated alopecia include self- or cage-mate-inflicted hair pulling or chewing (barbering) and

endocrinopathy-associated bilaterally symmetrical alopecia, seen most commonly with hyperadrenocorticism or cystic rete ovarii (see Section 3.3.2.2 and Section 3.8.2.1 for further information).

3.2.1.5 Group or Herd Management

Animal housing and management practices should be evaluated closely in simple cases of alopecia, looking for potential sources of abrasions or rough surfaces in which hair may be caught. Adequacy of diet should be ascertained, particularly with respect to vitamin C content.

3.2.2 Bacterial Dermatitis and Abscesses

Bacterial skin infection with or without abscessation is common, particularly in group-housed male guinea pigs, in which biting and fighting are seen frequently. Moist cervical and ventral dermatitis may also arise from dental malocclusion with subsequent excessive salivation (slobbers) or in animals that play with their water bottles or that are housed in damp, unsanitary conditions. Cheilitis with secondary bacterial infection may occur following local abrasion or contact with irritating substances. Abscessation of the cervical lymph nodes ("lumps") is seen occasionally and affected lymph nodes may fistulate.

3.2.2.1 Presenting Clinical Signs

Bacterial dermatitis presents as patchy nonpruritic alopecia with erythema, exudation, crusting, and ulceration. Abscesses may be palpable as fluctuant swellings, particularly in a cervical or submandibular location, or may disseminate systemically. Opportunistic bacteria residing within the oropharynx are thought to cause unilateral or bilateral abscesses in draining cervical lymph nodes secondary to abrasions of the oral or conjunctival mucosa, through bite wounds, or following direct translocation across the oral mucosa. Bacteria may also disseminate resulting in systemic abscessation.

3.2.2.2 Pathology

Bacteria are readily apparent within the superficial crust of affected areas and associated with suppurative superficial perivascular inflammation. Abscesses are variably sized and typically have a thick, fibrous capsule and contain abundant purulent material.

3.2.2.3 Laboratory Diagnostics

Bacteria isolated from skin infections in guinea pigs commonly include *Staphylococcus aureus* and *Streptococcus zooepidemicus*. *S. zooepidemicus* is isolated most frequently from abscesses; however, *S. aureus* may also induce abscessation. *Streptococcus moniliformis* is identified rarely.

3.2.2.4 Differential Diagnoses

Other causes of poor hair coat and alopecia should be explored, including hypovitaminosis C, mechanical abrasion from the cage or feeder, external parasitism, and dermatophytosis. Hair chewing (barbering or overgrooming) typically does not result in abraded skin.

3.2.2.5 Group or Herd Management

Bacterial dermatitis arises secondarily to other husbandry or health factors, such as malocclusion, and animal management should be evaluated (Figure 3.1C). Socially incompatible animals may need to be separated to minimize fighting, adverse stress, and trauma. Constant contact with wet or soiled bedding may initiate skin lesions, and the diet should be evaluated for adequacy of vitamin C content and fiber.

Methicillin-resistant *S. aureus* (MRSA) variants have been identified in guinea pigs on rare occasions and this may be a consideration for households with immunocom-

promised family members. Similarly, serious clustered family infections with *S. zooepidemicus* have been reported in households and definitively linked to subclinically infected guinea pigs using pulsed field gel electrophoresis patterns.

3.2.3 Dermatophytosis

Dermatophytes invade keratinized tissues, such as skin and hair, to establish an infection and subsequent pathology. The classification of *Trichophyton mentagrophytes* is complex and three species are known to exist, based on molecular rDNA sequencing methods: *Arthroderma vanbreuseghemii*, *A. benhamiae*, and *A. simii*. Of these, only *A. benhamiae* has been isolated from guinea pigs and it is known to be a zoonotic species.

Whereas indoor-housed pet guinea pigs may be subclinical carriers of *T. mentagrophytes* complex, clinical disease from cutaneous infection (ringworm) is uncommon. It is difficult to determine the true prevalence of the condition because of the wide variation in survey results and sometimes incomplete reporting of data sampling and testing methods. While some recent surveys of pet and pet store-housed animals suggest less than a 4% carrier rate, other surveys suggest higher rates of up to 40%. *Microsporum canis* and *M. gypseum* are isolated infrequently from lesions on affected animals. Overt dermatophytosis can occur in animals kept in overcrowded or unsanitary conditions, in animals with subclinical or clinical hypovitaminosis C, in animals with various ectoparasite infections or in pregnant animals. Otherwise, deep or systemic mycoses are rarely reported in guinea pigs.

3.2.3.1 Presenting Clinical Signs

Superficial mycotic infections present as nonpruritic to mildly pruritic, patchy foci of alopecia or areas of broken

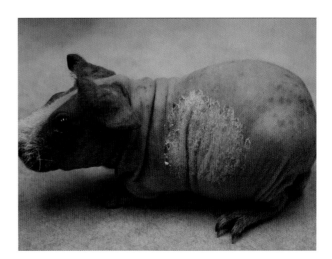

Figure 3.2 Dermatophytosis in a hairless guinea pig (skinny pig) characterized by a large scaling area of superficial dermatitis. *Source:* Courtesy of The Links Road Animal and Bird Clinic.

hair shafts with or without crusting, affecting the head, face, or thorax (Figure 3.2). Erythema and inflammation may occur in more chronic infections. Human caregivers may be affected in many cases, demonstrating similar pruritic circular lesions.

3.2.3.2 Pathology

Microscopically, fungal hyphae and arthrospores are seen to invade the stratum corneum and or are present within hair shafts. Mild neutrophilic inflammation may be present. Visualization of hyphae and spores can be enhanced with a PAS or a Gomori methenamine silver stain. Secondary bacterial infections may occur if there is cutaneous abrasion or ulceration.

3.2.3.3 Laboratory Diagnostics

T. mentagrophytes do not fluoresce under a Wood's lamp, as does *Microsporum* spp., and positive identification is best obtained through culture and biopsy with histopathology. Validated PCR assays may be used to identify species-specific DNA sequences of nuclear ribosomal internal transcribed spacer 1 (ITS1) regions.

3.2.3.4 Differential Diagnoses

Differential diagnoses for dermatophytosis include hair chewing and, alopecia secondary to mechanical abrasion, environmental or topical hypersensitivity reactions, or ectoparasitism.

3.2.3.5 Disease/Colony Management

Infection with *T. mentagrophytes* is potentially zoonotic and may spread to other household pets. Infectious arthrospores are shed into the environment and in households with multiple guinea pigs, all animals should be treated and the environment decontaminated. Spontaneous remissions have only been reported in approximately 7% of cases, suggesting that most animals should be treated.

3.2.4 External Parasites

Guinea pigs are host to a number of ectoparasites, and infestations are common amongst pets, although they are typically subclinical. Mixed infestations of mites and lice may be present on any one animal, and transmission is by direct contact with adult stages from other infested animals or by contact with immature forms that hatch from eggs present within the environment. Ectoparasitism is rare in commercially bred laboratory guinea pigs in North America. Except for cases of sarcoptic mange, clinical signs of ectoparasitism may be present only with very heavy infestations. Owners should be advised to conduct a thorough decontamination of the environment after clean-up to minimize opportunities for reinfestation.

Cutaneous myiasis (fly strike) occurs periodically in guinea pigs. In this condition, calliphorid flies lay eggs that hatch into larvae (maggots) that feed on necrotic tissue of the animal. Cutaneous myiasis is seen more commonly in older obese animals with fecal matting or poor grooming or on animals with wet or heavily soiled housing (see Rabbits Chapter 1, Section 1.2.4.1, for further discussion). Necrotic tissue may exude a foul odor and become infected with bacteria. In cases of extensive tissue damage, animals may die acutely of shock. The condition occurs more often under warm, humid ambient conditions.

3.2.4.1 Sarcoptic Mange

Trixacarus caviae is a burrowing mite that induces sarcoptic mange in guinea pigs. Infestations may be subclinical but usually result in severe pruritus and self-trauma. Shipping, pregnancy, hypovitaminosis C, and any condition lowering immune resistance may predispose animals to clinical disease. All ages may be infested, and lesions consist of areas of lichenification and erythema with scaling, crusting, hair loss, seborrhea, and hyperpigmentation. Whereas infestation may initially be limited to the head, neck, and dorsal thorax, the entire body may be affected in chronic disease (Figure 3.3A). The condition is diagnosed by deep skin scrapings or biopsy with histopathology, looking for the presence of characteristic sarcoptid mites and eggs.

Microscopically, there is marked orthokeratotic hyperkeratosis of affected areas with acanthosis and deep downgrowth of rete pegs, edema, and mixed leukocytic infiltrates. Secondary bacterial infections may occur in areas of ulceration. Mites, eggs, and associated dark pigmented debris are visualized superficially within burrows in the stratum corneum and hair follicles. The adult

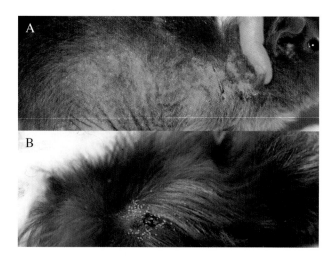

Figure 3.3 A: Sarcoptic mange secondary to *Trixacarus caviae* infestation in a guinea pig. B: *Gliricola porcelli* nits around the teat on the ventrum of a sow. *Source:* A: Courtesy of K. Korber. B: Courtesy of C. Wheler.

mites must be differentiated from other less common sarcoptid mites that are seen occasionally in guinea pigs, including *S. scabei* and *Notoedres cati*. *T. caviae* is smaller than either of these other mites (150 µm x 125 µm), with a more dorsal location of the anus in females, and simple dorsal setae.

The entire life cycle occurs on the host and once a positive diagnosis has been confirmed, other pet guinea pigs in a household should be treated, even if they have no clinical signs. The mites will infest humans and induce papillary urticaria, although humans are considered a nonviable host for further mite propagation.

Demodex caviae is a follicular mite of guinea pigs but infestation is subclinical. Mites may be found incidentally when collecting skin scrapings for *T. caviae* or during routine histologic examination of skin sections.

3.2.4.2 Fur Mites

Chirodiscoides caviae is a cavian fur mite that feeds on superficial debris and skin secretions of infested animals. Mites may be found anywhere on the body, but are found commonly deep within the pelage on the flanks and dorsum. While infestations are generally asymptomatic, pruritus, alopecia, scaling, and mild, self induced ulcerative dermatitis may occur with heavy infestations, and mites may be seen attached to the base of hairs with the unaided eye. Male mites may be carried on the backs of female mites, and the anterior set of legs is modified in both sexes into clasping structures. Adult mites are approximately 350–500 µm by 160 µm, and the long narrow eggs are cemented to individual hairs. Minimal inflammation is seen microscopically in infested animals. A recent prevalence study demonstrated that 32% of pet guinea pigs in southern Italy are infested with *C. caviae* and that prevalence is highest (67%) in animals originating from pet shops.

Cheyletiella parasitovorax also infests guinea pigs, resulting in scaling, and mild pruritus. Mites can be seen moving deep within the pelage. This mite is zoonotic, leading to mild urticaria, typically of the forearms, in human caregivers, and other pets may become infested.

Infestation of two guinea pigs with a nonfeeding nymphal stage (hypopus) of an astigmatic mite (*Acarus farris*) has been reported, resulting in subtotal truncal alopecia, scaling, and mild pruritus. Histopathologic changes were minimal suggesting that the hair loss was induced by mite hypersensitivity and local abrasion. Mites were present in the hay offered to these guinea pigs, and the dermatitis resolved rapidly with removal of the contaminated feed.

3.2.4.3 Lice, Fleas, and Ticks

Guinea pigs are host to two species of surface-dwelling sucking lice, *Gliricola porcelli* and, less commonly, *Gyropus ovalis*. Both species feed by abrading the skin. Lice infestations are common in pets and these parasites may induce mild pruritus and alopecia anywhere on the body, although clinical signs are often absent. Lice may be seen moving within the hair coat with the unaided eye, and eggs (nits) are found cemented to the base of hair shafts (Figure 3.3B). The entire life cycle occurs on the host and infestation is host-specific.

Ctenocephalides felis is found rarely on guinea pigs in households with infested cats or dogs, and may induce pruritus, patchy alopecia, and superficial abrasions.

Rhipicephalus sp. and *Amblyomma* sp. ticks may be transmitted to guinea pigs experimentally. Guinea pigs that graze out of doors should be examined for ticks if living in tick-infested areas.

Laboratory Diagnostics Except for *Trixacarus* and *Demodex* spp., most external parasites of guinea pigs are readily visualized with the unaided eye. Sucking lice and fur mites will move off the pelage as the cadaver cools and can be seen and collected if the body is placed on a dark surface. Eggs remain firmly cemented to hairs and can be collected with routine skin sections for microscopic evaluation. *Demodex* and *Trixacarus* spp. can be identified by microscopic evaluation of deep skin scrapings or via skin biopsies and histopathology.

Disease/Colony Management Transmission of mites and lice occurs by direct contact with other infested animals or through contact with subadult forms of the parasites that are hatched from eggs shed into the environment. Once an infestation has been detected, all guinea pigs in a home or breeding operation should be treated at the same time to break the cycle of infection, regardless of the presence of clinical signs consistent with infestation in any given animal. Several species of guinea pig parasites are zoonotic for human caregivers, and ectoparasites of other pet species may be transmitted to guinea pigs.

3.2.5 Mastitis

Bacterial mastitis can occur in nursing guinea pigs, and sows may present with mild to fulminant, acute or chronic disease. Affected animals may be depressed, dehydrated, anorectic, and pyrexic, with induration and swelling of the affected gland(s).

3.2.5.1 Pathology

Necrosis and suppuration may be seen within the affected glands, with hemorrhage, edema, and abscessation. A variety of pathogens has been isolated from affected sows, including alpha-hemolytic *Streptococcus* spp. *S. aureus*, *E. coli*, *Klebsiella pneumonia*, and *Proteus* sp.

3.2.5.2 Group or Herd Management

Sows may be predisposed to the condition by prolonged contact with wet, dirty bedding and coarse bedding materials, which may induce teat abrasions. Teats may also become lacerated during suckling of pups, providing a portal of entry for environmental bacteria. Affected breeding sows should be culled.

3.2.6 Pododermatitis

Ulcerative pododermatitis occurs commonly in guinea pigs and predisposing factors include housing on wire mesh floors or rough surfaces, coarse bedding material that induces footpad abrasions, obesity, persistent wet or dirty environmental conditions, and hypovitaminosis C, which may result in improper collagen formation in the skin and increased susceptibility to infections.

The palmar or plantar surfaces of one or more feet may be affected, and animals may be reluctant to walk. The affected limb or foot may be erythematous and edematous. Lesions may vary from superficial erosion to deep ulceration with frank hemorrhage or crusting, with or without accompanying suppurative osteomyelitis (Figure 3.4A). *S. aureus* may be isolated from more chronic lesions.

3.2.7 Cutaneous Masses and Neoplasia

Guinea pigs may have some natural resistance to tumors that is conferred by circulating Kurloff cells, which have natural killer (NK) cell-like activity, including tumor cell lytic properties. However, as guinea pigs have become more popular as pets and live to older ages, and as more tissue biopsies are submitted for microscopic assessment and cadavers for post mortem evaluation, increasing numbers and types of tumors have been recognized and characterized. Approximately 15% of all guinea pig tumors seen occur in the skin. Masses occur with equal incidence in males and females, and are more common in animals 3 years of age or older.

In guinea pigs, skin tumors are not thought to be virally-induced, and the more common masses seen include benign cutaneous growths, such as collagen nevi, trichofolliculoma and trichoepithelioma, benign and malignant mammary tumors, epitheliotropic lymphosarcoma, papillomas (Figure 3.5) and less commonly, benign and malignant adnexal tumors, lipomas/liposarcomas, fibrosarcomas, hemangiomas, squamous cell carcinomas (Figure 3.4B) and various sarcomas. Cutaneous masses must be differentiated from abscesses, and cytologic examination of fine needle

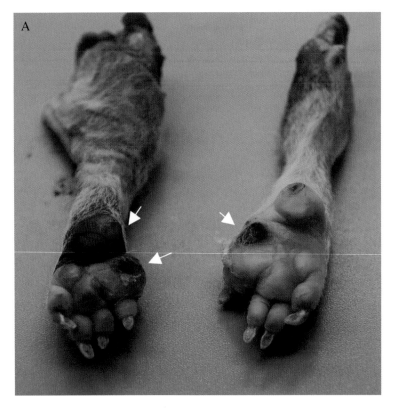
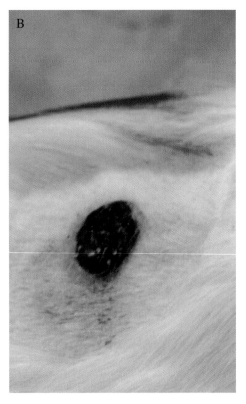

Figure 3.4 A: Bilateral hind paw ulcerative pododermatitis (arrows) in a guinea pig. These lesions commonly arise from housing mature animals in wire bottomed cages for extended periods of time. B: Squamous cell carcinoma on the side of a guinea pig. This mass was relatively well circumscribed and removed by surgical excision.

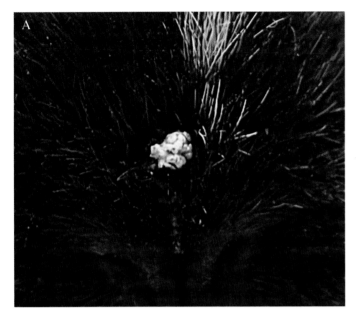

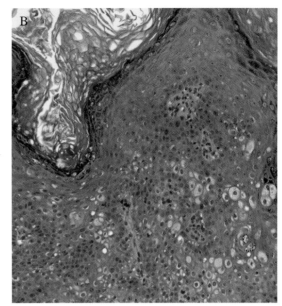

Figure 3.5 A: A small, squamous papilloma on the nose of a 3-year-old female guinea pig. B: The mass consists of multiple papillary projections covered by a squamous epithelium. Many of the epithelial cells have finely vacuolated cytoplasm. *Source:* A: Courtesy of The Links Road Animal and Bird Clinic.

aspirates or excisional biopsy may be used to differentiate among conditions.

3.2.7.1 Trichofolliculoma

Trichofolliculoma is the most common skin tumor seen in guinea pigs and may occur in either sex at any age. It is a benign mass that is currently classified as a cutaneous hamartoma with follicular differentiation. Masses are well circumscribed, hairless, variably-sized but can be quite large, exceeding 4–5 cm in diameter, firm, and may be sin-

gle or multiple in an individual animal. They may occur anywhere on the body, although the dorsum and caudal hip area are common sites. These tumors sometimes have a central pore, through which inspissated white or grayish cellular debris may be expressed (Figure 3.6). Animals may over-groom these masses, leading to superficial ulceration, hemorrhage, and crusting.

Microscopically, trichofolliculomas are seen to consist of densely packed abortive but well differentiated follicular structures, some with partial hair shafts, which may

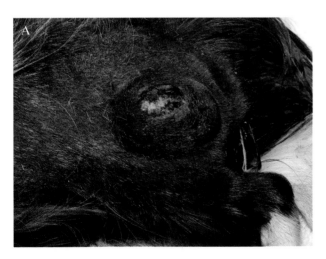

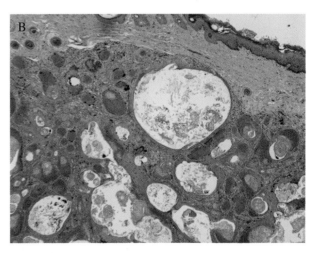

Figure 3.6 A: Trichofolliculoma on the hip of a guinea pig. Pale, greasy cellular debris can often be expressed from the central cavity of these tumors. B: Densely packed, well-differentiated follicular structures are noted microscopically. Although these tumors are benign, there can be significant inflammation present if the mass has ruptured. *Source:* A: Courtesy of The Links Road Animal and Bird Clinic.

be arranged around a primary follicle or central cyst lined by stratified squamous epithelium; however, no hairs are produced. Follicular masses may be dilated, cystic, and contain abundant central parakeratotic debris and hair fragments. There may be a mild, mixed inflammatory reaction superficially, particularly if there is concurrent ulceration. Untreated masses will eventually rupture and excision is usually curative, although other trichofolliculomas may arise spontaneously.

Trichofolliculomas must be differentiated from trichoepitheliomas, which occur with lower prevalence in guinea pigs. Trichoepitheliomas are also well circumscribed, unencapsulated masses consisting of multilobular aggregations of islands and nests of well differentiated basaloid cells organized around a central keratin-filled cyst within a moderate fibrovascular stroma. Cells differentiate towards the cyst center from basal to more keratinized squamous, although keratohyaline granules are absent in even the more differentiated squamous cells, which often have ghost nuclei. These are also benign masses but they can elicit intense excoriation if they rupture because of keratin-induced inflammation. Excision is generally curative.

3.2.7.2 Mammary Gland Tumors

Guinea pigs have only two inguinal mammary glands. Mammary tumors may occur in both male and female guinea pigs that are usually at least 3 years of age or older, and may involve one or both glands (Figure 3.7). Adenomas and adenocarcinomas must be differentiated from mammary gland hyperplasia, which can be seen in sows with cystic ovarian disease. Many of the masses appear to arise

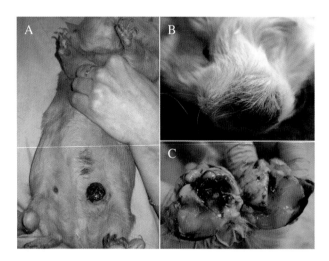

Figure 3.7 A: Mammary gland adenocarcinoma in a guinea pig. B: A large, soft, asymmetrical nasal mass on the face of a 2.5 year-old female guinea pig. C: The mass is gelatinous and fatty on cut section and consists of invading vacuolated, spindyloid cells within a myxoid stroma, most consistent with a liposarcoma. *Source:* A: Courtesy of The Links Road Animal and Bird Clinic.

from a ductal origin, based on cytokeratin expression in normal ductal and abnormal tumor cells, and also contain estrogen and progesterone receptors, indicating hormonal responsiveness. Masses may be solid or cystic in nature and benign masses consist of epithelial cells arranged in tubular, tubulopapillary, or lobular patterns. Very large masses may become ulcerated with an associated mixed, leukocytic inflammatory response. Malignant masses are more common in guinea pigs and demonstrate cellular atypia, increased cellularity and mitotic activity, and local invasion, making complete surgical excision difficult in many cases. Metastasis to local lymph nodes or the thoracic cavity generally occurs late in the course of the disease.

3.2.8 Other Integument Conditions

Fur chewing (barbering) is a common behavioral condition seen in singly or group-housed animals and, if hair shafts are chewed down to the skin surface, results in patchy areas of apparent hair loss anywhere on the body. While not harmful to the animal, minor skin abrasions from chewing may permit opportunistic bacterial colonization and subsequent abscessation. Causes of hair chewing are undetermined but boredom has been suggested as a possible cause. Fur chewing should be differentiated from other conditions causing nonpruritic alopecia, such as dermatophyte infection or mechanical abrasion.

A congenital, focal, superficial, cutaneous **vascular malformation** has been reported in an adult female guinea pig, with periodic hemorrhage and eventual vascular rupture and bleed-out, leading to death of the adult animal. There was no histologic evidence of neoplasia.

Allergic and irritant **contact dermatitis** resulting from exposure to a range of environmental antigens is reported anecdotally in pet guinea pigs. Detergents and disinfectants may be particularly irritating, and cages should be rinsed thoroughly after disinfection.

Sebaceous gland secretions may accumulate around the perianal folds and perineal area of male guinea pigs. Secretions are testosterone-dependent and may induce matting of hair in these areas.

3.3 Endocrine Conditions

Endocrine disorders are rare in guinea pigs and there have been no reports of spontaneous pituitary gland diseases or tumors. It is common for those not regularly conducting guinea pig necropsies to misinterpret the large size of the adrenal glands in this species. The guinea pig adrenal glands are normally bilobed and one-third to one half the length of the kidneys (Figure 3.8A).

Unencapsulated rests of thyroid follicular cells may be seen in the ventral cervical region of normal guinea pigs,

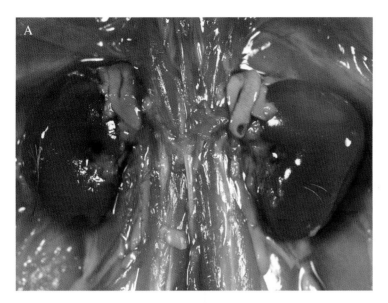
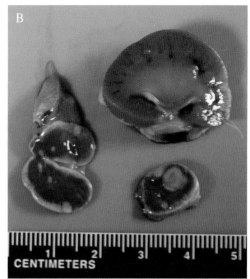

Figure 3.8 A: Normal adrenal glands in a guinea pig. Adrenal glands are large relative to other species; typically, one third to one half the length of the kidney. B: Adrenocortical nodules from a guinea pig, an incidental finding at necropsy.

adjacent to the thyroid glands. Parathyroid glands may be difficult to distinguish in guinea pigs. The parathyroid glands are found in close anterolateral proximity to the thyroid gland, rarely extending below its caudal border, but are less commonly embedded within the thyroid gland, as is seen for many other mammalian species. Up to eight parathyroid glands may be found in normal, healthy guinea pigs, and gland numbers and sizes are not bilaterally symmetrical.

The processes for calcium absorption and secretion are not understood as well for guinea pigs as they are for rabbits. Both species are dependent on adequate vitamin D levels in the diet. Guinea pigs appear to freely absorb calcium from their diet, as do rabbits, and excrete any surplus in their urine. Plasma calcium levels are not useful indicators of vitamin D toxicity in guinea pigs; hyperphosphatemia may be a better indicator.

3.3.1 Diabetes Mellitus

Guinea pigs may develop diabetes mellitus, and they are used as a research model for this condition. Spontaneous diabetes mellitus has been described in a guinea pig colony as a contagious, potentially virally-transmitted condition. Unaffected guinea pigs co-housed with affected animals developed glucosuria, cataracts, weight loss, polydipsia, polyuria, and islet cell degeneration after approximately 6–12 weeks. Microscopically, fatty degeneration and fibrosis of the pancreas were seen, with vacuolation of pancreatic islets. Beta cells appeared degranulated and contained PAS-positive glycogen-like electron-lucent material. Renal glomerular mesangial thickening and microangiopathy were variably present in chronically affected animals.

Type C retrovirus-like particles have been observed emerging from guinea pig chorioallantoic membranes inoculated with urine from affected animals; however, a specific virus has never been isolated and characterized. Interestingly, some picornaviruses are known to induce spontaneous type I diabetes mellitus in other species, for example, Coxsackie B4 virus infection of humans and encephalomyocarditis virus (mengovirus) infection of mice. Further work is required to characterize the pathogenesis of this condition in guinea pigs.

3.3.2 Endocrine Neoplasia

Endocrine tumors are uncommon in guinea pigs; however, tumors of the endocrine pancreas, adrenal glands, and thyroid gland have all been described. Note that an important and more common differential diagnosis for intact sows presenting with alopecia, polydipsia, and polyuria is ovarian cysts (i.e., cystic rete ovarii).

3.3.2.1 Pancreatic Islet Cell Tumor

Pancreatic islet cell tumor (PICT) or insulinoma has been reported on occasion in aging guinea pigs and there may be breed or strain predilections for developing this neoplasm. Tumors in guinea pigs are composed primarily of beta cells, and clinical signs are related to unregulated and excessive pulsatile secretion of insulin by the tumor. Animals may present with weakness and ataxia related to sudden hypoglycemia. Masses may be single or multiple with a medullary, trabecular or ribbon-like pattern of neoplastic cells supported by a fine fibrovascular stroma. Typically, the tumors are well differentiated but nonencapsulated, compressing the adjacent normal pancreatic tissue. Neoplastic cells vary widely in shape and size among animals, and mitotic figures are variable. There are no reported insulin or insulin:glucose reference ranges for guinea pigs.

3.3.2.2 Hyperadrenocorticism

Hyperadrenocorticism (Cushing's disease) is seen rarely in a guinea pigs, and is usually secondary to an adrenal gland mass. Clinical signs include bilaterally symmetrical alopecia, lethargy, obesity, hepatomegaly, polydipsia, and polyuria. Masses may be uni- or bilateral and are well circumscribed. Both adrenal cortical adenomas (Figure 3.8B) and carcinomas have been described in guinea pigs. Salivary cortisol levels may be elevated in affected animals but should not be used as the sole diagnostic criteria, since subclinical hypovitaminosis C may have the same effect.

3.3.2.3 Hyperthyroidism and Thyroid Gland Tumors

Thyroid hyperplasia, adenoma (Figure 3.9A), and carcinoma (Figure 3.9B) all occur relatively commonly in guinea pigs over 3 years of age, with a prevalence of up to 4.6%. Clinical signs noted in affected animals include hyperactivity, weight loss and wasting despite excellent appetite, polyuria and polydipsia, a palpable cervical mass, and diarrhea. Assessment of serum T_4 levels may be a useful diagnostic adjunct for surgical biopsy cases. In normal animals, serum thyroxine levels range from 14.2–66.9 nmol/L, with similar ranges reported for males and females, regardless of age.

Various patterns for thyroid gland tumors are seen including macrofollicular adenoma, papillary and cystadenomas, and small cell and follicular carcinomas, with almost an even mix of benign and malignant diagnoses. Adenomas are typically well differentiated, encapsulated with follicular, papillary or cyst-like patterns of epithelial

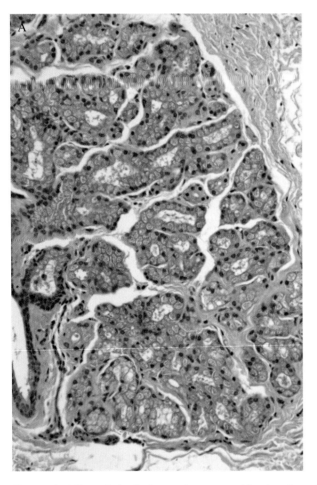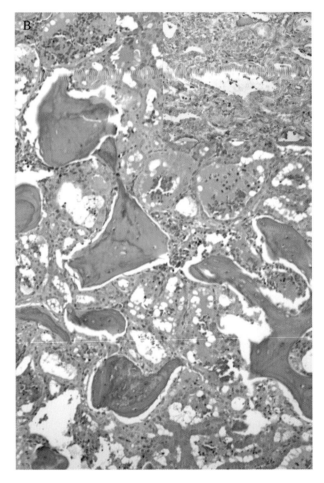

Figure 3.9 A: Thyroid gland adenoma in a 4-year-old male guinea pig with inappetence and weight loss. The nodule is composed of follicles surrounded by well differentiated cuboidal epithelium. B: Ossifying thyroid gland carcinoma in a guinea pig composed of less well differentiated cells without clear follicle formation. Multifocal bony spicules are present throughout. Inset: Moderate cytoplasmic immunolabeling for thyroglobulin is present (counter-stain: Mayer's hematoxylin).

cells, and compress the normal surrounding parenchyma. Malignant tumors are denser and may demonstrate capsular invasion as well as increased anisokaryosis, pleomorphism, and mitoses. Osseous metaplasia as well as cystic areas containing colloid-like proteinaceous material can be seen with both benign and malignant tumors as well as. Metastases are rare but have been noted in draining cervical lymph nodes, heart, and lungs. Parafollicular or C cell tumors are also seen sporadically (Figure 3.10).

3.3.3 Other Endocrine Conditions

Hyperparathyroidism has only been diagnosed anecdotally in guinea pigs, with several case reports of fibrous osteodystrophy suspected to result from underlying secondary hyperparathyroidism.

Fatty infiltration and degeneration of the pancreas, with or without mild accompanying fibrosis, is seen commonly in older, obese guinea pigs. This is usually an incidental histologic finding with no clinical correlate (Figure 3.11).

Metastatic mineralization of soft tissues may be seen with a dietary excess of phosphorus and a deficiency of magnesium or in cases of hypervitaminosis D. Hypervitaminosis D results commonly from over-supplementation of vitamin drops when attempting to administer adequate amounts of vitamin C to animals. Hypervitaminosis D with metastatic calcification has been reported in a colony of guinea pigs that were fed a diet inadvertently over-supplemented with vitamin D. A number of animals demonstrated nonspecific clinical signs prior to euthanasia, including poor body condition, lethargy, and feed refusal. Osteosclerosis, renal tubular mineralization, myocardial mineralization as well as calcification of other soft tissues were noted in many animals on gross and microscopic evaluation.

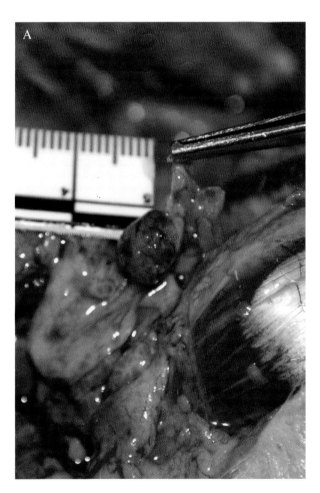
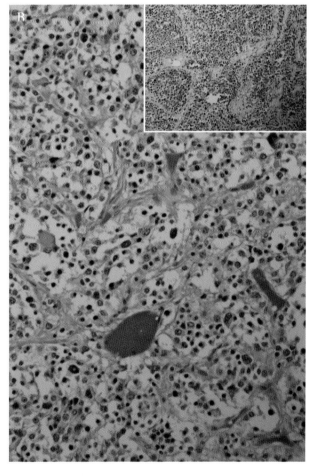

Figure 3.10 A: Parafollicular (C cell) tumor in a 4-year-old female neutered guinea pig that presented with tachypnea and gastrointestinal stasis. Two masses were found as well as evidence of metastasis to the submandibular lymph node. B: Cells were pleomorphic and there was loss of follicles. Strong positive cytoplasmic immunolabeling was present for synaptophysin and calcitonin (inset), with weaker labeling for chromogranin (counter-stain: Mayer's hematoxylin).

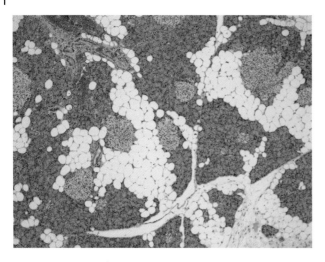

Figure 3.11 Fatty infiltration of the pancreas is seen commonly in older obese guinea pigs. Dense fatty infiltrates were also seen in the stomach wall (not shown).

3.4 Respiratory Conditions

As in other hystricomorph rodents, including chinchillas, the soft palate in guinea pigs is continuous with the base of the tongue, and a small opening, the palatal ostium, connects the oral cavity with the caudal pharynx. Vocal cords are poorly developed in guinea pigs. As in all rodents, all branches from the primary bronchi are bronchioles, distinguished by a lack of cartilage, and, in the guinea pig, submucosal glands. The pulmonary parenchyma has very little connective tissue in the guinea pig, but, in contrast to other rodents, guinea pigs have significant smooth muscle support around smaller bronchi and on the pleural surface. Guinea pigs have been used as models for respiratory sensitization and asthma because they manifest marked airway hyper-responsiveness following antigenic challenge. This may be due to the unique pulmonary musculature and large numbers of mast cells found in and around airways and on the pleural surface. Guinea pigs also have increased relative numbers of goblet cells in respiratory bronchi compared with other rodent species. The right lung of the guinea pig has four lobes (cranial, middle, accessory, and caudal), while the left lung has only three lobes (cranial, middle, and caudal).

Subclinical and clinical respiratory disease is common in pet guinea pigs that are purchased from pet stores and is primarily bacterial in nature. Clinical signs of disease may be subtle and nonspecific, including unexpected death, unkempt hair coat, decreased appetite, inactivity, oculonasal discharge, and sneezing.

3.4.1 Bordetellosis

Bordetella bronchiseptica is a small, motile, Gram-negative coccobacillus that is transmitted by direct contact with contaminated fomites or respiratory secretions and aerosols from clinically affected or carrier animals. Different strains exist, and those recovered from guinea pigs have a higher pathogenicity for this species than do *B. bronchiseptica* substrains isolated from other species, although infections may be subclinical. *B. bronchiseptica* has a predilection for colonizing ciliated epithelium, in which the bacteria intercalate between cilia, interfering with rhythmic ciliary movement and elimination of mucus, cellular debris, and other waste materials.

The bacterium is considered a primary pathogen for guinea pigs and peracute to chronic disease may be seen. There is no correlation between age and susceptibility to infection, with all age groups being susceptible. Some guinea pigs may become chronic carriers that periodically shed bacteria, while others may clear the infection completely, with few residual signs and long term resistance to reinfection.

3.4.1.1 Presenting Clinical Signs

Affected animals may have no clinical signs or may present with serous to purulent oculonasal discharge, head tilt, sneezing, lethargy, dyspnea, and decreased appetite. Some animals may be found dead with few premonitory signs following peracute infection.

3.4.1.2 Pathology

Grossly, patchy areas of hemorrhage and necrosis may be seen in anteroventral lung lobes of affected animals, spreading to caudal lobes in more fulminant and chronic cases, with serous to hemorrhagic pleural effusion. Concurrent otitis media is common and a serous to purulent exudate may be seen upon opening the tympanic bullae, with marked hyperostosis and subtotal lumenal occlusion in chronically affected animals.

Microscopically, there is a multifocal suppurative and necrotizing bronchitis and bronchiolitis, with epithelial hyperplasia and loss, goblet cell hyperplasia, and accumulation of degenerate neutrophils, sloughed epithelia, and other debris in airways (Figure 3.12). Parenchymal involvement may occur more chronically with thickening of alveolar septa, necrosis and consolidation of alveoli, hemorrhage, and a marked influx of alveolar macrophages, lymphocytes, and neutrophils. Perivascular lymphoid aggregates may be very prominent.

3.4.1.3 Laboratory Diagnostics

A definitive diagnosis is based on positive microbiologic culture results for *B. bronchiseptica* from exudate or tissue obtained from the nasopharynx, middle ear, or pulmonary parenchyma, combined with gross and microscopic findings consistent with a characteristic suppurative bronchopneumonia or otitis media. When nasal swabs are used to

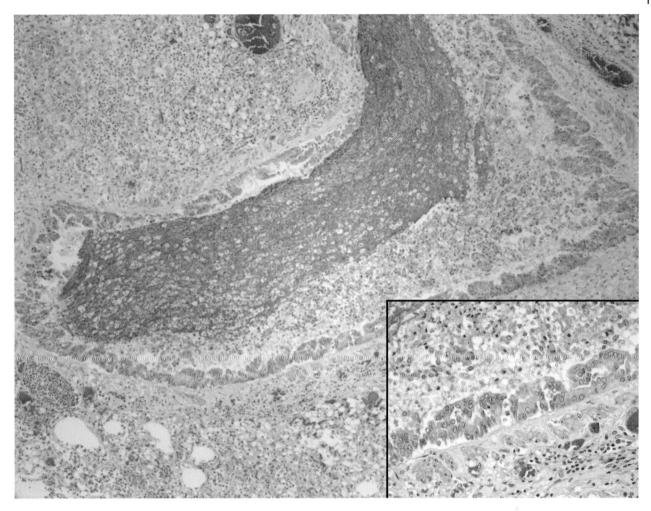

Figure 3.12 Photomicrograph of lung section from a guinea pig dying from *Bordetella bronchiseptica*-induced bronchopneumonia. Bronchioles are filled with suppurative exudate. Inset: The bronchiolar epithelium is jumbled and deciliated.

screen animal colonies for carriers, MacConkey agar is the preferred culture medium because it retards growth of contaminants. Serum ELISA testing can also be undertaken to prove exposure to the organism.

3.4.1.4 Disease/Colony Management

There is no commercial vaccine available to prevent this infection in guinea pigs, although autologous vaccine production has been attempted. Enzootically infected colonies may show few outward signs of disease; however, disease may recrudesce following stress, transportation, or changes in management practices. Animals with subclinical hypovitaminosis C may be more susceptible to infection, and underlying malnutrition should always be considered.

It is possible to eradicate *B. bronchiseptica* from breeding colonies using strict early weaning and isolation practices. In one study, newborn pups weaned and separated from infected dams within 4 days of birth remained free of infection into adulthood. Pups that were not separated until 3 weeks of age had a high rate of infection.

3.4.1.5 Differential Diagnoses

Other common causes of bacterial pneumonia in guinea pigs include *S. pneumonia*, *S. zooepidemicus*, and rarely, *Klebsiella pneumoniae*. Streptococcal infections tend to induce a more fibrinous reaction that involves the pleura. Adenoviral pneumonia is a potential differential diagnosis but tends to affect younger animals and cause high mortality. *B. bronchiseptica*, *S. pneumoniae*, *S. zooepidemicus*, and *P. aeruginosa* are the most common microbiologic isolates from cases of otitis media in guinea pigs. Other causes of head tilt include encephalitis caused by *Baylisascaris* spp. migration, trauma, and intracerebral abscess. Cardiovascular disease may also result in weakness and dyspnea.

3.4.2 Streptococcal Pneumonia

Streptococcus pneumoniae is a Gram-positive bacterium that grows in pairs or short chains. There are over 80 serotypes recognized; however, isolates of *S. pneumoniae* obtained from infected guinea pigs are of different serotypes than those routinely cultured from human cases of streptococcal infection, making human infection from diseased guinea pigs unlikely. Virulence factors vary by isolate and include a range of complement activating pneumolysins, neuraminidase, autolysin, and capsular and cell wall polysaccharides used for host cell attachment and immune cell evasion. The organism is carried subclinically in the oropharynx and upper respiratory tract of otherwise normal animals. Both the immune status of the host at the time of infection and the specific virulence factors of a given serotype determine the outcome of an infection.

Although less common as a cause of enzootic pneumonia in pet guinea pigs than *B. bronchiseptica*, sporadic epizootics may occur with *S. pneumoniae* infection. Death may be seen peracutely with few premonitory signs, and there is no age or sex predilection for infection. Bilateral purulent otitis media and fibrinopurulent pleuropneumonia, pericarditis, meningitis, and arthritis may occur following systemic infection. Pulmonary abscesses have also been reported. Similar findings may be associated with infection with *S. zooepidemicus*, although subcutaneous abscesses are a more common manifestation of infection with *S. zooepidemicus*. As for other respiratory infections, subclinical hypovitaminosis C may weaken immune system function, making animals more susceptible to infection and disease.

Bacteria are readily isolated from fibrinopurulent fluid or tissue from affected animals. Carrier states may be difficult to identify and several deep nasal swabs may be required for positive confirmation. The tympanic bullae should always be examined in cases of pneumonia in guinea pigs, for concurrent involvement.

3.4.3 Other Bacterial Respiratory Conditions

Mycoplasma pulmonis can be isolated occasionally from guinea pigs but affected animals show no clinical signs, suggesting that the infection is subclinical in this species. *Pasteurella pneumotropica* can be also isolated from the oropharynx of normal guinea pigs but clinical disease is not reported.

Sporadic and isolated cases of pulmonary abscessation have been seen in guinea pigs due to *S. aureus* or *P. aeruginosa* infection. Guinea pigs have been experimentally infected with cilia-associated respiratory bacillus (CARB), but natural disease has not been reported with this agent.

3.4.4 Viral Respiratory Diseases

Guinea pigs are commonly used as models for a number of human respiratory viruses, but viral disease in solitary pets is rare. Outbreaks may occur within exotic pet distribution centers or in breeding colonies in which there is mixing of animals of different ages.

3.4.4.1 Adenovirus Infections

Guinea pig adenovirus (GpAV) can infect colonies resulting in low morbidity and high mortality. Adenoviruses are enveloped DNA viruses that are host-specific and induce acute infections. Younger animals are most severely affected, dying peracutely or showing signs of inappetence, poor hair coat, depression, and dyspnea before death. Adult animals may present with a transient upper respiratory infection, characterized by mild rhinitis, which is quickly cleared. Gross examination of animals with dyspnea may reveal anteroventral pulmonary consolidation and hemorrhage with serous pleural exudate. Histologically, round to oval, large, smudgy, basophilic intranuclear inclusion bodies (approximately 70–90 nm in diameter) can be seen within the nasal mucosa, as well as within affected bronchiolar epithelial cells (Figure 3.13). Multifocally, airways are denuded and contain desquamated epithelial cells and necrotic cellular debris. Alveolar septa surrounding affected airways may be thickened with mixed lymphohistiocytic infiltrates and lesser numbers of neutrophils. The virus is transmitted by direct contact with infected animals or infected respiratory secretions. Specific PCR assays are available for viral detection in lung or feces.

A potential differential diagnosis for large basophilic intranuclear inclusion bodies in guinea pig tissues is

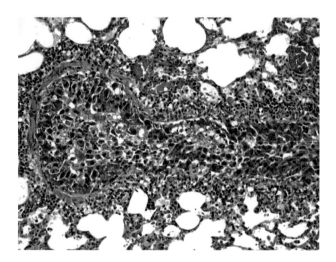

Figure 3.13 Acute adenoviral bronchopneumonia in a young adult guinea pig presenting with marked dyspnea. The bronchiolar epithelium is entirely eroded. Sloughed epithelial cells contain characteristic, smudgy, basophilic intranuclear inclusion bodies. The surrounding alveolar spaces are relatively unaffected.

cytomegalovirus (GpCMV) infection (see Section 3.6.2). Infection with guinea pig CMV is usually restricted to the salivary glands. GpCMV intranuclear inclusion bodies are approximately twice the size of those seen with GpAV. GpAV may be eliminated from colonies by Caesarian rederivation with fostering of pups onto naive dams.

3.4.4.2 Parainfluenza Virus Infections

Guinea pigs are susceptible to human parainfluenza virus-3 (PIV-3), but infections are subclinical with no histologic signs of disease and no reports exist of guinea pig to human transmission of the virus. More serious disease can be seen with secondary bacterial infection (Figure 3.14). A guinea pig-specific variant of the human virus has been identified and sequenced but is largely nonpathogenic. Animals may be protected by maternal antibodies until 2 weeks of age, after which they become susceptible to infection. There is no indication of cross-species transmission to humans or of viral persistence in the guinea pig host.

Similarly, guinea pigs can become infected with Sendai virus and pneumonia virus of mice, two other parainfluenza viruses that primarily affect mice, but infections are subclinical and rapidly cleared. Sendai virus is a type-1 parainfluenza virus (PIV-1). Guinea pigs infected with PIV-3 may test positive with PIV-1 serologic immunoassays because of cross-reactivity. Hemagglutination inhibition or PCR assays conducted using fresh or frozen tracheal tissue may be used to differentiate between PIV-3 and PIV-1 infection in guinea pigs.

3.4.5 Pulmonary Neoplasia

The most common tumor in the guinea pig is a bronchogenic adenoma, which is characterized as a well-circumscribed,

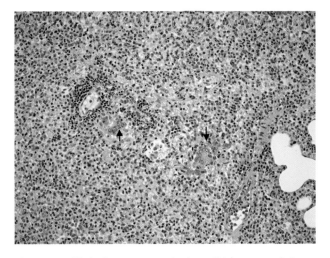

Figure 3.14 Marked, nonsuppurative interstitial pneumonia in a guinea pig with multifocal multinucleated syncytial cells (arrows). An underlying viral etiology, such as parainfluenza virus infection, was strongly suspected, and *Pasteurella multocida* was cultured from the tissue.

unencapsulated, single or multifocal pulmonary mass that compresses the adjacent normal parenchyma. Tumor cells are arranged in trabecular or papillary patterns within a fine fibrovascular stroma, and are well differentiated, with apical nuclei and rare mitoses. They are seen more commonly in animals older than 3 years of age. Care must be taken when evaluating these masses to ensure that they are bona fide tumors as infolding of bronchial mucosa caused by smooth muscle constriction during tissue fixation may create a histologic artifact of similar appearance.

Pulmonary adenocarcinoma has been reported in one older guinea pig, in addition to pulmonary metastases from a mammary adenocarcinoma. A papillary nasal adenocarcinoma was reported in a 4.5-year-old pet guinea pig.

3.4.6 Other Respiratory Conditions

Bony spicules of lamellar bone may be seen radiographically in the lungs and at necropsy, and are usually interpreted as incidental findings. The etiopathogenesis is unknown.

Pulmonary foreign body granulomas may be seen incidentally, generally a result of inhalation of food, bedding, or other organic material. In severe cases, granulomatous pneumonitis may occur.

Dyspnea may occur in guinea pigs for reasons unrelated to infectious pulmonary disease. Nonspecific stress, pregnancy toxemia, heat stress, and gastric torsion may all result in increased, shallow breathing or panting prior to death. Microscopic evaluation of tissues should be conducted to differentiate pulmonary from nonpulmonary causes of respiratory distress.

Allergic rhinitis is not well characterized in guinea pigs, but is reported clinically and attributed to environmental or bedding irritants, such as volatile softwood oils.

3.5 Musculoskeletal Conditions

Guinea pigs are not highly physically active animals and do not hop, jump, or climb. Further, they do not dig tunnels or burrows for shelter, and their nondomesticated counterparts have compact home ranges in the wild, compared with other small mammal species. Thus, guinea pigs have a relatively small muscle mass supporting their large gastrointestinal tract and appendicular skeleton. While any disease or condition affecting muscular or skeletal function may have a significant impact on a guinea pig's ability to ambulate, this may not be readily apparent to the caregiver or an observer because of the guinea pig's sedentary lifestyle.

3.5.1 Hypovitaminosis C

Hypovitaminosis C (scurvy) remains an important systemic condition of guinea pigs and may be challenging to definitively diagnose. Guinea pigs are unable to synthesize ascorbic acid, because they possess a mutated version of the final enzyme, L-gulono-γ-lactone oxidase, which is necessary for conversion of L-glucose to ascorbic acid. Ascorbic acid is a critical cofactor required in several biochemical pathways, including proline and lysine hydroxylation, which are required for type IV collagen cross-linking; carnitine, required for fatty acid transport; conversion of cholesterol to bile acids; renal vitamin D formation and intestinal vitamin D receptor binding; and various other amino acid and peptide synthesis reactions. Defective collagen production affects extracellular matrix composition in the skin, tendons, bony osteoid, dentin, and blood vessels, leading to vascular fragility and decreased tensile strength of various tissues. Reduced ascorbic acid also leads to hepatic accumulation of cholesterol and decreased bile acid production, affecting dietary lipid and fat soluble vitamin absorption. Because ascorbic acid is water-soluble, guinea pigs require the vitamin on a daily basis to maintain good health.

3.5.1.1 Presenting Clinical Signs

Clinical signs are nonspecific and may vary with animal age. Because subclinical hypovitaminosis C is widespread in pet guinea pigs, an underlying deficiency should be suspected in any animal presenting with poor hair coat, anorexia, dental disease, lethargy, diarrhea, weakness, lameness or increased susceptibility to infections (Figure 3.15).

3.5.1.2 Pathology

The classical signs of overt scurvy in juvenile animals include periarticular and subperiosteal swelling and

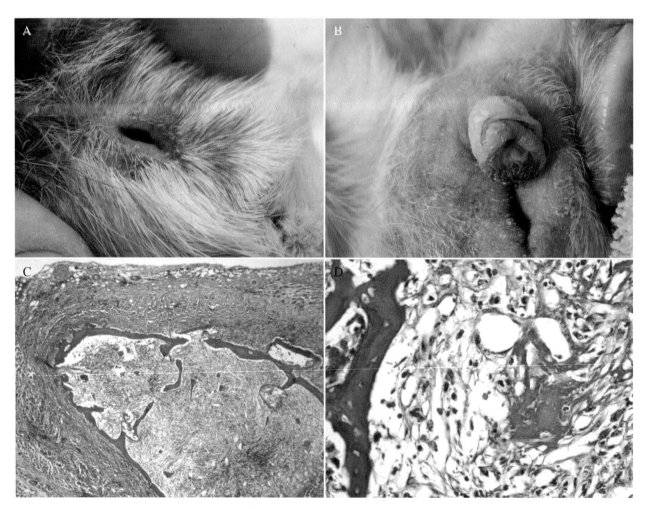

Figure 3.15 A: Skin lesions are common in guinea pigs with subclinical hypovitaminosis C. This animal has a nonexudative conjunctivitis. B: In addition, multifocal areas of patchy hyperkeratosis and scaling are noted, depicted are the penis perineal skin, and scrotum. C: Rib from a young guinea pig with hypovitaminosis C. Microscopically, proliferation of poorly differentiated mesenchymal cells is seen with microfractures and resultant hemorrhage. D: Photomicrograph of mesenchymal cells with nonmineralized osteoid.

hemorrhage, epiphyseal and costochondral junction swelling, hemorrhage into the urinary bladder and intestinal tract, and patchy hemorrhage of skeletal muscle and subcutaneous tissue. Post-mortem findings in subclinically affected adults may be less obvious and include thin or poor hair coat and watery intestinal content. Concurrent weakening of periodontal ligaments may result in loosening of teeth, pain upon eating, and molar overgrowth secondary to anorexia.

The epiphysis of a normal guinea pig should have numerous bony trabeculae extending to the metaphysis. Histologically, bony changes noted with hypovitaminosis C are characterized by epiphyseal thinning with loss of metaphyseal bony spicules and trabeculae, microfractures, and hemorrhage. Endochondral ossification fails to occur, with preservation of the calcified cartilaginous matrix (scorbutic lattice) beneath the zone of chondrocyte proliferation, and there is loss of osteoblast activity and proliferation of poorly differentiated fusiform mesenchymal cells. In severe cases, there is subtotal fibrous replacement of bony spicules and osteoid matrix. Bones are affected unequally.

Concurrent septicemia, respiratory disease, or gastrointestinal disease may be present, making a definitive diagnosis of hypovitaminosis C difficult, unless petechial hemorrhages or other hypovitaminosis C-related lesions are present.

3.5.1.3 Laboratory Diagnostics
Guinea pigs require 10–30 mg/kg of vitamin C daily, and more if they are suffering from infectious diseases of any kind. Tissue-level measurements are not conducted routinely for guinea pigs with suspected disease, and diagnosis of the condition is often based on dietary history, clinical signs, and gross and histologic findings.

3.5.1.4 Disease/Colony Management
Diets high in fat and cholesterol increase demands for ascorbic acid in guinea pigs, and fatty food treats should be avoided in this species as they may exacerbate vitamin C deficiencies. Tissue levels of ascorbate are higher if animals are fed vitamin C throughout the day, rather than as a single daily supplement. It takes approximately two weeks for early signs to be noted in a vitamin C-deficient animal and a week of supplementation for clinical signs to regress, enhancing diagnostic challenges. Although modern guinea pig diets are supplemented with microstabilized vitamin C, prolonged and improper food handling and storage may contribute to vitamin C loss from these diets. For this reason, clients are advised to purchase smaller quantities of food for their guinea pigs more often. Caution should also be exercised when providing vitamin C in the water in the form of multivitamin drops, as hypervitaminosis D may result, with subsequent metastatic calcification.

3.5.2 Other Nutritional Diseases

Osteodystrophy fibrosa (nutritional or secondary hyperparathyroidism) has been reported in pet guinea pigs fed a commercially available but calcium-deficient diet and in pet guinea pigs intentionally fed a low calcium diet to avoid urolithiasis. Animals were lame, off feed, and had radiographic and histologic evidence of healed compression fractures of the femur with osteopenia and myelofibrosis. Hyperplastic parathyroid glands were noted in several animals.

Metastatic calcification has been reported to occur spontaneously in guinea pigs fed high phosphorus, low magnesium diets or when owners provide excessive multivitamin supplementation, leading to hypervitaminosis D (Figure 3.16). Animals may present with an unkempt hair coat and a history of stiffness. Calcium deposits may occur around joints or in any tissue of the body, and nephrocalcinosis may be present in severely affected animals.

Experimentally, dietary deficiencies of combinations of vitamin E and selenium, vitamins C and E, and vitamin C and selenium, result in paresis and death of guinea pigs due to skeletal muscle degeneration and necrosis, and neuronal death with cystic degeneration of the spinal cord and midbrain. The pathogenesis in all cases may be related to oxidative stress. There are no reported cases of spontaneous diseases arising from vitamin E or selenium deficiencies in pet guinea pigs; however, animals fed selenium-deficient diets have lower circulating thyroxine levels.

3.5.3 Degenerative Bone Disease

Osteoarthritis occurs spontaneously in older guinea pigs, most commonly involving the femorotibial joints. There may be breed- or strain-related factors contributing to age at disease onset, with histologic changes noted as early as 3 months of age in Dunkin-Hartley strains. Microscopic changes seen include osteophyte production, subchondral osteosclerosis, femoral condyle cysts, and ligamentous mineralization.

3.5.4 Musculoskeletal Neoplasia

Osteosarcoma is rare but has been reported in several individual animals, generally in guinea pigs less than 2 years of age. Tumors arose in both flat and long bones in an equal proportion of cases and metastases to some or all of the lungs, liver, spleen, pancreas, heart, peritoneal and pleural cavities, and mesentery were noted in two thirds of cases. As for other species, tumors consist of poorly circumscribed, unencapsulated, expansile, multilobulated masses that are densely cellular with round to polygonal neoplastic cells arranged in clusters around mineralized homogenous matrix (osteoid). Anisocytosis, anisokaryosis, and mitoses are variable.

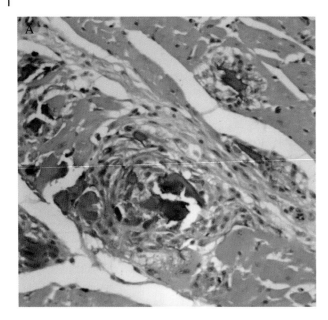
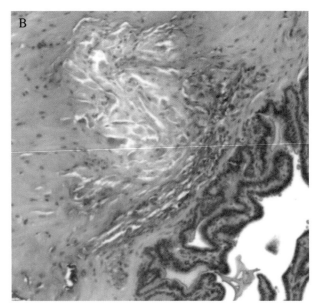

Figure 3.16 Soft tissue mineralization is seen commonly with renal failure or oversupplementation with vitamin D in the diet. Multifocal areas of myocardial (A) and seminal vesicle muscularis (B) mineralization are seen in this adult male guinea pig.

Other musculoskeletal masses are not reported.

3.5.5 Other Musculoskeletal Conditions

Fractures and **trauma** are not uncommon in pet guinea pigs and are due to inadvertent falls or crushing injuries. Iatrogenic **muscle necrosis** with sloughing may arise following intramuscular injection of irritating drugs, such as ketamine hydrochloride, or intramuscular injection of inappropriately large volumes of nonirritating drugs. Guinea pigs have a small muscle mass in their limbs compared with other companion animal species, and other routes of injection, such as subcutaneous, may be less problematic.

Splenic hemangiosarcoma has been reported in an 18-month-old guinea pig presenting with chronic inappetence.

3.6 Gastrointestinal Conditions

Guinea pigs are strict herbivores. The dental formula is 1/1, 1/1, and 3/3 for a total of 20 teeth, all of which grow constantly throughout the animal's life (elodont dentition). The premolars and molars are grossly indistinguishable, except by location, and are collectively referred to as cheek teeth. When examining the oral cavity postmortem for evidence of malocclusion, the occlusal surfaces of the cheek teeth should have an approximately 30^0 oblique slope. It is difficult to visualize the teeth because of the narrow oral cavity and large thick tongue.

In addition, the mouth commonly contains a wad of semi-chewed food in a healthy animal.

Guinea pigs have a simple monogastric stomach and, unlike many other rodent species, there is no nonglandular portion. They are coprophagic hindgut fermenters with a large, sacculated cecum. The proximal colon should never be empty in a healthy animal. Unlike rabbits but similar to chinchillas, guinea pigs use a mucus trap colonic separation mechanism in which mucus and bacteria are separated from fecal material in a furrow in the proximal colon and transported back to the cecum for further digestive functions. Guinea pigs are less efficient at digesting fiber than are rabbits and usually have pellets added to their diet to ensure complete nutrition. Guinea pigs ingest their cecotrophs; however, there is usually less of a visual distinction between these and the hard feces than there is in rabbits. The gut flora is primarily populated by Gram-positive bacteria, the majority of which consists of anaerobic *Lactobacillus* spp. Many of the intestinal disorders seen in guinea pigs occur secondary to disruptions in intestinal bacterial composition or gut motility, resulting in changes in bacterial flora (dysbiosis) and subsequent malabsorption or maldigestion.

Oral swabs are commonly collected from guinea pigs for microbiological monitoring of colony health. *Streptobacillus moniliformis*, the causative agent of rat bite fever in humans, has been periodically identified by serology and PCR from guinea pig colonies, sometimes leading to eradication of entire colonies to minimize the potential for transmitting a serious zoonotic disease. It is important that the 16S rRNA PCR amplicon used for detecting *S. moniliformis* be closely examined, as several nonpathogenic oral bacteria, including *Leptotrichia* spp. may be inadvertently amplified, giving a false positive result. Use of a more specific nested PCR assay or sequencing partially amplified fragments may be used as a confirmatory test.

3.6.1 Oral Conditions

Guinea pigs, like other hystricomorphs, have constantly erupting incisor, premolar, and molar teeth. In animals fed a diet with sufficient vitamin C, incisors will grow at a rate approaching 1 mm per day, and guinea pigs require roughage or objects to chew on to wear down their teeth surfaces. An oblique occlusal surface for molar teeth is normal in guinea pigs, as are alternating layers of enamel, dentine, and cementum.

3.6.1.1 Malocclusion

Overgrowth of incisors and cheek teeth are commonly seen in guinea pigs and may occur rapidly, leading to malocclusion. This condition is often accompanied by tongue entrapment and hypersalivation (slobbers) (Figure 3.17A). Guinea pigs are more susceptible to tongue entrapment compared with chinchillas and rabbits because of the more acute angle of their cheek teeth occlusal surfaces. Genetically determined primary malocclusion must be differentiated from malocclusion secondary to insufficient dietary fiber, inanition, or hypovitaminosis C. Secondary lacerations may be present on the buccal mucosa (maxillary arcade) or on the tongue (mandibular arcade) when malocclusion is present from any cause.

3.6.1.2 Other Oral Conditions

Hair or foreign body impaction with subsequent bacterial infection and gingivitis may occur in guinea pigs, although secondary abscessation and osteomyelitis are reportedly less common in this species than in rabbits.

Iatrogenic damage of incisors with vertical fracture and root abscessation can be seen following attempts to clip teeth in conscious animals with inappropriate tools.

Hyperdontia with **duplication of mandibular incisors** occurred as a spontaneous lesion in a young guinea pig, and was likely congenital in origin.

Fluorosis with subsequent enamel hypoplasia and impaired mineralization has been seen in a guinea pig colony that was inadvertently intoxicated by excessive fluoride levels in their drinking water. Animals became anorectic and developed malocclusion and secondary hypersalivation from tongue entrapment.

Spontaneous oral tumors are rare in guinea pigs. Sporadic oral papillomas are seen (Figure 3.17B). An **odontoma** of a maxillary tooth has been described in a 3.5-year-old neutered male guinea pig.

3.6.2 Salivary Gland Conditions

Cytomegalovirus is a species-specific betaherpesvirus. In the guinea pig, the virus (GpCMV) primarily targets

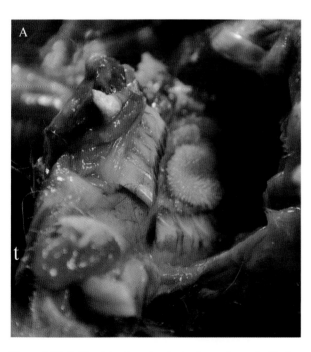 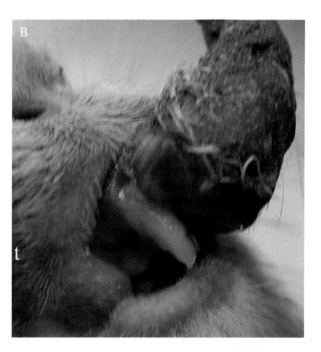

Figure 3.17 A: Cheek teeth malocclusion in a guinea pig. The tongue was entrapped under the mandibular cheek death, interfering with eating and swallowing. B: Oral papilloma growing above the upper incisors in a guinea pig (arrow). *Source:* B: Courtesy of The Links Road Animal and Bird Clinic.

the salivary glands, cervical lymph nodes, and kidneys. Subclinical infection is common in conventionally housed animals, and rare intranuclear inclusion bodies may be seen in ductal epithelial cells of salivary glands and renal tubular epithelial cells. Disseminated disease due to this virus is rare but has been reported. Affected animals were moribund or found dead with no premonitory signs, and had acute, multifocal necrosis of the kidney, liver, lung, spleen, cervical lymph nodes, and salivary glands, with syncytia and large basophilic intranuclear and occasionally intracytoplasmic inclusion bodies confirmed as viral in origin by electron microscopy. Immunosuppressed animals may be at greater risk of systemic disease after contracting infection with this virus. Transmission occurs by direct contact with infected animals as well as transplacentally. Colony infection status may be determined by serology. At least two other species-specific herpesviruses have been identified in guinea pigs but neither are betaherpesviruses and they do not infect the salivary gland.

Tumors of the salivary glands are rare with only one report of a *benign mixed salivary gland tumor* in a guinea pig.

3.6.3 Gastric Conditions

Gastric dilatation and volvulus may be seen in guinea pigs, with acute gastric rupture and death (Figure 3.18). Presenting signs include marked abdominal distension, tachypnea, and cyanosis. Splenic torsion, hepatic infarction, and gastric infarction may be present as sequelae. Ante-mortem gastric rupture may be distinguished from post-mortem gas accumulation and rupture by a hemorrhagic border in the gastric mucosa in the former condition. Breeding animals, animals repositioned during anesthesia, and animals that develop gastric stasis or ileus following anesthesia may be more at risk of developing this condition.

Gastric foreign body with puncture and subsequent peritonitis are seen sporadically. Staples and other small objects may be ingested by curious guinea pigs that are exercised on the floors of home offices. Clients should be advised to supervise animals closely when guinea pigs are exercised outside their cages.

Trichobezoars and phytobezoars occur in guinea pigs and are likely secondary to insufficient dietary fiber or inanition resulting from dental disease or other gastrointestinal conditions. Peruvian breed guinea pigs may be at increased risk for developing hair accumulations and provision of an adequate hay source to these animals is an important management tool to avoid this condition.

Soft tissue mineralization, including mineralization of the gastric muscularis, is seen sporadically in guinea pigs. Differential diagnoses include chronic renal failure or hypervitaminosis D from inappropriate levels of mineral supplements, feeding of rabbit pellets, which may contain higher levels of vitamin D than are required for

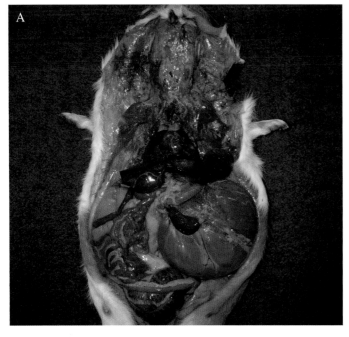
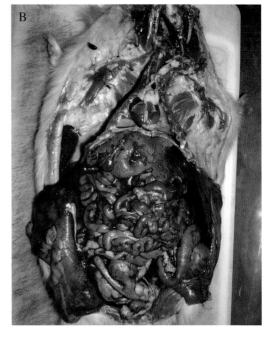

Figure 3.18 A: Marked gastric dilatation in a young guinea pig. The etiology was undetermined. B: Acute gastric rupture in a guinea pig. Staples were found in the stomach, likely resulting in perforation. The animal had been exercised on the floor of a home office.

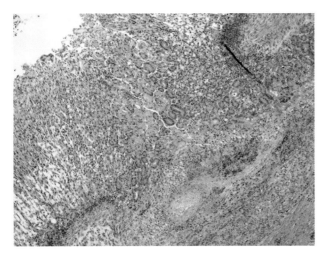

Figure 3.19 Section of stomach from a 4-month-old male hairless guinea pig (skinny pig) with a history of anorexia. There is locally extensive superficial mucosal hemorrhage and necrosis with marked fibrin exudation and large numbers of small pale basophilic coccoid bacteria, and herniation of the mucosa through the muscularis mucosa. *Streptococcus gallolyticus* was isolated from this case of acute bacterial gastritis.

guinea pigs, feed mill mixing errors or feeding plants high in vitamin D, such as *Solanum* spp.

Gastritis and gastric ulceration may also be seen sporadically (Figure 3.19).

3.6.4 Enteric Conditions

Gastrointestinal stasis and diarrhea are commonly reported for guinea pigs submitted for post-mortem evaluation, and these conditions are often related to loss of normal bacterial gut flora (dysbiosis) and opportunistic overgrowth or replacement by other pathogenic bacterial populations. A host of potential underlying noninfectious and infectious etiologies should be considered for these cases. The presenting clinical signs are similar in all cases, animals may have abdominal tympany and present with watery diarrhea, wasting, depression, and dehydration.

Initiating factors for dysbiosis with clostridial and Gram-negative bacterial overgrowth include adverse colony management stress, insufficient dietary fiber, carbohydrate overload or other dietary indiscretions inducing enteric content pH changes, and antibiotic toxicity. Young, pregnant, immunocompromised animals, and animals with hypovitaminosis C may be more susceptible to infections. Guinea pigs are highly susceptible to developing dysbiosis following treatment with antibiotics effective against Gram-positive organisms, for example, penicillins, cephalosporins, macrolides, tetracylines, and lincosamides, particularly when these agents are given orally. Long-term treatment with other antibiotics may also precipitate a change in flora with dysbiosis and opportunistic bacterial overgrowth.

3.6.4.1 Coliform Enteritis

A small number of coliform bacteria are normally present within the guinea pig intestinal tract. Disruption of flora may lead to proliferation of enteropathogenic *E. coli* within the small or large intestine, with ensuing watery diarrhea. There is some degree of host specificity for *E. coli*, and strains that are infectious for rabbits or other species may not be pathogenic for guinea pigs. Concurrent infections with enteric viruses or protozoa may exacerbate the severity of the condition. Although young animals are affected most commonly, different bacterial serotypes have differing pathogenicity, and any age group may be susceptible. Diarrhea may be transient to severe, leading to death.

Pathology   Depending on the infecting strain of *E. coli*, either the small or large intestine may be affected to a greater extent. Upon gross examination, distended loops of gut may be seen with watery, brown content. Histologically, characteristic small rod-shaped bacteria may be seen near the mucosal surface, and there may be mucosal edema with mild to marked neutrophilic infiltrates. Mucosal effacement and villus atrophy may be seen in more severe cases.

Laboratory Diagnostics   Microbiologic culture, bacterial serotyping, and *E. coli* toxin isolation may be used to identify pathogenic *E. coli* definitively, although, histopathologic examination of tissues and fecal culture usually suffice for routine diagnostic cases.

Differential Diagnoses   Other bacterial, viral, and protozoal induced enteropathies are potential differentials for coliform infections, and multiple pathogenic agents are often present concurrently. An underlying cause for dysbiosis and bacterial overgrowth should be sought.

Disease and Herd Management   Maintenance of good hygienic standards of animal husbandry, and prevention of contamination of food and water bowls with fecal droppings are important in controlling and preventing coliform infections. Sick guinea pigs should be isolated from healthy animals, and proper handwashing and sanitation procedures should be in place to minimize bacterial contamination between sick and healthy animals or their caregivers.

3.6.4.2 Clostridial Typhlitis

Fatal typhlitis due to clostridial infection and proliferation may occur in guinea pigs either spontaneously or following antibiotic treatment. In guinea pigs, both *C. perfringens* and *C. difficile* have been isolated from animals presenting with watery diarrhea. *C. difficile* elaborates two enterotoxins, A and B, which collectively disrupt tight junctions, leading to chemokine release, neutrophil infiltration, and direct enterocyte toxicity.

There are five strains of *C. perfringens*, each elaborating a unique spectrum of pathogenic toxins. Guinea pigs are reported to be predominantly infected with type E strains, which produce at least six toxins, including alpha and iota. Iota toxin promotes the secretion of water across gut epithelial cells into the intestinal lumen, promoting diarrhea and dehydration.

Presenting Clinical Signs Animals typically present with dehydration, anorexia, and watery diarrhea. All ages may be affected and animals may die peracutely in good body condition.

Pathology In guinea pigs, the cecum is predominantly affected and may appear grossly edematous and hyperemic with a watery brown-gray content and a "ground glass" appearance of the mucosal surface. Histologically, there is submucosal and lamina proprial edema with mucosal erosion and moderate mixed leukocytic infiltrates. A mucosal pseudomembrane composed of fibrinonecrotic debris has been reported in some animals.

Laboratory Diagnostics *C. difficile* and *C. perfringens* are Gram-positive, anaerobic, spore-forming rods. Cultures of cecal contents or feces may demonstrate the presence of one or both of these bacteria; however, definitive identification of disease requires evidence of toxin elaboration. Direct testing of cecal contents or feces for toxin production is done by enzyme immunoassay or PCR.

Disease and Herd Management Predisposing factors for dysbiosis should be evaluated, and sick animals should be quarantined from unaffected ones.

3.6.4.3 Salmonellosis

Several different serotypes of *Salmonella* spp. have been associated with outbreaks of enteritis, septicemia, and abortion storms in conventional colonies of guinea pigs with moderate to high mortality. In one outbreak from a commercial breeding operation, the ranch owners were both infected and subsequently developed watery diarrhea and fever. *S. enteriditis*, *S.* Typhimurium, *S. dublin*, and *S. ochiogu* have all been isolated from guinea pigs and infections may persist in subclinically infected carrier animals. Bacterial introduction into herds likely occurs through contaminated food or water sources, and younger or immunodeficient animals may be more susceptible to infection. Because salmonellosis remains an important public health concern and because of the demonstrated zoonotic potential, infected animals should not be treated and contaminated herds should be euthanatized.

3.6.4.4 Tyzzer's Disease

Sporadic and spontaneous cases of enteric Tyzzer's disease have been reported in guinea pigs. The disease is caused by *Clostridium piliforme*, a Gram-negative, motile, spore-forming, obligate intracellular bacterium. Hemorrhagic and necrotizing typhlocolitis and ileitis are seen in animals presenting with diarrhea and sudden death. Animals may carry bacterial spores subclinically, and bacteria can be transmitted by direct fecal contact as well as transplacentally. The disease is diagnosed based on the characteristic microscopic findings of bacteria, the presence of which is enhanced by silver staining, surrounding necrotic lesions. ELISA and PCR assays are also available.

3.6.4.5 Intestinal Spirochetosis

Brachyspira pilosicoli, the cause of colonic spirochetosis, is considered an emerging pathogen of animals and humans. Pathology is induced by spirochete adherence and intracellular uptake into or invasion of epithelial cells, leading to sloughing, attenuation, and mucosal erosion with secondary bacterial infections. There are several reports of intestinal spirochetosis in individually housed pet and group-housed herds of guinea pigs, although earlier reports did not further type the spirochetes observed. *B. pilosicoli* has been identified by PCR from one case of colonic spirochetosis in a pet guinea pig presenting with colorectal prolapse, and several human family members concurrently reported diarrhea that was not further investigated. Animals may present with watery diarrhea, depression, inappetence or sudden death. Watery to hemorrhagic typhlocolitis is seen at gross necropsy and a dense blanket of spirochetes is present along the apical membrane of the cecal enterocyte, causing loss of microvilli or within the apical epithelial cytoplasm (Figure 3.20). Animals may be co-infected with other pathogenic bacteria, such as *C. piliforme*, or various protozoa, but sole infections are also common. Koch's postulates have not yet been fulfilled for this organism in guinea pigs, and further research is needed to characterize the condition. Diagnosis is made by characteristic histologic lesions, confirmed with Warthin-Starry staining to visualize spirochetes, and a specific PCR assay. Because of the zoonotic potential, appropriate handwashing practices should be emphasized for clients with pet guinea pigs demonstrating diarrhea.

3.6.4.6 Viral Enteritis

Both coronavirus and rotavirus infections are reported to occur in guinea pig colonies, although neither virus has been well characterized. Rotaviral infection may be subclinical, and coronavirus-like infections are reported to induce wasting, intermittent diarrhea, and segmental ileitis. As for other species, these viruses may act in

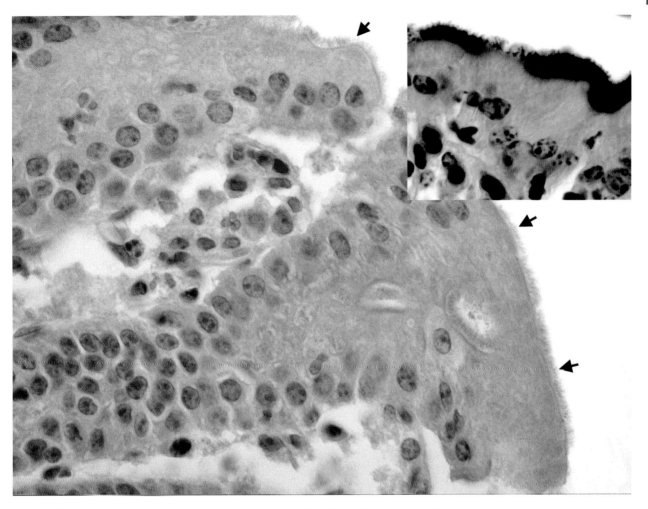

Figure 3.20 Colonic spirochetosis in a guinea pig due to natural infection with *Brachyspira pilosicoli*. The bacteria are seen densely blanketing the mucosal surface (arrows). Inset: The long slender spirochetes are readily visualized on the surface with a Warthin-Starry stain. *Source:* Courtesy of P. Helie.

concert with other enteric pathogens to induce diarrheal disease in young animals. There are no current commercial serologic tests available for either agent. Avoiding overcrowding and mixing of animals of different ages in breeding colonies and maintaining high standards of hygiene are nonspecific husbandry practices that are effective in reducing disease outbreaks with these viruses in other species.

3.6.4.7 Protozoal Enteritis

Intestinal cryptosporidiosis caused by *Cryptosporidium wrairi* is reported as a spontaneous cause of enteritis and sporadic death in young, conventionally housed guinea pigs. Small intestinal enterocyte sloughing with moderate villus blunting and fusion is seen in animals presenting with watery diarrhea, and numerous trophozoites can be seen adherent to the mucosal surface. Giemsa staining may enhance visualization of protozoa. Younger or immunocompromised animals may be at higher risk

for infection. Diagnosis is made by microscopic examination of tissues or intestinal mucosal scrapings with identification of protozoa. The organism may be infective for other animal species, such as mice and lambs, but has not been identified in humans to date. Regardless, excellent handwashing practices should be emphasized for clients, because there is no treatment for this condition. Animals with diarrhea should be housed separately from unaffected animals.

Eimeria caviae may induce mild colitis and diarrhea; however, infection is typically subclinical. Rare outbreaks of profuse watery diarrhea have been reported in guinea pigs purchased from pet stores. Typical sexual and asexual coccidial stages may be seen microscopically within the proximal colonic mucosa of affected animals. Initially, the mucosa may appear hyperplastic with increased mitoses in glands, followed later by sloughing of necrotic cells, mixed leukocytic mucosal infiltrates, and mucosal erosion and ulceration. Both young and older, immunocompromised animals may experience more severe infections. Previously infected animals demonstrate long-lasting immunity to reinfection but carrier animals may exist and shed organisms on an intermittent basis. Coccidiosis in animals typically occurs following stress from transportation, overcrowding, unsanitary housing conditions, or poor diet. When present, oocysts are readily identified from fecal smears or by flotation; however, death may occur before the prepatent period of 11 days has been surpassed. Speciation is not needed for treatment.

3.6.4.8 Other Enteric Conditions

Spontaneous proliferative enteritis is seen in guinea pigs and is associated with small, curved, argyrophilic intracellular bacteria in the apical cytoplasm of duodenal enterocytes. This is most consistent with *Lawsonia intracellularis* infection. *Citrobacter freundii*-induced intestinal hyperplasia has also been seen in an outbreak of septicemia in a guinea pig colony, and *Yersinia enterocolitica* has been isolated from laboratory guinea pigs presenting with enteritis. Other bacterial causes of enterocolitis are seen sporadically (Figure 3.21).

Cecal torsion or **omental torsion**, both with infarction and peracute death, have been reported sporadically in guinea pigs. The pathogenesis of these conditions is unknown.

Colonic and rectal impactions may occur in older male guinea pigs. The etiopathogenesis is unknown but may be related to obesity and colorectal atony. Without regular manual removal of fecoliths, animals may obstruct and die.

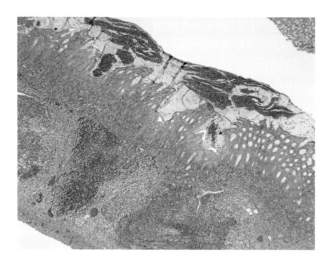

Figure 3.21 Colon from a 4-month-old female guinea pig submitted from a colony of 100 animals. Sudden deaths and abortions were occurring. Colonic hypertrophy and submucosal microabscesses were noted due to co-infection with *Listeria monocytogenes* and *Pseudomonas aeruginosa*.

Spontaneous, reactive **intestinal amyloidosis** may develop in guinea pigs with chronic systemic infections. Amyloid deposition is readily visualized most commonly in the lamina propria of the duodenum and jejunum, and may lead to malabsorption and diarrhea, although deposition may occur in other organs, such as the kidneys. Confirmation of amyloid fibrils may be seen by apple-green birefringence under polarized light in intestinal sections stained with Congo red.

Eggs and proglottid segments of *Hymenolepis diminuta* and *Rodentolepis nana* may be seen incidentally in intestinal sections at necropsy. The cestodes are largely nonpathogenic in guinea pigs and may be transmitted when animals inadvertently consume fleas, cockroaches, or other insects containing cysticercoid larvae.

Tumors of the gastrointestinal tract are uncommon. **Gastric leiomyoma** and **lipoma** have been reported.

3.6.5 Hepatobiliary Conditions

Severe hepatic lipidosis with ketosis, anorexia, and subsequent death may be seen in periparturient sows and obese boars (see Section 3.9.2 for more information).

Few reports exist of hepatobiliary masses in guinea pigs. Hepatic adenoma, hemangioma, and gall bladder papilloma have been noted.

3.7 Cardiovascular Conditions

Guinea pigs have marked coronary arterial collateralization, making spontaneous ischemic myocardial disease highly unlikely. The heart occupies a large portion of the central thorax and the bilayered pericardium is composed of a fibrous outer layer and an inner fine serosal layer. Pulmonary arteries are normally thick-walled (Figure 3.22A) and abundant mast cells may be in and around airways and pulmonary blood vessels.

3.7.1 Cardiomyopathy

Although clinical anecdotal reports of cardiomyopathy exist for guinea pigs and suspect cases are seen sporadically at post-mortem (Figure 3.22B), there are no published reports describing related pathology. Spontaneous pericardial effusion and tamponade are seen sporadically in pet guinea pigs (Figure 3.23A). Animals may be successfully treated by pericardial aspiration and the underlying pathogenesis for the effusion may never be determined.

3.7.2 Cardiac Rhabdomyomatosis

Rhabdomyomatosis is a common incidental finding at necropsy in some guinea pigs and may occasionally be

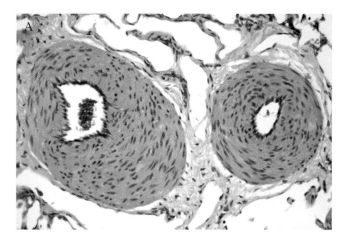
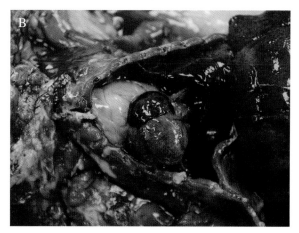

Figure 3.22 A: Pulmonary arteries in guinea pigs are normally thick-walled. B: Cardiac enlargement in a 4-year-old female neutered guinea pig that died of heart failure. The fine pale streaks noted on the epicardial surface are microscopically consistent with rhabdomyomatosis.

grossly visible as patchy pale streaks on the ventricular free walls or as discrete masses on the ventricular surface. Histologically, there is an irregular spongy appearance to affected areas of myocardium with enlarged vacuolated myofibers supported by a loose network of fibrils (Figure 3.23B). The nucleus of affected myocytes may be displaced to one side. In alcohol-fixed specimens, cytoplasmic vacuoles contain PAS-positive material that has been identified as glycogen. No associated abnormalities are seen in other organs, and despite large areas of the myocardium being affected, there is no associated cardiac functional abnormality.

3.7.3 Cardiac Neoplasia

Cardiac neoplasms are highly uncommon in guinea pigs with few well-characterized descriptions available. Isolated reports exist for fibrosarcoma, undifferentiated sarcoma, mesenchymoma, and leiomyosarcoma.

A primary leiomyosarcoma was diagnosed in a 3-year-old female guinea pig with a poor hair coat and depression that presented with dyspnea, tachycardia, and a heart murmur. The animal died shortly after presentation and a post-mortem was conducted. The tumor was only detected microscopically within the right ventricular septum. The

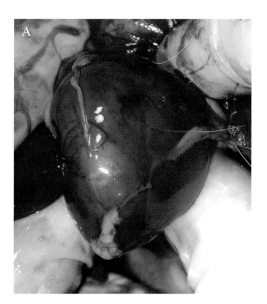
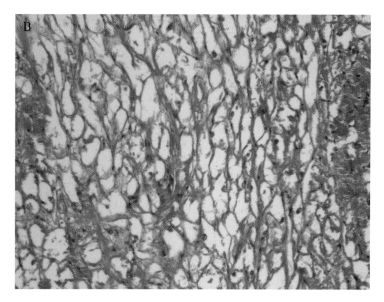

Figure 3.23 A: Pericardial effusion of unknown etiology in a guinea pig. B: Microscopic appearance of rhabdomyomatosis. The vacuolation of cardiomyofibers is consistent with glycogen accumulation. *Source:* A: Courtesy of The Links Road Animal and Bird Clinic.

mass was unencapsulated and poorly defined, consisting of bundles and streams of neoplastic cells dissecting between normal cardiomyocytes and supported by a moderate fibrovascular stroma. Some multinucleated cells were present, as were mild anisokaryosis and rare mitoses. There was mild associated lymphoplasmacytic and histiocytic inflammation and diffuse midzonal to centrilobular hepatic necrosis, consistent with chronic right-sided heart failure. Neoplastic cells were found to express vimentin and α-smooth muscle actin by immunohistochemistry.

3.7.4 Other Cardiovascular Conditions

Bacterial pericarditis may be seen in cases of pleuropneumonia in guinea pigs, induced by streptococcal or other bacterial species.

Metastatic mineralization of the pericardium, epicardium, or aorta with mild accompanying mononuclear leukocytic infiltration may be seen in cases of vitamin D intoxication, chronic renal failure, or nutritional hyperparathyroidism.

Heat stroke can occur in guinea pigs kept in overheated, poorly ventilated spaces. Animals may present with hypersalivation, tachypnea, prostration, and sudden death. Obese, aged, or pregnant animals may be at increased risk of developing the condition, and animals should never be left unattended in closed vehicles during hot weather. Histologic lesions are nonspecific and include multi-organ vascular congestion and acute, patchy myocardial necrosis and hemorrhage. Diagnosis is based on clinical history and consistent microscopic findings.

Multiple congenital malformations of the heart, including caudal vena cava duplication and incomplete atrial formation, were noted in a pregnant adult sow. Mild cardiac enlargement was also present but no cardiovascular compromise was seen.

3.8 Genitourinary Conditions

As in other rodents, the guinea pig kidney is unipapillate and bean-shaped. Guinea pigs produce thick, cloudy, pale yellow alkaline urine with an average pH of 9.0. The urethral opening is separate from the vaginal opening in sows. Boars have a thin os penis and two keratinaceous styles that project from the tip.

3.8.1 Urinary Tract Conditions

3.8.1.1 Chronic Renal Disease
Chronic renal disease is relatively common in older pet guinea pigs of both sexes and the etiopathogenesis is likely multifactorial, involving inappropriate dietary mineral content, high protein diets, overfeeding, and obesity.

Presenting Clinical Signs Animals with chronic renal disease may present with polydipsia and polyuria, a history of gradual weight loss and decreased appetite, weakness, depression, and anemia. In some cases, renal disease is subclinical and only noted at post-mortem.

Pathology Grossly, chronic renal disease or nephrosclerosis is characterized by fine pitting of the cortical surface and small, firm, pale kidneys (Figure 3.24). Microscopically, there is progressive arteriolar thickening induced by smooth muscle hypertrophy and arteriolar sclerosis, with diffuse to segmental interstitial fibrosis, mild interstitial lymphocytic infiltrates, tubular degeneration and dilatation, and hyaline

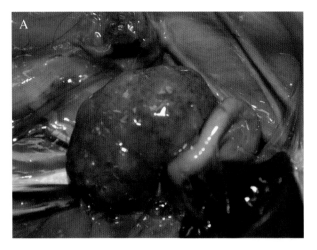
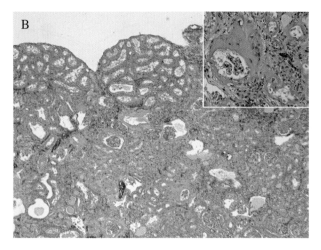

Figure 3.24 A: Chronic renal disease in a 4 year-old neutered, male guinea pig. Cortical irregularities are obvious. B: Microscopically, there is moderate to severe cystic dilatation of many cortical tubules, while other tubules have markedly thickened basement membranes (inset). There is concurrent interstitial and glomerular tuft fibrosis (nephrosclerosis). A mild lymphocytic interstitial infiltrate is present.

casts. Atrophy of severely affected nephrons with compensatory hypertrophy of tubules of scattered functional nephrons is observed occasionally. Glomeruli are relatively spared, with only occasional thickening of Bowman's capsule and mesangial tufts.

Laboratory Diagnostics   Blood urea nitrogen, creatinine, and phosphorus levels may be elevated and a nonregenerative anemia may be detected during a complete blood count. Mild hypertension occurs in advanced cases.

Disease/Herd Management   Primary renal disease should be distinguished from secondary renal disease resulting from other metabolic or urinary tract conditions. Diabetes mellitus more commonly results in glomerular tuft changes and microangiopathy. Renal amyloidosis results in thickening and enlargement of the mesangial tuft by pale, amorphous, eosinophilic proteinaceous material, which can be identified following Congo red staining by characteristic apple green birefringence under polarized light. Immune complex glomerulopathy also results in a thickened glomerular tuft and sclerosis of Bowman's capsule but Congo red staining is negative. Urolithiasis may result in intrarenal calculi and nonsuppurative interstitial inflammation and fibrosis in chronic cases. Metastatic calcification from inappropriate vitamin D or mineral supplementation may manifest as multifocal mineral deposits within renal tubular and collecting duct profiles, as well as mineralization of other soft tissues in the body. Intranuclear and intracytoplasmic inclusion bodies may be seen in renal tubular epithelial cells following cytomegalovirus infection but are interpreted as nonpathogenic unless accompanied by significant renal parenchymal necrosis. Mild fatty degeneration of renal tubular epithelial cells may occur in obese older animals and is an incidental finding.

3.8.1.2   Urolithiasis
Urolithiasis occurs in older guinea pigs and has a reported incidence of approximately 1–5%. Calculi may be found anywhere in the guinea pig urinary tract. Females may be more likely to develop this condition because of the shorter urethra, with increased potential for retrograde bacterial contamination. Feeding large quantities of foods containing high levels of oxalates, such as Swiss chard, beet root, and rhubarb leaves may induce calculi development and should be avoided. A case of fatal urolithiasis and acute renal failure was reported in a guinea pig following consumption of oxalate-containing leaves from a peace lily (*Spathiphyllum* sp.). Bacterial cystitis caused by *Streptococcus pyogenes*, *Corynebacterium renale*, and *E. coli* may be seen concurrently with urolithiasis in some animals. Bacterial infection may predispose guinea pigs to calculi formation because of ongoing inflammation and alterations in urinary pH, leading to mineral precipitation.

Affected animals may present with hematuria, dehydration, weight loss, and weakness. Urethral obstruction and anuria may occur in severe cases of urolithiasis with secondary hydroureter and hydronephrosis. In guinea pigs, uroliths are largely composed of calcium carbonate, with lesser contributions from calcium phosphate, calcium oxalate, or ammonium phosphate (struvite). Crystals may induce direct damage to renal tubular epithelial cells or bladder mucosa. The microscopic findings in cases of urolithiasis are highly dependent on the site and duration of the urolith, and whether there is a concurrent bacterial cystitis. Histologically, in longstanding uncomplicated cases with renal crystals, there may be a chronic interstitial nephritis with cystic dilation of tubules that contain microscopic crystals of various sizes. In cases with a concurrent bacterial cystitis, there may be erosion of the urinary bladder epithelium with transmural edema and hemorrhage, macroscopic uroliths, and an ascending pyelonephritis.

3.8.1.3   Cystitis
Urinary bladder infections are seen clinically following ascending infection with *E. coli* or *S. aureus*. They occur more frequently in female guinea pigs, and urolithiasis and diabetes mellitus may be present concurrently. A urinalysis and complete blood count should be conducted to rule out intercurrent disease.

3.8.1.4   Urinary Bladder and Renal Masses
Transitional cell carcinomas, squamous cell carcinomas, and hemangiopericytomas have been reported to occur spontaneously in the urinary bladder in certain inbred strains of guinea pigs over 3.5 years of age. The urinary bladder is an unusual location for hemangiopericytomas in any species and in all cases, these were incidental findings at necropsy. These masses were polypoid, projected from the interior surface of the urinary bladder, and consisted of small, oval pericytes with scant cytoplasm, which were noted to be invading surrounding muscle, lymph nodes, and blood vessels. Mitoses were abundant, and the border of the invading neoplastic cells was demarcated by a basal lamina. No immunohistochemistry was conducted; however, ultrastructural studies ruled out epithelial origin for these cells.

Renal tumors are otherwise rare in guinea pigs with a single report of renal lymphoma.

3.8.1.5   Other Renal Conditions
Renal cysts are uncommon in guinea pigs and may be congenital or acquired. **Congenital hydronephrosis** is occasionally seen.

Guinea pigs are commonly carriers of **Encephalitozoon cuniculi**, an obligate intracellular microsporidian organism, and are considered a reservoir host. Microsporidia are spore-forming parasites that are taxonomically classified as fungi. Transmission occurs through ingestion of infective spores shed in the urine but vertical transmission is suspected to occur in the guinea pig, as in rabbits. Infection is largely subclinical in immunocompetent animals and positive titers may be detected in guinea pig colonies via serologic testing. One report exists of multifocal cerebral necrosis with granulomatous encephalitis and chronic interstitial renal disease in a young adult guinea pig on a chronic lead ingestion study. No clinical signs were noted in this animal and the condition was only detectable microscopically. Gram-positive, rod-shaped microsporidial organisms may be found within a parasitophorous vacuole or free within inflammatory lesions.

3.8.2 Reproductive Tract Conditions

Accessory sex glands in male guinea pigs consist of large paired seminal vesicles and coagulating glands, a prostate gland, paired bulbourethral glands, and a rudimentary preputial gland. Boars also have paired perianal glands that can become impacted with secretions and debris. Similar to rabbits, the inguinal rings remain open following maturity in boars, allowing free movement of the testicles into the abdomen. Females have an intact vaginal closure membrane and if they are going to be used as breeding sows should be bred before 1 year of age, as their pubic symphysis may subsequently calcify. Older primiparous sows may experience dystocia during parturition because of complete pubic symphysis mineralization.

3.8.2.1 Cystic Rete Ovarii

Serous ovarian cysts, generally resulting from cystic rete ovarii, are commonly seen in sows 3 years of age and older. These cysts represent dilatation of an anastomosing network of rete tubules, which is a normal structure found within the hilus of most mammalian ovaries. The rete tubules play a role in primordial germ cell meiosis and formation of granulosa cells of the neonatal medullary follicles during embryogenesis, and the rete tubules may increase and decrease in size in various species during parturition, suggesting that they remain hormonally responsive. Typically, the rete ovarii become atrophic with age, although cystic rete ovarii are described in multiple species.

In guinea pigs, these ovarian cysts may be multiple and bilateral and may reach up to 2.5 cm or more in diameter (Figure 3.25). When unilateral, the right ovary is disproportionately involved. Large cysts grow into and compress the ovarian stroma, which is often barely recognizable as a

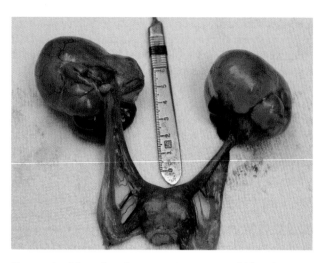

Figure 3.25 Bilateral cystic rete ovarii in a 3-year-old female guinea pig. *Source:* Courtesy of The Links Road Animal and Bird Clinic.

thin outer rim of tissue attached to the cyst. Parity does not appear to affect cyst size and animals may present with an enlarged, painful abdomen and bilaterally symmetrical alopecia. Histologically, cysts are lined by simple cuboidal to columnar ciliated epithelium and contain abundant low protein fluid (Figure 3.26).

Cystic endometrial hyperplasia, mucometra, endometritis, uterine adenoma, and uterine leiomyoma are seen with increased incidence in sows with cystic ovaries, likely reflecting underlying estrogenic stimulation.

3.8.2.2 Pregnancy Toxemia

Sows are susceptible to two forms of pregnancy toxemia: (1) a metabolic form related to overfeeding, and an obese prepartum body condition, similar to that seen in rabbits and ruminants, and (2) a circulatory form, reminiscent of preeclampsia in women. Metabolic pregnancy toxemia generally occurs within the last two weeks of pregnancy or the first two weeks following parturition. Older obese sows that become anorectic in late pregnancy are most at risk of developing the condition, and present with wasting, ketosis, hypoglycemia, and death. At necropsy, abundant abdominal fat stores and an enlarged pale, greasy liver may be seen, correlating histologically with marked hepatic lipidosis. The causes of reduced food consumption late in pregnancy may be multifactorial and can relate to changes in diet, dental disease, transportation stress, dysbiosis, or other management factors. Ketosis and death may also occur in obese boars with sudden decreased food consumption.

Animals with the circulatory form of pregnancy toxemia present with renal or uteroplacental ischemia due to compression of uterine and renal arteries by the enlarged gravid uterus. Sows may die peracutely with signs of disseminated intravascular coagulation.

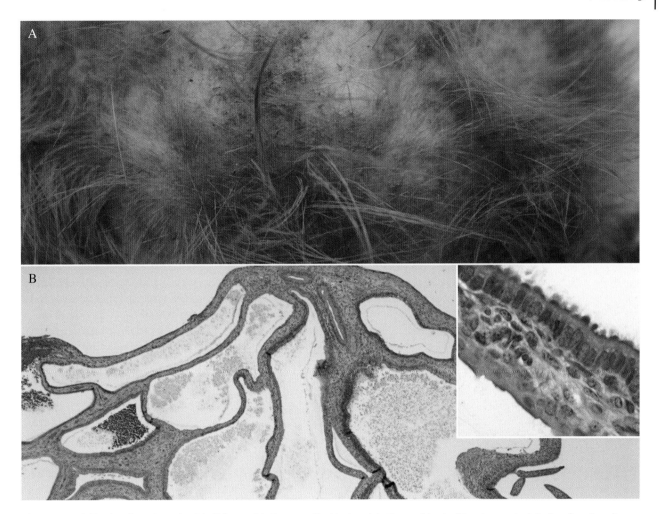

Figure 3.26 A: Patchy alopecia and epithelial petechiation over the hind end, both consistent with estrogen toxicity in a female guinea pig. B: Microscopically, these parovarian cysts may be single or multiloculated. They are lined by a ciliated, columnar epithelium (inset). *Source:* A: Courtesy of The Links Road Animal and Bird Clinic.

3.8.2.3 Reproductive Masses

Ovarian granulosa cell tumor and ovarian teratoma have been described in aged sows. Vaginal and endometrial stromal polyps (Figure 3.27), and uterine leiomyomas/-sarcomas are common incidental findings (Figure 3.28).

Testicular embryonal carcinoma has been described in a mature boar.

3.8.2.4 Other Reproductive Conditions

Vaginitis, **pyometra**, and **metritis** can occur in sows, regardless of breeding history. Animals may present with vaginal discharge, abdominal swelling and pain, depression, lethargy, reduced appetite, and pyrexia. *B. bronchiseptica* and *Streptococcus* spp. are most commonly isolated from clinical cases and may colonize the urogenital site during regular grooming. The same agents may induce **orchitis** and **epididymitis** in boars.

Normal parturition proceeds very rapidly in healthy sows with pups being born within minutes of each other. Sows with uterine inertia or fetal size mismatch may present with **dystocia** and, if untreated, may die from exhaustion.

Dystocia resulting from an **ectopic pregnancy** was reported in a 1-year-old sow that had been bred naturally. After giving birth to one dead pup, the animal continued with nonproductive straining. A subsequent laparotomy demonstrated three additional full-term but dead pups embedded in the gastric serosa and body wall. The sow died during recovery and no uterine anomalies or injuries were detected to account for the ectopic location of the three pups.

Prostatitis caused by *P. aeruginosa* infection, has been reported in a 1.5-year-old intact male.

Seminal vesicle impaction may be seen incidentally in aged boars.

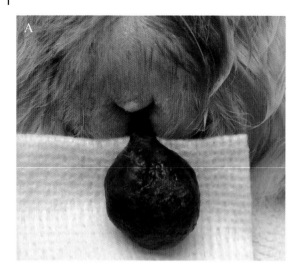

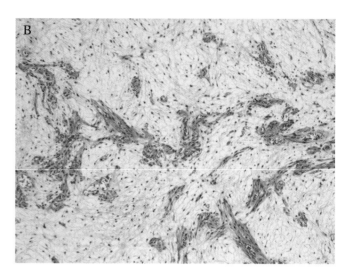

Figure 3.27 A: Vaginal polyps are common incidental findings in aging sows. B: Photomicrograph of the excised mass from A. Multiple small capillaries and arterioles are present throughout, consistent with the hemorrhagic gross appearance. The background consists of low numbers of fibroblasts set within a myxoid matrix. *Source:* A: Courtesy of The Links Road Animal and Bird Clinic.

3.9 Nervous System Conditions

There are few published reports of neurologic disorders in guinea pigs. Head tilt, circling, and head shaking may be seen with bacterial infections of the middle and inner ear. Common isolates include *S. zooepidemicus*, *S. pneumoniae*, *B. bronchiseptica*, *P. aeruginosa*, *Pasteurella* spp., and *Actinobacillus* spp. (see Section 3.4). Paresis or paralysis

may be seen with vertebral column or pelvic fractures, and weakness may be seen following any longstanding condition that induces inappetence or ketosis.

3.9.1 Rabies

A single case of rabies virus infection has been reported in a pet guinea pig in the United States that was bitten by a rabid raccoon while grazing outdoors. The guinea pig

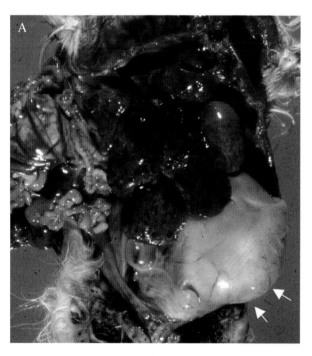

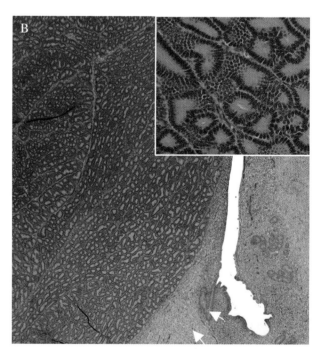

Figure 3.28 A: Uterine leiomyosarcoma (arrows) in an aged female guinea pig. B: A nodular uterine mass composed of well circumscribed clusters of well differentiated columnar epithelium with basally located nuclei arranged in tubuloacinar patterns. There was no evidence of necrosis or invasion, resulting in a diagnosis of endometrial adenoma.

subsequently bit the owner and was later euthanatized. Gross changes in the animal included a poor hair coat and body condition. There were no histologic changes consistent with rabies virus infection but tissue from the sublingual salivary gland was found to be positive for the raccoon rabies virus variant by fluorescent antibody testing. While a rare condition in guinea pigs, pathologists should be aware of the potential for rabies virus infection in pet guinea pigs that are exercised or housed outside, particularly in cases in which ante-mortem behavioral abnormalities are reported or where there has been human exposure through bites or scratches. There is no rabies vaccine currently approved for use in guinea pigs.

3.9.2 Cerebrospinal Parasitic Larval Migration

Baylisascaris procyonis larval migrans was reported in four guinea pigs housed strictly indoors. Animals presented with wasting, anorexia, and lateral recumbency prior to euthanasia. Histologically, multifocal patchy areas of cerebral malacia were seen with marked eosinophilic and granulomatous inflammation, gliosis, and necrosis. Nematode larva cross-sections consistent with *B. procyonis* were noted. Raccoon fecal contamination of the bags of wood shavings at the bedding distributor's storage facility was subsequently determined to be the source of the contamination. Eggs were presumably inhaled or ingested by the guinea pigs. Potential differential diagnoses for ataxia and head tilt in guinea pigs include otitis media and interna, head trauma, septicemia or other systemic disease, meningitis or brain abscess, all of which can readily be differentiated upon gross or histologic examination.

3.9.3 Cerebrospinal Masses

Ependymal cell hyperplasia within the lateral ventricles has been reported as a mild spontaneous condition of unknown etiology in Dunkin-Hartley guinea pigs.

A single case of teratoma of the pons has been reported in a guinea pig.

3.9.4 Other Conditions of the Brain and Spinal Cord

Pet guinea pigs may be asymptomatic carriers of **lymphocytic choriomeningitis virus** (LCMV), an arenavirus that can induce mild flu-like disease in immunocompetent humans, abortions in pregnant women, and encephalitis in immunocompromised people. Because most pet animals are not tested serologically, pathologists should use appropriate hygiene, including gloves and hand sanitation, when working with guinea pig carcasses. Viral transmission to humans occurs through direct contact with urine, blood, feces, or saliva. Routine testing is not currently recommended by the U.S. Centers for Disease Control and Prevention.

Spontaneous infection of guinea pigs with **Cryptococcus neoformans** and subsequent mild, chronic granulomatous meningitis has been described in Dunkin-Hartley guinea pigs. There were no clinical signs of infection prior to necropsy. The source of the infection was not determined.

Encephalitozoon cuniculi infection with subsequent granulomatous encephalitis can occur in guinea pigs, although infection is likely to be subclinical in immunocompetent animals (see Section 3.8.15).

There is a single report of **Parelaphostrongylus tenuis**-associated eosinophilic and lymphoplasmacytic choriomeningitis in a 2.5-year-old pet guinea pig. As part of its diet, the animal was fed grass clippings taken from a lawn frequented by white-tailed deer. Nematode larvae cross-sections were noted in the meninges, choroid plexus and spinal cord, and larval identification was confirmed by PCR.

3.10 Hematopoietic and Lymphoid Conditions

Guinea pig erythrocytes are larger than in other rodent species and in normal animals there is moderate anisocytosis, microcytosis, and polychromasia. Absolute cell counts are generally higher in males than in females. The guinea pig neutrophil is often referred to as a heterophil in the literature because of eosinophilic cytoplasmic granules, as seen in rabbits and some other rodent species, although functionally these cells behave like other mammalian neutrophils. The most abundant circulating white blood cells in normal guinea pigs are lymphocytes. Most guinea pigs are kept conventionally and have prominent perivascular lymphoid follicles in the lungs (Figure 3.29A).

Guinea pigs have a unique mononuclear cell, the Kurloff cell (sometimes termed the "Foa-Kurloff cell" after the two scientists who independently discovered the cell in the late nineteenth century), which is recognizable by a single large PAS- and toluidine blue-positive eosinophilic membrane-bound cytoplasmic inclusion, which is composed of mucopolysaccharide complexes. These cells can be found in many tissues in both male and female guinea pigs but are most numerous in the spleen, bone marrow, and thymus (Figure 3.29B). These cells are thought to have natural cytotoxic and NK cell activity.

3.10.1 Lymphosarcoma

Spontaneous multicentric lymphoblastic B cell leukemia is seen sporadically in guinea pigs. Most animals reported with this condition are young adults and animals present

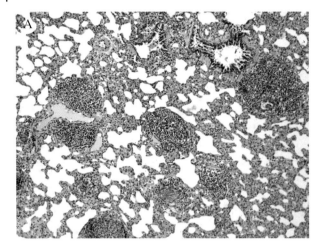
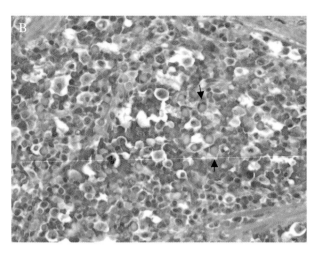

Figure 3.29 A: Perivascular lymphoid follicles in the lungs of a conventionally housed guinea pig. B: Kurloff cells (arrows) in the spleen. These cells have a prominent PAS-positive cytoplasmic inclusion and are thought to have cytotoxic activity.

with markedly enlarged lymph nodes in the cervical, axillary and inguinal areas, lethargy, anemia, and poor hair coat (Figure 3.30). White blood cell counts may be up to 500×10^9 cells/L in clinically affected animals, although some animals present as sudden death with no premonitory signs. The spleen, liver, and lymph nodes are also markedly enlarged with diffuse infiltration by lymphoblastic cells and lymph nodes may appear gray because of dense cellular infiltrates. Neoplastic infiltrates may also be present in other tissues. A type C retrovirus particle has been described in association with this condition; however, retroviral particles can also be

isolated from splenic follicles of clinically healthy guinea pigs, so the causative association is unclear.

Multicentric T cell lymphoblastic lymphoma has been described in a pet guinea pig with multiorgan and bilateral panocular involvement. The animal initially presented for unilateral corneal opacity that was unresponsive to topical treatments. Marked lymph node enlargement was noted upon palpation. No viral particles were identified by electron microscopy in any tissue.

A T cell-derived epitheliotropic lymphosarcoma has also been described in a pet guinea pig presenting with hair loss, and pruritic, erythematous, and scaling lesions

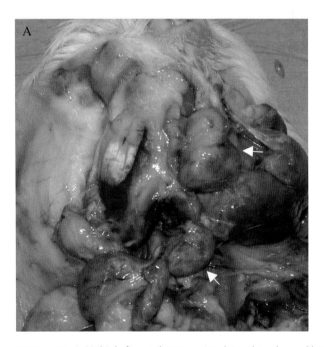
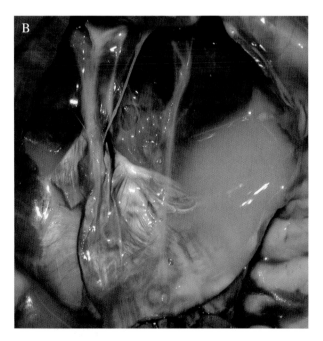

Figure 3.30 A: Multiple firm, pale masses involving the submandibular lymph nodes of a guinea pig, consistent microscopically with lymphosarcoma. B: Chylous effusion in a young guinea pig with lymphoma.. *Source:* A and B: Courtesy of C. Wheler.

on the ventral abdomen and hind legs. Dermal and epidermal infiltrates of small lymphocytes were abundant, with intraepithelial formation of Pautrier's microabscesses. Neoplastic cells were positively labeled with CD3 antibodies.

3.11 Ophthalmic Conditions

Conditions affecting the guinea pig eye and surrounding tissues are seen with regularity by clinical veterinarians, and in a recent survey, up to 45% of over 1000 guinea pigs of different breeds and backgrounds assessed by ophthalmic examination had some degree of ocular abnormality.

Guinea pigs have a rudimentary nictitating membrane formed by conjunctival folding at the medial canthus and lymphoid aggregates are common findings at the fornix of the eye. They have a large intraorbital lacrimal gland and zygomatic salivary gland, which impinge on the lateroventral and posteromedial aspects of the orbit, respectively. The guinea pig eye lacks a tapetum lucidum.

Unlike other rodent pups, newborn guinea pigs are born with open palpebrae.

3.11.1 Conditions of the Lacrimal Glands and Ducts

A white opaque discharge that contains high lipid content is normally produced by the lacrimal glands and is regularly groomed and removed by guinea pigs. Accumulations can be seen in animals that are not grooming or that are exposed to irritants within their environments.

3.11.2 Conditions of the Eyelid and Conjunctiva

Blepharitis and conjunctivitis with serous to suppurative discharge and local crusting may be seen in guinea pigs with hypovitaminosis C (Figure 3.31A). Differential diagnoses for this condition include bacterial conjunctivitis (Figure 3.31B), dermatophytosis, entropion, congenital trichiasis, retrobulbar abscesses, dental disease, high ammonia levels, and irritants in the bedding, such as pinenes. Conjunctivitis may occur in guinea pigs following infection with *B. bronchiseptica*, *P. pneumotropica*, *Listeria monocytogenes*, *S. aureus*, or *Chlamydia caviae* (inclusion body conjunctivitis).

Chlamydia spp. are obligate intracellular Gram-negative bacteria that may be seen in two forms, an elementary body (0.3 μm), which infects cells, and a reticulate body (up to 1.5 μm), which is the metabolically active intracellular form. *Chlamydia caviae* infection is enzootic in many guinea pig breeding herds and is a venereally transmitted disease. Pups are infected during passage through the vagina at parturition and may manifest signs of chemosis and mild conjunctivitis with increased ocular and nasal discharge, between 4 and 12 weeks of age (Figure 3.31C). Corneal scrapings or ocular histology demonstrate mild mixed neutrophilic/lymphocytic infiltrates and epithelial cells with intracytoplasmic reticulate bodies. Chlamydial inclusion bodies may be better visualized with Giemsa staining and diagnostic confirmation may also be obtained by PCR testing of conjunctival swabs.

Small, fatty, inferior, uni- or bilateral conjunctival masses ("pea eye") may be seen commonly in guinea pigs and are thought to represent extrusions of the lacrimal or salivary glands (Figure 3.31D). These must be distinguished from neoplasia. Bilateral firm, multifocal, proliferative conjunctival masses have been described in a 2.5-year-old male guinea pig with multicentric lymphoma. The masses consisted of dense infiltrates of neoplastic lymphocytes and no other evidence of ocular invasion was present.

Conjunctival dermoids occur in guinea pigs, sometimes with secondary irritation-induced keratitis and corneal ulceration. Corneoscleral and scleral dermoids have also been reported in guinea pigs.

Foreign bodies, such as hay awns, may induce conjunctival inflammation and hyperplasia.

A single report exists for a palpebral liposarcoma in a 1.5-year-old pet guinea pig that presented with unilateral chemosis and purulent ocular discharge. At post-mortem, the mass was determined to be well circumscribed, partially encapsulated, and multilobular but focally invasive into the underlying muscular tissue of the head. While most cells appeared to be adipocytes there was mild to moderate cellular atypia throughout and scant mitoses. Immunohistochemistry demonstrated positive labeling for vimentin and negative labeling for cytokeratin and melan-A

3.11.3 Conditions of the Cornea and Anterior Chamber

Chemosis with purulent and ulcerative keratoconjunctivitis has been seen in a group of hairless guinea pigs. Corneal sections demonstrated marked stromal edema with marked mixed leukocytic infiltrates, superficial epithelial ulceration, neovascularization and large numbers of Gram-positive bacterial rods. *L. monocytogenes* was subsequently cultured from conjunctival swabs. Clinical cases of *L. monocytogenes* infection are rare in guinea pigs, and the source of the infection was not determined.

Choroidal osseous choristomas have been seen incidentally in the eyes of male and female guinea pigs that were 3 years of age or older. Bony spicules were grossly visible in the anterior chamber and were attached to the

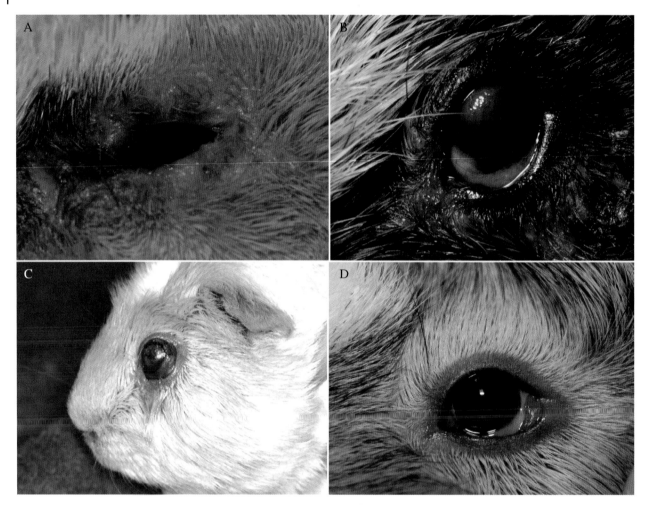

Figure 3.31 A: Conjunctivitis in a young guinea pig with hypovitaminosis C. B: Suppurative conjunctivitis in a guinea pig with a maxillary cheek tooth abscess and fistula. C: Chemosis and keratitis in a guinea pig infected with *Chlamydia caviae*. D: Conjunctival mass ('pea eye') in a guinea pig. *Source:* D: Courtesy of The Links Road Animal and Bird Clinic.

cornea and iris by fine vasculature. Bone marrow was present within some spicules and the iris was atrophic. There was no indication of previous trauma or other tumors in any of the cases.

Pinpoint corneal opacities are commonly seen in one or both eyes and may represent sites of previous trauma or corneal dystrophy.

A multi-organ and panophthalmic T cell lymphoblastic lymphoma was reported in a 2-year-old pet guinea pig that presented with lymphadenopathy and unilateral corneal thickening and ocular enlargement. Neoplastic lymphocytes were present in all parts of the eye and lymphocyte lineage was confirmed by immunohistochemistry, demonstrated by positive labeling for CD3.

3.11.4 Uveal and Lenticular Conditions

Cataracts with or without nuclear sclerosis are common findings in guinea pigs and may involve one or both eyes. Breed susceptibilities exist, suggesting a genetic compo-

nent to the condition. Animals with diabetes mellitus may also develop cataracts.

Lens subluxation occurs commonly in guinea pigs.

Panophthalmitis may occur in guinea pigs with systemic streptococcal infections.

Congenital anophthalmos and microphthalmos are seen sporadically and may result from inbreeding.

Unilateral or bilateral osseous choristoma or heterotopic bone formation is reported sporadically within the uvea of guinea pigs, sometimes associated with glaucoma.

Bibliography

Introduction

Asher, M., Spinelli de Oliviera, E., and Sachser, N. (2004) Social system and spatial organization of wild guinea pigs (*Cavia aperea*) in a natural population. *Journal of Mammology.* **85**(4), 788–796.

Donnelly, T.M. and Brown, C.J. (2004) Guinea pig and chinchilla care and husbandry. *Veterinary Clinics of North America: Exotic Animal Practice*, **7**, 351–373.

Harkness, J.E., Turner, P.V., Van deWoude, S., and Wheler, C.L. (2010) *Harkness and Wagner's Biology and Medicine of Rabbits and Rodents*, 5th edn. Wiley-Blackwell: Ames, IA.

Morales, E. (1995) *The Guinea Pig: Healing, Food and Ritual in the Andes*. University of Arizona Press: Tucson, AZ.

Pigière, F., Van Neer, W., Ancieau, C., and Denis, M. (2012) New archaeozoological evidence for the introduction of the guinea pig to Europe. *Journal of Archeological Science*, **39**(4), 1020–1024.

Alopecia

Bolognia, J.L., Murray, M.S., and Pawelek, J.M. (1990) Hairless pigmented guinea pigs: a new model for the study of mammalian pigmentation. *Pigment Cell Research*, **3**(3), 150–156.

Kim, J.H., Herrmain, F., and Sulzberger, M.B. (1962) The effect of plucking and of clipping on the growth of hair in guinea-pigs. *Journal of Investigative Dermatology*, **38**, 351–356.

Quarterman, J. and Humphries, W.R. (1983) The production of zinc deficiency in the guinea pig. *Journal of Comparative Pathology*, **93**, 261–270.

Reed, C. and O'Donoghue, J.L. (1979) A new guinea pig mutant with abnormal hair production and immunodeficiency. *Laboratory Animal Science*, **29**(6), 744–748.

Whiteway, C.E. and Robinson, R. (1989) Two recessive rex coat mutants in the guinea pig. *Journal of Heredity*, **80**(2), 163–165.

Zackheim, H.S. and Langs, L. (1962) The bald area of the guinea-pig. *Journal of Investigative Dermatology*, **38**, 347–349.

Bacterial Dermatitis

Fleming, M.P. (1976) *Streptobacillus moniliformis* isolations from cervical abscesses of guinea-pigs. *Veterinary Record*, **99**(13), 256.

Gruszynski, K., Young, A., Levine, S.J., et al. (2015) *Streptococcus equi* subsp. *zooepidemicus* infections associated with guinea pigs. *Emerging Infectious Diseases*, **21**(1), 156–158.

Rigby, C. (1976) Natural infections of guinea-pigs. *Laboratory Animals (UK)*, **10**(2), 119–142.

Walther, B., Wieler, L.H., Friedrich, A.W., et al. (2008) Methicillin-resistant *Staphylococcus aureus* (MRSA) isolated from small and exotic animals at a university hospital during routine microbiological examinations. *Veterinary Microbiology*, **127**(1–2), 171–178.

Walther, B., Wieler, L.H., Vincze, S., et al. (2012) MRSA variant in companion animals. *Emerging Infectious Diseases*, **18**(12), 2017–2020.

White, S.J., Bourdeau, P.J., and Meredith, A. (2003) Dermatologic problems in guinea pigs. *Compendium of Continuing Education*, **25**(9), 690–699.

Dermatophytoses

Chermette, R., Ferreiro, L., and Guillot, J. (2008) Dermatophytoses in animals. *Mycopathologia*, **166**, 385–405.

d'Ovidio, D., Grable, S.L., Ferrara, M., and Santoro, D. (2014) Prevalence of dermatophytes and other superficial fungal organisms in asymptomatic guinea pigs in Southern Italy. *Journal of Small Animal Practice*, **55**(7), 355–358.

Drouot, S., Mignon, B., Fratti, M., Roosje, P., and Monod, M. (2009) Pets as the main source of two zoonotic species of the *Trichophyton mentagrophytes* complex in Switzerland, *Arthroderma vanbreuseghemii* and *Arthroderma benhamiae*. *Veterinary Dermatology*, **20**(1), 13–18.

Hattori, N., Kaneko, T., Tamaki, K., Makimura, K., and Mochizuki, T. (2003) A case of kerion celsi due to *Arthroderma benhamiae* identified by DNA sequences of nuclear ribosomal internal transcribed spacer 1 regions. *Medical Mycology*, **41**(3), 249–251.

Kraemer, A., Hein, J., Heusinger, A., and Mueller, R.S. (2013) Clinical signs, therapy and zoonotic risk of pet guinea pigs with dermatophytosis. *Mycoses*, **56**(2), 168–72.

Kraemer, A., Mueller, R.S., Werckenthin, C., Straubinger, R.K., and Hein, J. (2012) Dermatophytes in pet guinea pigs and rabbits. *Veterinary Microbiology*, **157**(1–2), 208–213.

Lane, R.F. (2003) Diagnostic testing for fungal diseases. *Veterinary Clinics of North America: Exotic Animal Practice*, **6**, 301–314.

Lopez-Martinez, R., Mier, T., and Quirarte, M. (1984) Dermatophytes isolated from laboratory animals. *Mycopathologia*, **88**, 111–113.

Makimura, K., Mochizuki, T., Hasegawa, A., et al. (1998) Phylogenetic classification of *Trichophyton mentagrophytes* complex strains based on DNA sequences of nuclear ribosomal internal transcribed spacer 1 regions. *Journal of Clinical Microbiology*, **36**(9), 2629–2633.

Papini, R., Gazzano, A., and Mancianti, F. (1997) Survey of dermatophytes isolated from the coats of laboratory animals in Italy. *Laboratory Animal Science*, **47**(1), 75–77.

Pollock, C. (2003) Fungal diseases of laboratory rodents. *Veterinary Clinics of North America: Exotic Animal Practice*, **6**(2), 401–413.

Vangeel, I., Pasmans, F., Vanrobaeys, M., De Herdt, P., and Haesebrouck, F. (2000) Prevalence of dermatophytes in asymptomatic guinea pigs and rabbits. *Veterinary Record*, **146**, 440–441.

Parasitic Dermatitis

Brown, S.J., and Askenase, P.W. (1982) Blood eosinophil and basophil responses in guinea pigs parasitized by *Amblyomma americanum* ticks. *American Journal of Tropical Medicine and Hygiene*, **31**, 593–598.

Dorrestein, G.M. and Van Bronswijk, J.E.M.H. (1979) *Trixacarus caviae* Fain, Howell & Hyatt (1972 (Acari: Sarcoptidae) as a cause of mange in guinea pigs and papular urticaria in humans. *Veterinary Parasitology*, **5**, 389–398.

d'Ovidio, D., and Santoro, D. (2014) Prevalence of fur mites (Chirodiscoides caviae) in pet guinea pigs (*Cavia porcellus*) in southern Italy. *Veterinary Dermatology*, **25**(2), 135–137.

Fuentealba, C. and Hanna, P. (1996) Mange induced by *Trixacarus caviae* in a guinea pig. *Canadian Veterinary Journal*, **37**, 749–750.

Henderson, J.D. (1973) Treatment of cutaneous acariasis in the guinea pig. *Journal of the American Veterinary Medical Association*, **162**(4), 591–592.

Hirsjarvi, P., and Phyala, L. (1995) Ivermectin treatment of a colony of guinea pigs infested with fur mite (*Chirodiscoides caviae*). *Laboratory Animals (UK)*, **29**, 200–203.

Kummel, B.A., Estes, S.A., and Arlian, L.G. (1980) *Trixacarus caviae* infestation of guinea pigs. *Journal of the American Veterinary Medical Association*, **177**(9), 903–908.

Linek, M., and Bourdeau, P. (2005) Alopecia in two guinea pigs due to hypopodes of *Acarus farris* (Acaridae: Astigmata). *Veterinary Record*, **157**, 58–60.

Szabo, M.P.J., Aoki, V.L., and Sanches, F.P.S., et al: (2003) Antibody and blood leukocyte response in *Rhipicephalus sanguineus* tick-infested dogs and guinea pigs. *Veterinary Parasitology*, **115**, 49–59.

Wagner, J.E., Al-Rabiai, S., and Rings, R.W. (1972) *Chirodiscoides caviae* infestation in guinea pigs. *Laboratory Animal Science*, **22**(5), 750–752.

Mastitis

Gupta, B.N., Langham, R.F., and Conner, G.H. (1970) Mastitis in guinea pigs. *American Journal of Veterinary Research*, **31**(9), 1703–1707.

Kinkler, R.J. Jr, Wagner, J.E., Doyle, R.E., and Owens, D.R. (1976) Bacterial mastitis in guinea pigs. *Laboratory Animal Science*, **26**(2 Pt l), 214–217.

Pododermatitis

Blair, J. (2013) Bumblefoot: a comparison of clinical presentation and treatment of pododermatitis in rabbits, rodents, and birds. *Journal of Exotic Pet Medicine*, **16**, 715–735.

Cutaneous Masses

Allison, N., and Moeller, R. Jr. (1993) Complex adnexal tumor with sebaceous and apocrine differentiation in a guinea pig. *Veterinary Pathology*, **30**(3), 313–314.

Brackee, G., McPherson, S., Ostrow, R., Faras, A., and Gunther, R. (1995) Cutaneous papilloma arising from trichoepitheliomas in a guinea pig. *Contemporary Topics in Laboratory Animal Science*, **34**(6), 91–93.

Gibbons, P.M., and Garner, M.M. (2009) Mammary gland tumors in guinea pigs. *AEMV Proceedings*, Milwaukee, WI. p. 83.

Hammer, M., Klopfleisch, R., Teifke, J.P., and Löhr, C.V. (2005) Cavernous or capillary haemangioma in two unrelated guinea pigs. *Veterinary Record*, **157**, 252–253.

Jelinek, F. (2003) Spontaneous tumours in guinea pigs. *Acta Vet BRNO*, **72**, 221–228.

Kanfer, S., and Reavill, D.R. (2013) Cutaneous neoplasia in ferrets, rabbits, and guinea pigs. *Journal of Exotic Pet Medicine*, **16**, 579–598.

Martorell, J., Such, R., Fondevila, D., and Bardagi, M. (2011) Cutaneous epitheliotropic T-cell lymphoma with systemic spread in a guinea pig (*Cavia porcellus*). *Journal of Exotic Pet Medicine*, **20**(4), 313–317.

Mentre, V., and Bulliott, C. (2014) An erythematous mass on the lip of a guinea pig (*Cavia porcellus*). *Laboratory Animals (NY)*, **43**(1), 17–20.

Pouliot, N., Maghni, K., Blanchette, F., et al. (1996) Natural killer and lectin-dependent cytotoxic activities of Kurloff cells: target cell selectivity, conjugate formation, and Ca++ dependency. *Inflammation*, **20**(6), 647–671.

Pouliot, N., Maghni, K., Sirois, P., and Rola-Pleszczynski, M. (1996) Guinea pig Kurloff (NK-like) cells mediate TNF-dependent cytotoxic activity: analogy with NC effector cells. *Inflammation*. **20**(3), 263–280.

Quinton, J.F., Ollivier, F., and Dally, C. (2013) A case of well-differentiated palpebral liposarcoma in a Guinea pig (*Cavia porcellus*). *Veterinary Ophthalmology*, **16**(Suppl. 1), 155–159.

Rogers, J.B., and Blumenthal, H.T. (1960) Studies of guinea pig tumors. I. Report of fourteen spontaneous guinea pig tumors, with a review of the literature. *Cancer Research*, **20**, 191–197.

Steele, H. (2001) Subcutaneous fibrosarcoma in an aged guinea pig. *Canadian Veterinary Journal*, **42**(4), 300–302.

Suárez-Bonnet, A., Martín de Las Mulas, J., Millán, M.Y., et al. (2010) Morphological and immunohistochemical characterization of spontaneous mammary gland tumors in the guinea pig (*Cavia porcellus*). *Veterinary Pathology*, **47**(2), 298–305.

Vannevel, J., and Wilcock, B. (2005) Bile duct carcinoma and nasal adenocarcinoma in a guinea pig. *Canadian Veterinary Journal*, **46**(1), 72–73.

Zwart, P., van der Hage, M.H., Mullink, J.W., and Cooper, J.E. (1981) Cutaneous tumours in the guinea pig. *Laboratory Animals (UK).* **15**(4), 375–377.

Other Information

Osofsky, A., DeCock, H.E.V., Tell, L.A., Norris, A.J., and White, S.D. (2004) Cutaneous vascular malformation in a guinea pig (*Cavia porcellus*). *Veterinary Dermatology*, **15**, 47–52.

Schallreuter, K.U., Schulz, K.H., and Wood, J.M. (1986) Induction of contact dermatitis in guinea pigs by quaternary ammonium compounds: the mechanism of antigen formation. *Environmental Health Perspectives*, **70**, 229–237.

Diabetes Mellitus

Collins, B.R. (2008) Endocrine diseases of rodents. *Veterinary Clinics of North America: Exotic Animal Practice*, **11**, 153–162.

Horwitz, M.S., Bradley, L.M., Harbertson, J., Krahl, T., Lee, J., and Sarvennick, N. (1998) Diabetes induced by Coxsackie virus: Initiation by bystander damage and not molecular mimicry. *Nature Medicine*, **4**, 781–785.

Jordan, G.W., and Cohen, S.H. (1987) Encephalomyocarditis virus-induced diabetes mellitus in mice: A model of viral pathogenesis. *Review of Infectious Diseases*, **9**(5), 517.

Lang, C.M., Munger, B.L., and Rapp, R. (1977) The guinea pig as a model of diabetes mellitus. *Laboratory Animal Science*, **27**, 789–805.

Lee, K.J., Lang, C.M., and Munger, B.L. (1978) Isolation of virus-like particles from the urine of guinea pigs (*Cavia porcellus*) with spontaneous diabetes mellitus. *Veterinary Pathology*, **15**, 663–666.

Vannevel, J. (1998) Diabetes mellitus in a 3-year-old, intact, female guinea pig. *Canadian Veterinary Journal*, **39**, 503.

Other Endocrine Conditions

Brandao, J., Vergneau-Grosset, C., and Mayer, J. (2013) Hyperthyroidism and hyperparathyroidism in guinea pigs (*Cavia porcellus*). *Veterinary Clinics of North America: Exotic Animal Practice*, **16**, 407–420.

Enwonwu, C.O., Sawiris, P., and Chanaud, N. (1995) Effect of marginal ascorbic acid deficiency on saliva level of cortisol in the guinea pig. *Archives of Oral Biology*, **40**(8), 737–742.

Holcombe, H., Parry, N.M., Rick, M., et al. (2015) Hypervitaminosis D and Metastatic calcification in a colony of inbred strain 13 Guinea Pigs, *Cavia porcellus*. *Veterinary Pathology*, **52**(4), 741–751.

Mayer, J. and Wagner, R. (2009) Clinical aspects of hyperthyroidism in the guinea pig. *AEMV Proceedings*, Milwaukee, WI, pp. 69–73.

Mayer, J., Wagner, R., and Taeymans, O. (2010) Advanced diagnostic approaches and current management of thyroid pathologies in guinea pigs. *Veterinary Clinics of North America: Exotic Animal Practice*, **13**, 509–523.

Müller, K., Müller, E., Klein, R., and Brunnberg, L. (2009) Serum thyroxine concentrations in clinically healthy pet guinea pigs (*Cavia porcellus*). *Veterinary Clinical Pathology*, **38**(4), 507–510.

Schwarz, T., Stork, C.K., Megahy, I.W., et al. (2001) Osteodystrophia fibrosa in two guinea pigs. *Journal of the American Veterinary Medical Association*, **219**, 63–66.

Sparschu, G.L., and Christie, R.J. (1968) Metastatic calcification in a guinea pig colony: a pathological survey. *Laboratory Animal Care*, **18**(5), 520–526.

Thorson, L. (2014) Thyroid diseases in rodent species. *Veterinary Clinics of North America: Exotic Animal Practice*, **17**(1), 51–67.

Walter, W.G. and Baldwin, D.E. (1963) Observations on the parathyroid glands of guinea pigs affected with metastatic calcification. *Canadian Journal of Comparative Medicine and Veterinary Science*, **27**, 140–146.

Zeugswetter, F., Fenske, M., Hassan, J., and Künzel, F. (2007) Cushing's syndrome in a guinea pig. *Veterinary Record*, **160**, 878–880.

Endocrine Masses and Neoplasia

Gaschen, L., Ketz, C., Cornelkiae, V.M., Lang, J., Weber, U., Bacciarini, L., and Kohler, I. (1998) Ultrasonographic detection of adrenal gland tumor and ureterolithiasis in a guinea pig. *Veterinary Radiology & Ultrasound*, **39**(1), 43–46.

Gibbons, P.M., Garner, M.M., and Kiupel, M. (2013) Morphological and immunohistochemical characterization of spontaneous thyroid gland neoplasms in guinea pigs (*Cavia porcellus*). *Veterinary Pathology*, **50**(2), 334–342.

Hess, L.R., Ravich, M.L., and Reavill, D.R. (2013) Diagnosis and treatment of an insulinoma in a guinea pig (*Cavia porcellus*). *Journal of the American Veterinary Medical Association*, **242**(4), 522–526.

Rogers, J.B., and Blumenthal, H.T. (1960) Studies of guinea pig tumors. I. Report of fourteen spontaneous guinea pig tumors, with a review of the literature. *Cancer Research*, **20**, 191–202.

Vanneval, J.Y. and Wilcock, B. (2005) Insulinoma in 2 guinea pigs (*Cavia porcellus*). *Canadian Veterinary Journal*, **46**, 339–341.

Yoshida, A., Iqbal, Z.M., and Epstein, S.S. (1979) Spontaneous pancreatic islet cell tumours in guinea pigs. *Journal of Comparative Pathology*, **89**(4), 471–480.

Zarrin, K. (1974) Thyroid carcinoma of a guinea pig: a case report. *Laboratory Animals (UK)*. **8**, 145–148.

Bordetellosis

Baskerville, M., Baskerville, A., and Wood, M. (1982) A study of chronic pneumonia in a guinea pig colony with enzootic *Bordetella bronchiseptica* infection. *Laboratory Animals (UK)*. **16**(3), 290–296.

Boot, R. and Walvoort, H.C. (1986) Otitis media in guinea pigs: pathology and bacteriology. *Laboratory Animals (UK)*. **20**(3), 242–248.

Ganaway, J.R., Allen, A.M., and McPherson, C.W. (1965) Prevention of acute *Bordetella bronchiseptica* pneumonia in a guinea pig colony. *Laboratory Animal Care*, **15**, 156–162.

Wagner, J.E., Owens, D.R., Kusewitt, D.F., and Corley, E.A. (1976) Otitis media of guinea pigs. *Laboratory Animal Science*, **26**(6 Pt 1), 902–907.

Woode, G.M. and McLead, N. (1967) Control of acute *Bordetella bronchiseptica* pneumonia in a guinea-pig colony. *Laboratory Animals (UK)*. **1**, 91–94.

Yoda, H., Nakagawa, M., Muto, T., and Imaizumi, K. (1972) Development of resistance to reinfection of *Bordetella bronchiseptica* in guinea pigs recovered from natural infection. *Nihon Juigaku Zasshi*, **34**(4), 191–196.

Streptococcal Pneumonia

DeVelasco, E.A., Verheul, A.F., Verhoef, J., and Snippe, H. (1995) *Streptococcus pneumoniae*: virulence factors, pathogenesis, and vaccines. *Microbiology Reviews*, **59**(4), 591–603.

Keyhani, M. and Naghshineh, R. (1974) Spontaneous epizootic of pneumococcus infection in guinea pigs. *Laboratory Animals (UK)*. **8**, 47–49.

Petrie, G.F. (1933) The pneumococcal disease of the guinea pig. *Veterinary Journal*, **89**, 25–30.

Saito, M., Muto, T., Haruzono, S., Nakagawa, M., and Sato, M. (1983) An epizootic of pneumococcal infection occurred in inbred guinea pig colonies. *Jikken Dobutsu*, **32**(1), 29–37.

van der Linden, M., Al-Lahham, A., Nicklas, W., and Reinert, R.R. (2009) Molecular characterization of pneumococcal isolates from pets and laboratory animals. *PLoS ONE*, **4**(12), e8286.

Other Bacterial Infections

Bostrom, R.E., Huckins, J.G., Kroe, D.J., Lawson, N.S., Martin, J.E., Ferrell, J.F., and Whitney, R.A. Jr. (1969) Atypical fatal pulmonary botryomycosis in two guinea pigs due to *Pseudomonas aeruginosa. Journal of the American Veterinary Medical Association*, **155**(7), 1195–1199.

Schoondermark-van de Ven, E.M., Philipse-Bergmann, I.M., and van der Logt, J.T. (2006) Prevalence of naturally occurring viral infections, *Mycoplasma pulmonis* and *Clostridium piliforme* in laboratory rodents in Western Europe screened from 2000 to 2003. *Laboratory Animals (UK)*, **40**(2), 137–143.

Viral Respiratory Diseases

Blomqvist, G.A., Martin, K., and Morein, B. (2002) Transmission pattern of parainfluenza-3 virus in guinea pig breeding herds. *Contemporary Topics in Laboratory Animal Science*, **41**(4), 53–57.

Brennecke, L.H., Dreier, T.M., and Stokes, W.S. (1983) Naturally occurring virus-associated respiratory disease in two guinea pigs. *Veterinary Pathology*, **20**, 488–491.

Butz, N., Ossent, P., and Homberger, F.R. (1999) Pathogenesis of guinea pig adenovirus infection. *Laboratory Animal Science*, **49**(6), 600–604.

Colthoff, C.A., Mann, P., Guillard, E.T, Dyksu, M.J., and Swanson, G.L. (1998) Naturally developing virus-induced lethal pneumonia in two guinea pigs (*Cavia porcellus*). *Contemporary Topics in Laboratory Animal Science*, **37**, 54–57.

Hsiung, G.D., Bia, F.J., and Fong, C.K. (1980) Viruses of guinea pigs: considerations for biomedical research. *Microbiology Reviews*, **44**(3), 468–490.

Naumann, S., Kunstýr, I., Langer, I., Maess, J., and Hörning, R. (1981) Lethal pneumonia in guinea pigs associated with a virus. *Laboratory Animals (UK)*, **15**(3), 235–242.

Ohsawa, K., Yamada, A., Takeuchi, K., et al. (1998) Genetic characterization of parainfluenza virus 3 derived from guinea pigs. *Journal of Veterinary Medical Science*, **60**(8), 919–922.

Shankar, B.P. (2008) Adenovirus infection in guinea pig: a case study. *Veterinary World*. **1**(9), 280.

Simmons, J.H., Purdy, G.A., Franklin, C.L., et al. (2002) Characterization of a novel parainfluenza virus, cavid parainfluenza virus 3, from laboratory guinea pigs (*Cavia porcellus*). *Comparative Medicine*, **52**, 548–554.

Pulmonary Masses and Neoplasia

Franks, L.M. and Chesterman, F.C. (1962) The pathology of tumours and other lesions of the guinea pig lung. *British Journal of Cancer*, **16**, 696–700.

Greenacre, C.B. (2004) Spontaneous tumors of small mammals. *Veterinary Clinics of North America: Exotic Animal Practice*, **7**(3), 627–651.

Jelinek, F. (2003) Spontaneous tumours in guinea pigs. *Acta Vet. BRNO.* **72**, 221–228.

Lipschutz, A., Iglesias, R., Rojas, G., and Cerisola, H. (1959) Spontaneous tumourigenesis in aged guinea pigs. *British Journal of Cancer*, **13**, 486–496.

Rogers, J.B. and Blumenthal, H.T. (1960) Studies of guinea pig tumors. I. Report of fourteen spontaneous guinea pig tumors, with a review of the literature. *Cancer Research*, **20**, 191–102.

Vannevel, J. and Wilcock, B. (2005) Bile duct carcinoma and nasal adenocarcinoma in a guinea pig. *Canadian Veterinary Journal*, **46**(1), 72–73.

General Information

Borst, G.H., Zwart, P., Mullink, H.W., and Vroege, C. (1976) Bone structures in avian and mammalian lungs. *Veterinary Pathology*, **13**(2), 93–103.

Brewer, N.R. and Cruise, L.J. (1997) The respiratory system of the guinea pig: Emphasis on species differences. *Contemporary Topics in Laboratory Animal Science*, **36**(1), 100–108.

Kaufman, A.F. (1970) Bony spicules in guinea pig lung. *Laboratory Animal Care*, **20**(5), 1002–1003.

Knowles, J.F. (1984) Bone in the irradiated lung of the guinea pig. *Journal of Comparative Pathology*, **94**, 529–533.

Muto, T. (1984) Spontaneous organic dust pneumoconiosis in guinea pigs. *Japanese Journal of Veterinary Science*, **46**(6), 925–927.

Yarto-Jaramillo, E. (2011) Respiratory system anatomy, physiology, and disease: Guinea pigs and chinchillas. *Veterinary Clinics of North America: Exotic Animal Practice*, **14**, 339–355.

Hypovitaminosis C

Clarke, G.L., Allen, A.M., Small, J.D., and Lock, A. (1980) Subclinical scurvy in a guinea pig. *Veterinary Pathology*, **17**, 40–44.

Davis, J.A. (1993) Dyspnea and diarrhea in guinea pigs. *Laboratory Animals (NY)*, **22**(1), 20–21.

Eva, J.K., Fifield, R., and Rickett, M. (1976) Decomposition of supplementary vitamin C in diets compounded for laboratory animals. *Laboratory Animals (UK)*, **10**, 157–159.

Frikke-Schmidt, H., Tveden-Nyborg, P., Muusfeldt Birck, M., and Lykkesfeldt, J. (2011) High dietary fat and cholesterol exacerbates chronic vitamin C deficiency in guinea pigs. *British Journal of Nutrition*, **105**, 54–61.

Holloway, D.R., and Rivers, J.M. (1984) Long-term effects of inadequate and excessive dietary ascorbate on bile acid metabolism in the guinea pig. *Journal of Nutrition*, **114**, 1370–1376.

Nishikimi, M., Kawai, T., and Yagi, K. (1992) Guinea pigs possess a markedly different gene for L-gulono-gamma-lactone oxidase, the key enzyme for L-ascorbic acid biosynthesis missing in this species. *Journal of Biological Chemistry*, **267**(30), 21967–21972.

Sergeev, I.N., Arkhapchev, Y.P., and Spirichev, V.B. (1990) Ascorbic acid effects on vitamin D hormone metabolism and binding in guinea pigs. *Journal of Nutrition*, **120**, 1185–1190.

Tsuchiya, H. and Bates, C.J. (1994) Ascorbic acid deficiency in guinea pigs: contrasting effects of tissue ascorbic acid depletion and of associated inanition on status indices related to collagen and vitamin D. *British Journal of Nutrition*, **72**, 745–752.

Nutritional Diseases

Burk, R.F., Christensen, J.M., Maguire, M.J., et al. (2006) A combined deficiency of vitamins E and C causes severe central nervous system damage in guinea pigs. *Journal of Nutrition*, **136**(6), 1576–1581.

Cammack, P.M., Zwahlen, B.A., and Christensen, M.J. (1995) Selenium deficiency alters thyroid hormone metabolism in guinea pigs. *Journal of Nutrition*, **125**(2), 302–308.

Hawkins, M.G. (2010) Secondary nutritional hyperparathyroidism with fibrous osteodystrophy in 3 guinea pigs. *AEMV Proceedings*, San Diego, CA. P 121.

Hill, K.E., Montine, T.J., Motley, A.K., et al. (2003) Combined deficiency of vitamins E and C causes paralysis and death in guinea pigs. *American Journal of Clinical Nutrition*, **77**, 1484–1488.

Hill, K.E., Motley, A.K., Li, X., May, J.M., and Burk, R.F. (2001) Combined selenium and vitamin E deficiency causes fatal myopathy in guinea pigs. *Journal of Nutrition*, **131**, 1798–1802.

Hill, K.E., Motley, A.K., May, J.M., and Burk, R.F. (2009) Combined selenium and vitamin C deficiency causes cell death in guinea pig skeletal muscle. *Nutrition Research*, **29**(3), 213–219.

Schwarz, T., Störk, C.K., Megahy, I.W., Lawrie, A.M., Lochmüller, E-M., and Johnston, P.E.J. (1991) Osteodystrophy fibrosa in two guinea pigs. *Journal of the American Veterinary Medical Association*, **219**(1), 63–66.

Sparschu, G.L. and Christie, R.J. (1968) Metastatic calcification in a guinea pig colony: a pathological survey. *Laboratory Animal Care*, **18**(5), 520–526.

Wickham, N. (1958) Calcification in soft tissues associated with dietary magnesium deficiency in guinea pigs. *Australian Veterinary Journal*, **34**, 244–248.

Degenerative Conditions

Bendele, A.M., White, S.L., and Hulman, J.F. (1989) Osteoarthrosis in guinea pigs: histopathologic and scanning electron microscopic features. *Laboratory Animal Science*, **39**(2), 115–121.

Jimenez, P.A., Glasson, S.S., Trubetskoy, O.V., and Haimes, H.B. (1997) Spontaneous osteoarthritis in Dunkin Hartley guinea pigs: histologic, radiologic, and biochemical changes. *Laboratory Animal Science*, **47**(6), 598–601.

Neoplasia

Brunetti, B., Bo, P., and Sarli, G. (2013) Pathology in practice. *Journal of the American Veterinary Medical Association*, **243**(6), 801–803.

Cook, R.A., Burk, R.L., and Herron, A.J. (1982) Extraskeletal osteogenic sarcoma in a guinea pig. *Journal of the American Veterinary Medical Association*, **181**(11), 1423–1424.

Hong, C.C., and Liu, P.I. (1981) Osteogenic sarcoma in 2 guinea pigs. *Laboratory Animals (UK)*. **15**(1), 49–51.

Thompson, J.J., Burgmann, P.M., Brash, M., DeLay, J., and Regan, K. (2016) Spontaneous splenic hemangiosarcoma in a guinea pig (*Cavia porcellus*). *Journal of Exotic Pet Medicine*, **25**(2), 139–143.

Oral Conditions

Boot, R., Van de Berg, L., Reubsaet, F.A., and Vlemminx, M.J. (2008) Positive *Streptobacillus moniliformis* PCR in guinea pigs likely due to *Leptotrichia* spp. *Veterinary Microbiology*, **120**(3–4), 395–399.

Capello, V. (2008) Clinical technique: Treatment of periapical infections in pet rabbits and rodents. *Journal of Exotic Pet Medicine*, **17**(2), 124–131.

Capello, V. (2010) Maxillary cheek tooth elodontoma in a guinea pig. *AEMV Proceedings*, Seattle, WA. pp. 93–102.

Dalldorf, G. and Zall, C. (1930) Tooth growth in experimental scurvy. *Journal of Experimental Medicine*, **52**(1), 57–64.

Gupta, B.N. (1978) Duplication of lower incisors in a guinea pig. *Veterinary Pathology*, **15**, 683–684.

Hard, G.C., and Atkinson, F.F.V. (1967) 'Slobbers' in laboratory guinea-pigs as a form of chronic fluorosis. *Journal of Pathology*, **94**, 95–102.

Jekl, V., Hauptman, K., and Knotek, Z. (2008) Quantitative and qualitative assessments of intraoral lesions in 180 small herbivorous mammals. *Veterinary Record*, **162**, 442–449.

Reiter, A.M. (2008) Pathophysiology of dental disease in the rabbit, guinea pig, and chinchilla. *Journal of Exotic Pet Medicine*, **17**(2), 70–77.

Salivary Gland Conditions

Bhatt, P.N., Percy, D.H., Craft, J.L., and Jonas, A.M. (1971) Isolation and characterization of a herpeslike (Hsiang-Kaplow) virus from guinea pigs. *Journal of Infectious Diseases*, **123**(2), 178–189.

Connor, W.S., and Johnson, K.P. (1976) Cytomegalovirus infection in weanling guinea pigs. *Journal of Infectious Diseases*, **134**(5), 442–449.

Hsiung, G.D., Bia, F.J., and Fong, C.K. (1980) Viruses of guinea pigs: considerations for biomedical research. *Microbiology Reviews*, **44**(3), 468–90.

Koestner, A. and Buerger, L. (1965) Primary neoplasms in the salivary glands of animals compared to similar tumors in man. *Veterinary Pathology*, **2**, 201–226.

Schoondermark-van de Ven, E.M., Philipse-Bergmann, I.M., and van der Logt, J.T. (2006) Prevalence of naturally occurring viral infections, *Mycoplasma pulmonis* and *Clostridium piliforme* in laboratory rodents in Western Europe screened from 2000 to 2003. *Laboratory Animals (UK)*, **40**(2), 137–143.

Van Hoosier, G.L., Giddens, Jr W.E., Gillett, C.S., and Davis, H. (1985) Disseminated cytomegalovirus disease in the guinea pig. *Laboratory Animal Science*, **35**(1), 81–84.

Gastric Conditions

Bennett, R., and Russo, E. (1985) What is your diagnosis? Soft tissue density mass in the stomach consistent with trichobezoar or phytobezoar. *Journal of the American Veterinary Medical Association*, **186**, 812–814.

Holcombe, H., Parry, N.M., Rick, M., Brown, D.E., Albers, T.M., Refsal, K.R., Morris, J., Kelly, R., and Marko, S.T. (2015) Hypervitaminosis D and metastatic calcification in a colony of inbred Strain 13 guinea pigs, *Cavia porcellus*. *Veterinary Pathology*, **52**(4), 741–751.

Jäpelt, R.B., and Jakobsen, J. (2013) Vitamin D in plants: a review of occurrence, analysis, and biosynthesis. *Frontiers in Plant Science*, **4**, 136.

Jensen, J.A., Brice, A.K., Bagel, J.H., Mexas, A.M., Yoon, S.Y., and Wolfe, J.H. (2013) Hypervitaminosis D in guinea pigs with α-mannosidosis. *Comparative Medicine*, **63**(2), 156–162.

Keith, J.C. Jr, Rowles, T.K., Warwick, K.E., and Yau, E.T. (1992) Acute gastric distention in guinea pigs. *Laboratory Animal Science*, **42**(4), 331–332.

Mitchell, E.B., Hawkins, M.G., Gaffney, P.M., and Macleod, A.G. (2010) Gastric dilatation-volvulus in a guinea pig (*Cavia porcellus*). *Journal of the American Animal Hospital Association*, **46**(3), 174–180.

Reavill, D. (2014) Pathology of the exotic companion mammal gastrointestinal system. *Veterinary Clinics of North America: Exotic Animal Practice*, **17**(2), 145–164.

Theus, M., Bitterli, F., and Foldenauer, U. (2008) Successful treatment of a gastric trichobezoar in a Peruvian guinea pig (*Cavia aperea porcellus*). *Journal of Exotic Pet Medicine*, **17**(2), 148–151.

Enteric Conditions

Angus, K.W., Hutchison, G., and Munro, H.M. (1985) Infectivity of a strain of *Cryptosporidium* found in the guinea-pig (*Cavia porcellus*) for guinea-pigs, mice and lambs. *Journal of Comparative Pathology*, **95**(2), 151–165.

Boot, R., Angulo, A.F., and Walvoort, H.C. (1989) *Clostridium difficile*-associated typhlitis in specific pathogen free guinea pigs in the absence of antimicrobial treatment. *Laboratory Animals (UK)*. **23**(3), 203–7.

Boot, R., and Walvoort, H.C. (1984) Vertical transmission of *Bacillus piliformis* infection (Tyzzer's disease) in a guinea pig: case report. *Laboratory Animals (UK)*, **18**, 195–199.

Cheney, C.P., Schad, P.A., Formal, S.B., and Boedeker, E.C. (1980) Species specificity of in vitro *Escherichia coli* adherence to host intestinal cell membranes and its correlation with in vivo colonization and infectivity. *Infection and Immunity*, **28**(3), 1019–1027.

Chrisp, C.E., Reid, W.C., Rush, H.G., et al. (1990) Cryptosporidiosis in guinea pigs: an animal model. *Infection and Immunity*, **58**(3), 674–679.

De Castro, L., De Araujo, H.P., Fialho, A.M., Gouvea, V.S., and Pereira, H.G. (1988) Serological evidence of rotavirus infection in a guinea pig colony. *Mem Instituto Oswaldo Cruz*, **83**(4), 411–413.

DeCubellis, J., and Graham, J. (2013) Gastrointestinal disease in guinea pigs and rabbits. *Veterinary Clinics of North America: Exotic Animal Practice*, **16**(2), 421–435.

Duhamel, G.E. (2001) Comparative pathology and pathogenesis of naturally acquired and experimentally induced colonic spirochetosis. *Animal Health Research Review*, **2**(1), 3–17.

Ellis, P.A., and Wright, A.E. (1961) Coccidiosis in guinea-pigs. *Journal of Clinical Pathology*, **14**(4), 394–396.

Elsheika, H., Brown, P., and Skuse, A. (2009) Death and diarrhea in guinea pigs (*Cavia porcellus*), *Eimeria caviae* infection. *Laboratory Animals (NY)*, **38**(6), 189–191.

Elwell, M.R., Chapman, A.L., and Frenkel, J.K. (1981) Duodenal hyperplasia in a guinea pig. *Veterinary Pathology*, **18**(1), 136–139.

Farrar, W.E. Jr, and Kent, T.H. (1965) Enteritis and coliform bacteremia in guinea pigs given penicillin. *American Journal of Pathology*, **47**(4), 629–642.

Fish, N.A., Fletch, A.L., and Butler, W.E. (1968) Family outbreak of salmonellosis due to contact with guinea pigs. *Canadian Medical Association Journal*, **99**(9), 418–420.

Helie, P. (2000) Intestinal spirochetosis in a guinea pig with colorectal prolapse. *Canadian Veterinary Journal*, **41**, 134.

Jaax, G.P., Jaax, N.K., Petrali, J.P., Corcoran, K.D., and Vogel, A.P. (1990) Coronavirus-like virions associated with a wasting syndrome in guinea pigs. *Laboratory Animal Science*, **40**(4), 375–378.

John, P.C., Gowal, K.N., Jayasheela, M., and Saxena, S.N. (1988) Natural course of salmonellosis in a guinea pig colony. *Indian Veterinary Journal*, **65**, 200–204.

Lawson, G.H.K. and Gebhart, C.J. (2000) Proliferative enteropathy. *Journal of Comparative Pathology*, **122**, 77–100.

Lipschutz, A., Iglesias, R., Rojas, G., and Cerisola, H. (1959) Spontaneous tumourigenesis in aged guinea pigs. *British Journal of Cancer*, **13**, 486–496.

Madden, D.L., Horton, R.E., and McCullough, N.B. (1970) Spontaneous infection in ex-germfree guinea pigs due to *Clostridium perfringens*. *Laboratory Animal Care*, **20**(3), 454–455.

McLeod, C.G., Stookey, J.L., Harrington, D.G., and White, J.D. (1977) Intestinal Tyzzer's disease and spirochetosis in a guinea pig. *Veterinary Pathology*, **14**(3), 229–235.

Muto, T., Noguchi, Y., Suzuki, K., and Zaw, K.M. (1983) Adenomatous intestinal hyperplasia in guinea pigs associated with *Campylobacter*-like bacteria. *Japanese Journal of Medical Science and Biology*, **36**(6), 337–342.

Ocholi, R.A., Chima, J.C., Uche, E.M.I., and Oyetunde, I.L. (1988) An epizootic infection of *Citrobacter freundii* in a guinea pig colony: short communication. *Laboratory Animals (UK)*. **22**, 335–336.

Onyekaba, C.O. (1983) Clinical salmonellosis in a guinea pig colony caused by a new *Salmonella serotype, Salmonella ochiogu*. *Laboratory Animals (UK)*, **17**(3), 213–216.

Rogers, J.B. and Blumenthal, H.T. (1960) Studies of guinea pig tumors. I. Report of fourteen spontaneous guinea pig tumors, with a review of the literature. *Cancer Research*, **20**, 191–102.

Shrubsole-Cockwill, A.N., Cockwill, K.R., and Parker, D.L. (2008) Omental torsion in a guinea pig (*Cavia porcellus*). *Canadian Veterinary Journal*, **49**(9), 898–900.

Simpson, L.L., Stiles, B.G., Zepeda, H.H., and Wilkins, T.D. (1987) Molecular basis for the pathological actions of *Clostridium perfringens* iota toxin. *Infection and Immunity*, **55**(1), 118–122.

Vannevel, J. and Wilcock, B. (2005) Bile duct carcinoma and nasal adenocarcinoma in a guinea pig. *Canadian Veterinary Journal*, **46**(1), 72–73.

Vanrobaeys, M., De Herdt, P., Ducatelle, R., et al. (1998) Typhlitis caused by intestinal *Serpulina*-like bacteria in domestic guinea pigs (*Cavia porcellus*). *Journal of Clinical Microbiology*, **36**(3), 690–694.

Voth, D.E. and Ballard, J.D. (2005) *Clostridium difficile* toxins: mechanism of action and role in disease. *Clinical Microbiology Reviews*, **18**(2), 247–263.

Zwicker, G.M., Dagle, G.E., and Adee, R.R. (1978) Naturally occurring Tyzzer's disease and intestinal spirochetosis in guinea pigs. *Laboratory Animal Science,* **28**(2), 193–198.

General Gastrointestinal References

Capello, V. (2008) Diagnosis and treatment of dental disease in pet rodents. *Journal of Exotic Pet Medicine,* **17**(2), 114–123.

Crecelius, H.G. and Rettger, L.F. (1943) The intestinal flora of the guinea pig. *Journal of Bacteriology,* **46**(1), 1–13.

Johnson-Delaney, C.A. (2006) Anatomy and physiology of the rabbit and rodent gastrointestinal system. *AEMV Proceedings,* pp. 9–17.

Kararli, T.T. (1995) Comparison of the gastrointestinal anatomy, physiology, and biochemistry of humans and commonly used laboratory animals. *Biopharmaceutical Drug Disposition,* **16**(5), 351–380.

Kohles, M. (2014) Gastrointestinal anatomy and physiology of select exotic companion mammals. *Veterinary Clinics of North America: Exotic Animal Practice,* **17**(2), 165–178.

Cardiovascular Conditions

Brewer, N.R. and Cruise, L.J. (1994) The guinea pig heart: some comparative aspects. *Contemporary Topics in Laboratory Animal Science,* **33**(6), 64–67.

Dzyban, L.A., Garrod, L.A., and Besso, J. (2001) Pericardial effusion and pericardiocentesis in a guinea pig (*Cavia porcellus*). *Journal of the American Animal Hospital Association,* **37**, 21–26.

Harris, A.M., Horton, A.L., Terpolilli, R.N., Van Stee, E.W., and Back, K.C. (1976) Anomalous cardiovascular structures in a guinea pig. *Veterinary Pathology,* **13**, 157–158.

Heatley, J.L. (2009) Cardiovascular Anatomy, Physiology, and Disease of Rodents and Small Exotic Mammals. *Veterinary Clinics of North America: Exotic Animal Practice,* **12**, 99–113.

Kobayashi, T., Kobayashi, Y., Fukuda, U., Ozeki, Y., Takahashi, M., Fujioka, S., and Fuchikami, J. (2010) A cardiac rhabdomyoma in a guinea pig. *Journal of Toxicologic Pathology,* **23**(2), 107–110.

McConnell, R.F., and Ediger, R.D. (1968) Benign mesenchymoma of the heart in the guinea pig: a report of four cases. *Veterinary Pathology,* **5**, 97–101.

Rae, M.V. (2004) Epizootic streptococcic myocarditis in guinea pigs. *Journal of Infectious Diseases,* **59**, 236–241.

Rogers, J.B., and Blumenthal, H.T. (1960) Studies of guinea pig tumors. I. Report of fourteen spontaneous guinea pig tumors, with a review of the literature. *Cancer Research,* **20**, 191–102.

Rooney, J.R. (1961) Rhabdomyomatosis in the heart of the guinea pig. *Cornell Veterinarian,* **51**, 388–394.

Vink, H.H. (1969) Rhabdomyomatosis (nodular glycogenic infiltration) of the heart in guinea-pigs. *Journal of Pathology,* **97**(2), 331–334.

Vogler, B.R., Vetsch, E., Wernick, M.B., Sydler, T., and Wiederkehr, D.D. (2012) Primary leiomyosarcoma in the heart of a guinea pig. *Journal of Comparative Pathology,* **147**(4), 452–454.

Chronic Renal Disease

Jenkins, J.R. (2010) Diseases of geriatric guinea pigs and chinchillas. *Veterinary Clinics of North America: Exotic Animal Practice,* **13**, 85–93.

Takeda, T. and Grollman, A. (1970) Spontaneously occurring renal disease in the guinea pig. *American Journal of Pathology,* **60**(1), 103–117.

Urolithiasis and Cystitis

Boll, R.A., Suckow, M.A., and Hawkins, E.C. Bilateral ureteral calculi in a guinea pig. *Journal of Small Animal Exotic Medicine,* **578**, 60–63.

Fehr, M. and Rappold, S. (1997) Urolithiasis bei Meerschweinchen. *Tierärztliche Praxis.* **5**, 543–547.

Hawkins, M.G., Ruby, A.L., Drazenovich, T.L., and Westropp, J.L. (2009) Composition and characteristics of urinary calculi from guinea pigs. *Journal of the American Veterinary Medical Association,* **234**(2), 214–220.

Holowaychuk, M.K. (2006) Renal failure in a guinea pig (*Cavia porcellus*) following ingestion of oxalate containing plants. *Canadian Veterinary Journal,* **47**, 787–789.

Okewole, P.A., Odeyemi, P.S., Oladunmade, M.A., et al. (1991) An outbreak of *Streptococcus pyogenes* infection associated with calcium oxalate urolithiasis in guinea pigs (*Cavia porcellus*). *Laboratory Animals (UK).* **25**, 184–186.

Peng, X., Griffiths, J.W., and Lang, C.M. (1990) Cystitis, urolithiasis and cystic calculi in aging guinea pigs. *Laboratory Animals (UK).* **24**, 159–163.

Quesenbery, K.E. (1994) Guinea pigs. *Veterinary Clinics of North America: Exotic Animal Practice,* **24**, 67–88.

Spink, R.R. (1978) Urolithiasis in a guinea pig. *Veterinary Clinics of North America: Exotic Animal Practice,* **73**, 501–502.

Stuppy, D.E., Douglass, P.R., and Douglass, P.J. (1979) Urolithiasis and cystotomy in a guinea pig. *Veterinary Medicine Small Animal Clinician,* **74**, 565–567.

Wood, M. (1981) Cystitis in female guinea pigs. *Laboratory Animal Science,* **15**, 141–143.

General Urinary Tract Infections

Capella-Gutiérrez, S., Marcet-Houben, M., and Gabaldón, T. (2012) Phylogenomics supports microsporidia as the earliest diverging clade of sequenced fungi. *BMC Biology,* **10**, 47.

Fisher, P.G. (2006a) Exotic mammal renal disease: causes and clinical presentation. *Veterinary Clinics of North America: Exotic Animal Practice*, **9**, 33–67.

Fisher, P.G. (2006b) Exotic mammal renal disease: Diagnosis and treatment. *Veterinary Clinics of North America: Exotic Animal Practice*, **9**, 69–96.

Illanes, O.G., Tiffani-Castiglioni, E., Edwards, J.F., and Shadduck, J.A. (1993) Spontaneous encephalitozoonosis in an experimental group of guinea pigs. *Journal of Veterinary Diagnostic Investigation*, **5**(4), 649–651.

Wan, C., Franklin, C., Riley, L.K., Hook, R.R., and Besch-Williford, C. (1996) Diagnostic exercise: granulomatous encephalitis in guinea pigs. *Laboratory Animal Science*, **46**, 228–230.

Wasson, K. and Peper, R.L. (2000) Mammalian microsporidiosis. *Veterinary Pathology*, **37**(2), 113–128.

Cystic Ovarian Disease

Eppig, J.J., and Handel, M.A. (2012) Origins of granulosa cells clarified and complexified by waves. *Biology of Reproduction*, **86**(2), 34.

Keller, L.S.F., Griffith, J.W., and Lang, C.M. (1987) Reproductive failure associated with cystic rete ovarii in guinea pigs. *Veterinary Pathology*, **24**, 335–339.

Löffler, S., Horn, L.C., Weber, W., and Spanel-Borowski, K. (2000) The transient disappearance of cytokeratin in human fetal and adult ovaries. *Anatomy and Embryology (Berlin).* **201**(3), 207–215.

Nielsen, T.D., Holt, S., Ruelokke, M.L., and McEvoyo, F.J. (2003) Ovarian cysts in guinea pigs: influence of age and reproductive status on prevalence and size. *Journal of Small Animal Practice.* **44**, 257–260.

Pilny, A. (2014) Ovarian cystic disease in guinea pigs. *Veterinary Clinics of North America: Exotic Animal Practice*, **17**(1), 69–75.

Quattropani, S.L. (1977) Serous cysts of the aging guinea pig ovary. *Anatomical Record*, **188**(3), 351–359.

Wenzel, J.G., and Odend'hal, S. (1985) The mammalian rete ovarii: a literature review. *Cornell Veterinarian*, **75**(3), 411–425.

Renal and Reproductive Masses

Burns, R.P., Paul-Murphy, J. and Sicard, G.K. (2001) Granulosa cell tumor in a guinea pig. *Journal of the American Veterinary Medical Association*, **218**(5), 726–728.

Field, K.J., Griffith, J.W., and Lang, C.M. (1989) Spontaneous reproductive tract leiomyomas in aged guinea-pigs. *Journal of Comparative Pathology*, **101**(3), 287–294.

Hoch-Ligeti, C., Congdon, C.C., Deringer, M.K., Strandberg, J.D., and Stewart, H.L. (1980) Hemangiopericytoma and other tumors of urinary tract of guinea pigs. *Toxicologic Pathology*, **8**, 1–8.

Rogers, J.B. and Blumenthal, H.T. (1960) Studies of guinea pig tumors. I. Report of fourteen spontaneous guinea pig tumors, with a review of the literature. *Cancer Research*, **20**, 191–102.

Saraiva, A.L., Payan-Carreira, R., and Pires, M. (2010) Adenoma of the uterus in a guinea pig. *ESVP/ECVP Proceedings*, **143**(4), 317.

Pregnancy Toxemia

Bishop, C.R. (2002) Reproductive medicine of rabbits and rodents. *Veterinary Clinics of North America: Exotic Animal Practice*, **5**(3), 507–535.

Foley, E.J. (1942) Toxemia of pregnancy in the guinea pig. *Journal of Experimental Medicine*, **75**(5), 539–546.

Pritt, S. (1996) Pregnancy toxemia in guinea pigs (*Cavia porcellus*), A case report and discussion. *ASLAP Newsletter*, **29**(3), 15–17.

Seidl, D.C., Hughes, H.C., Bertolet, R., and Lang, C.M. (1979) True pregnancy toxemia (preeclampsia) in the guinea pig (*Cavia porcellus*). *Laboratory Animal Science*, **29**(4), 472–478.

Other Reproductive Conditions

Martinho, F. (2006) Dystocia caused by ectopic pregnancy in a guinea pig (*Cavia porcellus*). *Veterinary Clinics of North America: Exotic Animal Practice*, **9**(3), 713–716.

Samii, V.F., Dumonceaux, G., and Nyland, T.G. (1996) Radiographic diagnosis – Prostatitis in a guinea pig. *Veterinary Radiology and Ultrasound*, **37**(5), 357–358.

Rabies Virus Infections

Eidson, M., Matthews, S.D., Willsey, A.L., et al. (2005) Rabies virus infection in a pet guinea pig and seven pet rabbits. *Journal of the American Veterinary Medical Association*, **227**(6), 932–935.

Fitzpatrick, J.L., Dyer, J.L., Blanton, J.D., Kuzmin, I.V., and Rupprecht, C.E. (2014) Rabies in rodents and lagomorphs in the United States, 1995-2010. *Journal of the American Veterinary Medical Association*, **245**(3), 333–337.

Lackay, S.N., Kuang, Y., and Fu, Z.F. (2008) Rabies in small animals. *Veterinary Clinics of North America: Small Animal Practice*, **38**(4), 851–860.

Cerebrospinal Parasitic Larval Migration

Van Andel, R.A., Franklin, C.L., Besch-Williford, C., et al. (1995) Cerebrospinal larva migrans due to *Baylisascaris procyonis* in a guinea pig colony. *Laboratory Animal Science*, **45**(1), 27–30.

Cerebrospinal Masses

Betty, M.J. (1977) Ependymal hyperplasia in the lateral ventricle of a guinea pig. *Journal of Comparative Pathology*, **87**, 185–194.

Rogers, J.B., and Blumenthal, H.T. (1960) Studies of guinea pig tumors. I. Report of fourteen spontaneous guinea pig tumors, with a review of the literature. *Cancer Research*, **20**, 191–102.

Other Neurologic Conditions

Betty, M.J. (1977) Spontaneous cryptococcal meningitis in a group of guinea pigs caused by a hyphae-producing strain. *Journal of Comparative Pathology*, **87**, 377–382.

Centers for Disease Control and Prevention. (2005) Interim guidance for minimizing risk for human lymphocytic choriomeningitis virus infection associated with rodents. *Morbidity and Mortality Weekly Reports*, **54**(30), 747–749.

Hotchin, J. (1971) The contamination of laboratory animals with lymphocytic choriomeningitis virus. *American Journal of Pathology*, **64**(3), 747–767.

Meredith, A.L., and Richardson, J. (2015) Neurological diseases of rabbits and rodents. *Journal of Exotic Pet Medicine*, **24**, 21–33.

Southard, T., Bender, H., Wade, S.E., Grunenwald, C., and Gerhold, R.W. (2013) Naturally occurring *Parelaphostrongylus tenuis*-associated choriomeningitis in a guinea pig with neurologic signs. *Veterinary Pathology*, **50**(3), 560–562.

Lymphosarcoma

Debout, C., Caillez, D., and Izard, J. (1987) A spontaneous lymphoblastic lymphoma in a guinea-pig. *Pathologie-Biologie (Paris)*. **35**(9), 1249–1252.

Hong, C.C., Liu, P.I., and Poon, K.C. (1980) Naturally occurring lymphoblastic leukemia in guinea pigs. *Laboratory Animal Science*, **30**(2 Pt 1), 222–226.

Kitchen, D.N., Carlton, W.W., and Bickford, A.A. (1975) A report of fourteen spontaneous tumors of the guinea pig. *Laboratory Animal Science*, **25**(1), 92–102.

Koebrich, S., Grest, P., Favrot, C., and Wilhelm, S. (2011) Epitheliotropic T-cell lymphoma in a guinea pig. *Veterinary Dermatology*, **22**(2), 215–219.

Opler, S.R. (1967) New oncogenic virus producing acute lymphatic leukemia in guinea pigs. *Proceedings of the 3rd International Symposium on Comparative Leukeumia Research, Paris, France*, **31**, 81–88.

Opler, S.R. (1967) Pathology of cavian viral leukemia. *American Journal of Pathology*, **51**, 1135–1151.

Rogers, J.B. and Blumenthal, H.T. (1960) Studies of guinea pig tumors. I. Report of fourteen spontaneous guinea pig tumors, with a review of the literature. *Cancer Research*, **20**, 191–202.

Steinberg, H. (2000) Disseminated T-cell lymphoma in a guinea pig with bilateral ocular involvement. *Journal of Veterinary Diagnostic Investigation*, **12**, 459–462.

General Hematology

Kittas, C., Parsons, M.A., and Henry, L. (1979) A light and electron microscope study on the origin of Foà-Kurloff cells. *British Journal of Experimental Pathology*, **60**(3), 276–285.

Pouliot, N., Maghni, K., Blanchette, F., et al. (1996) Natural killer and lectin-dependent cytotoxic activities of Kurloff cells: target cell selectivity, conjugate formation, and Ca++ dependency. *Inflammation*, **20**(6), 647–671.

Pouliot, N., Maghni, K., Sirois, P., and Rola-Pleszczynski, M. (1996) Guinea pig Kurloff (NK-like) cells mediate TNF-dependent cytotoxic activity: analogy with NC effector cells. *Inflammation*, **20**(3), 263–280.

Thrall, M.A. (2012) *Veterinary Hematology and Clinical Chemistry*, 2nd edn. Wiley-Blackwell, Ames, IA.

Zimmerman, K., Moore, D.M., and Smith, S.A. (2015) Hematological assessment in pet guinea pigs (*Cavia porcellus*), blood sample collection and blood cell identification. *Veterinary Clinics of North America: Exotic Animal Practice*, **18**(1), 33–40.

Conditions of the Eyelid and Conjunctiva

Allgoewer, I., Ewringmann, C.P., and Pfleghaar, S. (1999) Lymphosarcoma with conjunctival manifestation in a guinea pig. *Veterinary Ophthalmology*, **2**(2), 117–119.

Bettelheim, F.A., Churchill, A.C., and Zigler, Jr J.R. (1997) On the nature of hereditary cataract in strain 13/N guinea pigs. *Current Eye Research*, **16**, 917–924.

Deeb, B.J., DiGiacomo, R.F., and Wang, S.P. (1989) Guinea pig inclusion conjunctivitis (GPIC) in a commercial colony. *Laboratory Animal (UK)*, **23**(2), 103–106.

Gupta, B.N. (1972) Scleral dermoid in a guinea pig. *Laboratory Animal Science*, **22**, 919–921.

Lutz-Wohlgroth, L., Becker, A., Brugnera, E., et al.(2006) Chlamydiales in guinea-pigs and their zoonotic potential. *Journal of Veterinary Medicine A: Physiology, Pathology, Clinical Medicine*, **53**(4), 185–193.

Pannekoek, Y., Dickx, V., Beeckman, D.S.A., Jolley, K.A., et al. (2010) Multi locus sequence typing of *Chlamydia* reveals an association between *Chlamydia psittaci* genotypes and host species. *PLoS ONE*, **5**(12), e14179.

Quinton, J.F., Ollivier, F., and Dally, C. (2013) A case of well-differentiated palpebral liposarcoma in a Guinea pig (*Cavia porcellus*). *Veterinary Ophthalmology*, **16**(Suppl. 1), 155–159.

Rank, R.G., Hough, A.J., Jacobs, R.F., Cohen, C., and Barron, A.L. Chlamydial pneumonitis induced in newborn guinea pigs. *Infection and Immunity*, **48**(1), 153–158.

Stephens, R.S., Myers, G., Eppinger, M., and Bavoil, P.M. (2009) Divergence without difference: phylogenetics and taxonomy of Chlamydia resolved. *FEMS Immunology and Medical Microbiology*, **55**, 115–119.

Strik, N.I., Alleman, A.R., and Wellehan, J.F. (2005) Conjunctival swab cytology from a guinea pig: it's elementary! *Veterinary Clinical Pathology*, **34**(2), 169–171.

Wappler, O., Allgoewer, I., and Schaeffer, E.H. (2002) Conjunctival dermoid in two guinea pigs: a case report. *Veterinary Ophthalmology*, **5**(3), 245–248.

Conditions of the Cornea and Anterior Chamber

Brooks, D.E., McCracken, M.D., and Collins, B.R. (1991) Heterotopic bone formation in the ciliary body of an aged guinea pig. *Laboratory Animal Science*, **40**, 88–90.

Colgin, L.M., Nielsen, R.E., Tucker, F.S., and Okerberg, C.V. (1995) Case report of listerial keratoconjunctivitis in hairless guinea pigs. *Laboratory Animal Science*, **45**(4), 435–436.

Griffith, J.W., Sassani, J.W., Bowman, T.A., and Lang, C.M. (1988) Osseous choristoma of the ciliary body in guinea pigs. *Veterinary Pathology*, **25**, 100–102.

Otto, G., Lipman, N.S., and Murphy, J.C. (1991) Corneal dermoid in a hairless guinea pig. *Laboratory Animal Science.*, **41**, 171–172.

General Ophthalmic Conditions

Kern, T.J. (1997) Rabbit and rodent ophthalmology. *Seminars in Avian and Exotic Pet Medicine*, **6**(3), 138–145.

Sandmeyer, L.S., Parker, D., and Grahn, B.H. (2011) Diagnostic ophthalmology. *Canadian Veterinary Journal*, **52**(7), 801–802.

Steinberg, H. (2000) Disseminated T-cell lymphoma in a guinea pig with bilateral ocular involvement. *Journal of Veterinary Diagnostic Investigation*, **12**, 459–462.

Williams, D. (2007) Rabbit and rodent ophthalmology. *European Journal of Comparative Animal Practice*, **17**(3), 242–252.

Williams, D. and Sullivan, A. (2010) Ocular disease in the guinea pig (*Cavia porcellus*), a survey of 1000 animals. *Veterinary Ophthalmology*, **13**(Suppl 1), 54–62.

4

Chinchillas

4.1 Introduction

Chinchillas are members of the suborder Hystricomorpha within the order Rodentia. There are two species of chinchilla: *Chinchilla lanigera* and *C. brevicaudata*. *C. lanigera* is more commonly encountered in small mammal pet practice and is the smaller of the two species with more rounded ears and a longer tail.

Chinchillas originated from the Andes mountains in South America, where they live in social colonies in rock crevices or burrows, and feed upon fibrous grasses and shrubs. Because of their very thick, dense hair coat, chinchillas are well adapted to cold, dry temperatures but they are very sensitive to high heat and humidity. In captivity, chinchillas may suffer from heat prostration if temperatures exceed 27°C and humidity is high (i.e., greater than 50–60%). They do not hibernate and are crepuscular to nocturnal in nature. Chinchillas live much longer than most pet rodents with a lifespan of 12–20 years.

Historically, raising and breeding of chinchillas on farms were solely for the production of high quality luxurious fur; however, with the increased interest in these animals as pets and for research, chinchilla breeders also raise chinchillas to meet these demands.

Chinchillas are gentle, docile animals that are relatively easy to handle. The range of hearing in chinchillas is also similar to humans and they are susceptible to acoustic injury. They suffer less from middle ear infections than other small rodent species.

4.2 Integument Conditions

The fur of the chinchilla is very fine, silky, and dense and each compound hair follicle contains 50–60 fine wool hairs and a central guard hair. Chinchillas demonstrate fewer photoperiod-dependent cycles of molting compared with fur-bearing carnivores, such as mink, and the first molt in an adult chinchilla can occur at any time of the year. Chinchilla hair grows in waves with multiple cycles each forming their own pattern. These cycles are altered by physiologic events, including lactation and pregnancy, such that when hair is lost or removed, the amount of time required for regrowth is unpredictable and asychronous.

Patchy to generalized hair loss is seen with many conditions, including fur slip, fur chewing, nutritional deficiencies, dermatophytosis, trauma, bacterial infections, and nutritional deficiencies.

4.2.1 Fur Slip

Fur slip is a predator avoidance mechanism and occurs when chinchillas are frightened or roughly handled. In these situations, when the fur is grasped, a patch of hair is released allowing the animal to escape. This leaves a clean, smooth area of skin and the hair can take several months to regrow, depending on the stage of the hair growth cycle when hair loss occurs. Microscopically, the skin appears normal, but no hair shafts are present in follicles.

4.2.2 Fur Chewing

Fur chewing or barbering results when chinchillas chew their own or a conspecific's hair. The condition is seen more often in female chinchillas. When self-chewing occurs, a "lion's mane" appearance may result, with all the hair within reach on the lower body chewed to a short length. Chinchillas can also chew the fur of conspecifics resulting in a moth-eaten appearance to the haircoat. Microscopically, hair shafts are seen to end abruptly at the level of the epidermis and there is no infiltrate, crusting or hyperkeratosis.

Why fur chewing occurs is unknown and in the past some have suggested that it is a hereditary or learned behavioral disorder or that it arises because of nutritional imbalances. Recent studies have suggested that poor environmental conditions, environmental stressors, such as loud noises, boredom, overcrowding, lack of access to dust baths on a regular basis, and low fiber diets are contributing factors. Elevated urinary cortisol metabolites may be detected in females that demonstrate severe fur chewing behavior. Differential diagnoses for

Pathology of Small Mammal Pets, First Edition. Patricia V. Turner, Marina L. Brash and Dale A. Smith.
© 2018 John Wiley & Sons, Inc. Published 2018 by John Wiley & Sons, Inc.

fur chewing include fur slip, dermatophytosis, and various nutritional deficiencies.

4.2.3 Dermatophytosis

Dermatophyte infections (ringworm) are common in group-housed chinchillas and are often subclinical in nature, particularly in immature and geriatric animals, likely because of incomplete immunocompetence. *Trichophyton mentagrophytes* is the most commonly isolated species but *Microsporum canis* and *Microsporum gypseum* infections have also been described.

4.2.3.1 Presenting Clinical Signs
Affected animals present with patchy, scaling alopecia affecting the nose, feet, ears, and tail, although lesions can appear anywhere on the body (Figure 4.1). Close examination of the skin reveals broken hairs and variable amounts of erythema.

4.2.3.2 Pathology
Histopathology of affected skin is diagnostic, characterized by a multinodular pyogranulomatous folliculitis and furunculosis. Arthrospores encircle hair shafts and fungal hyphae are seen within the hairs.

4.2.3.3 Laboratory Diagnostics
Histochemical stains, such as periodic acid Schiff (PAS) or Gomori's methenamine silver (GMS) are useful for

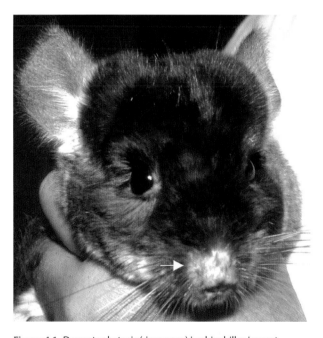

Figure 4.1 Dermatophytosis (ringworm) in chinchillas is most commonly caused by *Trichophyton mentagrophytes*. The characteristic patchy, scaling alopecic lesions generally affect the nose (arrow), feet, ears, and tail, but can be located anywhere on the body.

demonstrating the fungal arthrospores. Skin scrapings and plucked hair taken from the lesion margins can be cultured and examined microscopically following potassium hydroxide digestion. *T. mentagrophytes* does not fluoresce with ultraviolet light, *M. gypseum* rarely fluoresces, and *M. canis* is more likely to fluoresce.

4.2.3.4 Differential Diagnoses
Differential diagnoses for dermatophytosis include trauma, fur chewing, bacterial dermatitis, and nutritional deficiencies.

4.2.3.5 Disease/Colony Management
Hay, contaminated bedding, fomites found on brushes and within dust baths, and carrier and infected animals are potential sources of infection. Infectious spores can be carried from one animal to another on the hands and clothing of people handling the chinchillas. Dermatophytosis is a zoonotic condition and if an animal within a group is suspected or known to have the condition, animals should be handled with gloves.

4.2.4 Skin Trauma and Subcutaneous Abscesses

Abscessed bite wounds often occur in group-housed animals and can frequently be the result of fighting during breeding, as females are larger than males and can be aggressive during breeding. Other causes of skin trauma include abrasions or lacerations from poorly built or maintained cages or other sharp-edged equipment that comes into contact with animals (Figure 4.2).

Bacteria, including *Streptococcus pneumoniae, S. pyogenes, S. zooepidemicus, Staphylococcus aureus,* and *Pseudomonas aeruginosa* can be recovered from subcutaneous abscesses, and secondary lymphadenitis and septicemia can be sequelae.

4.2.5 External Parasites

Because of the chinchilla's dense haircoat, ectoparasites are not commonly noted on clinical examination. Fur mites (*Cheyletiella* sp.) have been described in anecdotal reports and if chinchillas are housed with cats and dogs, fleas can transfer onto chinchillas. If the infestation is significant, consequences include dull hair coat with patchy alopecia and intense pruritus. Careful examination of the skin for fleas and flea excreta is needed to confirm infestation.

4.2.6 Pododermatitis

Pododermatitis occurs less often in chinchillas than in guinea pigs, and is associated with lack of mobility, constant exposure to wire or other abrasive flooring, obesity, and poor sanitation. Constant trauma of the foot results in reddening, swelling, ulceration, and crusting of the soft footpads. There is often extension of the inflammation to

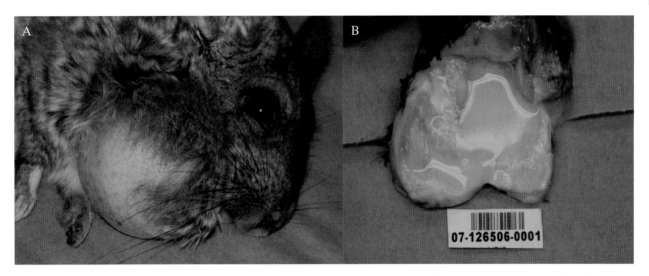

Figure 4.2 A: Large subcutaneous facial abscess from which *S. zooepidemicus* was isolated. These abscesses can develop from bite wounds or other causes of skin trauma, including sharp-edged caging and equipment. B: The subcutaneous abscess has a thick capsule and contains abundant thick creamy purulent exudate.

involve bone resulting in osteomyelitis. *Staphylococcus* spp. or *Streptococcus* spp. are typically isolated from these lesions.

4.2.7 Agalactia

There are several potential causes of agalactia, including chinchillas bred at too young an age, females in poor body condition, because of underlying disease, such as metritis, poor nutrition or inadequate quantities of feed given in addition to the demands of a large litter, damaged teats from trauma from nursing kits, and bacterial mastitis as a sequela to primary infection or secondary infection from injuries sustained from nursing kits.

4.2.8 Bacterial Mastitis

In cases of bacterial mastitis, the mammary glands are swollen, firm, discolored, and painful, and the affected female will be pyrexic, anorexic, listless, and uninterested in her pups. Bacterial etiologies for mastitis in chinchillas include *Staphylococcus* spp. and *Streptococcus* spp.

4.2.9 Seborrhea and Matted Fur Coats

Chinchillas require frequent dust baths to absorb skin oils and they can develop matted fur from normal sebaceous secretions if they are deprived of regular dust baths or if they are kept in inappropriate environments, such as warm humid conditions with temperatures above 24°C and 50% humidity.

4.2.10 Nutritional Deficiencies

Feeding diets too high in protein can result in the growth of fine and gently coiled or wavy hair, termed cotton fur.

Typical chinchilla diets contain 15–18% protein. Poor hair coats with reduced hair growth, dry scaly skin, and hair loss are seen with dietary deficiencies of various fatty acids, including linoleic, linolenic, arachidonic, and pantothenic acids. Zinc deficiency can also lead to alopecia and parakeratotic hyperkeratosis.

4.2.11 Cutaneous Neoplasia

Skin tumors are uncommonly reported in chinchillas, despite their long lifespan; however, because these animals were initially bred for fur production, the lack of data in this regard may be the result of non-reporting rather than low incidence (Figure 4.3).

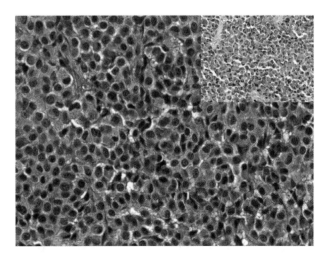

Figure 4.3 Biopsy from a 9 year-old, male chinchilla presenting with a skin mass. A mast cell tumor was diagnosed with typical metachromatic granules seen with a toluidine blue stain (inset). Source: Courtesy of C.A. Schiller.

4.2.12 Other Skin Conditions

Chinchillas have large delicate pinnae that are easily traumatized and secondary bacterial infection with abscessation can result with *Staphylococcus* spp. often being isolated. Frostbite can occur with exposure to extreme cold.

4.3 Endocrine Conditions

Endocrine disorders are relatively uncommon in chinchillas.

4.3.1 Diabetes Mellitus

Diabetes mellitus is the most common endocrine condition reported in chinchillas and is highly correlated with obesity. Clinical signs include inappetence, progressive weight loss, depression, polyuria, polydipsia, and bilateral cataracts. Ante-mortem diagnostic testing demonstrates hyperglycemia, glycosuria, and ketonuria. At necropsy, the pancreas may be atrophic and wispy with microscopic evidence of pancreatic islet vacuolation as well as hepatic lipidosis. Differential diagnoses include urinary disease, cystitis, stress or pain, inappetence, hepatic lipidosis, and hyperthyroidism.

4.3.2 Hyperthyroidism

Hyperthyroidism is rarely reported in chinchillas. In one case, a 6-year-old female chinchilla presented with a history of rapid and progressive weight loss, poor body condition, focal scurfy alopecia of one forelimb, soft feces, yeast stomatitis, and unilateral seromucoid ocular discharge. Serum T_4 levels were elevated on repeated measurement, although no apparent changes could be identified in the thyroid glands by palpation or sonography. Following initiation of treatment, a clear correlation was noted between the decreasing T_4 level and improvement in body weight, however, no follow-up pathology was ever conducted.

In some animals, fur chewing has been associated with elevated thyroid gland activity as measured by thyroid ^{131}I release rates and thyroid hormone secretion rates. These chinchillas also have histologic evidence of thyroid gland hyperplasia, characterized by small follicles lined by columnar epithelium containing reduced amounts of colloid.

4.3.3 Chronic Adrenocortical Hyperplasia

Animals that chew hair may have elevated plasma cortisol levels and adrenocortical hypertrophy. Histologic examination of skin sections from affected chinchillas demonstrate changes that are consistent with chronic hyperadrenocorticism, including orthokeratotic hyperkeratosis, epithelial atrophy, follicular and sebaceous gland atrophy, follicular hyperkeratosis with comedo formation, and calcinosis cutis. These animals also have microscopic evidence of adrenocortical hyperplasia. Interestingly, evaluation of the haired skin from "non-chewer" conspecifics may demonstrate mild epidermal hyperkeratosis but no follicular or sebaceous gland changes are usually seen, and the adrenal glands show milder adrenocortical hyperplasia.

Adrenal gland enlargement may occur in a variety of stress-inducing conditions in chinchillas (Figure 4.4). In one study, necropsies were conducted on culled breeder or pet chinchillas that died or were euthanized for clinical illness. Some 84% of these animals had cheek teeth elongation and close to a third had concurrent adrenocortical hyperplasia, suggesting high levels of corticosteroids in these animals possibly resulting from chronic dental disease and associated pain. This suggests that adrenocortical hyperplasia as a sequela to stress, including heat stress and other disease processes, and the condition may be more common in chinchillas than has been reported.

4.4 Respiratory Conditions

The oral cavity of the chinchilla is a small narrow chamber and the soft palate extends to the base of the tongue. There is a small opening in the soft palate, the palatal ostium, which connects the oropharynx with the pharynx. Because the larynx lies dorsally within the oropharynx, closely associated with the nasopharynx, the chinchilla is an obligate nasal breather.

Chinchillas may be more prone to bacterial respiratory disease as a result of these unique anatomic features and adaptations for increased airflow. Bacterial conditions of the respiratory tract are common in both pet and farmed chinchillas. Historical summaries of diagnoses from post-mortems conducted on farmed chinchillas indicate that conditions of the respiratory and gastrointestinal tracts accounted for 88% of the diagnoses.

Reduced activity levels, hunched posture, an unkempt hair coat, and inappetence are frequent nonspecific signs that may be present with respiratory disease.

4.4.1 Conditions of the Upper Respiratory Tract

4.4.1.1 Bacterial Rhinitis and Sinusitis

Predisposing factors for outbreaks of respiratory disease in chinchillas include excessive humidity, overcrowding, poor ventilation, constant drafts, recent transportation, and contact with infected conspecifics, as well as other animals, including rabbits, cats, and dogs, which may serve as carriers of *Streptococcus* spp. including *S. pneumoniae* and

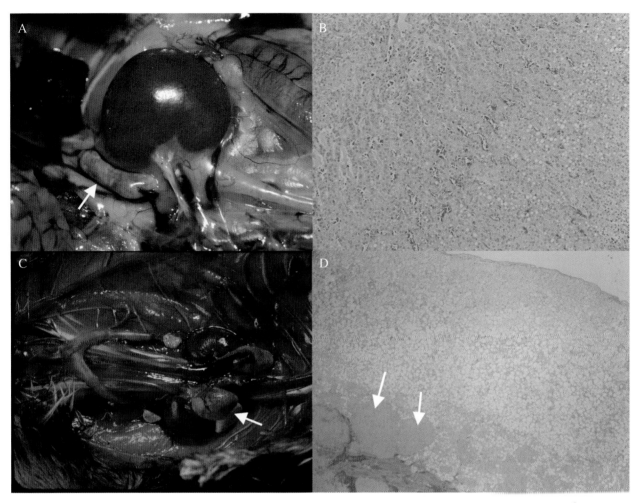

Figure 4.4 A: Normal left adrenal gland (arrow). Note size in comparison with the left kidney. B: Histology of normal adrenal gland. Note the width of the adrenal cortex and the appearance of the adrenal cortical cells. C: Markedly hypertrophied adrenal gland (arrow). Compare the relative size to the kidney. D: Hypertrophied adrenal gland. Note the expanded cortex and the marked adrenal cortical cytoplasmic vacuolation. Clusters of ceroid-laden macrophages (arrows) are present at the adrenal corticomedullary junction.

S. pyogenes, *Pasteurella multocida*, and *Bordetella bronchiseptica*. Sinusitis and rhinitis more often affect young or stressed chinchillas and can progress to pneumonia and death if untreated.

Presenting Clinical Signs Clinical signs in chinchillas with rhinitis and sinusitis include sneezing, dyspnea, serous to mucopurulent oculonasal discharge, and matting of the fur on the forelimbs as a result of increased grooming.

Pathology In affected animals, nasal and sinus cavities contain mucoid to mucopurulent exudate and microscopically, mucus, proteinaceous fluid, neutrophils, and colonies of bacteria are present, with mild to moderate sloughing of nasal epithelial cells.

Differential Diagnoses Differential diagnoses for rhinitis and sinusitis include malocclusion and tooth root abscesses.

Laboratory Diagnostics Laboratory testing includes bacterial culture and susceptibility testing of the nasal exudate.

4.4.1.2 Foreign Body Rhinitis

Young chinchillas can inhale foreign material, including components of the dust bath, such as cornstarch, leading to foreign body rhinitis. As a preventative measure, breeders will often reduce or eliminate cornstarch from the dust bath while the dams are lactating.

4.4.2 Conditions of the Lower Respiratory Tract

4.4.2.1 Aspiration Pneumonia

Aspiration pneumonia can occur in hand-reared infant chinchillas that are overfed, and it can also develop as a result of iatrogenic misdosing of oral medications.

4.4.2.2 Bacterial Pneumonia

Upper respiratory tract infections of chinchillas can extend to involve the lungs with subsequent septicemia and systemic dissemination, resulting in secondary otitis media/interna and meningoencephalitis. Common bacteria inducing bronchopneumonia in chinchillas include *S. aureus*, *S. pneumoniae*, *S. pyogenes*, *S. zooepidemicus*, *Klebsiella pneumoniae*, *Bordetella bronchiseptica*, *Pasteurella multocida*, and *Pseudomonas aeruginosa*. Streptococcal pneumonia originating from human handlers has also been reported in an adult chinchilla.

Clinical signs in affected chinchillas may include depression, dyspnea, diarrhea, fever, anorexia, dehydration, lethargy, and sudden death. Peracute septicemia is especially common in chinchillas with Gram-negative bacterial infections. The acute forms of respiratory disease include suppurative to fibrinous bronchopneumonia (Figure 4.5), often in conjunction with suppurative rhinitis, otitis media, and meningoencephalitis. With chronic disease, hematogenous dissemination and subcutaneous abscesses have been described. In young chinchillas, *P. aeruginosa* can cause an acute hemorrhagic pneumonia.

Farmed chinchilla infected with *K. pneumoniae* demonstrated pulmonary congestion and consolidation, pleural effusion, cardiac enlargement, gastroenteritis, and subcapsular renal petechiation. Histologic lesions consisted of marked pulmonary congestion and edema, and suppurative pneumonia. Immunization with an autogenous bacterin has been effective in controlling the disease in some breeding operations.

A single chinchilla housed with ten others and reported to be smaller than others in the group, was

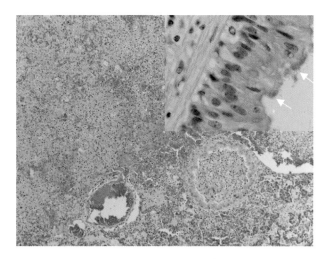

Figure 4.5 Acute fibrinohemorrhagic and suppurative bronchopneumonia caused by *Bordetella bronchiseptica*. Clinical signs included dyspnea and mucoid nasal discharge followed by increased mortality. At post-mortem, lungs were dark red. Inset: Large numbers of coccobacilli colonize the tips of the cilia of the tracheal epithelium (arrows).

diagnosed with *Mycobacterium genavense*-associated multinodular granulomatous pneumonia with bullous emphysema and multifocal necrohemorrhagic hepatitis following a 4-week history of progressive weight loss. The animal had received medical treatment for paraphimosis and had been castrated three months prior. Mortality from this small colony was investigated over the next two years and further mycobacterial lesions were not identified. The source of the infection was not discovered. *M. genavense* infections pose a zoonotic risk, especially for immunocompromised humans.

4.4.2.3 Mycotic Pneumonia

Mycotic pneumonia is rarely seen in chinchillas and fungal organisms are generally considered to be opportunistic, inducing infections in animals secondary to other conditions, such as primary bacterial infections. In one case, 17 chinchillas from a group of 130 died within a 1-month period with clinical signs including anorexia and weight loss, constipation, and tachypnea. No oculonasal discharge was noted. Deaths occurred within 2–4 days following the development of respiratory signs. Of this group, one chinchilla evaluated had emphysematous lungs with multifocal hemorrhages and a marked bronchopneumonia. The spleen was enlarged with generalized prominent white nodules, the liver had extensive areas of focal necrosis, and the gastrointestinal tract was empty. Histologically, the lungs demonstrated extensive proliferation of type II pneumocytes with focal areas of consolidation and a fibrinous pleuritis. Organisms consistent with *Histoplasma capsulatum* were observed in multinucleated giant cells, macrophages, and endothelial cells. Multifocal granulomatous hepatitis, splenitis, lymphadenitis, and nephritis were also noted. *P. multocida* was also recovered from the lung of this animal. *H. capsulatum* was isolated from the hay samples fed to animals and was considered to be the source of the infection. The hay originated from an area known to be endemic for histoplasmosis.

4.4.2.4 Pulmonary Adenomatosis

In one case, several farm-raised chinchillas presented with dyspnea, lethargy, gradual weight loss, anorexia, rhinitis, conjunctivitis, and loss of facial fur. The disease had an insidious onset and animals were ill for 1–6 weeks prior to euthanasia. On gross examination, chinchillas were in poor body condition with poor quality pelts. Pinpoint white foci were noted throughout the pulmonary parenchyma and livers were normal in size but sometimes had an orange tinge.

Histologically, multifocal alveoli were lined by uniformly arranged cuboidal to columnar epithelial cells with papillary formations consistent with pulmonary adenomatosis and these cells were continuous with the bronchiolar epithelium. There was a concurrent non-suppurative, interstitial pneumonia sometimes with marked pulmonary edema. It was hypothesized that chronic irritation of the bronchiolar and alveolar epithelial cells from irritants from the dust bath resulted in proliferative changes with eventual development of adenomatosis.

4.4.2.5 Toxoplasmosis

Toxoplasma gondii infections in chinchillas are moderately common. Clinical signs include sudden death, depression, hunched posture with drooping of the ears and head, tachypnea, ataxia, and convulsions. Upon gross examination, lesions include pleural effusion, patchy pulmonary consolidation, miliary white hepatic foci, and mild splenomegaly. Microscopically, interstitial pneumonitis is seen with numerous *T. gondii* trophozoites contained within macrophages as well as free within alveoli. In addition, pyogranulomatous hepatitis with numerous *T. gondii* pseudocysts and multifocal granulomatous encephalitis with variable numbers of pseudocysts are seen. Immunohistochemistry can be used to confirm infection.

4.4.3 Pulmonary Neoplasia

Despite the long life span of chinchillas, occurrences of pulmonary neoplasia are rare. One case of pulmonary adenocarcinoma has been reported.

4.5 Musculoskeletal Conditions

Chinchillas are active, agile animals and unlike their close relative, the guinea pig, chinchillas are able to synthesize ascorbic acid from dietary intermediates. Musculoskeletal conditions are rarely reported.

4.5.1 Nutritional Deficiencies

Clinical signs in these cases may be nonspecific and can include lethargy, depression, weakness, incoordination progressing to difficulty or inability to rise, and recumbency. In other species with nutritional deficiencies, the myocardium can be involved and if lesions are severe, cardiac insufficiency may be a presenting sign. Differential diagnoses include ionophore toxicosis.

Degenerative myopathy secondary to vitamin E deficiency has been reported in one case.

4.5.2 Parasitic Myositis

Cysts of the second larval stage of *Taenia serialis* have been identified in subcutaneous tissues and fascia in multiple chinchillas housed in laboratory settings as well as in commercial fur operations. The significance of this infestation depends primarily on location of the cysts. In one case, multiple coenuri were present on the mandibular ramus and interfered with food consumption. Lameness was the presenting clinical sign in two other animals with cysts in the axillary connective tissue and the subscapularis fascia, respectively. Coenuri were identified morphologically via characterization of the protoscolices. Cystic structures should be differentiated from abscesses.

The definitive host of *T. serialis* includes dogs, foxes, and coyotes. It was presumed, in all cases, that the chinchilla feed or, possibly, the bedding material was contaminated with feces from dogs infected with *T. serialis*. Historically, fresh grass cuttings have been fed in some research facilities for enrichment and were considered to be the most likely source of *T. serialis* contamination. Pet chinchillas allowed access to the outside or fed diets supplemented with grass clippings, hay, and other roughage, may be at increased risk for this condition.

4.5.3 Traumatic Injury

Traumatic fractures of the tibia are common in chinchillas because the bone is long and slender and attached to a vestigial fibula. Fractures can occur following entrapment of the leg in a cage component or toy, as a consequence of improper restraint if a chinchilla is caught by a hind leg, or if a chinchilla is accidently dropped.

4.5.4 Intoxication

4.5.4.1 Vitamin D Intoxication

Vitamin D toxicosis (see Section 4.9.3 for a fuller discussion) is seen rarely on chinchilla farms, usually in association with inadvertent vitamin over-supplementation. Microscopically, abundant intensely basophilic mineral matrix is deposited on the surface of bone trabeculae and is pathognomonic for vitamin D intoxication. Other possible bony lesions include osteocyte necrosis within both cortical and trabecular bone resulting in empty lacunae, resorption of cortical bone, new periosteal bone production, and mineralization of soft tissues (see Figure 4.13 on p. 220).

4.5.4.2 Salinomycin Intoxication

Salinomycin intoxication of farmed chinchillas has occurred following an inadvertent feed mill mixing error. Affected animals were depressed, off their feed, recumbent, and found dead 8 days after being presented with the contaminated feed. Skeletal muscle myofiber swelling, degeneration, and necrosis were noted microscopically. In this case, the salinomycin level in the feed was 37 ppm.

4.5.5 Bacterial Arthritis

Septicemia caused by *Streptococcus pneumoniae, S. pyogenes*, and other *Streptococcus* spp., can result in bacterial localization in joints with resultant septic arthritis. Secondary osteoarthritis can develop from severe pododermatitis as a result of intralesional extension of infection and inflammation induced by *Staphylococcus* sp. or *Streptococcus* spp.

4.5.6 Musculoskeletal Neoplasia

Lumbar osteosarcoma has been reported in a mature male chinchilla presenting with a chronic history of progressive weight loss, depression, anorexia, and tail tip alopecia. On examination, the chinchilla was reluctant to move and demonstrated hind leg stiffness that quickly progressed to paralysis. The animal also demonstrated self-trauma to the tail tip. A 3-cm diameter fixed, firm mass was palpated in the ventral region of the last lumbar vertebra and the inguinal lymph nodes were enlarged. Survey radiographs identified an irregular opaque mass attached to the ventral border of the seventh lumbar vertebra that also extended into the subtending vertebral canal. Microscopically, the mass was confirmed to be an osteosarcoma with intravascular invasion but no evidence of distant metastasis. Other musculoskeletal tumors have not been reported in chinchillas.

4.6 Gastrointestinal Conditions

Chinchillas consume most of their daily food at dawn or dusk and because they are hind-gut fermenters, sufficient grass hay needs to be provided to encourage normal gastrointestinal motility. Like other small rodents, they are unable to vomit. Feeding of high carbohydrate foods and treats should be minimized to prevent formation of dental caries and to prevent acidosis and dysbiosis. Chinchillas are coprophagic and consume fecal pellets directly from their anus. This is thought to enhance extraction of various dietary components, such as B vitamins and certain amino acids. The use of narrow spectrum antibiotics, such as penicillins and cephalosporins, particularly when given orally, can result in the development of enterotoxemia. Dietary changes should be phased in over several days to lessen the impact on the intestinal microflora.

Gastrointestinal problems are seen commonly in pet chinchillas, often a result of inappropriate diet and lack of sufficient exercise.

4.6.1 Dental Conditions

Chinchillas have hypsodont dentition, such that the incisors grow continuously, the molars have long, continually growing, crowns with no anatomic root, and there is a gap (diastema) between the incisors and the molars. Provision of materials for gnawing, such as autoclaved softwood, pumice stones, small branches, and pieces of bark, in addition to daily access to grassy hay, helps to prevent destructive gnawing behaviors as well as maintaining the teeth in proper alignment. Branches from trees such as cedar, plum, redwood, cherry, and oleander should be avoided because of toxicity.

4.6.1.1 Presenting Clinical Signs
Dental abnormalities are common in chinchillas and animals present with a wide range of clinical signs, including dysphagia, weight loss, emaciation, tooth grinding, ptyalism, epiphora, proptosis, mandibular swelling, and incisor and cheek teeth malocclusions. The fur around the mouth is often moistened and matted giving rise to the common name of the 'condition, slobbers.' More subtle signs of dental disease include flattening of the hair around the eyes, changes in the profile of the skull, changes in size and consistency of fecal pellets, and alterations in behavior and food preferences. Often dental disease is unnoticed in the early stages.

4.6.1.2 Pathology
Dental abnormalities are observed in over 50% of chinchillas presenting for veterinary care. In the majority of these cases, lesions are secondary to coronal elongation of the cheek teeth or to the absence of an opposing tooth somewhere along the dental arcade. A congenital absence or pathologic loss of teeth and malocclusion secondary to skeletal abnormalities are infrequently observed in chinchillas.

Food material can accumulate in the expanded interproximal spaces between the cheek teeth resulting in caries, odontoclastic resorption, and periodontitis. Spikes and spurs can develop on the lingual or buccal aspects of cheek teeth, resulting in gingival and glossal erosions and ulcerations (Figure 4.6). When elongation of cheek tooth roots occurs, roots can penetrate into the periorbital soft tissues as well as into the orbit, resulting in proptosis. Elongation of roots within the maxilla and mandible may also result in bony remodelling with profile distortion, osteomyelitis, and abscessation. Other consequences of chronic dental disease include compression or obliteration of the lacrimal canal and the associated duct with resultant chronic epiphora.

4.6.1.3 Differential Diagnoses
Clinical signs associated with upper respiratory tract infections such as rhinitis, sinusitis, and conjunctivitis can mimic some of the signs associated with dental disease.

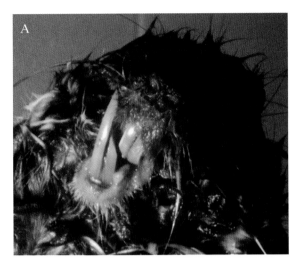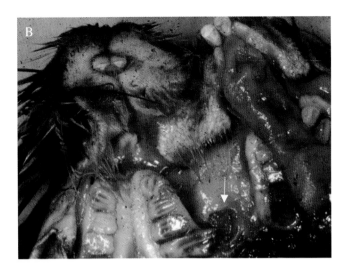

Figure 4.6 A: Incisor malocclusion with marked salivation. B: Malocclusion, as seen in this post mortem specimen, can result from elongation and lateral displacement of the molar teeth. In this case, craterous buccal ulcers have developed. Dental spikes and spurs can also cause gingival, buccal, and glossal erosions or ulcerations.

4.6.1.4 Disease/Colony Management

Skulls from wild-caught chinchillas generally only demonstrate mild dental disease and they have shorter cheek teeth compared with skulls from domesticated chinchillas. Cheek tooth elongation is thought to be associated with insufficient tooth wear highlighting the critical requirement of fiber for captive chinchillas. Appropriate diets that are high in fiber encourage more normal chewing movements and increase tooth wear, thereby improving the dental health of captive chinchillas. Daily provision of free-choice, good quality, grassy hay, small amounts of pelleted feed, and very small amounts of fibrous vegetables and fruits are recommended to maintain dental integrity.

4.6.2 Esophageal Choke

Esophageal choke can occur in chinchillas of all ages, especially in animals that consume their food rapidly. Raisins, pieces of fruits or nuts, and bedding are examples of potential offending materials, but females can also choke on pieces of placenta, which are normally consumed post-partum. The onset of clinical signs is sudden and the owner may report that the chinchilla suddenly started to salivate or retch, pawed at its face or became dyspneic. When material is lodged in the upper portion of the esophagus or is in the pharynx, asphyxiation may result.

A foreign body that is wedged across the roof of the mouth or between the teeth will produce similar clinical signs.

4.6.3 Gastric Tympany

Bloat is associated with over-consumption of clover hay, kale, cabbage, feeding excessive carbohydrates, and sudden dietary changes. The condition is most common in nursing females. The signs are sudden in onset and an affected animal will have a distended, taut abdomen, and demonstrate lateral recumbency with exaggerated respiratory efforts. If unrelieved, animals may die of shock, asphyxiation or gastric rupture.

4.6.4 Gastrointestinal Stasis

Gastrointestinal stasis may occur in chinchillas fed inappropriate diets or provided with insufficient opportunities for exercise. Stasis may result in accumulation of hair within the stomach and trichobezoar formation. Affected animals are lethargic and inappetent. Differential diagnoses include diaphragmatic hernia and intestinal obstruction.

4.6.5 Enteritis

Diarrhea is a common presenting sign in chinchillas and both infectious and noninfectious causes are prevalent. The most common causes of diet-induced diarrhea include sudden changes in diet, insufficient dietary fiber, excessive intake of lush green feed, such as cabbage, kale, lettuce and immature clover, and excessive amounts of protein. Animals will have diarrhea and mild bloating but will otherwise be bright and alert. Differential diagnoses include antibiotic-induced dysbiosis, and various bacterial and parasitic causes of enteritis.

4.6.5.1 Yersiniosis

Yersinia infections are caused by Gram-negative pleomorphic coccobacilli, and most recently have been linked to *Yersinia enterocolitica*, but historically were associated with *Y. pseudotuberculosis*. The clinical signs and pathologic lesions of *Y. enterocolitica* and *Y. pseudotuberculosis* infections are similar and require bacterial culture for differentiation. Bacteria are thought to enter via contaminated feed or through the introduction of infected animals.

Presenting Clinical Signs Chinchillas may present with listlessness, anorexia, progressive weight loss, slimy or mucus-coated soft fecal pellets, diarrhea, weakness, and death.

Pathology The liver, spleen, and less frequently, the kidney, may contain multifocal, pale necrotic foci throughout the parenchyma. The intestinal tract is usually severely inflamed with small mucosal erosions and ulcers extending into the intestinal muscularis. Mesenteric lymph nodes are enlarged and congested, and lung lesions are rare.

Laboratory Diagnostics *Yersinia* spp. can be recovered from samples of heart blood or affected tissues using selective media, such as cefsulodin-irgasan-novobiocin (CIN) agar.

Colony/Herd Management *Yersinia enterocolitica* biogroup 3, serogroups O:1, 2, and 3 are associated with chinchilla infections and can also cause infections in humans. Infected animals should be quarantined from healthy, unexposed animals and should be handled after all other husbandry tasks have been completed. Humans infected with *Y. enterocolitica* usually present with gastrointestinal signs, but in cases of immunosuppression or iron overload, septicemia can occur.

4.6.5.2 Listeriosis

Listeria monocytogenes, a Gram-positive, rod-shaped bacillus, is a common disease agent in chinchilla breeding operations. Three clinical forms of listeriosis are recognized in domestic animals, including septicemia, which occurs principally in monogastric animals, encephalitis or abortion, which occur principally in adult ruminants, and a visceral form. Chinchillas are highly susceptible to visceral septicemia and acquire the infection by ingestion of feed, such as pellets, meal, or hay contaminated with infected rodent, chicken or ruminant feces. *L. monocytogenes* can also be introduced into a herd through infected chinchillas. Transmission occurs by orofecal contamination with subsequent hepatic dissemination, causing multifocal necrosis and abscessation. From the liver, there is hematogenous spread to other organs, including lymph nodes, lung, spleen, kidney, adrenal glands, uterus, and placenta. Involvement of the brain also occurs but the actual route of cerebral infection is debated.

Presenting Clinical Signs Clinical signs in infected chinchillas include sudden death, depression, torticollis,

anorexia, progressive weight loss, constipation, and tenesmus, which may result in intestinal intussusception or rectal prolapse. Less frequently, diarrhea, abortion, and vaginal discharge are seen.

Pathology Post-mortem findings include multifocal, pale, miliary foci on the hepatic capsular surface and throughout the parenchyma (Figure 4.7) as well as within mesenteric lymph nodes. Similar foci are also seen on the serosal surfaces of the small and large intestines, particularly on the cecum.

Microscopically, foci of necrosis and microabscessation are present throughout the liver, mesenteric lymph nodes, and Peyer's patches, as well as on the intestinal serosa. Similar lesions are seen less frequently within the spleen, lung, uterus, placenta, and brain of affected animals. Intralesional Gram-positive bacteria are abundant.

Laboratory Diagnostics *Listeria monocytogenes* can be cultured readily from affected tissues.

Differential Diagnoses Differential diagnoses for listeriosis in chinchillas include pseudomoniasis, yersiniosis, and salmonellosis. With pseudomoniasis, the primary lesions are found in the cecum and colon and the liver is less frequently involved.

Disease/Colony Management Following infection with *Listeria*, bacteria are passed in the feces. Thus, equipment, cages, feed, water, and dust baths contaminated with infected feces are important means by which the infection is spread to other chinchillas. Not all animals respond to treatment with antimicrobials and apparently recovered animals may remain carriers and shed *Listeria* for extended periods. Listeriosis is a zoonotic condition with transmission of bacteria from infected animals as well as from contaminated equipment and the environment. Human caregivers should wash their hands carefully after handling known infected equipment or animals.

4.6.5.3 Pseudomoniasis

Acute or chronic *Pseudomonas aeruginosa* infections can also be seen sporadically in pet and farmed chinchillas. In acute outbreaks, otitis media and interna may occur as well as conjunctivitis, uveitis, rhinitis, and septicemia. Septicemia is common in neonates and post-parturient or pregnant females. Localized *Pseudomonas* sp. infections can also occur in the skin, resulting in subcutaneous abscesses, as well as in other sites, such as the gastrointestinal tract, liver, lungs or urogenital tract.

Presenting Clinical Signs When the upper respiratory system is involved, clinical signs include purulent oculonasal discharge, otitis externa, facial paralysis, torticollis, circling,

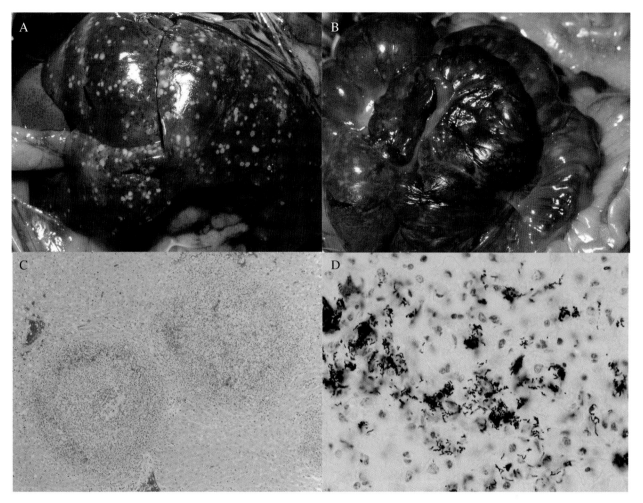

Figure 4.7 A: Characteristic lesions of hepatic listeriosis include numerous small white foci found speckling the capsular surface and throughout the liver parenchyma. B: Similar small white foci are visible through the cecal serosa and the cecal content is dry. The small intestinal and colonic serosa may be similarly affected. C: Scattered randomly throughout the liver are microabscesses containing central necrotic cellular debris, fibrin, numerous neutrophils surrounded by fewer lymphocytes and macrophages. D: Numerous Gram-positive rod-shaped bacteria are present within foci of hepatic necrosis. Brown and Brenn.

and rolling. With gastrointestinal disease, animals may present with lethargy, inappetence, depression, diarrhea, weight loss, intestinal intussusception, rectal prolapse, and sudden death with no premonitory signs. Inguinal dermal pustules with dermatitis, cellulitis, and acute mesenteric lymphadenitis were seen in a laboratory-reared chinchilla following apparent recovery from initial signs of conjunctivitis, corneal and oral ulcers, mild diarrhea, anorexia, and weight loss. Urogenital infections include purulent vaginal discharge, and preputial and penile ulceration. Pregnant females may abort prior to death.

Pathology   At necropsy, lesions are extensive and often involve multiple systems, including mucopurulent to purulent rhinitis and conjunctivitis, uveitis, caseous yellow exudate in external ear canals, and purulent exudate in tympanic bullae. Lungs from affected animals may be wet,

and mottled red and white, with frothy to serosanginous fluid in the trachea. Enteritis presents as gas- or fluid-filled loops of bowel with microabscesses within the cecal and colonic walls (Figure 4.8). The liver is less frequently affected. Secondary intestinal intussusception and rectal prolapse may be seen as well as fibrinous peritonitis, suppurative vaginitis, and ulcerative or suppurative balanoposthitis.

Microscopically, lesions include fibrinosuppurative otitis media and interna, and meningitis. Pulmonary lesions are often reflective of septicemia or acute hemorrhagic pneumonia in the case of chinchilla kits. Cecal and colonic lesions include multifocal areas of mucosal to transmural necrosis.

Laboratory Diagnostics   *Pseudomonas aeruginosa* is readily cultured from affected tissues.

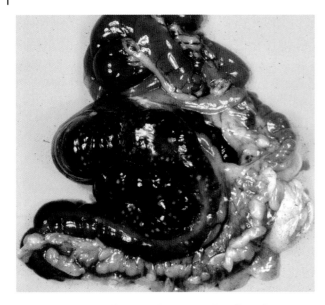

Figure 4.8 In chinchillas, pseudomoniasis also affects the intestinal tract with microabscesses visible through the serosal surface of the cecum and colon. However, in contrast to listerosis, the liver is less frequently involved. Culture of affected organs is necessary to differentiate between the two conditions.

Differential Diagnoses Differential diagnoses for pseudomoniasis in chinchillas include listeriosis, yersiniosis, and salmonellosis. With listerosis, involvement of the liver is a common finding.

Disease/Colony Management *Pseudomonas aeruginosa* is a ubiquitous opportunistic pathogen found widely in the environment. It has poor susceptibility to most antibiotics, making eradication by treatment difficult. *P. aeruginosa* has been recovered from 20% of swabs taken from water bottles of clinically normal pet and laboratory chinchillas. Thus, acidification of the water supply and regular flushing and disinfection of water bottles and automatic water lines are important preventive measures. Historically, vaccination of chinchillas with polyvalent bacterins has been successful. *P. aeruginosa* is a common environmental contaminant and presents a low potential zoonotic risk except in immunosuppressed individuals.

4.6.5.4 Salmonellosis
Salmonella spp. infections occur sporadically in both pet and farmed chinchillas and are associated with a variety of serovars. All serovars have public health significance and induce serious disease in chinchillas. For example, an established chinchilla breeding operation introduced a new male of unknown health status that became ill soon after arrival. All of the females co-housed with this new animal died, as well as the male. Clinical signs in these animals included intermittent diarrhea with emaciation, followed by rapid clinical decline and death. At necropsy,

acute enteritis was the predominant finding with some animals also demonstrating cecal mucosal ulceration. *Salmonella* Dublin was isolated from liver, small intestine, and fecal samples, and the newly introduced breeding male was suspected to be the source of the infection as there was no evidence of food contamination.

In other cases, *S.* Arizonae was recovered from a chinchilla with septicemia, and *S.* Pullorum was recovered from a chinchilla with abscesses in the lung, liver and diaphragm. The only clinical sign seen in the latter case was reduced feed intake for the week prior to death. Outbreaks of disease associated with *S.* Enteritidis have been reported on several chinchilla farms. Sudden death with no obvious clinical signs is the typical history, and post-mortem findings include catarrhal gastroenteritis, splenomegaly, multifocal splenic and hepatic necrosis, and hemorrhagic metritis in some females. *Salmonella* Typhimurium has been recovered from the heart blood of ranched chinchillas experiencing a spike in mortality, with most chinchillas found dead overnight and a few animals showing anorexia and diarrhea 1 or 2 days before death. Animals of all ages were affected and lesions included gastric and cecal mucosal necrosis and colonic intussusception in animals that died acutely, and colonic mucosal abscesses and impaction in other animals that survived for longer periods. More recently, a chinchilla farm experienced an outbreak of *S.* Typhimurum that lasted for a week, resulting in the loss of 35% of animals. At post-mortem examination, animals were in poor body condition with nodular gastritis and duodenitis, multifocal hepatic necrosis, splenomegaly, and hemorrhagic pneumonia. The source of the infection was not confirmed but the facility was not well maintained and had poor biosecurity as wild rodents were present in the barn. Wild vermin may be a source of contamination.

4.6.5.5 Coliform Enteritis
Young, farmed chinchillas approximately 6 months-old presented with acute mortality and upon post-mortem examination, the small intestine fluid content was whereas the cecal content was dry. A proportion of the animals also had rectal prolapse. Microscopically, aggregations of numerous coccobacilli were noted in close proximity to mildly attenuated and exfoliating enterocytes and there was villus blunting and fusion. The lamina propria was congested and contained numerous neutrophils and fewer pyknotic cells, some of which were seen to be migrating into the superficial epithelium (Figure 4.9). *Escherichia coli* was isolated from the small intestines, and were positive for Pool 1 N, O, and K isolates, which are most commonly associated with neonatal diarrhea of piglets and calves. No further analyses were conducted.

Attaching and effacing *eae* adhesin-positive *E. coli* enteritis and septicemia were reported in one of a group of three laboratory-housed chinchillas. The histologic ileal and colonic lesions demonstrated carpeting of enterocytes

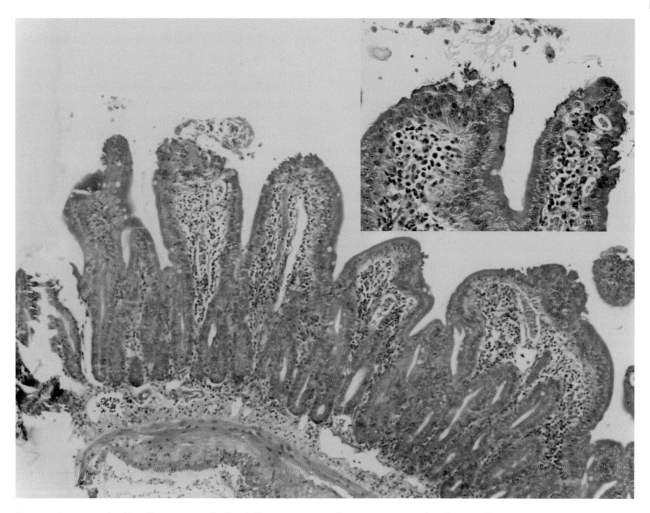

Figure 4.9 Intestinal colibacillosis in juvenile chinchillas. Microscopically, numerous coccobacilli are in close proximity to mildly attenuated epithelium at the tips and along the sides of atrophic, blunted and fused villi with degeneration and exfoliation of superficial epithelial cells. Numerous neutrophils and fewer pyknotic cells are present within the congested lamina propria and are migrating into the superficial epithelium. Inset: The surface of epithelial cells at the tips and sides of villi is scalloped and colonized by clusters of short bacterial rods, characteristic of *E. coli*.

with mats of Gram-negative bacilli and moderate numbers of neutrophils within the lamina propria. Additional lesions included suppurative nephritis, neutrophilic interstitial pneumonia with microvascular fibrinous thrombosis, erosive gastritis, and hepatic lipidosis.

4.6.5.6 Antibiotic-Induced Dysbiosis and Enterotoxemia

Use of narrow spectrum antibiotics, including amoxicillin, ampicillin, cephalosporins, clindamycin, erythromycin, lincomycin, and penicillins, may lead to the development of enterotoxemia and hemorrhagic typhlitis in chinchillas. This is thought to occur as a result of increased populations of Gram-negative bacteria and overgrowth of clostridial organisms in the hind gut, including *Clostridium difficile.*

Clostridial spores may be found in contaminated feed and may induce disease. A chinchilla farm experienced severe diarrhea with rectal prolapse and subsequent death within 24–48 hours, resulting in 20% morbidity and mortality. Necropsy findings in affected animals included large intestinal mucosal erosion and inflammation, and hepatosplenomegaly. Microscopic lesions included centrilobular hepatic necrosis, proliferation of the splenic white pulp, and large intestinal mucosal edema, congestion, and necrosis. *Clostridium perfringens* A enterotoxin was detected by ELISA in the gastric content and the bacterium was isolated from the feed, producing large amounts of enterotoxin in vitro.

4.6.5.7 *Bacillus cereus* Enterotoxemia

A group of farmed chinchillas experienced severe diarrhea and sudden death, and at post-mortem examination, severe typhocolitis was observed. *Bacillus cereus* and a related enterotoxin were recovered from the feed and intestinal content, and were determined to be morphologically and biochemically similar to those isolated from the animals.

4.6.5.8 Coccidiosis

Intestinal coccidiosis has been reported infrequently in farmed chinchillas and is caused by *Eimera chinchillae* The agent can infect other rodents, contradicting generally accepted principles of host specificity of *Eimeria* spp. Presenting clinical signs include diarrhea, rectal prolapse, and sudden death. In affected chinchillas, post-mortem examination demonstrated cecal and colonic distension with semi-solid ingesta and gas, erythema and thickening of the cecal and anterior colonic mucosa, and mucosal speckling with miliary pale foci. The rectum contained small numbers of mucus-coated fecal pellets and coccidial oocysts were identified in the droppings. Oocysts are oval, subspherical or spherical, and measure 13–22 μm by 11–18 μm with a single-layered light brown wall that is 0.7–1μm thick (Figure 4.10). The oocysts sporulate within three days of being produced.

4.6.5.9 Giardiasis

Historically, *Giardia chinchillae* was considered to be a primary pathogen of chinchillas, as infected animals presented with diarrhea and increased mortality, however, *Giardia* organisms have also been found in apparently healthy animals. Given that chinchillas with giardiasis commonly have concomitant bacterial infections, such as pseudomoniasis, the significance of this organism as a primary pathogen has been unclear. Recent investigations support the concept that *G. chinchillae* is an opportunistic pathogen. *G. chinchillae* trophoblasts most commonly reside in the upper small intestine and were seen in intestinal scrapings of >82% of normal, healthy chinchillas in one study, and in fecal smears from >64% of culled chinchillas in another study. Only one of these animals had abnormal fecal pellets. No other parasitic or bacterial

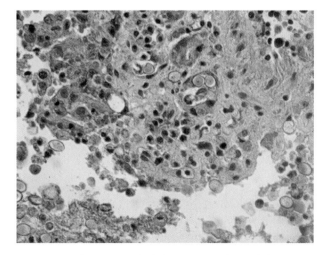

Figure 4.10 Characteristic, light brown-stained coccidial oocysts are noted within the small intestinal epithelial cells as well as found free within the intestinal lumen.

pathogens were detected in this animal and there was no evidence of abdominal discomfort.

Pet chinchillas have also been tested for the presence of *Giardia duodenalis* using a sedimentation flotation technique and a subset of the *Giardia* isolates were characterized. Multiple isolates were identified, including A and B forms, which are considered zoonotic. Juvenile and show chinchillas were more likely to be positive for *G. duodenalis*.

4.6.5.10 Intestinal Nematodiasis and Cestodiasis

Intestinal nematodes are not thought to be important pathogens in chinchillas. In one report, chinchillas had lost weight and were dull and listless with no change in fecal consistency. Nematode eggs were subsequently identified on fecal flotation and female *Ostertagia* worms were found in the stomach as well as one male *Trichostrongylus colubriformis* worm in the small intestine. These chinchillas responded well to treatment with parasiticides and the source of the infections was thought to be alfalfa hay cut from pastures grazed occasionally by sheep and goats.

Cestodes can cause rare problems in young chinchillas. Post-mortem examinations conducted on a group of young, emaciated chinchillas identified numerous *Rodentolepis* sp. tapeworms within the small intestines. A farm visit indicated that the recently weaned chinchillas were in very poor condition but were eating well and passing normal fecal droppings. Unweaned and adult chinchillas appeared normal. Tapeworm segments were not being excreted but eggs were identified by fecal flotation.

R. nana has three life cycle variations. With the direct life cycle, ova bearing proglottids are passed in the feces by one definitive host and ingested by another. Because chinchillas are coprophagic, they may reinfect themselves. The second type of life cycle is an internal autoinfection cycle in which the ova release hexacanth larvae into the intestinal lumen without ever leaving the intestine. The third type of life cycle is indirect, in which ova bearing proglottids are passed in the feces from a definitive host to an intermediate host, such as beetles, cockroaches, or fleas and then the intermediate host bearing cysticeroids is ingested by the next definitive host. In the case mentioned above, fleas or grain beetles were considered as potential intermediate hosts or feed contaminated with droppings from infested rats or mice.

4.6.5.11 Cryptosporidiosis

Cryptosporidiosis may occur in both pet and farmed chinchillas. An 8 month-old chinchilla developed severe diarrhea shortly after being purchased from a pet store and died despite aggressive antibiotic and fluid treatment. The stomach, small intestine, and colon were distended with gas and yellow fluid. Histologically, large numbers of 2–5 μm spherical bodies were seen on the

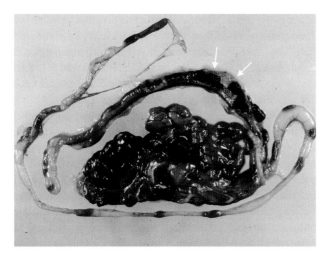

Figure 4.11 Small and large intestines from a chinchilla with constipation. Note the scant amount of small intestinal content and the reduced cecal size. There are reduced numbers of widely spaced fecal pellets in the distal colon. The colonic mucosa is tightly wrapped around the dried dark content (arrows).

luminal surface of the stomach, duodenum, jejunum, ileum, and colon, and confirmed as *Cryptosporidia* sp. by transmission electron microscopy. There was mild to moderate villus atrophy with irregular foci of epithelial necrosis, and lamina proprial infiltrates of neutrophils, lymphocytes, and macrophages. Sinus histiocytosis was noted in mesenteric lymph nodes as well as lesser numbers of neutrophils. Coliform bacteria were also isolated from the small intestine, lungs, and liver. Based on the clinical findings, lack of response to treatment, and the presence of large numbers of protozoal organisms, cryptosporidial infection was deemed the likely cause of the gastroenteritis.

4.6.6 Other Intestinal Conditions

Fecal pellets of chinchillas should be plentiful, about 1-cm in length, rice-shaped, and plump and dry to the touch when fresh. A history of scant, hard fecal pellet production with or without frank blood may be indicative of **cecal** or **colonic impaction** (Figure 4.11). **Rectal prolapse** may occur whenever chinchillas strain to defecate (Figure 4.12). Impaction may be caused by insufficient dietary fiber. Other causes of constipation include dehydration, lack of exercise, obesity, intestinal obstruction, chronic bacterial enteritis, and intestinal compression and ischemia secondary to a large gravid uterus. Differential diagnoses for colonic impaction include gastric foreign bodies and intestinal accidents, such as torsion and intussusception.

Intestinal intussusception can occur following outbreaks of bacterial gastroenteritis or intestinal parasitism, and typically, the colon is affected. Animals with an intussusception may be hypothermic, have a distended abdomen, and refuse to eat or use a dustbath, and they may demonstrate abnormal postures because of the acutely painful abdomen. Tenesmus is not usually present unless the intussuscepted intestine prolapses rectally. In one report of intestinal torsion, there was 360° rotation of the distal 20 cm of the small intestine through a rent in the mesocolon. The affected bowel was severely congested and dilated with gas and serosanguinous fluid.

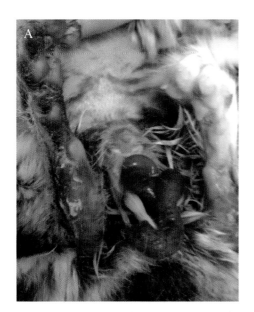
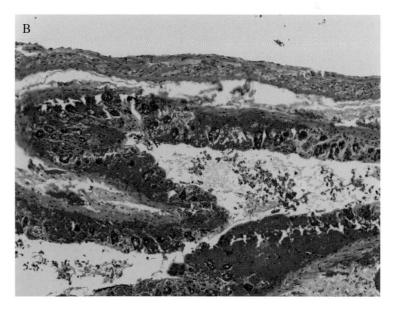

Figure 4.12 A: Colonic intussusception and prolapse in a mature female chinchilla following treatment for intestinal stasis and constipation. The small intestine was dilated with dark green watery content. B: Photomicrograph of colon demonstrating marked transmural and luminal hemorrhage and submucosal edema. *Source:* A: Courtesy of B. Lee-Chow

Chronic **sodium carbonate intoxication** from accidental replacement of sodium bicarbonate with sodium carbonate in the feed eventually resulted in depopulation of a chinchilla farm. Within the first two weeks of introducing the contaminated feed, animals became lethargic with reduced feed intake and exhibited exaggerated responses to stimulation. With longer-term consumption, progressive hair loss and fur chewing were seen as well as discoloration of the teeth, abortions, vaginal hemorrhage, polyuria, production of feces containing undigested content and mucus, and sudden death. Postmortem lesions included highly alkaline abdominal fluid, marked mesenteric congestion, and gastric erosion, ulceration and hemorrhage with occasional gastric perforation. The small and large intestines were largely empty, livers were enlarged and dotted with subcapsular petechial hemorrhages, and the kidneys and adrenal glands were enlarged. There was alkaline pleural effusion and lungs were wet and congested.

4.6.7 Hepatic and Pancreatic Conditions

4.6.7.1 Hepatic Lipidosis
Hepatic lipidosis is common in obese chinchillas. The condition can also develop during periods of fasting, anorexia secondary to intercurrent disease, or in cases of severe dental disease with resultant anorexia. It is a nonspecific sign and should be interpreted based on other post-mortem findings.

4.6.7.2 *Listeria ivanovii* Septicemia
Atypical species of *Listeria* can sporadically induce hepatitis in chinchillas. In one case, a pet female chinchilla of unknown age and in poor body condition died shortly after purchase. At necropsy, generalized, miliary pale foci were seen throughout the liver, and the intestinal content was scant and mucoid in nature. Abundant *Saccharomyces*-like yeast cells were seen in cecal smears. Microscopically, acute multifocal hepatic necrosis was noted together with infiltrating neutrophils. Vacuolated hepatocytes contained Gram-positive, intracytoplasmic rod-shaped bacteria and there was activation of the splenic white pulp. *Listeria ivanovii* was cultured from the liver.

4.6.7.3 Sarcocystosis
Various protozoal parasites can infect chinchillas, resulting in hepatitis. A 7 month-old pet chinchilla, one of a group of seven, died unexpectedly. Microscopically, acute interstitial pneumonitis and multifocal hepatitis were seen with numerous protozoa in various stages of development, including schizonts and merozoites. Schizonts were positively labeled via immunohistochemistry for antibodies against *Sarcocytis cruzi* but were negative for *Toxoplasma gondii* and *Neospora caninum*. Protozoal

organisms were antigenically and structurally identical to *S. canis* from dogs. The source of infection was not identified and it was unlikely that the chinchilla was exposed to food or water contaminated with feces from an infected carnivore. The possibility that the chinchilla became subclinically infected at an early age could not be discounted. The other six chinchillas remained healthy.

4.6.7.4 Hepatic Alveolar Echinococcosis
Echinococcus multilocularis is a zoonotic tapeworm identified around the world. Hydatid cysts have been reported sporadically in both farmed and pet chinchillas and may be an incidental finding at post-mortem or may induce clinical disease. The significance to the animal depends primarily on the location that is affected. In a recent European case, a 6-year-old pet chinchilla presented with clinical signs of anorexia, tachypnea, and an enlarged, firm, and painful abdomen. The animal was euthanized and a post-mortem examination was conducted.

The liver capsule had numerous 1–5 vesicles 5-mm in diameter, which upon microscopic examination were noted to have outer laminated walls, an inner germinal epithelium, and internal protoscolices. An immunofluorescence assay using an *E. multilocularis*-specific monoclonal antibody labeled the outer walls positive. PCR testing confirmed the diagnosis of the larval stage (hydatid cyst) of the tapeworm *E. multilocularis*. Definitive hosts for *E. multilocularis* include foxes, coyotes, and domestic dogs. Rodents are intermediate hosts and must be eaten by a carnivore to transmit the infection. Infections of intermediate and aberrant hosts occur through ingestion of eggs in feces-contaminated feed. The chinchilla in this case was fed pellets and hay, but on occasion, also received branches from trees and shrubs, which may have been contaminated. Humans are considered aberrant hosts but may develop potentially serious and even life-endangering hydatid cysts following ingestion of infective eggs from a definitive canid host.

4.6.7.5 Aflatoxicosis
Aflatoxins are a group of naturally occurring, carcinogenic mycotoxins produced by *Aspergillus* fungi, including *A. flavus* and *A. parasiticus*, which can grow on a wide variety of feed ingredients including grains, silages, and forages. In one case, a chinchilla producer experienced catastrophic on-farm mortality losing all 200 animals following consumption of an oat-based commercial pelleted feed. At necropsy, livers were markedly enlarged by up to 71%, friable, and pale yellow with multiple grey foci. Histologically, marked diffuse hepatic lipidosis and necrosis were seen. Thin layer chromatography analysis of the feed revealed approximately 212 ppb of aflatoxin B_1. The safe limit of AFB_1 in chinchilla feed is estimated to be 10 ppb.

4.6.7.6 Acute Necrotizing Pancreatitis

Pancreatitis occurs sporadically and obese pet chinchillas receiving excessive fatty or high carbohydrate treats may be at increased risk. Affected animals may be found dead suddenly with few prodromal signs. At necropsy, findings include abundant subcutaneous and abdominal fat stores often with multifocal hemorrhages and acute fat necrosis, and an enlarged pale, friable liver. Histologically, acute necrotizing and hemorrhagic pancreatitis, peripancreatic and subcutaneous fat necrosis, and marked hepatic lipidosis may be seen.

4.6.8 Gastrointestinal Neoplasia

4.6.8.1 Salivary Gland Neoplasms

Salivary gland neoplasms are uncommonly reported in chinchillas. In one case, a 12 year-old female chinchilla presented with a slow-growing nonpainful fluctuant mass in the right submandibular region. The animal had lost some weight, but was still bright and alert with intermittent dysphagia, facial pruritus, and mild peripheral lymph node enlargement. The animal's condition deteriorated quickly and it was euthanized. The submandibular mass was approximately 6 x 4 x 2.5 cm, mottled pale yellow with numerous fluid-filled cysts, and involved the submandibular lymph nodes with additional metastases to liver, lung, and spleen. Microscopically, the mass was composed of nodular, unencapsulated populations of spindloid to polygonal cells contiguous with salivary gland epithelium and surrounded by moderate amounts of fibrous tissue with large pseudocytic spaces containing abundant pale eosinophilic fluid that stained mildly positive with PAS and Alcian blue. Neoplastic emboli were present within lymphatic vessels and populations of similar cells formed streams, bundles, and small pseudocysts in the submandibular lymph node, liver, lungs, and spleen. Immunohistochemistry demonstrated strong positive cytoplasmic labeling of neoplastic cells for vimentin and pan-cytokeratin. Co-expression of vimentin and cytokeratin, lack of α-SMA, S100, and myosin labeling, and close contact with the salivary gland were the basis for diagnosing this mass as an undifferentiated salivary gland carcinoma.

4.6.8.2 Gastric Neoplasms

Gastric adenocarcinoma was identified in a 5 year-old female chinchilla reported to be anorectic and lethargic for a short period of time before dying. Interestingly, a PCR assay for *Helicobacter pylori* was positive on the gastric tissue but the organism was not identified in the tissues by immunohistochemistry or with silver stains.

4.6.8.3 Hepatic Neoplasms

Hepatic adenocarcinomas are reported sporadically in chinchillas.

4.7 Cardiovascular Conditions

The left coronary artery is the primary supply of blood to cardiac tissue in chinchillas as the right coronary artery is absent. Cardiac ganglia are located on the ventral surface of the right atrial epicardium in a more exposed position than in other mammals.

4.7.1 Cardiomyopathy

Cardiac disease, including cardiomyopathy, cardiomegaly, valvular abnormalities, and ventricular septal defects can be seen periodically at post-mortem in chinchillas. Affected animals may present with heart murmurs and clinical signs of heart failure, such as dyspnea.

4.7.2 Pericarditis and Endocarditis

Pericarditis can be a sequela to severe bacterial conjunctivitis, rhinitis, bronchopneumonia, and septicemia. *B. bronchiseptica, K. pneumoniae, Staphylococcus* sp., *S. pneumoniae*, and other *Streptococcus* spp., may be cultured from infected animals. Vegetative valvular endocarditis has been associated with *S. pneumoniae, S. pyogenes*, and *S. zooepidemicus* infections in chinchillas.

4.7.3 Vitamin D Intoxication

Vitamin D toxicosis is seen in pet and farmed chinchillas following overuse of vitamin supplements. At post-mortem examination, great vessels are rigid with chalky white streaking of the walls, and there may be fine pale stippling of the diaphragm, trachea, lung, heart, and gastric muscularis (Figure 4.13). Mineralization may also be seen in the renal cortices, contributing to a gritty feel upon sectioning. Microscopically, lesions include mineralization of arterial walls and soft tissues including the endocardium and myocardium, pulmonary alveolar basement membranes, gastric and intestinal mucosa, and renal glomerular and tubular basement membranes. An abundant intensely basophilic matrix is deposited on the surface of bone trabeculae, and is considered to be pathognomonic for vitamin D intoxication. Other bony lesions include osteocyte necrosis, resorption of cortical bone, and new periosteal bone production. Other potential intoxications or conditions that may result in metastatic calcification include accidental poisoning with cholecalciferol rodenticides, dietary imbalances of calcium and phosphorus, and chronic renal disease.

4.7.4 Heat Prostration

Because of their dense fur coats, chinchillas can withstand very cold conditions, provided they are housed in an environment that is dry and free from drafts. This same dense hair coat makes chinchillas particularly susceptible to heat prostration, particularly in conjunction with high relative

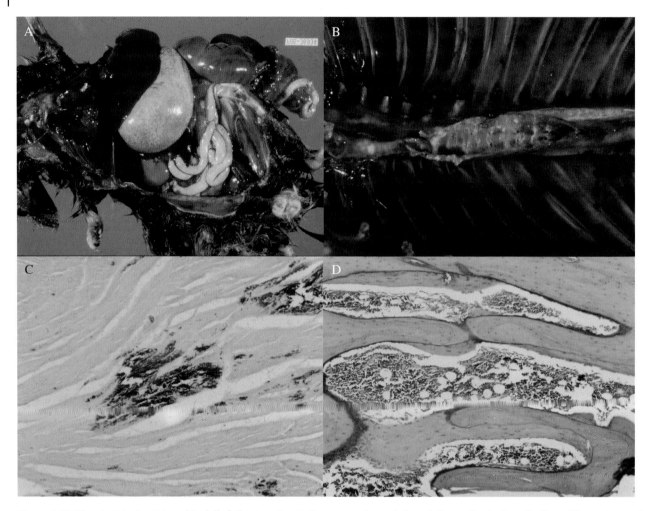

Figure 4.13 Vitamin D toxicosis in a chinchilla following vitamin D over-supplementation. A: Generalized mineralization of the gastric and intestinal walls and white stippling of the heart and lungs. B: Chalky white streaking of the aortic wall contributes to a hard consistency C: Multifocal areas of myocardial mineralization. Von Kossa. D: Photomicrograph of bone demonstrating thick, dark, basophilic matrix deposits on the surface of the trabecular bone. This lesion is considered pathognomonic for vitamin D toxicity.

humidity. Direct exposure to sunlight, insufficient water during hot, humid days, and inadequate ventilation of housing or during transportation are all predisposing factors. Chinchillas with excessive fat stores are considered to be more at risk. Clinical signs include panting with excessive salivation, recumbency, hyperthermia, bloody diarrhea, and engorgement of ear veins and mucosa with blood. At post-mortem, lesions include marked pulmonary congestion (Figure 4.14), distension of blood vessels with dark blood, pale straw-colored fluid in the pericardial sac, and subcutaneous edema along the lateral sides of the body wall seen upon reflection of the skin.

4.8 Genitourinary Conditions

Chinchillas have an elongated renal papilla, which is thought to assist with the production of concentrated urine. In the wild, chinchillas ingest daily water indirectly through consumption of a variety of herbs and grasses. Domesticated chinchillas consume 25–50 mL of water per day. Sanitation of water bottles and waterers is critical as they can be a source of *Pseudomonas aeruginosa* colonization. The normal urine pH is 8–9.

Chinchillas have lengthy gestation periods, a long estrus cycle, give birth to precocial young, and have a vaginal closure membrane that only opens at estrus and during parturition.

4.8.1 Idiopathic Penile Prolapse

In this condition, the penis is prolapsed but is not enlarged or engorged (Figure 4.15). The condition is thought to be associated with overexcitement brought about by separating a chinchilla from its mate or from over-exhaustion because of too many females in the same pen. It is also reported in males not exposed to females.

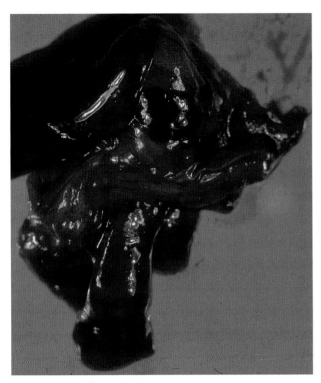

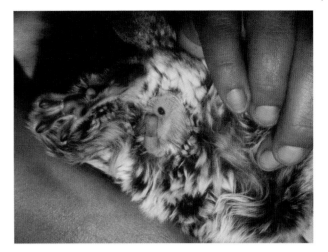

Figure 4.15 Penile prolapse in a chinchilla. The penis is neither enlarged nor engorged. The condition is seen in males with and without exposure to females and may be associated with fur accumulation around the penis.

Figure 4.14 A: Clinical presentation of heat stroke can include excessive salivation, recumbency, hyperthermia, bloody diarrhea, and engorgement of ear veins and mucosa with blood. Lesions include marked pulmonary congestion and edema (depicted). Blood vessels may be distended with dark coloured blood. The pericardial sac may contain pale straw colored fluid and there may be subcutaneous edema along the lateral sides of the body.

4.8.2 Paraphimosis

Male chinchillas can develop paraphimosis because of balanoposthitis or from accumulation of hair around the penis (penile fur ring) resulting in swelling of the distal penis and urethral obstruction. Affected males may have a clinical history of stranguria, dysuria, or pollakiuria, and overgrooming of the genital areas.

4.8.3 Balanoposthitis

Ulcerative and suppurative balanoposthitis is one of the manifestations of *Pseudomonas aeruginosa* infection and with chronicity, perigenital abscesses can form.

4.8.4 Chronic Renal Failure

Chronic renal failure occurs sporadically in chinchillas, as in other rodents, but is less common. Histologic findings are as for the guinea pig.

4.8.5 Oxalate Nephrosis

Oxalate nephrosis has been seen in a group of commercial female chinchillas with a history of progressive weakness

culminating in death. Microscopically, lesions were confined to the renal cortex, with moderate to marked tubular deposits of oxalate crystals, moderate hydropic degeneration and regeneration of tubular epithelial cells, protein casts, and interstitial inflammatory cell infiltrates. Oxalate crystals can be identified by their distinctive microscopic appearance, as they are pale yellow, variably-shaped crystals that are birefringent under polarized light. Common dietary sources are plants containing high levels of oxalic acid include chard, kale, rhubarb, spinach, and beetroot.

4.8.6 Urolithiasis

Urinary calculi are typically found in the urinary bladder and urethra of chinchillas leading to anuria or changes in urination, such as stranguria, hematuria, or dysuria (Figure 4.16). If the calculi are located in the upper urinary tract, the only clinical signs present may be depression, anorexia, and weight loss with no obvious changes in urination patterns. Differential diagnoses for this condition include constipation and paraphimosis due to a penile fur ring or balanoposthitis. Calculi are composed primarily of calcium carbonate.

4.8.7 Pyelonephritis

Pyelonephritis is infrequently reported in chinchillas. Acute pyelonephritis has been associated with *Streptococcus zooepidemicus* vaginitis (Figure 4.17). Chronic unilateral pyelonephritis with ureteral dilation has also been described.

4.8.8 Fetal Resorption and Abortion

Fetal resorption occurs relatively commonly in chinchillas, and dead fetuses can be resorbed or become

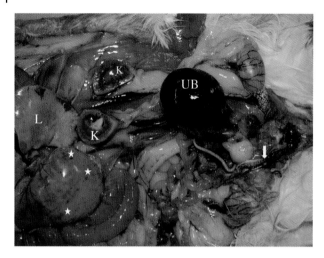

Figure 4.16 A mature chinchilla was found dead. The previous day the chinchilla had taken a dust bath and ate some hay but no pellets. The owner checked for a penile fur ring, and found blood dripping from the penis. At post mortem examination, a small olive green calculus (arrow), composed of both calcium and magnesium carbonate was noted obstructing the distal urethal lumen, 3-cm from the penis tip. Note the very distended hemorrhagic urinary bladder (UB) that also contains small calculi. There is bilateral hydroureter and hydronephrosis (K). Pinpoint gastric mucosal ulcers (stars) and hepatic lipidosis (L) are also seen.

mummified and remain in the uterus. Causes of early pregnancy termination are numerous, and include rough handling during palpation, jumping, falling, fighting or shipping, startling or frightening the female, especially in latter part of gestation, poor body condition due to disease or inadequate nutrition, unbalanced diets, heat stress, and pyrexia or illness from septicemia. Bacterial agents associated with fetal loss include *Pseudomonas aeruginosa*, *Staphylococcus aureus*, *Streptococcus pyogenes*, *S. pneumoniae*, *Salmonella* spp., *Pasteurella multocida*, and *Listeria monocytogenes*. Aborted fetuses may not be found as they are ingested by the dam.

4.8.9 Uterine Conditions

Retained placentas or fetuses, trauma during parturition or an unsanitary environment may lead to vaginitis, pyometra or metritis in chinchillas. Affected animals are usually depressed, anorectic, and agalactic, and the vulva is swollen and hyperemic with mucopurulent to purulent malodorous vaginal discharge that may soil the perianal region. Secondary septicemia may occur. Agents isolated from cases of metritis in chinchillas include *Streptococcus* spp., *Staphylococcus aureus*, *Pseudomonas aeruginosa*, *Listeria monocytogenes*, and *Proteus vulgaris* or *P. mirabilis* (Figure 4.18). Mucoid vaginal discharge with secondary mucometra (Figure 4.19) and chronic endometritis and cystic endometrial hyperplasia (Figure 4.20) are also reported.

4.8.10 Dystocia

Chinchillas are amenable to caesarian section in order to correct conditions such as primary uterine inertia, dystocia and retained fetuses.

4.8.11 Trophoblastic Embolism

Pulmonary trophoblastic emboli are seen in pregnant and post-parturient chinchillas and are considered an incidental finding. The trophoblastic cells are large, 100 µm to > 400 µm with multiple large nuclei, and they are found in clusters of 1–6 cells within alveolar septal capillaries (Figure 4.21). Sometimes groups of cells can be so large that they are visible as small, raised pulmonary nodules. Rodents, like humans, have hemochorial placentation, such that the maternal blood is in direct contact with the fetal chorionic epithelium. This circumstance allows migration of trophoblastic cells directly into the maternal bloodstream. Trophoblastic cells are also seen in the myometrium. These cells migrate from the developing placenta and can persist long after the pregnancy has completed.

4.8.12 Neoplasia

Urogenital neoplasms are uncommon in chinchillas. Uterine leiomyomas and leiomyosarcomas are reported sporadically.

4.9 Nervous System Conditions

Many neurologic conditions of chinchillas present with similar clinical signs, including sudden death, depression, torticollis, ataxia (Figure 4.22), recumbency, and anorexia. Differential diagnoses include bacterial, fungal and parasitic otitis media and interna, meningitis, encephalitis, nutritional deficiencies, and lead toxicity. For all cases, the diagnostic plan is similar and includes gross examination, histology, and potentially bacterial and fungal culture, virus isolation, and toxicology.

4.9.1 Listeriosis

Listeriosis (see Section 4.6.5.2 for a more complete description) is caused by *Listeria monocytogenes*, a common disease of farmed chinchillas. Chinchillas are highly susceptible to the visceral septicemic form of the disease and the route of infection is typically via the intestine with later dissemination to the liver and a resultant septicemia. Involvement of the brain also occurs as a sequela to septicemia. When the brain is involved, neural lesions include fibrinosuppurative meningitis, and foci of parenchymal necrosis and microabscessation with intralesional Gram-positive bacilli. The more characteristic hepatic

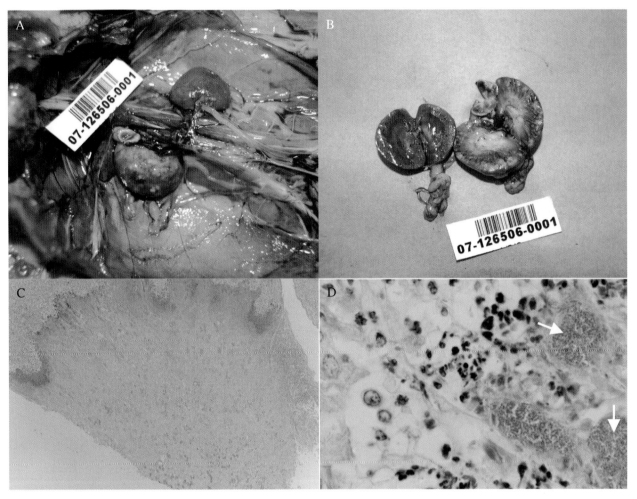

Figure 4.17 Acute unilateral pyelonephritis. A: The right kidney is moderately enlarged with numerous white, raised, subcapsular foci. B: The affected kidney has renal papillary pallor, alternating pale and red cortical streaking, and raised abscesses within the outer cortex. This chinchilla also had a *S. zooepidemicus*-associated suppurative vaginitis and metritis. C: Microscopically, there is renal papillary necrosis demarcated from normal tissue by a band of necrotic neutrophils and inflammatory cellular debris. D: Colonies of coccoid bacteria fill medullary tubular lumens (arrows).

and intestinal lesions of listerosis may also be seen in these animals or in other affected animals from the same group, which will assist in selecting relevant diagnostic tests and differential diagnoses.

4.9.2 Bacterial Otitis Media and Interna, Meningitis, Encephalitis

Otitis media and interna are frequently seen in young chinchillas secondary to bacterial infection. Potential bacterial agents include *Bordetella bronchiseptica*, *Streptococcus pneumoniae*, *S. pyogenes*, *S. zooepidemicus*, *Klebsiella pneumoniae*, *Pasteurella multocida*, *Pseudomonas aeruginosa*, and *Staphylococcus aureus*. Mucopurulent or caseous exudate can be found within the external ear canal if the tympanic membrane has ruptured as well as within the tympanic bulla (Figure 4.23). Inflammation can progress to involve the inner ear, meninges and brain, and affected animals will present with ataxia,

torticollis, circling, and rolling. Microscopically, fibrino-suppurative exudate and bacteria can be seen within the tympanic bullae and meninges with extension into the cerebral parenchyma.

4.9.3 Mycotic Meningitis

Cryptococcosis has been reported sporadically in chinchillas. In one case, an aged animal presented with a short history of lethargy, anorexia, and mild, intermittent rear leg tremors. Granulomatous meningitis and optic neuritis were noted with large numbers of yeast organisms typical of *Cryptococcus* spp.

4.9.4 Cerebral Nematodiasis

Chinchillas are susceptible to infection with raccoon round-worm larvae (*Baylisascaris procyonis*) and outbreaks of cerebral nematodiasis have occurred between farms sharing

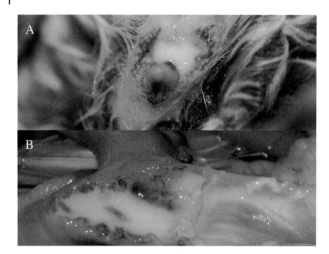

Figure 4.18 This chinchilla had delivered a dead pup approximately two weeks before being found dead. In addition to thick white opaque vulvar discharge (A), there is suppurative vaginitis and metritis (B) with *S. zooepidemicus* isolated by bacterial culture.

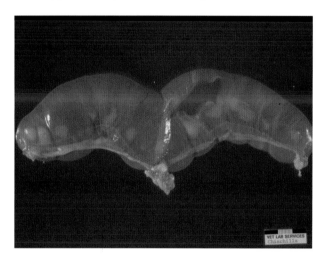

Figure 4.19 Bilateral mucometra in a chinchilla.

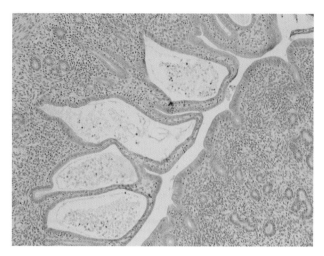

Figure 4.20 This mature, nulliparous chinchilla presented with blood staining of the perivaginal fur and spotting of blood in the cage with no evidence of hematuria. The animal underwent ovariohysterectomy and tissues were submitted for microscopic evaluation. Chronic suppurative and hemorrhagic endometritis with cystic endometrial hyperplasia (demonstrated in image) were diagnosed. The etiology of the endometritis was not determined. *Source:* Courtesy of J. Davies.

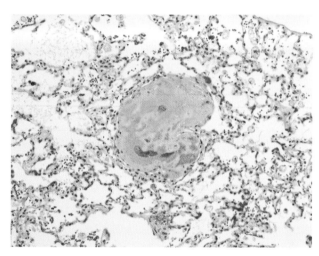

Figure 4.21 Large pulmonary trophoblastic emboli within alveolar septal capillaries are seen in pregnant and post partum chinchillas and are considered an incidental finding.

the same equipment, feed, and storage facilities. Affected animals developed acute progressive ataxia, torticollis, paralysis, incoordination, and tumbling. The clinical signs progressed and animals became recumbent, comatose, and died or were euthanized. At necropsy, no gross lesions were seen. Microscopically, foci and tracks of malacia with swollen and degenerating axons and neurons were seen in midbrain, medulla, and cerebellar peduncles with varying amounts of eosinophilic and lymphohistiocytic meningeal and perivascular infiltrates. Cross-sections of ascarid larvae with prominent lateral alae were present in close proximity to areas of parenchymal necrosis. A presumptive diagnosis of *B. procyonis* larval migration and encephalitis was based on the fact that the hay for the three farms was stored at one location where raccoons were known to reside and the ranch owner had noticed raccoon feces on the hay. Sourcing

and maintaining bedding and feed ingredients in biosecure facilities will reduce the risk of contamination with raccoon feces containing *B. procyonis* eggs.

4.9.5 Cerebral Coccidiosis

A large *Frenkelia microti* tissue cyst with no associated inflammatory response was identified in the cerebrum of a retired breeding female chinchilla. This animal exhibited no clinical signs and at necropsy, no lesions were observed. Coccidia of the genus *Frenkelia* have an obligatory two-

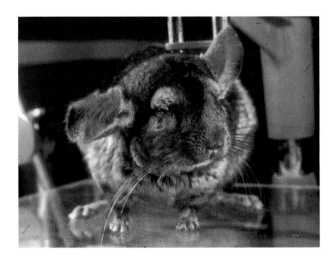

Figure 4.22 Chinchilla exhibiting torticollis. Many neurologic conditions of chinchillas present with similar clinical signs, including torticollis. Differential diagnoses include bacterial, fungal, and parasitic otitis media and interna, meningitis, and encephalitis. This animal had cerebral nematodiasis, likely secondary to *Baylisascaris procyonis* infection and larval migration.

host life cycle, which includes a rodent intermediate host and a raptor definitive host. The chinchilla likely became infected by ingesting food contaminated with feces from an infected hawk.

4.9.6 Toxoplasmosis

Toxoplasma infections in chinchillas are moderately common (see Section 4.4.2.5. for a fuller discussion of the organism). When the cerebrum is involved, clinical signs include sudden death, depression, hunched posture, tachypnea, ataxia, and inability to stand. Typical microscopic lesions include a granulomatous encephalitis with intralesional *Toxoplasma* sp. bradyzoites.

4.9.7 Herpesvirus Infections

Systemic disease, uveitis, and sudden death with non-suppurative encephalitis were reported in pet chinchillas infected with human herpesvirus-1. Microscopic cerebral lesions included neuronal necrosis, microgliosis and lymphocytic perivascular cuffing with numerous intranuclear inclusions, both eosinophilic Cowdry Type A and large, amphophilic, homogeneous viral inclusions in neurons and astroglia. Herpesvirus was confirmed by transmission electron microscopy and the virus was recovered and shown to have near 100% sequence homology with human herpes simplex virus Type 1 (HHV-1). Ocular infection was considered to be the originating site of the infection with subsequent spread to the brain. The source of infection was not determined but close contact with a human shedding HHV-1 was considered the most likely.

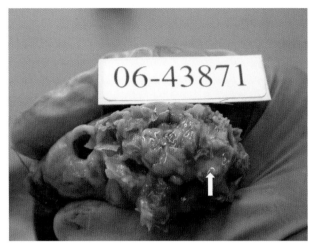

Figure 4.23 This chinchilla was noted to be listless, and had mucoid nasal discharge and dyspnea prior to death. On post-mortem examination, the right tympanic bulla contains purulent exudate (arrow). In addition, cloudy white mucoid exudate was noted in the distal tracheal lumen, the cranial lung lobes were dark purple, and the remainder of the lungs were mottled purple-pink. Microscopically, fibrinosuppurative bronchopneumonia was present and large numbers of *Bordetella bronchiseptica* were isolated from the middle ear and the lung.

4.9.8 Rabies

Rabies virus infection has been reported in one feral chinchilla in the United States. It is an unlikely etiologic agent of central nervous system disease in chinchillas, but one that should be included in the differential diagnoses, particularly if the animal had access to the outdoors prior to the onset of clinical signs.

4.9.9 Other Nervous System Conditions

Dietary B vitamin deficiencies (thiamine, vitamin B_1; pyridoxine, vitamin B6; and pantothenic acid, vitamin B5) may result in neurologic signs in chinchillas. Clinical signs include tremors, circling, convulsions or paralysis, and sudden death.

Calcium deficiency can result in convulsions, especially in young, rapidly growing animals or pregnant or lactating females. No microscopic changes are expected in acute cases.

Chinchillas that are allowed to have free run of their environment are more likely to come in contact with **lead** with reported clinical signs of convulsions, seizures and blindness.

Cabin pressurization problems during air transport resulted in a group of chinchillas dying during transit. At necropsy, the lungs were edematous and mottled red-black, and the tympanic bullae contained blood. Microscopically, the tympanic membranes were congested and frank blood filled the tympanic bullae (Figure 4.24). The lungs from affected animals were edematous and congested.

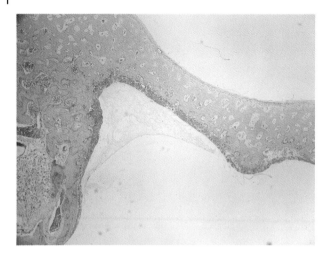

Figure 4.24 Cabin pressurization problems during air transport resulted in a group of chinchillas dying during transit. Congestion and hemorrhage were seen within the external ear canals at post mortem examination. Microscopically, there is congestion and hemorrhage within the middle and inner ears.

4.10 Hematopoietic and Lymphoid Conditions

Lymphosarcoma is uncommonly reported in chinchillas and presents as hepatosplenomegaly and peripheral lymph node enlargement. Nodules and aggregates of neoplastic lymphocytes may also be present within the kidneys and pulmonary parenchyma (Figure 4.25). Hemangiosarcoma has been reported rarely in chinchillas.

4.11 Ophthalmic Conditions

In one retrospective study of clinical ocular disorders of chinchillas, lenticular abnormalities were most common,

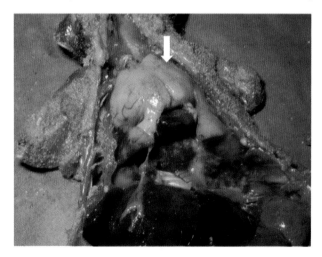

Figure 4.25 Lymphosarcoma in a juvenile chinchilla. Thymic enlargement obscures the heart arrow and pulmonary and renal involvement were also present.

with cataracts being most frequently identified. As in other species, there is an association between elevated blood glucose levels and cataract development, warranting dietary assessment and additional testing including blood glucose and fructosamine levels to rule out diabetes mellitus. In addition to other causes, congenital defects resulting in cataract formation have been reported. Lenticular luxation and loss were less common. Although seen infrequently, lenticular sclerosis is also considered to be a normal age-related change in chinchillas.

4.11.1 Conjunctivitis

In a retrospective study of clinical ocular disorders, conjunctival disease was the third most common condition reported. Foreign body conjunctivitis in both nursing and adult chinchillas can develop secondary to excessive exposure to dust baths. Catarrhal conjunctivitis can be seen in environments with dirty or poor quality bedding, inadequate cage ventilation, and elevated ammonia levels. Conjunctivitis in chinchillas can also have a primary bacterial etiology and agents include *S. aureus*, *Streptococcus* spp., and *P. aeruginosa* cultured from affected animals, and is also seen in conjunction with respiratory disease. Infected conjunctivae are hyperemic and swollen with serous to purulent ocular discharge (Figure 4.26). Where the ocular discharge is serous and no other ophthalmic clinical signs are present, underlying dental disease should be considered.

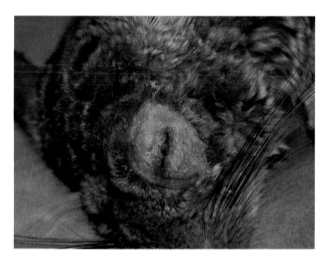

Figure 4.26 Conjunctivitis in chinchillas can result from excessive dust bathing or the use of unsuitable dust, dirty or poor quality bedding, inadequate cage ventilation, and elevated ammonia levels. The condition can be primary with a bacterial etiology, including *Staphylococcus aureus*, *Streptococcus* spp., and *Pseudomonas aeruginosa* or conjunctivitis can occur secondary to respiratory disease. In severe cases, the eyelids are glued closed from the mucopurulent ocular discharge and there is periocular alopecia, as in this case.

4.11.2 Other Conditions of the Eye

In one retrospective study of clinical ocular disorders, corneal disease ranked second with corneal erosions and ulcerations most frequently diagnosed possibly from trauma or irritation from unsuitable dust bathing material. One aged chinchilla had bilateral lipid keratopathy; thyroid function was not evaluated but cholesterol and triglyceride levels were within normal reference ranges.

Secondary stromal abscesses may result from trauma-induced corneal ulceration. Stromal abscesses are usually contaminated with either *Staphylococcus* sp. or *Pasteurella* sp., and appear as a white plaque on the cornea in conjunction with neovascularization and anterior uveitis.

Hypopyon has been seen in a chinchilla associated with *Pseudomonas aeruginosa* infection (Figure 4.27).

Human herpesvirus infections may induce keratitis, mild lymphohistiocytic uveitis, lymphocytic retinitis with partial to complete retinal detachment, and mild lymphocytic optic neuritis (see Section 4.9.7 for a more complete discussion).

An **intraorbital *Taenia coenuris*** resulted in slowly progressive exophthalmos in an adult male chinchilla. This chinchilla had been kept indoors, but was provided with dandelions from the backyard. Microscopically, a single cyst with multiple invaginated protoscolices, each bearing a prominent scolex with refractile hooks, suckers and numerous calcareous corpuscles, consistent with *Taenia* coenurus, was identified within the orbit. Dogs are definitive hosts of *T. serialis* and it is likely that either the hay or the dandelions fed to the chinchilla were contaminated with feces infected with *T. serialis*.

Retrobulbar hemorrhage from retroorbital sinus blood collection is another cause of exopthalmos reported in chinchillas. Elongation of premolar and molar teeth roots as a consequence of insufficient wear can lead to penetration of periorbital soft and bony tissues and the orbit resulting in **ocular proptosis**. Roots can also invade into alveolar bone causing remodelling, bony distortion, and compression or obliteration of the lacrimal canal and duct with resultant **epiphora**.

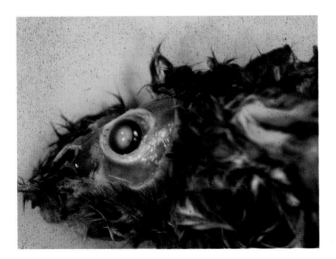

Figure 4.27 Hypopyon has been associated with *Pseudomonas aeruginosa* infection in a chinchilla.

Bibliography

Introduction

Donnelly, T.M. and Brown, C.J. (2004) Guinea pig and chinchilla care and husbandry. *Veterinary Clinics of North America: Exotic Animal Practice*, **7**(2), 351–373.

Fox, J.G., Anderson, L.C., Loew, F.M., and Quimby, F.W. (2002) *Laboratory Animal Medicine*, 2nd edn. Academic Press, San Diego.

Harkness, J.E., Turner, P.V., VandeWoude, S., and Wheler, C.L. (2010) *Harkness and Wagner's Biology and Medicine of Rabbits and Rodents*, 5th edn. Wiley-Blackwell, Ames, IA, pp. 58–65.

Heffner, R.S. and Heffner, H.E. (1991) Behavioral hearing range of the chinchilla. *Hearing Research*, **52**(1), 13–16.

Hoefer, H.L. (1994) Chinchillas. *Veterinary Clinics of North America: Exotic Animal Practice*, **24**(1), 103–111.

Hoefer, H.L., and Crossley, D.A. (2002) *Chinchillas, in BSAVA Manual of Exotic Pets* (eds. A. Meredith and S. Redrobe), 4th edn. British Small Animal Veterinary Association, Quedgeley, pp. 65–72.

Johnson-Delaney, C. (2010) *Guinea pigs, chinchillas, degus and duprasi, in BSAVA Manual of Exotic Pets* (eds. A. Meredith and S. Redrobe), 4th edn. British Small Animal Veterinary Association, Quedgeley, pp. 28–62.

Miller, J.D. (1970) Audibility curve of the chinchilla. *Journal of Acoustic Society of America*, **48**(2), 513–523.

Yarto-Jaramillo, E. (2011) Respiratory system anatomy, physiology, and disease: guinea pigs and chinchillas. *Veterinary Clinics of North America: Exotic Animal Practice*, **14**(2), 339–355.

Integument General

Chase, H.B. and Eaton, G.J. (1959) The growth of hair follicles in waves. *Annals of New York Academy of Sciences*, **83**, 365–368.

Lanszki, J., Allain, D., Thebault, R-G., and Szendro, Z. (2002) The effect of melatonin treatment on fur maturation period and hair follicle cycle in growing chinchillas. *British Society of Animal Science*, **75**, 49–55.

Plikus, M.V. and Chuong, C.M. (2008) Complex hair cycle domain patterns and regenerative hair waves in living rodents. *Journal of Investigative Dermatology*, **128**(5), 1071–1080.

Wilcox, H.H. (1950) Histology of the skin and hair of the adult chinchilla. *Anatomical Record*, **108**(3), 385–397.

Fur Slip, Fur Chewing, Barbering

Bowden, R.S.T. (1962) The nutrition of chinchillas: observations on pelleted diets, hay roughage, and fur chewing. *Journal of Small Animal Practice*, **3**, 141–149.

Eidmann, S. (1992) *Studies on the Etiology and Pathogenesis of Fur Damage in the Chinchilla* (p. 162). Tierärztliche Hochschule, Hannover, Germany.

Harkness, J.E., Turner, P.V., VandeWoude, S., and Wheler, C.L. (2010) *Harkness and Wagner's Biology and Medicine of Rabbits and Rodents*, 5th edn. Wiley-Blackwell, Ames, IA, pp. 58–65.

Lapinski, S., Lis, M.W., Wójcik, A., Migdal, L., and Guja, I. (2014) Analysis of factors increasing the probability of fur chewing in chinchilla (*Chinchilla lanigera*) raised under farm conditions. *Annals of Animal Science*, **14**(1), 189–195.

Ponzio, M.F., Busso, J.M., Ruiz, R.D., and Fiol de Cuneo, M. (2007) A survey assessment of the incidence of fur-chewing in commercial chinchilla (*Chinchilla lanigera*) farms. *Animal Welfare*, **16**, 471–479.

Dermatophytosis

Canny, C.J. and Gamble, C.S. (2003) Fungal diseases of rabbits. *Veterinary Clinics of North America: Exotic Animal Practice*, **6**(2), 429–433.

Donnelly, T.M., Rush, E.M., and Lackner, P.A. (2002) Ringworm in small exotic pets. *Seminars in Avian and Exotic Pet Medicine*, **9**(2), 82–93.

Marshall, K.L. (2003) Fungal diseases in small mammals: therapeutic trends and zoonotic considerations. *Veterinary Clinics of North America: Exotic Animal Practice* **6**(2), 415–427.

Pollock, C. (2003) Fungal diseases of laboratory rodents. *Veterinary Clinics of North America: Exotic Animal Practice*, **6**(2), 401–413.

Skin Trauma, Subcutaneous Abscesses, Pododermatitis

Doerning, B.J, Brammer, D.W., and Rush, H.G. (1993) *Pseudomonas aeruginosa* infection in a *Chinchilla lanigera*. *Laboratory Animals*, **27**(2), 131–133.

Donnelly, T.M. and Brown, C.J. (2004) Guinea pig and chinchilla care and husbandry. *Veterinary Clinics of North America: Exotic Animal Practice*, **7**(2), 351–373.

Hoefer, H.L. and Crossley, D.A. (2002) *Chinchillas, in BSAVA Manual of Exotic Pets* (eds. A. Meredith and S. Redrobe), 4th edn. British Small Animal Veterinary Association, Quedgeley, pp. 65–72.

Hoppmann, E. and Wilson Baron, H. (2007) Rodent dermatology. *Journal of Exotic Pet Medicine*, **16**(4), 238–255.

Jenkins, J.R. (1992) Husbandry and common diseases of the chinchilla (*Chinchilla lanigera*). *Journal of Small Exotic Animal Medicine*, **2**(1), 15–17.

Johnson-Delaney, C. (2010) *Guinea pigs, chinchillas, degus and duprasi, in BSAVA Manual of Exotic Pets* (eds. A. Meredith and S. Redrobe), 4th edn. British Small Animal Veterinary Association, Quedgeley, pp. 28–62.

External Parasites

Hoefer, H.L. and Crossley, D.A. (2002) *Chinchillas, in BSAVA Manual of Exotic Pets* (eds. A. Meredith and S. Redrobe), 4th edn. British Small Animal Veterinary Association, Quedgeley, pp. 65–72.

Hoppmann, E. and Wilson Baron, H. (2007) Rodent dermatology. *Journal of Exotic Pet Medicine*, **16**(4), 238–255.

Orcutt, C.J. (2008) *Diseases of guinea pigs and chinchillas, in Proceedings of the 145th American Veterinary Medical Association*, New Orleans, Louisiana. July 19–22.

Richardson, V.C.G. (2003) *Diseases of Small Domestic Rodents* (pp. 1–53). Blackwell, Oxford.

Agalactia, Mastitis

Hoefer, H.L. and Crossley, D.A. (2002) *Chinchillas, in BSAVA Manual of Exotic Pets* (eds. A. Meredith and S. Redrobe), 4th edn. British Small Animal Veterinary Association, Quedgeley, pp. 65–72.

Kennedy, A.H. (1952) *Chinchilla Diseases and Ailments*. Clay Publishing Co., Bewdley.

Richardson, V.C.G. (2003) *Diseases of Small Domestic Rodents* (pp. 1–53). Blackwell, Oxford.

Seborrehea and Nutritional Deficiencies

Donnelly, T.M. (2004) Disease problems of chinchillas. in *Ferrets, Rabbits and Rodents: Clinical Medicine and Surgery* (eds. K.E. Quesenberry and J.W. Carpenter), 2nd edn. Saunders, St. Louis, MO.

Kennedy, A.H. (1952) *Chinchilla Diseases and Ailments*. Clay Publishing Co., Bewdley/

Richardson, V.C.G. (2003) *Diseases of Small Domestic Rodents* (pp. 1–53). Blackwell, Oxford.

Diabetes Mellitus

Marlow, C. (1995) Diabetes in a chinchilla. *Veterinary Record*, **56**, 136.

Keeble, E. (2001) Endocrine diseases in small mammals. *In Practice*, **23**, 570–585.

Hyperthyroidism

Fritsche, R., Simova-Curd, S., Clauss, M., and Hatt, J.M. (2008) Hyperthyroidism in connection with suspected diabetes mellitus in a chinchilla (*Chinchilla lanigera*). *Veterinary Record*, **163**(15), 454–456.

Adrenocortical Hyperplasia

Brenon, H.C. (1953) Postmortem examinations of chinchillas. *Journal of American Veterinary Medicine Association*, **123**(919), 310.

Crossley, D.A. (2001) Dental disease in chinchillas in the UK. *Journal of Small Animal Practice*, **42**, 12–19.

Crossley, D.A. (2003) Dental disease in chinchillas. PhD thesis. The University Dental Hospital of Manchester. http://www.vetdent.eu/cpd/cpddownloads/ thesis1-002-96dpi.pdf (accessed September 2013).

Leader, R.W. and Holte, R.J.A. (1955) Studies on three outbreaks of listeriosis in chinchillas. *Cornell Veterinarian*, **45**(1), 78–84.

Roos, T.B. and Shackelford, R.M. (1955) Some observations on the gross anatomy of the genital system and two endocrine organs and body weights in the chinchilla. *Anatomical Record*, **123**(3), 301–311.

Yarto-Jaramillo, E. (2011) Respiratory system anatomy, physiology, and disease: guinea pigs and chinchillas. *Veterinary Clinics of North America: Exotic Animal Practice*, **14**(2), 339–355.

Rhinitis and Sinusitis

Donnelly, T.M., and Brown, C.J. (2004) Guinea pig and chinchilla care and husbandry. *Veterinary Clinics of North America: Exotic Animal Practice*, 7(2), 351–373.

Johnson-Delaney, C.A., and Orosz, S.E. (2009) The respiratory system: exotic companion mammals. *AEMV Proceedings*, Milwaukee, WI.

Orcutt, C.J. (2008) Diseases of guinea pigs and chinchillas. *Proceedings of the 145th American Veterinary Medicine Association*, New Orleans, LA.

Pneumonia and Pulmonary Adenomatosis

Bartoszcze, M., Matras, J., Palec, S., Roszkowski, J., and Wystup, E. (1990) *Klebsiella pneumoniae* infection in chinchillas. *Veterinary Record*, **127**(5), 119.

Boussarie, Didier. (2002) Carte d'identité chinchilla. *Proceedings of the 27th World Small Animal Veterinary Association*. Grenada, Spain.

Helmboldt, C.F., Jungherr, E.L., and Caparo, A.C. (1958) Pulmonary adenomatosis in the chinchilla. *American Journal of Veterinary Research*, **19**(71), 270–276.

Huynh, M., Pingret, J.L., and Nicolier, A. (2014) Disseminated *Mycobacterium genavense* infection in a chinchilla (*Chinchilla lanigera*). *Journal of Comparative Medicine*, **151**: 122–125.

Johnson-Delaney, C.A., and Orosz, S.E. (2009) The respiratory system: exotic companion mammals. *AEMV Proceedings*, Milwaukee, WI.

McAllister, R.A. (1964) An outbreak of toxoplasmosis in an Ontario chinchilla herd. *Canadian Journal of Comparative Medicine and Veterinary Science*, **28**(3), 53–56.

Orcutt, C.J. (2008) Diseases of guinea pigs and chinchillas. *Proceedings of the 145th American Veterinary Medicine Association*, New Orleans, LA.

Owens, D.R., Menges, R.W., Sprouse, R.F., Stewart, W., and Hooper, B.E. (1975) Naturally occurring histoplasmosis in the chinchilla (*Chinchilla lanigera*). *Journal of Clinical Microbiology*, **1**(5), 486–488.

Pridham, T.J. (1966) Pseudomonas infection in the chinchilla. *Fur Trade Journal of Canada*, Mar, 8–9.

Pridham, T.J., Budd, J., and Karstad, L.H. (1966) Common diseases of fur bearing animals. II. Diseases of chinchillas, nutria, and rabbits. *Canadian Veterinary Journal*, **7**(4), 84–87.

Richardson, V.C.G. (2003) *Diseases of Small Domestic Rodents*. Blackwell, Oxford, pp. 1–53.

Trautwein, G., and Helmboldt, C.F. (1967) Experimental pulmonary talcum granuloma and epithelial hyperplasia in the chinchilla. *Veterinary Pathology*, **4**(3), 254–267.

Wallach, J.D., and Boever, W.J. (1983) *Diseases of Exotic Animals: Medical and Surgical Management*. W.B. Saunders, Philadelphia, PA, pp. 135–195.

Neoplasia

Boussarie, D. (2002) Carte d'identité chinchilla. *Proceedings of the 27th World Small Animal Veterinary Association*, Grenada, Spain.

Bracken, F.K. and Olsen, O.W. (1950) Coenurosis in the chinchilla. *Journal of American Veterinary Medical Association*, **116**(879), 440–442.

Greenacre, C.B. (2004) Spontaneous tumors of small mammals. *Veterinary Clinics of North America: Exotic Animal Practice*, **7**(3), 627–651.

Hoefer, H.L. and Crossley, D.A. (2002) *Chinchillas, in BSAVA Manual of Exotic Pets* (eds. A. Meredith and S. Redrobe), 4th edn. British Small Animal Veterinary Association, Quedgeley, pp. 65–72.

Johnson-Delaney, C. (2010) *Guinea pigs, chinchillas, degus and duprasi, i in BSAVA Manual of Exotic Pets* (eds. A. Meredith and S. Redrobe), 5th edn. British Small Animal Veterinary Association, Quedgeley, pp. 28–62.

Simova-Curd, S., Nitzl, D., Pospischil, A., and Hatt, J.M. (2008) Lumbar osteosarcoma in a chinchilla (*Chinchilla laniger*). *Journal of Small Animal Practice*, **49**(9), 483–485.

Teague Self, J., and Murphy, C.E. (1954) Hydatid disease in chinchillas. *NCBA Research Bulletin*, Oct.(2).

Thompson, K. (2007) *Bones and joints, in Jubb, Kennedy, and Palmer's Pathology of Domestic Animals* (ed. G.M. Maxie), 5th edn. Elsevier Saunders, Edinburgh.

Van Vleet, J.F. and Valentine, B.A. (2007) *Muscle and tendon, in Jubb, Kennedy, and Palmer's Pathology of Domestic Animals* (ed. G.M. Maxie), 5th edn. Elsevier Saunders, Edinburgh.

Wallach, J.D. and Boever, W.J. (1983) *Diseases of Exotic Animals: Medical and Surgical Management.* W.B. Saunders, Philadelphia, PA.

Dental Conditions

Capello, V. (2009) Chinchilla dental health. *Exotic DVM.* **11**(3), 28.

Crossley, D.A. (2001) Dental disease in chinchillas in the UK. *Journal of Small Animal Practice,* **42**(1), 12–19.

Crossley, D.A., Dubielzig, R.R., and Benson, K.G. (1997) Caries and odontoclastic resorptive lesions in a chinchilla (*Chinchilla lanigera*). *Veterinary Record,* **27**, 141(13), 337–339.

Crossley, D.A., Jackson, A., Yates, J., and Boydell, I.P. (1998) Use of computed tomography to investigate cheek tooth abnormalities in chinchillas (*Chinchilla lanigera*). *Journal of Small Animal Practice,* **39**(8), 385–389.

Crossley, D.A. and Miguélez, M.M. (2001) Skull size and cheek-tooth length in wild-caught and captive-bred chinchillas. *Archives of Oral Biology,* **46**(10), 919–928.

Derbaudrenghien, V., Van Caelenborg, A., Hermans, K, Gielen, I., and Martel, A. (2010) Dental pathology in chinchillas. *Vlaams Diergeneeskundig Tijdschrift,* **79**, 345–358.

Esophageal and Gastrointestinal Conditions

Cousens, P.J. (1963) The chinchilla in veterinary practice. *Journal of Small Animal Practice,* **14**, 199–205.

Dall, J. (1962) Diseases of the chinchilla. *Journal of Small Animal Practice,* **4**, 207–212.

Donnelly, T.M. (2004) *Disease problems of chinchillas, in Ferrets, Rabbits and Rodents: Clinical Medicine and Surgery* (eds. K.E. Quesenberry and J.W. Carpenter), 2nd edn. Saunders, St. Louis, MO.

Johnson-Delaney, C.A., and Orosz, S.E. (2009) The gastrointestinal system: Exotic companion mammals. *AEMV Proceedings,* Milwaukee, WI, Aug 8, pp. 25–41.

Kennedy, A.H. (1952) *Chinchilla Diseases and Ailments.* Clay Publishing Co., Bewdley.

McGreevy, P.D. and Carn, V.M. (1988) Intestinal torsion in a chinchilla. *Veterinary Record,* **122**(12), 287.

Wojtacka, J., Szarek, J., Babinska, I., et al. (2014) Sodium carbonate intoxication on a chinchilla (*Chinchilla lanigera*) farm: a case report. *Veterinary Medicine,* **59**(2), 112–116.

Bacterial Enteritides

Bartoszce, M., Nowakowska, M., Roszkowski, J., et al. (1990) Chinchilla deaths due to *Clostridium perfringens* A enterotoxin. *Veterinary Record,* **126**(14), 341–342.

Bottone, E.J. (1999) *Yersinia enterocolitica*: overview and epidemiologic correlates. *Microbes and Infection,* **4**, 323–333.

Cavill, J.P. (1967) Listeriosis in chinchillas (*Chinchilla lanigera*). *Veterinary Record,* **80**(20), 592–594.

Churria, C.D.G., Vigo, G.B., Origlia, J., et al. (2014) Diagnosis of an outbreak of *Salmonella* Typhimurium in chinchillas (*Chinchilla lanigera*) by pulsed-field gel electrophoresis. *Revista Argentina de Microbiología,* **46**(3), 205–209.

Czernomysy-Furowicz, D., Furowicz, A.J., and Peruzynska, A. (2000) Feed intoxication in chinchilla induced by *Bacillus cereus* enterotoxin. *Scientifur.* **24**(1), 31–36.

Dall, J. (1962) Diseases of the chinchilla. *Journal of Small Animal Practice,* **4**, 207–212.

Diaz, L.I., Lepherd, M., and Scott, J. (2013) Enteric infection and subsequent septicemia due to attaching and effacing *Escherichia coli* in a chinchilla. *Comparative Medicine,* **63**(6), 503–507.

Doerning, B.J., Brammer, D.W., and Rush, H.G. (1993) *Pseudomonas aeruginosa* infection in a *Chinchilla lanigera. Laboratory Animals,* **27**(2), 131–133.

Finley, G.G. and Long, J.R. (1977) An epizootic of listeriosis in chinchillas. *Canadian Veterinary Journal,* **18**(6), 164–167.

Hirakawa, Y., Sasaki, H., Kawamoto, E. et al. (2010) Prevalence and analysis of Pseudomonas aeriuginosa in chinchillas. *BMC Veterinary Research,* **6**, 52–60.

Hubbert, W.T. (1972) Yersiniosis in mammals and birds in the United States. *American Journal of Tropical Medical Hygiene,* **21**(4), 458–463.

Keagy, H.F. and Keagy, E.H. (1951) Epizootic gastroenteritis in chinchillas. *Journal of the American Veterinary Medical Association,* **117**(886), 35–37.

Kimpe, A., Decostere, A., Hermans, K., Baele, M., and Haesebrouck, F. (2004) Isolation of *Listeria ivanovii* from a septicaemic chinchilla (*Chinchilla lanigera*). *Veterinary Record,* **154**(25), 791–792.

Langford, E.V. (1972a) *Pasteurella pseudotuberculosis* infections in Western Canada. *Canadian Veterinary Journal,* **13**(4), 85–87.

Langford, E.V. (1972b) *Yersinia enterocolitica* isolated from animals in the Fraser Valley of British Columbia. *Canadian Veterinary Journal,* **13**(5), 109–113.

Larrivee, G.P. and Elvehjem, C.A. (1954) Disease problems in chinchillas. *Journal of the American Veterinary Medical Association,* **124**(927), 447–455.

Leader, R.W., and Baker, G.A. (1954) A report of two cases of *Pasteurella pseudotuberculosis* infection in the chinchilla. *Cornell Veterinarian,* **44**(2), 262–267.

Lusis, P.I., and Soltys, M.A. (1971) Immunization of mice and chinchillas against *Pseudomonas aeruginosa. Canadian Journal of Comparative Medicine,* **35**(1), 60–66.

Mountain, A. (1989) *Salmonella arizona* in a chinchilla. *Veterinary Record*, **125**(1), 25.

Naglić, T., Seol, B., Bedeković, M., Grabarević, Z., and Listes, E. (2003) Outbreak of *Salmonella enteritidis* and isolation of *Salmonella sofia* in chinchillas (*Chinchilla lanigera*). *Veterinary Record*, **152**(23), 719–720.

Orcutt, C.J. (2008) Diseases of guinea pigs and chinchillas. Proceedings of the 145th American Veterinary Medical Association, New Orleans, Louisiana, July 19–22.

Pridham, T.J. (1966) *Pseudomonas* infection in the chinchilla. *The Fur Trade Journal of Canada*, Mar, 8–9.

Pridham, T.J., Budd, J., and Karstad, L.H. (1966) Common diseases of fur bearing animals. II. Diseases of chinchillas, nutria, and rabbits. *Canadian Veterinary Journal*, 7(4), 84–87.

Watson, W.A. and Watson, F.I. (1966) An outbreak of *Salmonella dublin* infection in chinchillas. *Veterinary Record*, **78**(1), 15–17.

Wideman, W.L. (2006) *Pseudomonas aeruginosa* otitis media and interna in a chinchilla ranch. *Canadian Veterinary Journal*, **47**(8), 799–800.

Wilkerson, M.J., Melendy, A., and Stauber, E. (1997) An outbreak of listeriosis in a breeding colony of chinchillas. *Journal of Veterinary Diagnostic Investigation*, **9**(3), 320–323.

Gastrointestinal Parasitism

Cousens, P.J. (1963) The chinchilla in veterinary practice. *Journal of Small Animal Practice*, **4**, 199–205.

de Vos, A.J. and van der Westhuizen, I.B. (1968) The occurrence of *Eimeria chinchilla* n. sp. (Eimeriidae) in *Chinchilla lanigera* (Molina, 1782) in South Africa. *Journal of South African Veterinary Medical Association*, **39**(1), 81–82.

Goltz, J.P. (1980) Giardiasis in chinchillas. Thesis. University of Guelph.

Harkness, J.E., Turner, P.V., VandeWoude, S., and Wheler. C.L. (2010) *Harkness and Wagner's Biology and Medicine of Rabbits and Rodents*. 5th edn. Wiley-Blackwell, Ames, IA, pp. 266–269.

Levecke, B., Meulemans, L., Dalemans, T., et al. (2011) Mixed *Giardia duodenalis* assemblage A, B, C and E infections in pet chinchillas (*Chinchilla lanigera*) in Flanders (Belgium). *Veterinary Parasitology*, **177**(1–2), 166–170.

Macnish, M.G., Morgan, U.M., Behnke, J.M., and Thompson, R.C. (2002) Failure to infect laboratory rodent hosts with human isolates of *Rodentolepis* (= *Hymenolepis*) *nana*. *Journal of Helminthology*, **76**(1), 37–43.

Pellérdy, L.P. (1974) *Coccidia and Coccidiosis*. 2nd edn. Parey, Berlin.

Percy, D.H. and Barthold, S.W. (2007) *Pathology of Laboratory Rodents and Rabbits*. 3rd edn. Blackwell, Ames, IA, pp. 179–205.

Shelton, G.C. (1954a) Giardiasis in the chinchilla. I. Observations on morphology, location in the intestinal tract, and host specificity. *American Journal of Veterinary Research*, **15**(54), 71–74.

Shelton, G.C. (1954b) Giardiasis in the chinchilla. II. Incidence of the disease and results of experimental infections. *American Journal of Veterinary Research*, **15**(54), 75–78.

Stampa, S., and Hobson, N.K. (1966) Control of some internal parasites of chinchillas. *Journal of the American Veterinary Medical Association*, **49**(7), 929–931.

Teague Self, J., and Murphy, C.E. (1954) Hydatid disease in chinchillas. *NCBA Research Bulletin*, Oct, (**2**).

Yamini, B., and Raju, N.R. (1986) Gastroenteritis associated with a *Cryptosporidium* sp in a chinchilla. *Journal of the American Veterinary Medical Association*, **189**(9), 1158–1159.

Hepatic Conditions and Pancreatitis

Brooks, A., Skelding, A., Stalker, M., et al. (2013) Alveolar hydatid disease (*Echinococcus multilocularis*) in a dog from southern Ontario. *AHL Newsletter*, **17**(1), 8.

Charles, J.A. (2007) *Pancreas, in Jubb, Kennedy, and Palmer's Pathology of Domestic Animals* (ed. M.G. Maxie), 5th edn. Elsevier Saunders, Edinburgh.

Dubey, J.P., Chapman, J.L., Rosenthal, B.M., Mense, M., and Schueler, R.L. (2006) Clinical *Sarcocystis neurona*, *Sarcocystis canis*, *Toxoplasma gondii*, and *Neospora caninum* infections in dogs. *Veterinary Parasitology*, **137**(1–2), 36–49.

González Pereyra, M.L., Carvalho, E.C., Tissera, J.L., et al. (2008) An outbreak of acute aflatoxicosis on a chinchilla (*Chinchilla lanigera*) farm in Argentina. *Journal of Veterinary Diagnostic Investigation*, **20**(6), 853–856.

Hoefer, H.L. and Crossley, D.A. (2002) *Chinchillas, in BSAVA Manual of Exotic Pets* (eds. A. Meredith and S. Redrobe), 4th edn. British Small Animal Veterinary Association, Quedgeley, pp. 65–72.

Huynh, M., Pingret, J.L., and Nicolier, A. (2014) Disseminated *Mycobacterium genavense* infection in a chinchilla (*Chinchilla lanigera*). *Journal of Comparative Medicine*, **151**, 122–125.

McAllister, R.A. (1964) An outbreak of toxoplasmosis in an Ontario chinchilla herd. *Canadian Journal of Comparative Medicine and Veterinary Science*, **28**(3), 53–56.

Pridham, T.J., Budd, J., and Karstad, L.H. (1966) Common diseases of fur bearing animals. II. Diseases of chinchillas, nutria, and rabbits. *Canadian Veterinary Journal*, 7(4), 84–87.

Rakich, P.M., Dubey, J.P., and Contarino, J.K. (1992) Acute hepatic sarcocystosis in a chinchilla. *Journal of Veterinary Diagnostic Investigation*, **4**(4), 484–486.

Staebler, S., Steinmetz, H., Keller, S., and Deplazes, P. (2007) First description of natural *Echinococcus multilocularis* infections in chinchilla (*Chinchilla lanigera*) and Prevost's squirrel (*Callosciurus prevostii borneoensis*). *Parasitology Research*, **101**(6), 1725–1727.

Toft, J.D. and Ekstrom, M.E. (1980) Identification of metazoan parasites in tissue sections. In: *The Comparative Pathology of Zoo Animals*. Proceedings of a Symposium at the Natural Zoology Park (eds.R.J. Montali and G. Migaki). Smithsonian Institution Press, Washington, DC, pp. 369–378.

Gastrointestinal Neoplasia

Nobel, T.A. and Neumann, F. (1963) Carcinoma of the liver in a nutria (*Myocastor coypus*) and a chinchilla (*Chinchilla lanigera*). *Refu Vet*, **20**, 161–162.

Reavill, R. (2014) Pathology of the exotic companion animal gastrointestinal system. *Veterinary Clinics of North America: Exotic Animal Practice*, **17**(2), 145–164.

Smith, J.L., Campbell-Ward, M., Else, R.W., and Johnston, P.E. (2010) Undifferentiated carcinoma of the salivary gland in a chinchilla (*Chinchilla lanigera*). *Journal of Veterinary Diagnostic Investigation*, **22**(1), 152–155.

General Gastrointestinal References

Brenon, H.C. (1953) Postmortem examinations of chinchillas. *Journal of the American Veterinary Medical Association*, **123**(919), 310.

Donnelly, T.M., and Brown, C.J. (2004) Guinea pig and chinchilla care and husbandry. *Veterinary Clinics of North America: Exotic Animal Practice*, **7**(2), 351–373.

Harkness, J.E., Turner, P.V., VandeWoude, S., and Wheler. C.L. (2010) *Harkness and Wagner's Biology and Medicine of Rabbits and Rodents*. 5th edn. Wiley-Blackwell, Ames, IA. pp. 58–65.

Cardiomyopathy, Cardiac Abnormalities

Donnelly, T.M. (2004) *Disease problems of chinchillas, in Ferrets, Rabbits and Rodents: Clinical Medicine and Surgery* (eds. K.E. Quesenberry and J.W. Carpenter), 2nd edn. Saunders, St. Louis, MO.

Hoefer, H.L., and Crossley, D.A. (2002) Chinchillas. In: *BSAVA Manual of Exotic Pets* (eds. A. Meredith and S. Redrobe), 4th edn. British Small Animal Veterinary Association, Quedgeley, pp. 65–72.

Kuder, T., Nowak, E., Szczurkowski, A., and Kuchinka, J. (2003) A comparative study on cardiac ganglia in midday gerbil, Egyptian spiny mouse, *Chinchilla lanigera* and pigeon. *Anatomia, Histologia, Embryologia*, **32**(3), 134–140.

Linde, A., Summerfield, N.J., Johnston, M., et al. (2004) Echocardiography in the chinchilla. *Journal of Veterinary Internal Medicine*, **18**(5), 772–774.

Ozdemir, V., Cevik-Demirkan, A., and Turkmenoglu, I. (2008) The right coronary artery is absent in the chinchilla (*Chinchilla lanigera*). *Anatomia, Histologia, Embryologia*, **37**(2), 114–117.

Pignon, C., Sanchez-Migallon Guzman, D., Sinclair, K. et al. (2012) Evaluation of heart murmurs in chinchillas (*Chinchilla lanigera*, 59 cases (1996-2009). *Journal of the American Veterinary Medical Association*, **241**(10), 1344–1347.

Pericarditis and Endocarditis

Boussarie, D. (2002) Carte d'identité chinchilla. *Proceedings of the 27th World Small Animal Veterinary Association*. Grenada, Spain.

Wallach, J.D. and Boever, W.J. (1983) *Diseases of Exotic Animals: Medical and Surgical Management*. W.B. Saunders, Philadelphia, PA, pp. 135–159.

Vitamin D Intoxication and Heat Prostration

Donnelly, T.M. (2004) *Disease problems of chinchillas, in Ferrets, Rabbits and Rodents: Clinical Medicine and Surgery* (eds. K.E. Quesenberry and J.W. Carpenter), 2nd edn. Saunders, St. Louis, MO.

Hoefer, H.L. (1994) Chinchillas. *Veterinary Clinics of North America: Small Animal Practice*, **24**(1), 103–111.

Kennedy, A.H. (1952) *Chinchilla Diseases and Ailments*. Clay Publishing Co., Bewdley.

Reproductive Conditions

Billington, W.D. and Weir, B.J. (1967) Deportation of trophoblast in the chinchilla. *Journal of Reproductive Fertility*, **13**(3), 593–595.

Boussarie, D. (2002) Carte d'identité chinchilla. *Proceedings of the 27th World Small Animal Veterinary Association*. Grenada, Spain.

Doerning, B.J., Brammer, D.W., and Rush, H.G. (1993) *Pseudomonas aeruginosa* infection in a *Chinchilla lanigera*. *Laboratory Animals*, **27**(2), 131–133.

Donnelly, T.M. (2004) Disease problems of chinchillas. In: *Ferrets, Rabbits and Rodents: Clinical Medicine and Surgery* (eds. K.E. Quesenberry and J.W. Carpenter), 2nd edn. Saunders, St. Louis, MO.

Granson, H.J., Carr, A.P., Parker, D., and Davies, J.L. (2011) Cystic endometrial hyperplasia and chronic endometritis in a chinchilla. *Journal of the American Veterinary Medical Association*, **239**(2), 233–236.

Hawkins, M.G., and Graham, J.E. (2007) Emergency and critical care of rodents. *Veterinary Clinics of North America: Exotic Animal Practice*, **10**(2), 501–531.

Kennedy, A.H. (1952) *Chinchilla Diseases and Ailments*. Clay Publishing Co., Bewdley.

Pridham, T.J. (1966) *Pseudomonas* infection in the chinchilla. *Fur Trade Journal of Canada*, Mar. 8–9.

Prior, J.E. (1986) Caesarean section in the chinchilla. *Veterinary Record*, **119**(16), 408.

Richardson, V.C.G. (2003) *Diseases of Small Domestic Rodents*. Blackwell, Oxford.

Silva Ilha, M.R., Soares Bezerra Jr, P., Wilhelm Dilger Sanches, A., and Severo Lombardo de Barros, C. (2000) Trophoblastic pulmonary embolism in chinchillas (*Chinchilla lanigera*). *Ciencia Rural*. **30**(5), 903–904.

Sims, E. (1990) Caesarian section in a chinchilla. *Veterinary Record*, **126**(19), 490.

Stephenson, R.S. (1990) Caesarean section in a chinchilla. *Veterinary Record*, **126**(15), 370.

Tvedten, H.W. and Langham, R.F. (1974) Trophoblastic emboli in a chinchilla. *Journal of the American Veterinary Medical Association*, **165**(9), 828–829.

Weir, B.J. (1966) Aspects of reproduction in Chinchilla: Proceedings of the Ann Soc Study Fertility, Cambridge. *Journal of Reproductive Fertility*, **12**, 405–422.

Wilkerson, M.J., Melendy, A., and Stauber, E. (1997) An outbreak of listeriosis in a breeding colony of chinchillas. *Journal of Veterinary Diagnostic Investigation*, **9**(3), 320 233.

Urinary Tract Conditions

Donnelly, T.M. (2004) Disease problems of chinchillas. In: *Ferrets, Rabbits and Rodents: Clinical Medicine and Surgery* (eds. K.E. Quesenberry and J.W. Carpenter), 2nd edn. Saunders, St. Louis, MO.

Goudas, P., and Lusis, P. (1970) Case report. Oxalate nephrosis in chinchilla (*Chinchilla lanigera*). *Canadian Veterinary Journal*, **11**(12), 256–257.

Hawkins, M.G., and Graham, J.E. (2007) Emergency and critical care of rodents. *Veterinary Clinics of North America: Exotic Animal Practice*, **10**(2), 501–531.

Holowaychuk, M.K. (2006) Renal failure in a guinea pig (*Cavia porcellus*) following ingestion of oxalate containing plants. *Canadian Veterinary Journal*, **47**(8), 787–789.

Johnson-Delaney, C. (2010) Guinea pigs, chinchillas, degus and duprasi. In: *BSAVA Manual of Exotic Pets* (eds A. Meredith and S. Redrobe), 5th edn. BSAVA. Quedgeley, pp. 28–62.

Jones, R.J., Stephenson, R., Fountain, D., and Hooker, R. (1995) Urolithiasis in a chinchilla. *Veterinary Record*, **136** (15), 400.

Lucena, R.B., et al. (2012) Doenças de chinchilas (*Chinchilla lanigera*). *Pesquina Vet. Bras.* **32**(6), 529–535.

Osborne, C.A., Albasan, H., Lulich, J.P., Nwaokorie, E., Koehler, L.A., and Ulrich, L.K. (2008) Quantitative analysis of 4468 uroliths retrieved from farm animals, exotic species, and wildlife submitted to the Minnesota Urolith Center: 1981–2007. *Veterinary Clinics of North America: Exotic Animal Practice*, **39**(1), 65–78.

Sanford, S.E. (1988) Oxalate nephropathy associated with seizures in mink. *Canadian Veterinary Journal*, **29**(12), 1005–1006.

Spence, S., and Skae, K. (1995) Urolithiasis in a chinchilla. *Veterinary Record*, **136**(20), 524.

Sportono, A.E., Zuleta, C.A., Valladares, J.P., Deane, A.L., and Jiminez, J.E. (2004) *Chinchilla lanigera*. *American Society of Mammals*, **758**, 1–9.

Stephenson, R.S. (1990) Caesarean section in a chinchilla. *Veterinary Record*, **126**(15), 370.

Bacterial, Fungal and Parasitic Diseases

Bicknese, E., White, A., Pessier, A., and Pye, G.W. (2010) Cryptococcal meningitis and optic nerve neuritis in a chinchilla (*Chinchila lanigera*). *AEMV Proceedings*, San Diego.

Dubey, J.P., Clark, T.R., and Yantis, D. (2000) *Frenkelia microti* infection in a chinchilla (*Chinchilla lanigera*) in the United States. *Journal of Parasitology*, **86**(5), 1149–1150.

Finley, G.G. and Long, J.R. (1977) An epizootic of listeriosis in chinchillas. *Canadian Veterinary Journal*, **18**(6), 164–167.

Orcutt, C.J. (2008) Diseases of guinea pigs and chinchillas. *Proceedings of the 145th American Veterinary Medical Association*, New Orleans, LA.

Richter, C.B., and Kradel, D.C. (1964) Cerebrospinal nematodosis in Pennsylvania groundhogs (*Marmota monax*). *American Journal of Veterinary Research*, **25**, 1230–1235.

Sanford, S.E. (1991) Cerebrospinal nematodiasis caused by *Baylisascaris procyonis* in chinchillas. *Journal of Veterinary Diagnostic Investigation*, **3**(1), 77–79.

Wallach, J.D. and Boever, W.J. (1983) *Diseases of Exotic Animals: Medical and Surgical Management*. W.B. Saunders, Philadelphia, pp. 135–195.

Wilkerson, M.J., Melendy, A., and Stauber, E. (1997) An outbreak of listeriosis in a breeding colony of chinchillas. *Journal of Veterinary Diagnostic Investigation*, **9**(3), 320–323.

Viral Diseases

Goudas, P. and Giltoy, J.S. (1970) Spontaneous herpes-like viral infection in a chinchilla (*Chinchilla lanigera*). *Journal of Wildlife Diseases*, **6**(3), 175–179.

Krebs, J.W., Mondul, A.M., Rupprecht, C.E., and Childs, J.E. (2001) Rabies surveillance in the United States during 2000. *Journal of the American Veterinary Medical Association*, **219**(12), 1687–1699.

Wohlsein, P., Thiele, A., Fehr, M., et al. (2002) Spontaneous human herpes virus type 1 infection in a chinchilla (*Chinchilla lanigera* f. dom.). *Acta Neuropathology*, **104**(6), 674–678.

Deficiencies, Toxicities and Trauma

Hoefer, H.L. and Chinchillas. (1994) *Veterinary Clinics of North America: Small Animal Practice*, **24**(1), 103–11.

Hoefer, H.L. and Crossley, D.A. (2002) Chinchillas. In *BSAVA Manual of Exotic Pets* (eds. A. Meredith and S. Redrobe), 4th edn, British Small Animal Veterinary Association. Quedgeley, pp. 65–72.

Kennedy, A.H. (1952) *Chinchilla Diseases and Ailments.* Clay Publishing Co., Bewdley.

Morgan, R.V., Moore, F.M., Pearce, L.K., and Rossi, T. (1991) Clinical and laboratory findings in small companion animals with lead poisoning: 347 cases (1977–1986). *Journal of the American Veterinary Medical Association*, **199**(1), 93–97.

Richardson, V.C.G. (2003) *Diseases of Small Domestic Rodents.* Blackwell Publishers, Oxford.

Hematopoietic and Lymphoid Conditions

Donnelly, T.M. (2004) Disease problems of chinchillas. In: *Ferrets, Rabbits and Rodents: Clinical Medicine and Surgery* (eds. K.E. Quesenberry and J.W. Carpenter), 2nd edn. Saunders, St. Louis, MO.

Greenacre, C.B. (2001) Spontaneous tumors of small mammals. *Veterinary Clinics of North America: Exotic Animal Practice*, 7(3), 627–651.

Newberne PM, and Seibold HR. (1953. Malignant lymphoma in a chinchilla. *Veterinary Medicine*, **48**, 428–429.

Ophthalmic Conditions

Brookhyser, K.M., Aulerich, R.J., and Vomachka, A.J. (1977) Adaptation of the orbital sinus bleeding technique to the chinchilla (*Chinchilla lanigera*). *Laboratory Animal Science*, 27(2), 251–254.

Derbaudrenghien, V., Van Caelenberg, A., Hermans, K., Gielen, I., and Martel, A. (2010) Dental pathology in chinchillas. *Vlaams Diergeneeskundig Tijdschrift*, **79**, 345–358.

Donnelly, T.M. (2004) Disease problems of chinchillas. In: *Ferrets, Rabbits and Rodents: Clinical Medicine and Surgery* (eds. K.E. Quesenberry and J.W. Carpenter), 2nd edn. Saunders, St. Louis, MO.

Holmberg, B.J., Hollingsworth, S.R., Osofsky, A., and Tell, L.A. (2007) *Taenia coenurus* in the orbit of a chinchilla. *Veterinary Ophthalmology*, **10**(1), 53–59.

Kern, T.J. (1997) Rabbit and rodent ophthalmology. *Seminars in Avian and Exotic Pet Medicine*, **6**(3), 138–145.

Mauler, D., Lübke-Becker, A., and Eule, C. (2009) Ocular findings in healthy chinchillidae. *Veterinary Ophthalmology*, **12**(6), 387.

Müller, K., Mauler, D.A., and Eule, J.C. (2010) Reference values for selected ophthalmic diagnostic tests and clinical characteristics of chinchilla eyes (*Chinchilla lanigera*). *Veterinary Ophthalmology*, **13**(Suppl 1), 29–34.

Müller, K., and Eule, J.C. (2014) Ophthalmic disorders observed in pet chinchillas (*Chinchilla lanigera*). *Journal of Exotic Pet Medicine*, **23**(2), 201–205.

Montiani-Ferreira, F. (2009) Major ophthalmic disorders in exotic animals. *Proceedings of 34th World Small Animal Vet Association*, São Paulo, Brazil.

Peiffer, R.L., and Johnson, P.T. (1980) Clinical ocular findings in a colony of chinchillas (*Chinchilla lanigera*). *Laboratory Animals (UK)*. 14(4), 331–5.

Teague Self, J., and Murphy, C.E. (1954) Hydatid disease in chinchillas, *NCBA Research Bulletin*, Oct (**2**).

Van der Woerdt, A. (2004) Ophthalmologic diseases in small pet animals. In: *Ferrets, Rabbits and Rodents: Clinical Medicine and Surgery* (eds. K.E. Quesenberry and J.W. Carpenter), 2nd edn. Saunders, St. Louis, MO.

Wideman, W.L. (2006) *Pseudomonas aeruginosa* otitis media and interna in a chinchilla ranch. *Canadian Veterinary Journal*. 47(8), 799–800.

Wohlsein, P., Thiele, A., Fehr, M., Haas, L., Henneicke, K., Petzold, D.R., and Baumgärtner, W. (2002) Spontaneous human herpes virus type 1 infection in a chinchilla (*Chinchilla lanigera f. dom.*). *Acta Neuropathol.* **104**(6), 674–678.

5

Rats

5.1   Introduction

Wild rats have had a close but often uneasy relationship with man for thousands of years. They are highly intelligent and resourceful omnivorous animals that can subsist on a wide range of foods and successfully adapt to live in almost any space fit for human habitation, including seagoing vessels and airplanes. While there are many species of rats worldwide, in Western Europe and North America, most domesticated rats have been derived from the Brown Norway rat (*Rattus norvegicus*) or brown rat, which likely migrated to Europe from Asia in the mid to late 1600s. The brown rat eventually dominated and outcompeted the smaller, indigenous black rat (*Rattus rattus*), which is best known for transmitting bubonic plague throughout Europe via *Yersinia pestis*-infected fleas that they carried. Today, the black rat is found more commonly in subtropical and tropical regions.

Rats have been feared and maligned for centuries as purveyors of pestilence and disease, and consequently have been hunted, trapped, and killed as vermin, for sport, and for food. Despite this, because they are small and relatively easy to keep, and are also highly inquisitive and charming animals, it is inevitable that many were domesticated and kept as pets from very early times. As for mice, rats with different coat colors have always been kept as unusual specimens and bred by hobbyists, eventually leading to the formation of fancy rat clubs in the United Kingdom and Europe in the nineteenth century and in the United States in the twentieth century. There are seven varieties of rats recognized by the American Fancy Rat and Mouse Association today (http://www.afrma.org/), each of which is organized into six subgroups based on body markings and coat color.

The use of rats in research, and in particular, the use of albino rats, increased exponentially in the early twentieth century. They remain the rodent model of choice for many toxicology and psychology studies, and their use may increase further with development of specific genetic engineering technologies that permit study of various biologic mechanisms in a larger rodent model.

Depending on the study outcomes, some of these animals may be adopted out to homes as pets once research projects have been completed. In addition to being kept as pets and used in research, hundreds of thousands of rats are bred each year for use as feeder animals for various species that are kept in private and public collections, including captive reptiles, birds, and small carnivores. While some rat species, such as the giant pouched Gambian rat (*Cricetomys gambianis*), are used today as working animals for bomb and explosives sniffing as well as human tuberculosis infection detection, these are completely different species from the brown rat. There may be some overlap in diseases experienced by domesticated brown rats and these more exotic rat species; however, a discussion of specific disease conditions of exotic species of rats is beyond the scope of this book.

The diverse sources of rats received for pathologic investigation must be considered by the pathologist and will assist in interpretation of disease conditions and in making appropriate colony and public health recommendations. Traditionally, pet rats came from pet stores supplied by local breeders or by fancy rat hobbyists; settings in which animals are housed conventionally (that is, in open-topped cages breathing shared room air) but typically in modest numbers, and in which background infectious diseases and parasites are common. Today, many of these animals may be sent to large, exotic animal distribution centers by rodent breeders before being shipped to pet stores around the country. Infections more common in other rodents may be transmitted to rats under these settings and transportation stress may exacerbate underlying infectious disease. Rats acquired from research facilities are usually specific pathogen-free inbred or outbred animals. While these rats may be free of many infectious and parasitic diseases common in conventionally raised animals, inbred rats can be more susceptible to developing certain tumors as they age. For that reason, some references pertinent to laboratory rats have been provided as a resource in this chapter. Feeder rat breeding is often conducted on a

Pathology of Small Mammal Pets, First Edition. Patricia V. Turner, Marina L. Brash and Dale A. Smith.
© 2018 John Wiley & Sons, Inc. Published 2018 by John Wiley & Sons, Inc.

massive scale involving tens of thousands of animals with less attention paid to environmental hygiene and management than in research facilities. Feeder rat breeders are likely to tolerate moderate disease and mortality levels not accepted by fancy rat or laboratory rat breeders. Wild rodents are common pests in these operations and may spread infectious diseases to colony animals that are not commonly seen in captive rats, thus some knowledge of wild rat diseases is also required. Finally, rat rescue societies are becoming increasingly common and the unknown background and history of these animals make it imperative for the pathologist to consider diseases and conditions more common in feral animals, including those with important public health implications.

When submitting rat specimens for pathology investigations samples should be sent as soon after death as possible. Cadavers may be sent chilled (never frozen!) or if shipping will be delayed, the thoracic and abdominal cavities can be opened and the body or selected tissues placed in formalin at a ratio of 10 parts neutral buffered formalin to 1 part tissue. Plastic containers of formalinized specimens should always be sealed in a bag or other waterproof outer wrapping, and then securely padded and packaged in a box to prevent leakage during shipment.

5.2 Integument Conditions

Pet and show rats come with a wide variety of coat colors and hair types, including rex, wavy, and hairless. The rex (*Re*) hair coat has been recently evaluated in rats and linked to a keratin mutation on chromosome 7. Rex is a dominant mutation and hair follicles in these animals are dilated, and hairs have an irregular cuticular pattern, resulting in short, wavy hairs and vibrissae of reduced diameter. Hairless varieties of pet rats also exist and have increased sensitivity to changes in ambient temperature and mechanical irritation. These animals have early hair loss (hypotrichosis), abnormally keratinized hairs, and are immunocompetent. They have different underlying mutations than those seen in nude, athymic (immunodeficient) rats found in research settings.

Interestingly, as for other domestic species, coat color is linked to temperament in rats, with milder, more docile temperaments generally linked to mutations or dilutions of the wild-type agouti coat. This occurs because proteins expressed by the agouti locus are melanocortin receptor antagonists, which affects coat color, satiation and body weight, and aspects of behavior.

Rats have several different hair types, including at least three types of guard hairs and a fine undercoat hair. Hair growth in rats occurs in waves from head to tail and ventral to dorsal, with different rates noted for different

hair types. Longer guard hairs grow faster and for a longer period of time than do shorter hairs. There are also sex, age, and breed-related differences in hair growth patterns in rats.

5.2.1 Alopecia

Nonpruritic spontaneous alopecia is uncommon in pet rats, except in animals with hereditary hypotrichosis, in which permanent hair loss is expected. Hair chewing (barbering) of self or others may be seen in singly- or group-housed rats and is histologically identified by normal follicular structures and an intact epithelium with hair broken off at the skin surface, and a lack of underlying inflammation. Immune-mediated alopecia areata is reported in certain strains of rats in research environments but has not been described in pets. Dietary deficiencies are uncommon in well-tended animals fed a balanced, pelleted commercial diet. Poor hair coat and scaliness with or without greying of fur (loss of pigmentation) may occur in rats with zinc or vitamin B deficiencies, and a dietary history should be obtained, if suspected. Mechanical loss of hair from abrasion on feeders or cage materials can be seen and can lead to abscessation if the epithelium is penetrated. Epidermal atrophy with dermal fibrosis may be seen in rats undergoing treatment with various oncology chemotherapeutics.

Differential diagnoses for alopecia with pruritus include external parasitism, dermatophytosis, bacterial dermatitis, hyperadrenocorticism (see Section 5.3), neoplasia, and hypersensitivity reactions. A biopsy of the affected section will often assist with determining the etiology of the alopecia.

5.2.2 Bacterial Dermatitis and Abscesses

5.2.2.1 Ulcerative Dermatitis

Ulcerative dermatitis may be seen sporadically in rats, occasionally as an epizootic with moderate morbidity. Animals may be mildly pruritic and present with irregular areas of ulceration and crusting, generally over the neck and shoulder area. Evaluation of microscopic sections demonstrates deep erosion or ulceration of the affected skin, which is overlain by a serocellular crust containing dense colonies of Gram-positive coccoid bacteria. *Staphylococcus aureus* is commonly isolated from these lesions. As for humans and other animal species, *S. aureus* is a common inhabitant of the skin of rats, generally producing no clinical signs. It is thought that the initiating factor in ulcerative dermatitis is self-excoriation or other trauma with secondary bacterial contamination from the toenails or surrounding skin. This bacterium has recently been demonstrated to produce a delta toxin, which leads to mast cell degranulation in the skin of

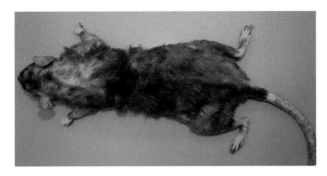

Figure 5.1 Seborrhea (yellow oily appearance to skin and tail) with flaking skin in an aged rat.

humans and mice, contributing to severe atopic dermatitis in both species. It is unknown whether this reaction occurs in rats, but if so, it may contribute to the refractory nature of staphylococcal skin infections in rats.

Differential diagnoses for cutaneous ulcerations include mechanical abrasion and fighting injuries. Mild pruritus may also be seen with some ectoparasites and in cases of dermatophytosis. Rarely, perianal itching may occur secondary to heavy pinworm infestation (see Section 5.6.4.5).

5.2.2.2 Abscesses and Other Bacterial Skin Conditions

Abscesses are uncommon in rats but may occur secondarily to traumatic skin lesions, for example, from injury or fighting (Figure 5.2). Abscesses appear as firm to fluctuant localized swellings, usually on the head and upper torso areas. Preputial and clitoral gland abscesses are

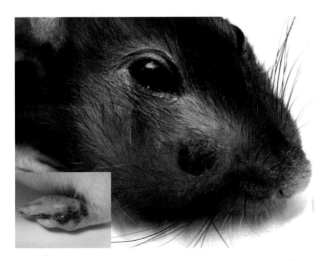

Figure 5.2 Facial abscess in a pet rat. These are less commonly associated with tooth root abscesses and more often the result of fighting or infected microabrasions from cage or feeder irregularities. Inset: Severe staphylococcal foot infection arising from a cagemate's bite. *Source:* Courtesy of The Links Road Animal and Bird Clinic.

seen from time to time in rats. These may be ventral soft or firm swellings near the genital papilla and may arise secondarily to local trauma or bite wounds. More common bacterial agents cultured from cutaneous abscesses of pet rats include *Staphylococcus aureus*, *Streptobacillus moniliformis*, *Corynebacterium kutscheri*, and *Pasteurella pneumotropica*. The first three of these agents may induce a gangrenous pododermatitis, characterized by painful and marked swelling and erythema of the affected extremity with subsequent ischemia and coagulation necrosis. The inciting injury may not always be obvious, and all four feet may be affected.

5.2.3 Dermatophytosis

Dermatophytosis (ringworm) is not seen commonly in rats as a clinical condition. The disease is caused by infection with the saphrophytic zoophilic organism, *Trichophyton mentagrophytes*, a keratinophilic fungus. Subclinical infection can occur, and the condition may manifest following stress or immunosuppression. Animals present with patchy alopecia and nonpruritic to mildly pruritic scaling lesions on the head or back or on the limbs. Skin scrapings or biopsies of affected areas will demonstrate broken hairs and hair shafts and follicles infiltrated by fungal hyphae and arthrospores. The condition is zoonotic, and arthroconidia may persist within the environment.

Differential diagnoses include mechanical trauma, parasitic alopecia, and barbering. Rats do not appear to be significant carriers of dermatophytes compared with other small mammal species, such as chinchillas and guinea pigs.

5.2.4 External Parasites

Dermatologic problems are the primary reason for client presentation of small mammal pets for veterinary examinations, and, of those visits, over 40% are for pruritus. Over 86% of exotic animal pruritus cases are reported to be due to parasitic infestations, demonstrating the high prevalence of these infestations in the pet rodent population. External parasites are also very common in commercial feeder breeding operations, and infestations may be very heavy at times, causing severe debilitation and even death of infant animals from anemia. Rats are susceptible to a number of specific mites, fleas, lice, and ticks, but may be infested with parasites from other companion animal species. Cuterebriasis has rarely been reported in rats that spend time outdoors (see Rabbits, Chapter 1, 1.2.4.4).

5.2.4.1 Fur and Ear Mites

Radfordia ensifera (suborder Prostigmata) is a common fur mite of rats and feeds on superficial secretions and skin debris without piercing the skin. The prepatent period for this mite is approximately one week, and the life cycle occurs entirely on the host, although eggs may be shed into the environment. Although some infestations may be asymptomatic, a hypersensitivity reaction commonly develops towards mite allergens, resulting in mild to intensive pruritus with alopecia, erythema, focal erosions or ulcerations, and secondary bacterial infections. In heavy infestations, the mite can be visualized by pressing a piece of cellophane tape on the dorsum and then examining for mites and eggs. Otherwise, combing or nontraumatic scraping and evaluation of the collected skin debris are used for diagnosis. Skin biopsies may be nondiagnostic because the mite lives on the skin surface and may be dislodged during trimming or fixation. Histologic examination occasionally demonstrates mites on the skin surface with or without accompanying inflammation in the underlying skin. The mite is not zoonotic.

Notoedres muris is a burrowing mange mite found most frequently on the pinnae, nose, and tail, where it induces proliferative, nodular, and disfiguring dermatitis with intense pruritus (Figure 5.3). Lesions on the tail of albino animals may appear as numerous pinpoint raised red papules. Diagnosis requires deep skin scrapings or biopsy, examination of which demonstrates marked parakeratotic hyperkeratosis with mites, eggs, and excreta embedded in deep epithelial tunnels. There is generally a moderate mixed, predominantly neutrophilic infiltrate in the surrounding stratum corneum, as well as in the underlying dermis.

Ornithonyssus bacoti, the tropical rat mite, is a hematophagous mite that is found worldwide and has a temperature-dependent life cycle (e.g., approximately

10 days at 25°C). The mite can live off the host for periods of up to 10 days. The mite is relatively long-lived, up to 26 weeks, and is uncommon in pet rats but may be found on other rodent species, including wild rodents and pet mice. Large populations of these mites have been found sporadically in research facilities, for example, laboratory mouse breeding colonies infested with wild vermin. The mite occasionally will infest humans with moderate resultant pruritus and even debilitation, depending on arachnid density and age of the infested human host. Environmental management is important in eliminating these mites because females drop off the host after a blood meal, and eggs, intermediate forms, and adults may be found in the environment. *O. bacoti* are barely discernible to the unaided eye and are mobile, with four pairs of legs, like other rat mites, but the legs are longer and these mites have more obvious mouthparts (chelicerae and pedipalp) compared with surface dwelling fur mites or burrowing mange mites. Cellophane tape imprints of the dorsal pelage and skin scrapings may or may not be useful for detection of these mites because of their opportunistic life cycle. Experimentally, the mite has been shown to transmit rodent and human rickettsial organisms; however, these infections have not been documented to occur naturally in rats.

Other mites seen rarely on rats include *Sarcoptes scabei* and *Trixacarus* spp. *Laelaps echidnina*, the spiny rat mite, is found commonly on wild rats and rarely in house mice but the mite is not reported on pet rats. The potential for these mites to be seen in commercial feeder rat operations has not been studied.

Differential diagnoses for mite infestations include other ectoparasitic infestations, ulcerative dermatitis, and various hypersensitivity reactions. *Notoedres muris* infestations may appear grossly similar to auricular chondritis lesions, although the former are typically more discrete, with crusting.

5.2.4.2 Lice, Fleas and Ticks

Polyplax spinulosa is an anopluran, hematophagean louse found occasionally on pet and wild rats. Infested animals may present with alopecia, pruritus, excoriations, crusting, and in severe infestations, anemia and debilitation (Figure 5.4). *P. spinulosa* has an obligate 26-day life cycle on the rat host, although hairs with attached nits occasionally may be shed into the environment, and adults more commonly are infested than are preweaned pups. Transmission between rats occurs through direct contact or via contact with infested bedding materials and infestations are highly host specific but not zoonotic. *P. spinulosa* may be seen with the unaided eye as long, slender, white, dorsoventrally flattened arachnids up to 1.5 mm in length, and moving within the hair coat. Eggs (nits) are cemented to the base of the hair shaft and

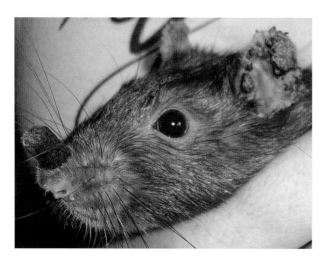

Figure 5.3 *Notoedres muris* infestation in a rat causing crusting and disfiguration of the ears. A large keratinized papilloma is present on the nose of this animal. *Source:* Courtesy of D. Ducommun.

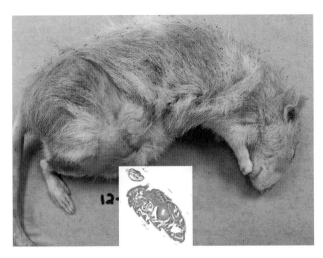

Figure 5.4 Severe *Polyplax spinulosa* (inset) infestation (seen as dark spots on the tips of hairs in this animal) with debilitation in a female rat. Heavy parasitic burdens may result in anemia, as in this animal.

hatch approximately 6 days after being laid. As per fur mites, lice will move off an animal's pelage within 30 minutes of death and may be seen in the debris within the bag or container in which the animal was submitted. Lice and eggs can be found on skin biopsies in heavy infestations. *P. spinulosa* has been shown to transmit *Mycoplasma haemomuris* (*Haemobartonella muris*), a bacterium that infects erythrocytes and induces murine hemobartonellosis.

Fleas may be seen occasionally on pet rats and are moderately common on wild rats. Affected animals may present with pruritus, hair loss, and excoriations with crusting. Fleas and their eggs may be found within the nesting material and animal environment, necessitating thorough decontamination when infestations are discovered. The northern rat flea, *Nosopsyllus fasciatus*, is prevalent in North American and Western European feral rats, mice and other rodents, and may transmit murine typhus (*Rickettsia typhi*) and plague-inducing organisms (*Yersinia pestis*), both of which induce serious infections in humans. The fleas may also bite other pet species. Flea species from pet rodents are rarely typed and it is difficult to know which species are more prevalent. Wild rodents should always be excluded from commercial rat feeder operations to minimize parasite and other disease agent transmission between feral and domestic animals and human caregivers.

Ticks are rarely seen on pet rats and are transmitted by direct contact to animals that spend time outdoors in infested areas. More commonly, ticks may be acquired from purchased bedding, typically wood shavings, that have been contaminated at source. Although there are no published reports of Lyme disease in pet rats, rats are experimentally susceptible to *Borrelia burgdorferi*

infection, and wild rodents are considered to be a natural reservoir for the spirochete in North America.

5.2.4.3 Laboratory Diagnostics

Small pet rodents are commonly treated by their owners using parasiticidal products intended for other larger pet species, instead of being presented to veterinarians for a further evaluation and diagnosis. Thus, the exact nature of the infestation may be difficult for the pathologist to determine retrospectively. The approach to diagnostic investigation for all rat ectoparasites is similar to that for other small mammal pet species, involving a thorough examination of the pelage, combings, and superficial scrapings of the skin. Detection of burrowing mite infestations requires deeper scrapings, as for cats and dogs. Microscopic evaluation of skin biopsies or post mortem specimens may or not be diagnostic for many superficially dwelling rodent ectoparasites and may show only nonspecific focal to multifocal ulcerations with serocellular crusting and mixed, predominantly neutrophilic superficial infiltrates.

5.2.4.4 Colony Management

Thorough environmental decontamination should always be recommended for ectoparasite infestations. This can be very difficult to achieve in extensive feeder rat breeding operations, in which cages may be placed on unfinished wood surfaces in buildings with dirt floors. Ensuring that housing and holding areas are constructed of watertight, readily sanitizable, impervious materials, and that cracks and gaps are sealed, will assist with this process. With the exceptions noted in the previous section, most rat ectoparasites are highly host-specific and infest other animals and humans only on a temporary basis. Rats are susceptible to ectoparasite infestations from wild rodents and from other pet species.

5.2.5 Mastitis

Mastitis is an uncommon condition of lactating female rats and presents as single or multiple painful, erythematous indurations on the ventral or ventrolateral aspect of the body. Lesions may range from acute and necrotizing to chronic and granulomatous, with mineralization and necrosis of the overlying skin. Organisms isolated from affected animals include coagulase positive *Staphylococcus aureus* and *Pasteurella pneumotropica*.

5.2.6 Pododermatitis

Pododermatitis with subsequent erosion or ulceration may occur in rats, particularly in heavy animals housed on wire, on rough, abrasive surfaces or in animals maintained in unhygienic conditions. As per other species, hyperkeratosis of the foot pad may precede erosion

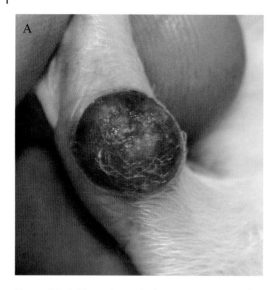
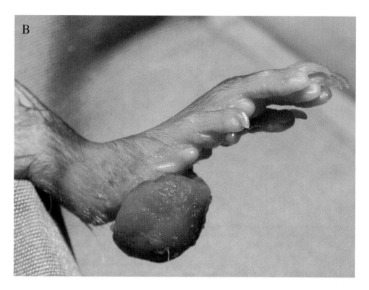

Figure 5.5 A: Ulcerative pododermatitis is commonly seen in larger, heavier animals housed on wire bottom floors. B: Fibroma on the foot of a rat prior to surgical excision. *Source:* A and B: Courtesy of The Links Road Animal and Bird Clinic.

and ulceration (Figure 5.5A). Secondary infections with opportunistic bacteria, such as *Staphylococcus aureus*, may occur, making these lesions difficult to resolve in the long term.

5.2.7 Cutaneous Masses and Neoplasia

Older rats may exhibit a variety of skin and associated adnexal masses. Mammary tumors are the most common tumor of female rats, with an incidence up to 57% (higher in certain inbred strains of rats used in biomedical research). Virus-induced mammary tumors are less common in rats than in mice. Common nonviral non-neoplastic cutaneous or adnexal masses seen in rats include mammary gland fibroadenoma, clitoral and preputial gland adenoma, keratoacanthoma (Figure 5.6A), trichoepithelioma, fibroma (Figure 5.5B), lipoma and hibernoma, hemangioma, Zymbal's gland adenoma, basal cell tumor (Figure 5.6B), histiocytoma, and hemangiopericytoma. Malignant cutaneous masses include mammary gland adenocarcinoma, squamous cell carcinoma, malignant melanoma, Zymbal's gland adenoma and adenocarcinoma, and fibrosarcoma. There is a single report of epitheliotropic lymphoma (mycosis fungoides) in a rat, and the condition is considered uncommon in this species.

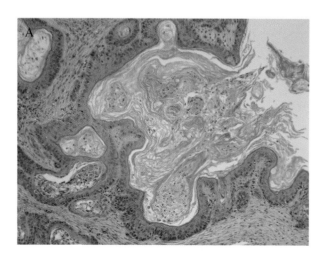
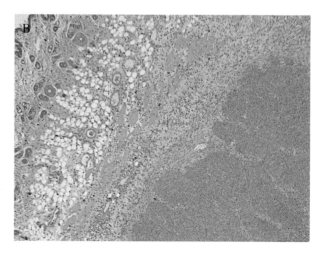

Figure 5.6 A: Tissue from a periorbital mass in a rat. The multiloculated keratin-filled cysts have an irregular outer wall composed of squamous epithelium with a prominent basal cell layer, stratum spinosum and granular cell layer and superficial layer of keratinizing epithelium and there are mild mixed, subepithelial inflammatory cell infiltrates. These findings are consistent with a keratoacanthoma. B: Basal cell tumor presenting as a neck mass in a rat. Microscopically, the well encapsulated, multilobular dermal mass is composed of polygonal cells arranged in cords and islands with no evidence of invasion.

Virus-induced squamous papillomas may be seen in rats, often on the pinna, and may be solitary or multiple. Rats have a unique papilloma virus, classified as a Pipapillomavirus, which is host specific and not transmissible to humans. Lesions are self-limiting and often resolve without treatment.

Cowpox is reported to be transmitted from pet rats to humans in Europe, inducing a localized maculopapular rash and vesicles with subsequent ulceration and scarring in human caregivers in contact with infected animals. Definitive diagnosis is made by PCR confirmation of virus in exudates. Lesions in infected rats have not been well described but include dry crusty lesions on the extremities, respiratory disease, and death. A consistent history of animal acquisition from pet stores shortly before illness in the pet rats and humans suggests that rats may acquire the virus during holding at exotic animal distributors or at large, extensive breeding operations. The natural reservoir for cowpox virus is thought to be wild rodents, which may be asymptomatic and yet shed the virus for prolonged periods. In addition, feral rats have been shown to be susceptible experimentally to foot and mouth disease virus infection. Wild rodents should always be excluded from rodent breeding facilities and distribution centers.

5.2.7.1 Mammary Gland Tumors

Tumors of the mammary gland may be benign or malignant, with the former being more common in female rats and malignant tumors predominating in males. Susceptibility to mammary gland tumors is heritable with high incidence in certain strains and lines. Tumors are seen predominantly in female rats over one year of age, with an incidence of <3% reported in aged males. Tumor induction and growth are strongly hormonally responsive. Significantly fewer tumors are seen in ovariectomized rats and fewer tumors are seen in nulliparous animals. Higher circulating prolactin levels have been documented in female rats with mammary gland tumors and mammary tumors are also common in rats with concurrent prolactin-secreting pituitary adenomas. Dietary restriction leads to a reduction in mammary tumors in female rats, likely secondary to occurrence of pituitary gland hyperplasia and the associated reductions in circulating prolactin levels. Mammary gland tissue is extensive in an adult animal and masses may be found anywhere on the ventrum to ventrolateral aspect, ranging up the side of the neck and tail head.

Cystic hyperplasia is a frequent change seen in the mammary glands of older rats and is characterized by single or multiple dilated glands or ducts lined by flattened epithelium and containing fluid and precipitated protein within the lumen. Glandular hyperplasia, periductal fibrosis, and mild inflammation may also be present.

There are many types of mammary tumors in rats and they are classified according to involvement of epithelial components, stroma or both. Fibroadenomas are the most common form of mammary gland tumor in rats (Figure 5.7). Diagnostic features include firm, well-defined, encapsulated, multilobular masses composed of proliferating, well differentiated ductal and lobular structures separated by dense fibrous connective tissue. Proteinaceous secretory exudate may be present within acini and ducts. These tumors may grow very large and ulcerate but are readily removed at surgery. They may recur in intact animals or in animals with prolactin-secreting pituitary tumors, which occur more commonly in intact females, thus concurrent ovariohysterectomy or ovariectomy are recommended for long-term management.

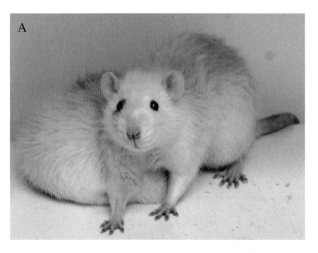
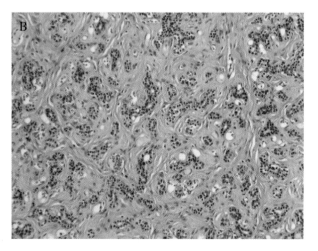

Figure 5.7 A: Mammary fibroadenomas in a pet rat. Tumors can become very large and interfere with locomotion. B: Microscopically, the encapsulated mass is composed of well differentiated acinar cells separated by a dense fibrovascular stroma. *Source:* A: Courtesy of The Links Road Animal and Bird Clinic.

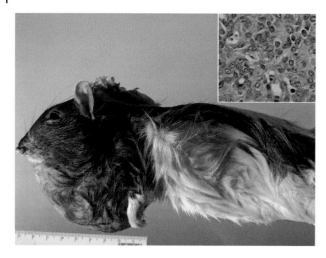

Figure 5.8 Cervical soft tissue sarcoma in a rat. Inset: Microscopically, the unencapsulated mass is composed of whorls, streams, and bundles of spindle cells within a mild to moderate fibrovascular stroma. Neoplastic cells have well-defined cell borders, moderate amounts of eosinophilic cytoplasm, single round to oval-shaped nuclei, up to five-fold anisocytosis and anisokaryosis, and up to 16 mitoses/ten 400x fields.

Mammary carcinomas and adenocarcinomas occur significantly less commonly in female rats (<17%) than benign tumors, but they constitute the majority of mammary tumors seen in male rats. These tumors may become very large and ulcerate, with necrosis, hemorrhage, and mineralization seen microscopically. Although generally well circumscribed, late in their growth cycle, these tumors can invade locally into the mammary fat pad, surrounding skin, and muscle. The lungs are the most common site of metastases.

Differential diagnoses for mammary gland masses include abscesses, fibromas or fibrosarcomas (Figure 5.8), lymphosarcomas, and lipomas. Cervical tumors should be differentiated from salivary gland masses. Multiple mammary gland tumors may be present in the same individual, and both benign and malignant tumors may be present concurrently. Surgical excision with histopathologic characterization of all masses is recommended for prognostication.

5.2.7.2 Keratoacanthoma

Keratoacanthomas are moderately common, benign epithelial tumors of aging rats and may be seen on the face, legs or trunk. The masses appear as horn-like proliferations or as firm to ulcerated masses with a central channel from which keratinaceous debris may be expressed (see Figures 5.6A). Histologically, the affected epithelium may be overlain by a thick, irregular, keratinaceous proliferation or they can appear crater-like with one or more cystic spaces containing keratin and exfoliated cellular

debris communicating with a central pore. The epithelial lining may be thickened, folded, and hyperkeratotic with marked keratohyaline granule accumulation, and if self-induced trauma occurs, there may be concurrent locally extensive inflammation. Unlike keratoacanthomas in humans, it is rare for these tumors to progress to squamous cell carcinomas in rats.

5.2.7.3 Squamous Cell Carcinoma

Squamous cell carcinoma is an invasive malignant tumor that involves the epithelium, dermis, and other adnexal structures. These tumors may be found anywhere on the body, as well as in association with internal epithelial tissues. Jumbling and irregularity of epithelial cell layers are common with focal to coalescing nests of pleiomorphic malignant cells present in the dermis and hypodermis. Keratin production may be scant or abundant with multifocal keratin pearl formation. Larger masses may become necrotic with associated inflammation. Mitoses are variable, and more aggressive tumors can metastasize to local lymph nodes and lungs.

5.2.7.4 Zymbal's Gland Hyperplasia and Neoplasia

Zymbal's glands are modified sebaceous (holocrine) glands subtending the epithelium within the ventrolateral aspect of the external ear canal. The paired structures are best viewed microscopically via a transverse section through the decalcified skull just rostral to the external ear canals. Glandular hyperplasia, adenoma, and (adeno-) carcinoma may be uni- or bilateral, and identified clinically as localized swellings on the side of the face with or without ulceration, bleeding from the ear, head tilt or head shaking (Figure 5.9). Cystic hyperplasia of the glands can be seen at times with occasional discharge of inspissated sebaceous debris into the external ear canal. Malignancies are classified on the basis of predominantly involving glandular (adenocarcinoma) or ductal (carcinoma) structures and tumors are generally locally invasive with a poor prognosis. A marked inflammatory response with fibroplasia and necrosis can be seen in traumatized or ulcerated tumors.

5.2.7.5 Melanoma

Melanomas, both pigmented and amelanotic, occur sporadically in aging rats, and are described using criteria as for other small companion animals. Amelanotic melanoma is seen as a single firm pale mass, most frequently on the pinnae, palpebrae, perianal skin, and scrotum of rats. Tumors (Figure 5.10) are well circumscribed but unencapsulated and may invade surrounding tissue. Neoplastic cells are spindloid, with abundant pale eosinophilic cytoplasm, and form interlacing perivascular bundles. Anaplasia and mitoses occur variably. Whereas the incidence of this tumor type is low, it has been misdiagnosed

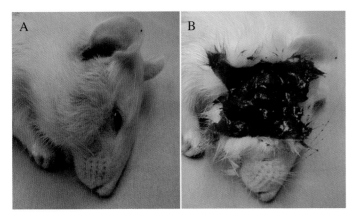
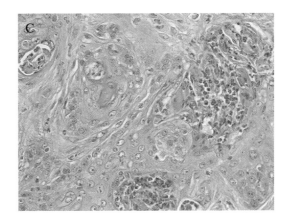

Figure 5.9 A: Facial swelling in a rat with a Zymbal's gland tumor. Hemorrhagic exudate can be seen in the external ear canal. B: The invasive and hemorrhagic nature of the mass is seen with skin reflection. C: These tumors often incite marked neutrophilic infiltrates and necrosis. *Source:* A and B: Courtesy of L. Martin.

historically as a fibroma or Schwannoma. In up to 19% of reported cases of amelanotic melanoma, the tumor metastasized to the lungs, making accurate diagnosis critical for long-term prognosis. Both immunohistochemistry for S-100 protein labeling and electron microscopy to confirm the presence of intracytoplasmic premelanosomes have been used to confirm suspect cases.

5.2.8 Other Skin Conditions

Seborrhea and red discoloration of the pelage are common in aging male rats and may be related to reduced grooming. The hair coat may appear greasy with an accumulation of yellow scales on the skin and tail (Figure 5.1).

Tail necrosis (ringtail) can be seen as a spontaneous condition in preweaned and young weaned rats. It is characterized grossly as one or more annular constrictions of the tail, often with erythema and edema, followed

later by dry necrosis of the portion distal to the annular constriction, likely due to ischemic necrosis (Figure 5.11). The pathogenesis is not completely understood but the condition has been correlated with low environmental humidity, low ambient temperatures, animal hydration status, and genetics. For both rats and mice, the tail has an important thermoregulatory function, with sympathetic nerve-mediated vasoconstriction that is closely linked to the core body temperature. Experimentally, complete occlusion of blood flow to the tail occurs when rectal temperatures approach 37°C. If this condition is prolonged, it is quite possible that tail ischemia might occur. Microscopically, epidermal acanthosis and hyperkeratosis are seen overlying areas of annular construction early in the course of the disease, followed by vascular dilatation, and regional necrosis with focal, predominantly suppurative infiltrates. The condition is seen more commonly in winter months and

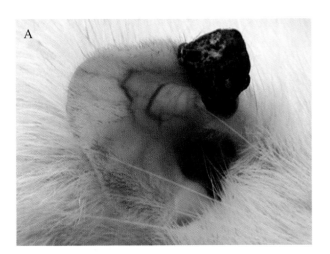
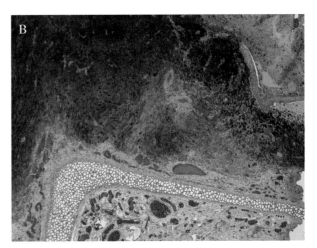

Figure 5.10 A: Highly pigmented melanoma of the pinna. B: The mass is relatively well localized, unencapsulated, and composed of highly pigmented spindle cells. *Source:* A: Courtesy of The Links Road Animal and Bird Clinic.

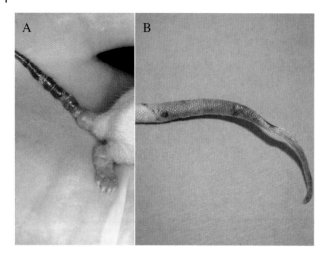

Figure 5.11 A: Tail necrosis in a preweaned rat pup. The pathogenesis of the condition is unknown but it tends to occur more commonly in cold, dry environments. B: Tail necrosis may also result from perivascular injection of irritating substances or excessive application of heat to the tail. *Source* B: Courtesy of C. Wheler.

not all animals in a litter are affected. Re-evaluation of husbandry conditions should be advised when the condition is seen.

Tail degloving injuries (tail slip) may occur when animals are restrained by the distal half of the tail. This is an escape mechanism for a prey species and may be treated by amputation of the exposed tissue.

Auricular chondritis can be seen as a spontaneous, non-pruritic condition of rats. Lesions are usually bilateral and may be initiated by ear tag placement, with subsequent involvement of the contralateral untagged ear. Affected ears are erythematous and uniformly thickened (cauliflower ear) or have multifocal, small, pale, firm, subcutaneous nodules on their edges. Microscopically, chondrolysis is seen with multifocal to coalescing granulomatous inflammation, nodular cartilage proliferation, and osseous metaplasia. The overlying epidermis is normal. In ear-tagged animals, lesions may spontaneously resolve with removal of the ear tag. Differential diagnoses include fibromas, amelanotic melanoma, and chondroma.

Cutaneous hypersensitivity reactions are anecdotally reported in rats and may occur in response to contact with irritating substances within the environment, including air fresheners, detergents, and volatile oils from softwood shavings used as bedding. Histology findings are nonspecific and may consist of mild edema, alopecia, and superficial nonsuppurative perivascular inflammation.

5.3 Endocrine Conditions

Rats are susceptible to a range of endocrine-related diseases and tumors; however, these are recognized infrequently and often not treated in pet animals. Increased age, unlimited daily caloric intake, and obesity underpin many of these conditions, as for other species. The pathogenesis of metabolic disease is likely related to altered gene expression patterns for lipid and glucose regulation in animals with unrestricted access to food. Sex and strain or breed are also important disease predisposition determinants for endocrine conditions; however, genetic background can be much more difficult to ascertain in pet rats.

Pancreatic islets in rats and other rodents may be variably sized, with up to eight-fold variation in volume. There is no compression of surrounding parenchyma by these normal islets. They are not correlated with a change in function or hormonal secretion variation and are interpreted as incidental.

5.3.1 Diabetes Mellitus

Diabetes mellitus is reported uncommonly in pet rats and affected animals demonstrate increased drinking, urination, and glucosuria. There are several research rat strains, including the BB and fatty Zucker, which develop the condition spontaneously. Whereas disease onset may occur acutely or be more chronic in nature with an insidious onset, histologic changes in rats with diabetes mellitus often include chronic nonsuppurative interstitial and islet pancreatic inflammation. The disease can rapidly be fatal if left untreated.

5.3.2 Endocrine Neoplasia

5.3.2.1 Pituitary Gland Masses

Glandular hypertrophy or hyperplasia and adenomas are very common in the pars distalis of the anterior pituitary gland, especially in aged nulliparous female rats, where the reported incidence exceeds 60% for certain strains. Breeding females delays the incidence and onset of tumor development. Adenomatous masses tend to expand slowly, resulting in compressive lesions in surrounding neural structures. Owners may report sudden behavioral changes, blindness, seizures, ataxia, paresis or paralysis in animals that appeared otherwise healthy. Lesions may be nodular or diffuse and are often visible grossly as soft, enlarged, hemorrhagic masses on the base of the brain (Figure 5.12). Histologically, areas of hypertrophy consist of well circumscribed, noncompressive, focal to uniform enlargements of parenchymal cells with distinct cell borders and clear cytoplasm, arranged as sheets. Hyperplastic areas may consist of focal dense aggregates of small parenchymal cells. Adenomas are usually unencapsulated but well circumscribed, and are surrounded by a rim of compressed parenchyma. There are several variations seen but all are considered benign, with no evidence of invasion or metastasis. Adenomas

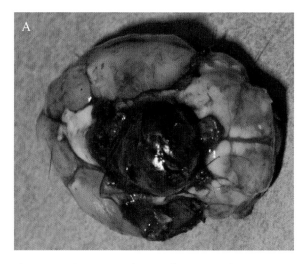 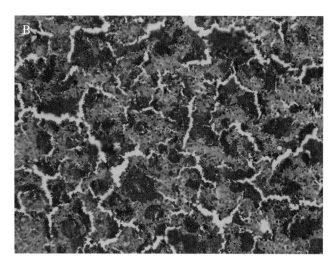

Figure 5.12 A: Pituitary adenoma from an aged rat. B: Microscopically, these tumors are generally benign and consist of polyhedral or ovoid cells arranged in sheets or cords, sometimes surrounded by blood-filled channels. *Source:* Courtesy of L. Tatiersky.

are usually highly cellular and consist of oval or polyhedral cells with large round nuclei arranged in sheets or cords, within a fine fibrovascular stroma. Occasionally, abundant dissecting blood-filled channels are seen throughout the masses. The majority of these adenomas secrete prolactin (also detectable via immunohistochemistry) and this suggestion has been correlated positively with elevated serum prolactin levels as well as with findings of secondary mammary gland fibroadenomas. Some tumors may induce a secondary hydrocephalus following cerebrospinal fluid outflow obstruction. There is no treatment for animals with these tumors other than supportive care.

A mixed pituitary adenoma/gangliocytoma has been reported in a two year-old rat as an incidental finding at necropsy.

5.3.2.2 Adrenal Gland Masses

Adrenal cortical hyperplasia and benign adrenal cortical adenomas are common incidental findings at necropsy, generally found in animals at least 18 months of age. Adenomas may be nodular or diffuse, resulting in compression of other parts of the gland. Masses are largely composed of cells from the zona fasciculata and zona reticularis and the cell populations may be uniform or mixed. Areas of hemorrhage or necrosis may be seen in larger tumors. Carcinomas of the adrenal cortex are reported infrequently in rats.

Pheochromocytomas are also moderately common tumors noted at post mortem. Affected glands may be enlarged or nodular. Most tumors are benign and induce compressive effects on the adjacent cortex. Adrenal medullary ganglioneuroma and neuroblastoma are described rarely in rats.

5.3.2.3 Thyroid and Parathyroid Gland Masses

As in other species, prolonged dietary iodine deficiency or fed goitrogens can lead to thyroid gland hyperplasia, so a dietary history should be obtained whenever thyroid gland masses are observed. Thyroid gland adenomas are very common in certain stocks of laboratory rats but are uncommon in pet rats. These tumors may be encapsulated and consist of colloid-containing follicles of varying sizes lined by densely packed cuboidal epithelium. Papillary infoldings of epithelium may be seen and there is compression of the surrounding thyroid tissue or parathyroid gland. Follicles are sometimes dilated and filled with foamy macrophages or cholesterol clefts. Parafollicular C cell adenomas are reported rarely in pet rats. Thyroid carcinomas are much less common and in these tumors, neoplastic cells penetrate the walls of follicles and may proliferate, replacing colloid. Pulmonary metastases are infrequent.

Parathyroid gland hyperplasia or adenoma is rarely reported in pet rats, however, parathyroid gland hyperplasia with increased serum parathyroid hormone (PTH) levels is commonly noted in laboratory rats with renal disease. Increased gland volume may be seen as early as six months of age in some strains of rats. The condition does not cause changes in serum phosphate or calcium levels, although parathyroid gland hyperplasia is temporally correlated with changes in renal function. Glands may be markedly enlarged, compressing adjacent thyroid tissue.

Other differential diagnoses for cervical swellings include lymphosarcomas, salivary gland tumors, abscesses, and mammary gland tumors.

5.3.2.4 Pancreatic Islet Cell Tumors

Pancreatic islet cell tumors are seen on occasion in pet rats. Tumors present as focal to multifocal pale nodules

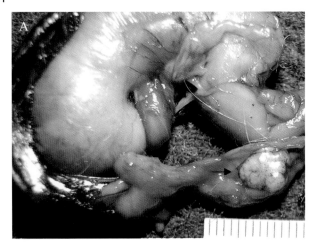
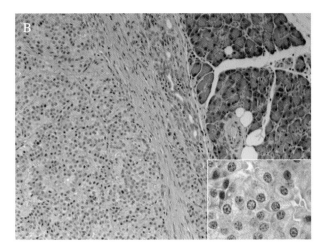

Figure 5.13 A: Pancreatic islet cell tumor (arrow) in an aged rat. B: The mass is encapsulated and compressing the surrounding normal pancreatic tissue. Inset: Tumor cells are polygonal with abundant granular cytoplasm. Tumor cells were immunopositive for both insulin and glucagon.

within the pancreatic mass (Figure 5.13). Microscopically, the masses are encapsulated and consist of packets of polygonal cells with abundant pale eosinophilic, granular cytoplasm and a large central nucleus arranged in nests, separated by a fine, fibrovascular stroma. Metastases have not been reported, and neoplastic cells are largely immunopositive for insulin and glucagon.

5.3.3 Other Endocrine Conditions

Accessory adrenocortical tissue can be found in the perirenal fat or anywhere within the abdominal cavity and the tissue lacks the trilayer of zones seen in normal adrenocortical tissue. This tissue is considered to be congenital and incidental in nature. Lipofuscinosis, focal post-necrotic mineralization, and adrenocortical extramedullary hematopoiesis are also considered incidental findings of the adrenal gland in otherwise healthy animals.

Ectopic thyroid and **parathyroid tissue** can be seen rarely in rats, as well as **ultimobranchial gland cysts**, which are remnants of ultimobranchial bodies from the embryo. These findings are considered to be congenital in origin with no impact on animal health.

Fatty or cystic degeneration of endocrine glands with or without associated hemorrhage is a common aging lesion noted microscopically in rats and is considered incidental.

Pancreatic islet cell hyperplasia, **acinar fibrosis**, and **ductal hyperplasia** with interstitial lymphocytic infiltrates occur spontaneously in aging rats and are usually determined to be an incidental finding.

Severe, lymphoplasmacytic thyroiditis with follicular hyperplasia was noted in a 4-month-old male, Wistar rat presenting with a 1-week history of inappetence and

weight loss (Figure 5.14). The microscopic findings in this case were consistent with autoimmune thyroiditis, a lesion that is seen spontaneously in up to 42% of BB Wistar rats. There was no histologic evidence of diabetes mellitus in this case.

5.4 Respiratory Conditions

Respiratory conditions are common causes for presentation of pet rats to veterinarians and are widespread in breeding colonies of feeder rats. There is a range of primary and opportunistic bacterial, parasitic, fungal, and viral agents that may induce upper and lower respiratory

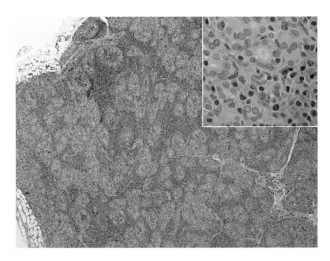

Figure 5.14 Lymphoplasmacytic thyroiditis and follicular hyperplasia in a 4-month-old male Wistar rat (inset represents a higher magnification of the tissue). The animal presented with inappetence and weight loss of short duration.

disease, and co-infections are common. No discussion of respiratory disease is complete without evaluation of rat husbandry and management practices, as suboptimal housing and cleaning schedules may make animals more susceptible to opportunistic infections. Poor ventilation and hygiene permit accumulation of ammonia and CO_2, which can irritate the nasal and respiratory mucosa. Dusty bedding or food and pungent volatile oils in softwood bedding are other common respiratory irritants. Volatile oils can be removed by kiln drying or autoclaving bedding material before use.

Rats have four lung lobes on the right side and a single lobe on the left side. The rat trachea and bronchi are lined by columnar ciliated epithelium admixed with goblet cells and globule leukocytes and only the extrapulmonary bronchi are supported by cartilage, such that bronchiectasis is common with chronic pulmonary infections. Rats are obligate nose breathers and any nasal discharge or crusting that interferes with air exchange can induce cyanosis and respiratory distress, exacerbating underlying disease.

5.4.1 Bacterial Diseases

5.4.1.1 Mycoplasmosis

Mycoplasma pulmonis is a minute pleiomorphic bacterium lacking a cell wall that is usually classified with Gram-positive organisms because of genetic homology. Mammalian *Mycoplasma* organisms typically infect mucosa of the respiratory and urogenital tracts; however, other sites can be infected, including joints, eyes, and mammary glands. *M. pulmonis* is the most common bacterial cause of respiratory disease in pet and commercial feeder rat populations. Infections are generally chronic and subclinical, and because veterinary care may not be sought until after the infection has become deep-seated, treatment is often intermittent and palliative. While largely host-specific, this organism can cross-infect other species, including humans, and owners should be aware of the zoonotic potential.

Presenting Clinical Signs Sneezing, dyspnea, and rhinitis are characteristic clinical signs, as is otitis media with or without an accompanying head tilt. Animals may have a serous to mucopurulent oculonasal discharge, and porphyrin accumulations around the eyes or nares are seen frequently. The organism colonizes the luminal surface of the epithelium and disturbs cilia-associated particulate clearance, leading to secondary infections by opportunistic microorganisms. Chronically infected animals may demonstrate weight loss, a ruffled hair coat, and chattering.

Pathology The gross changes evident will depend on the chronicity of the infection and may range from inapparent infection to anteroventral pulmonary consolidation and hemorrhage with abscessation. Microscopically, there is suppurative peribronchial and perivascular inflammation, with chronic pyogranulomatous bronchitis and bronchiolitis, syncytial giant cell formation in respiratory epithelium, squamous metaplasia of bronchiolar epithelium, bronchiectasis, and accumulation of neutrophils, mucous, and necrotic cellular debris in terminal airways (Figure 5.15). Peribronchiolar lymph nodes are enlarged. Chronic suppurative rhinitis and otitis media can be present. Because *M. pulmonis* acts as a B-cell mitogen, marked peribronchiolar lymphoplasmacytic infiltrates are common. *M. pulmonis* also may cause perioophoritis and salpingitis with reduced fertility.

Laboratory Diagnostics PCR and bacterial culture remain the most reliable means of detecting the organism. Serology has been used, but infected animals may be slow to seroconvert and may appear as false negatives early in the course of infection.

Disease/Colony Management Transmission of *M. pulmonis* occurs by direct contact with infected animals or contaminated fomites, but transplacental transmission may also occur. Poor hygiene with elevated ammonia levels, overcrowding, poor ventilation, and dusty bedding and food may all exacerbate existing infections. Mice may also be clinically infected with the organism and transmit the disease to colony animals. Feral rodents should always be eliminated from feeder rat breeding colonies.

Differential Diagnoses The clinical signs and gross and histologic lesions associated with cilia-associated

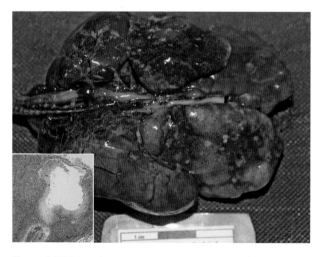

Figure 5.15 *Mycoplasma* pneumonia in a young rat from a breeder-feeder colony. Multifocal areas of abscessation are seen. Inset: Microscopically, there is erosion of bronchiolar epithelium (depicted) and airways are filled with fibrin, cellular debris, and neutrophils. Surrounding parenchyma is consolidated.

respiratory bacillus (CARB) are almost identical to those seen with *M. pulmonis* infection, and co-infection with both organisms is common. Histopathology or PCR may be used to determine whether CARB/*F. rodentium* is also present. Other bacterial agents, such as *Streptococcus pneumoniae* and *Corneybacterium kutscheri*, may induce pneumonia in rats, but can be identified readily by bacterial culture and typical microscopic changes.

5.4.1.2 *Filobacterium rodentium* or Cilia-Associated Respiratory Bacillus

Cilia-associated respiratory bacillus (CARB) is a Gram-negative, argyrophilic, motile, filamentous, nonspore-forming bacterium. 16S rRNA sequence determination has indicated that the rat bacterium is of *Flavobacter/Flexibacter* origin, and it has recently been renamed *Filobacterium rodentium*. Natural infection is host- and species-specific. Whereas the rat and mouse strains of

F. rodentium may be similar, clinical disease is much more common in rats. The organism is transmitted by direct contact between infected animals.

Inapparent infections may occur and when clinical respiratory disease is present, it is indistinguishable grossly from *M. pulmonis* infection (Figure 5.16). Animals are commonly co-infected with both agents and may demonstrate a spectrum of severity, from mild rhinitis through to severe chronic bronchopneumonia. Histologically, the bacterium is visualized in terminal airways with a Warthin-Starry or Steiner silver stain, where it is seen to intercalate between cilia, interfering with beating movements. Because bronchiolar epithelial lining is commonly denuded in chronic infections, it can be difficult to ascertain the presence of the organism at times.

F. rodentium cannot be cultured by traditional methods, although co-culture on embryonated chick eggs or using other cell lines is possible. Histopathology or PCR

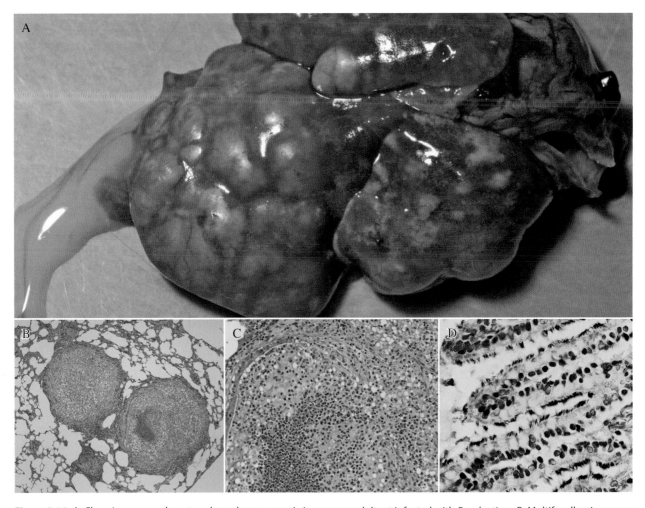

Figure 5.16 A: Chronic pyogranulomatous bronchopneumonia in a young adult rat infected with *F. rodentium*. B: Multifocally, airways are occluded with sloughed necrotic cells, mucous, and neutrophils. C: The peribronchiolar smooth muscle and bronchiolar lining have been eroded, permitting the infection to spill over into the surrounding alveolar spaces. D: Long filamentous bacteria intercalate between cilia on the surface of epithelial cells lining a bronchiole. Warthin-Starry stain. *Source:* B, C and D: Courtesy of L. Tatiersky.

have been traditionally used for definitive diagnosis. Serologic monitoring of animals by ELISA is also possible; however, false negatives may occur.

5.4.1.3 Streptococcal Respiratory Infections

Streptococci are Gram-positive, non-spore-forming, facultatively anaerobic, encapsulated, spherical bacteria, which grow in pairs or short chains. Traditional classification schemes have largely used hemolytic properties and cell wall carbohydrate characteristics (Lancefield groupings) to classify the bacteria; however, more recent schemes use 16S rRNA analysis and separate lactococcal and enterococcal strains from the streptococci. *S. pneumoniae*, an α-hemolytic bacterium, has been associated with clinical disease in young rats.

Presenting Clinical Signs Animals with clinical streptococcal infections may present with head tilt secondary to otitis media, serosuppurative oculonasal discharge, hunched posture, poor hair coat, sneezing, and peracute death. Outbreaks of streptococcal pneumonia have been reported rarely in rat colonies and disease tends to be sporadic and opportunistic.

Pathology *S. pneumoniae* may induce severe fibrinopurulent pleuropneumonia with consolidation and necrosis via hematogenous spread of the organism from the oropharynx (Figure 5.17A). Airways are filled with neutrophils, fibrin, and sloughed cellular debris. Pairs of coccoid bacteria (diplococci) are readily apparent in and around necrotic areas. Fibrinosuppurative pericarditis, peritonitis, periorchitis, salpingitis, meningitis, and otitis media may be seen concurrently. Cervical lymphadenitis with dehydration has been reported in a colony of rats infected with Group G streptococcal bacteria.

Laboratory Diagnostics Both α- and β-hemolytic streptococcal strains may infect rats and bacteria may be cultured from gross lesions of clinically affected animals, as well as from the oropharynx and middle ear of asymptomatic animals. Most cases of clinical disease have been associated with *S. pneumoniae* infection. Subclinical carriage is uncommon in laboratory rat colonies but the extent has not been surveyed in pet or feeder rat colonies.

Disease and Colony Management Streptococcal disease in rats is largely opportunistic in nature, and predisposing factors should be considered when outright disease occurs, such as intercurrent disease, transportation, new colony introductions, and suboptimal husbandry and management. It is likely that bacteria are initially transmitted from human caregivers to animals. There are no documented cases of *S. pneumoniae* or β-hemolytic strains being transmitted from rats to humans. Streptococcal isolates obtained from two pet rats in Europe were reported to have multi-drug resistance, reinforcing the need for separation of sick human caregivers from pets. Mice also may be infected with streptococcal bacteria and feral mice and rats should be excluded from breeding colonies to minimize bacterial transmission. Bacteria are susceptible to most common disinfectants, and proper cage cleaning and hygiene procedures will eliminate the bacteria.

Differential Diagnoses Many other Gram-positive and Gram-negative bacterial agents may induce rhinitis, otitis media, lymphadenitis, and embolic abscessation in rats, however, the finding of fibrinosuppurative pleuropneumonia at necropsy is almost pathognomonic for *S. pneumoniae* infection. Other common causes of

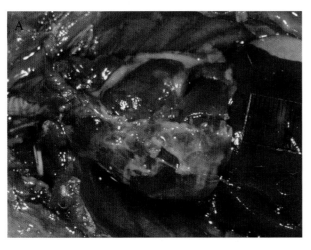
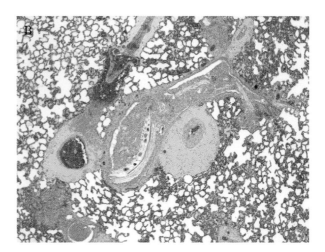

Figure 5.17 A: Fibrinosuppurative pleuropneumonia, caused by peracute *Streptococcus pneumoniae* infection in a rat found dead with no history of illness. B: Aspiration pneumonia in a rat post-anesthesia. Inhaled foreign plant material (arrow) is present in a large airway and is surrounded by marked, mixed, predominantly neutrophilic infiltrates. There is also marked perivascular edema.

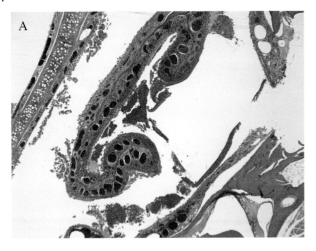
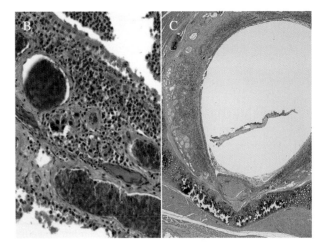

Figure 5.18 A: Marked, fibrinosuppurative and erosive nasal sinusitis with osteolysis (B) in a pet rat with marked nasal discharge and dyspnea. C: A fibrinosuppurative tracheitis is also present. *Klebsiella pneumoniae* was cultured from nasal tissues.

pneumonia in rats include *M. pulmonis, Filobacterium rodentium* (CARB), and *Corynebacterium kutscheri.* Aspiration pneumonia is uncommon in rats but may occur if food or bedding particles are aspirated during recovery from anesthesia (Figure 5.17B).

5.4.1.4 Other Bacterial Respiratory Conditions

Corynebacterium kutscheri is a Gram-positive, nonmotile, nonhemolytic, non-spore-forming short rod that may induce opportunistic respiratory (pseudotuberculosis) or systemic disease in rats, generally following exposure to environmental stressors, nutritional deficiency, or in animals co-infected with other pathogens. Affected animals may evince nonspecific signs of respiratory disease and stress including weight loss, chattering, poor hair coat, sneezing, mucopurulent oculonasal discharge, lethargy, dyspnea, and swollen joints. The organism induces disease following hematogenous dissemination. Grossly, there may be widespread abscessation throughout the body or multifocal to coalescing umbilicated lesions within the lungs, consisting of a central area of caseous necrosis surrounded by a more acutely affected zone of inflammation and hemorrhage. Organisms are abundant and readily visualized in routine sections and cultured. The bacterium may be detected in the oral cavity or gastrointestinal tract. The bacterium has been reported to induce local tissue necrosis and abscessation in a young girl bitten by a clinically unaffected pet rat.

A number of Gram-negative bacteria may normally be cultured from the oro- and nasopharynx of otherwise healthy rats, such as *Bordetella bronchiseptica, Klebsiella pneumoniae,* and *Pastuerella pneumotropica*; however, these agents are considered to be secondary or opportunistic agents and not primary pathogens. *K. pneumoniae* has been noted to induce submandibular,

cervical, and inguinal lymph node abscessation in rats (Figure 5.18). *Pseudomonas aeruginosa* may induce severe necrotizing pneumonia with concurrent vasculitis in immunocompromised and irradiated laboratory rats, but *Pseudomonas* sp. has not been reported to induce natural disease in pet rats.

5.4.2 Pneumocystosis

Pneumocystis carinii is a ubiquitous, species-specific, fungal organism that only recently has been identified as a causative agent of nonsuppurative pneumonia and even death in immunocompetent laboratory rats. This agent caused significant confusion before it was fully classified the condition and was originally thought to be caused by an unidentified virus, giving rise to the name "rat respiratory virus" (RRV) for the putative agent, which may still be seen in historical literature. After many years of research, Koch's postulates have been fulfilled for this condition by *P. carinii*.

Infection is seen most commonly in young adult animals, approximately 10–13 weeks of age, and is usually subclinical, although affected animals may die unexpectedly during anesthesia for unrelated procedures. Gross lesions consist of random, multifocal, 1–4 mm, flat to raised, gray foci on the pleural surface of the lungs. Microscopically, lesions are initially perceived as mixed lymphoplasmacytic and histiocytic to lymphocytic perivascular infiltrates with focal alveolitis and hyperplasia of type II pneumocytes (Figure 5.19). The lesions usually resolve in older animals with residual mild perivascular lymphoid cuffing and multifocal alveolar macrophage aggregates. Confirmation of suspected cases is achieved best by specific PCR assay on fresh frozen lung tissue, as the traditional argyrophilic *Pneumocystis* spp. cyst forms may not be present in

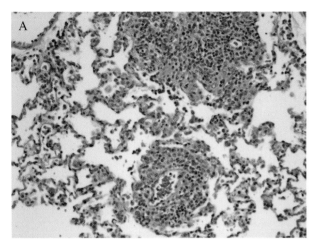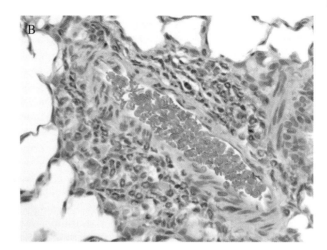

Figure 5.19 A: Perivascular and peribronchiolar histiocytic and lymphoplasmacytic cuffing in an immunocompetent rat dying acutely during anesthesia. The presumptive diagnosis was pneumocystosis. B: Contrast the changes in 5.19A with the marked perivascular eosinophilia that can be seen occasionally in the lungs after intravenous injection of substances in rats.

tissue sections from infected immunocompetent animals. The prevalence of infection and disease in pet and feeder rat populations is unknown.

5.4.3 Viral Respiratory Diseases

There are few well-characterized primary viral respiratory diseases of rats. Most of the viral agents induce subclinical disease but may predispose animals to other bacterial infections or exacerbate underlying co-infections. Sialodacryoadenitis virus (SDAV) is a coronavirus of rats that has primary tropism for salivary glands (see Section 5.6.2.2) but this virus may induce nonsuppurative rhinitis, tracheobronchitis, and dacryoadenitis in some infected animals. SDAV also may potentiate underlying disease induced by *M. pulmonis* or *F. rodentium* (CARB).

Sendai virus, a paramyxovirus of mice, may induce transient infection with few overt clinical signs in rats. Microscopically, a nonsuppurative interstitial pneumonia with lymphoplasmacytic peribronchiolar and perivascular cuffing has been reported in a colony of otherwise normal rats. Serologic assay or PCR of fresh frozen lung tissue are used for diagnosing virus exposure and presence, respectively. Similar transient and subclinical infections can occur in rats infected with Pneumonia Virus of Mice (PVM), another mouse paramyxovirus. As per Sendai virus, PVM can be disseminated by wild rodent reservoirs. Similar diagnostic tests are available for monitoring exposure and infection.

5.4.4 Pulmonary Neoplasia

Spontaneous pulmonary tumors are described rarely in aging pet rats. Both alveolar adenoma and bronchogenic carcinoma are reported in aged laboratory rats of

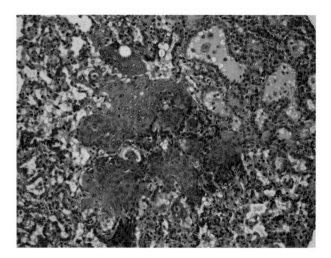

Figure 5.20 Metastatic squamous cell carcinoma in the lungs of a rat.

different stocks and strains, with microscopic characteristics as for other companion animal species. The lungs are a common site for metastasis of other carcinomas (Figure 5.20).

5.4.5 Other Respiratory Conditions

Amorphous eosinophilic inclusions are seen occasionally within the nasal epithelium of aging rats. The etiology is unknown and they are interpreted as proteinaceous in composition and incidental in nature. **Ectasia of laryngeal and tracheal submucosal glands** may occur sporadically in aged rats.

Subpleural **alveolar histiocytosis** is seen in older rats and consists of subpleural aggregates of macrophages, some of which may contain hemosiderin, foamy cytoplasmic material or cholesterol clefts (Figure 5.21).

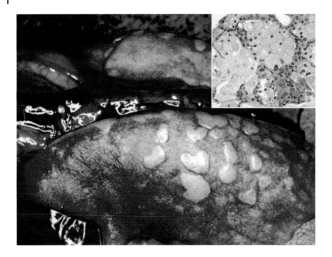

Figure 5.21 Alveolar histiocytosis in an aged rat characterized by pale raised plaques on the pleural surface. Inset: Microscopically, the plaques correspond to subpleural aggregations of foamy macrophages within alveolar spaces. These lesions are considered an incidental finding in aged rats.

Without other signs of inflammation, these findings are interpreted as incidental.

Pulmonary alveolar ectasia can be seen incidentally in aged rats and differentiated from emphysema by lack of destruction of alveolar walls.

Mild, patchy **pulmonary congestion and hemorrhage** are seen commonly in rats euthanatized by CO_2 inhalation.

Chronic pyogranulomatous bronchopneumonia, characterized by raised, gray, multifocal to coalescing nodules containing branching, thick-walled yeast cells (5–25 um diameter) admixed with abundant neutrophils and histiocytes, has been reported in a young, male colony rat. ***Blastomyces dermatitidis* infection** was subsequently confirmed by PCR assay. The infected animal was hunched, lethargic, and dyspneic prior to euthanasia and was the only animal in the group with clinical signs. *Blastomyces* spp. is a dimorphic fungus and common soil inhabitant. Infection in this animal may have resulted from inadvertent food or bedding contamination.

The **rat lungworm**, *Angiostrongylus catonensis*, a metastrongyloid nematode, infects wild rats and has not been reported in pet rats to date. It bears mention because it is a sporadic and serious cause of eosinophilic meningitis/meningoencephalitis in the aberrant human host and infection might be postulated to occur in feral rescue rats. The life cycle is complex and adult female worms lay their eggs within pulmonary arteries of rats. The first stage larvae move into alveoli after hatching and are swallowed and eliminated in the feces, where they are ingested or penetrate land snails, the intermediate host. Rats are infected when they ingest infected intermediate hosts. After several stages of molting and

migration, the larvae migrate back to the pulmonary arteries and become sexually mature, approximately 35 days after ingestion. Stage one larvae appear in the feces approximately 42 days after ingestion of third stage larvae. Infections in humans occur when they eat soil contaminated by infected molluscs, they ingest raw or undercooked snails or slugs or when they ingest raw or undercooked paratenic hosts, such as frogs and freshwater shrimp, or vegetables contaminated with larvae excreted by intermediate hosts. Clinical signs result from death of the migrating larvae in the brain and sporadic outbreaks of the infection are reported in parts of the south-eastern United States, the Caribbean, Hawaii, and parts of South America and Asia.

5.5 Musculoskeletal Conditions

Musculoskeletal conditions are rarely described in pet rats. Despite this, ataxia is a common presenting sign and it is often secondary to pituitary tumor growth with compression of the motor cortex. Spontaneous arthritis of older animals is described anecdotally but the histopathology has not been characterized. Fractures secondary to inadvertent falls or trauma may occur in rats but are less common than in guinea pigs. Hind leg neurogenic muscular atrophy is reported in sedentary, aged rats of both sexes.

Some animals with congenital bone anomalies are bred specifically by hobbyists. Popular pet breeds, such as the Dumbo rat, which has foreshortened maxillary, mandibular, and zygomatic bones and a low ear position, have a distinctive flattened appearance to their head. This is due to a differential expression of the Msx1 and Dsx1 genes during embryonic development, which are important for craniofacial bone formation. These rats have no other reported anatomic or phenotypic abnormalities.

Tailless or Manx rats also are produced as fancy rat breeds. There are a number of mutations that may result in taillessness, some of them autosomal lethal and dominant. Anecdotally, some offspring from tailless rat breedings may be born with vertebral and pelvic anomalies, which are otherwise highly uncommon congenital conditions in rats.

5.5.1 Infectious Musculoskeletal Conditions

Erysipelothrix rhusiopathiae was isolated from two rats displaying spontaneous chronic polyarthritis. It is unknown how the animals acquired these infections, but in addition to fibrinopurulent polyarthritis, the rats had chronic vegetative valvular endocarditis, myocarditis, and suppurative nephritis.

5.5.2 Musculoskeletal Neoplasms

Primary bone and muscle tumors are rare in rats. Osteosarcoma, rhabdomyosarcoma, and vertebral T-cell lymphoma with spinal cord impingement and secondary paresis have all been noted.

5.5.3 Other Musculoskeletal Conditions

Osteochondrosis lesions can be seen in older male animals of certain fast growing strains, such as Sprague–Dawley rats. Animals may appear clinically normal but retain cartilaginous cores bilaterally in the humeral head or medial femoral condyles. Histologically, cartilaginous flaps, endochondral bony cysts, and chondrocyte degeneration with fibrous tissue proliferation may occur.

Spontaneous hypertrophic osteopathy has been reported as a single case in a 34-month-old rat. The animal presented with bilateral metatarsal swellings, tenderness, and paresis in addition to multiple extrapulmonary tumors.

Osteosclerosis with no associated clinical signs was seen in two 18 month-old female rats. The pathogenesis of this condition is unclear. Whether underlying secondary hyperparathyroidism was present in these animals was not reported.

5.6 Gastrointestinal Conditions

Compared to rabbits and other rodents, rats have a very robust gastrointestinal system and generally experience few conditions and diseases, provided that they are fed a well-balanced and nutritionally complete diet. Rats are omnivorous, coprophagic, monogastric, and are unable to vomit, although passive regurgitation may occur in animals with over-distended stomachs. The inability of rodents to vomit is thought to be due to several factors, including the relatively long esophagus, the shape of the stomach, reduced muscularity of the diaphragm, compared with emetic species, and an absent brainstem reflex relay, compared with emetic species. Rats have constantly growing incisors (elodont) but fixed and rooted (brachyodont) molars. Rats have three pairs of salivary glands; the parotid and submandibular glands produce a serous secretion whereas the sublingual glands produce a mixed seromucoid secretion. The salivary glands continue to develop postnatally and androgen-dependent sexual dimorphism may be seen microscopically when evaluating glands from adult male versus female rats. Adult male rats have a 1:1 ratio of acinar cells to granular convoluted tubules (which develop from salivary ducts), whereas females generally have a 2:1 ratio.

The rat stomach is divided into a large nonglandular portion, which has a keratinized stratified squamous epithelial surface separated from the smaller glandular component by a limiting ridge. Both stomach compartments should be evaluated microscopically. Hyperkeratosis and bacterial overgrowth are seen commonly in the nonglandular stomach of rats suffering from inanition. Lactobacilli may be found in the distal esophagus and nonglandular stomach of healthy rats and also constitute a large proportion of enteric bacteria in healthy rats. The cecum is not as large proportionately as the ceca of guinea pigs and chinchillas, and rats are not as efficient at digesting fiber. The large intestine is not sacculated. The entire intestine and colon can be sectioned efficiently and examined using a "Swiss roll" technique, in which the gut is carefully opened along its length, rolled, and fixed before embedding. Rats do not possess a gall bladder and have consistent liver lobation, with four recognizable lobes. Liver weights may be dramatically altered by overnight fasting and are best reported relative to overall body weights.

5.6.1 Oral Conditions

Dental disease other than malocclusion is uncommon in rats, but the oral cavity should always be closely examined at post-mortem for evidence of malocclusion, trauma or neoplasia. Incisor malocclusion may result in excessive salivation, weight loss, and nonspecific signs of stress, such as chromodacryorrhea (Figure 5.22). Dental or mandibular fractures may be noted following trauma, attempts to trim incisors with inappropriate tools or may occur secondarily to neoplasia. Periapical abscesses of the cheek teeth may present as facial or retrobulbar swellings. Mineralization of the tongue and other oral

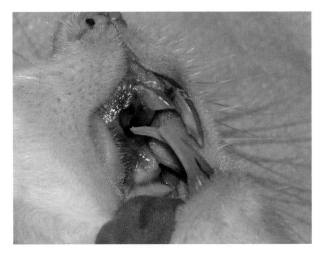

Figure 5.22 Malocclusion in a rat with laceration of the soft palate. *Source:* Courtesy of C. Wheler.

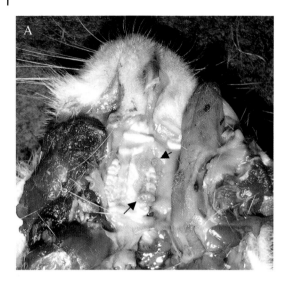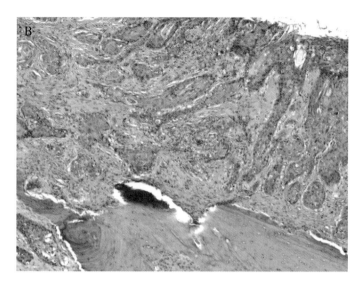

Figure 5.23 A: Oral squamous cell carcinoma in a 4-year-old rat. Neoplastic tissue is seen surrounding the molars and invading the soft palate (arrows). B: Microscopically, the tumor is seen eroding through the hard palate (depicted) and facial bones. *Source:* B: Courtesy of H. Adissu.

soft tissues may rarely be seen in animals with significant renal disease.

Spontaneous dental tumors are very rare in rats and reports include ameloblastoma, odontoma, and ameloblastic odontoma. Squamous cell carcinoma of the oral cavity is uncommon, but when present may result in secondary pathologic fractures (Figure 5.23). These tumors are highly invasive locally and by the time they are detected may extend into the nasal cavities. Often a marked fibrous reaction surrounds invading cords of neoplastic cells.

5.6.2 Salivary Gland and Esophageal Conditions

Spontaneous bacterial sialoadenitis is not reported in rats, although several Gram-negative bacteria may induce a suppurative cervical lymphadenitis in rats that can extend locally to involve the salivary glands. Foreign body-induced sialitis can occur following perforation of the esophagus by ingested materials, such as wood slivers.

5.6.2.1 Bacterial Conditions of the Salivary Gland and Oropharynx

Streptobacillus moniliformis a pleomorphic, filamentous, Gram-negative bacteria that may induce rat bite fever in humans, can be isolated occasionally from the salivary glands, oropharynx, and middle ear of apparently normal rats. Both wild and pet rats may be natural reservoirs for this agent, and all human rat bite wounds should be washed thoroughly with soap to minimize bacterial transmission. This is a serious zoonotic disease for humans in that it can produce localized abscesses, relapsing fever, septic polyarthritis, and even death if left untreated. Known carriers should be culled from breeding colonies, and feral rodents should be excluded from breeding colonies to minimize bacterial contamination and bite risks.

The organism is fastidious and difficult to culture, requiring microaerophilic conditions. PCR assays, while highly specific, are not readily available to confirm infections.

5.6.2.2 Viral Conditions of the Salivary Gland and Oropharynx

Several viruses may infect the salivary glands of pet and wild rats, including rat coronaviruses, cytomegalovirus, and polyoma virus. Clinical disease is only seen with coronavirus infection in immunocompetent animals. Both polyoma and cytomegalovirus infection may result in minimal to mild, nonsuppurative sialadenitis and residual intraductal intranuclear inclusion bodies.

A number of rat coronavirus isolates, including sialodacryoadenitis virus (SDAV) and Parker's rat coronavirus, may induce significant but transient disease of the salivary and lacrimal glands of rats. Animals present with marked cervical swelling, photophobia, and sneezing. Chromodacryorrhea, a poorly kempt hair coat, and weight loss may also be seen. Infection results in marked swelling, edema, and necrosis of the serous (parotid and submandibular), salivary, and lacrimal (exorbital and Harderian) glands. Mild serous rhinitis, tracheobronchitis, and alveolitis may also occur in some animals. Microscopically, there is marked intra- and interlobular edema with necrosis and sloughing of salivary gland acinar and ductular epithelial cells, mixed, predominantly lymphoplasmacytic inflammatory cell infiltrates, and squamous metaplasia of surviving cells (Figure 5.24). Similar changes are seen in the lacrimal glands, and temporary loss of normal lacrimal gland secretions may lead to keratitis. With supportive care, most immunocompetent rats will clear the virus and make a full recovery within one month of infection. Antibodies in recovered

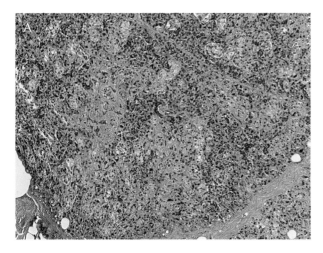
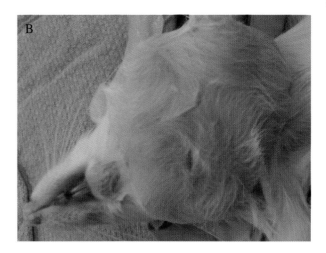

Figure 5.24 A: Acute sialoadenitis in a pet rat with cervical swelling. A coronavirus infection was suspected. B: A fast-growing, fluctuant cervical mass in an adult rat that was consistent microscopically with a salivary gland carcinoma.

individuals may be detected by serology, and PCR assays are available to detect viral antigens. Host resistance to coronaviruses is short-lived and not cross-protective to different strains, and, because the virus mutates rapidly, reinfection of colonies is common. To eliminate the virus from breeding colonies, cessation of all breeding must occur for 8–12 weeks with no new colony introductions during this period. Alternatively, depopulation and repopulation with clean breeding stock may be used.

5.6.2.3 Neoplasia of the Salivary Glands
Salivary gland carcinoma (Figure 5.24B), adenocarcinoma, and squamous cell carcinoma are uncommon in rats, and present as firm, multilobulated, cervical swellings. These masses have diverse morphology and can grow quickly and demonstrate marked anaplasia, pleiomorphism, cystic and hemorrhagic areas, and necrosis. Local invasion of lymph nodes and surrounding soft tissue is common, but metastases are rare. Other more common tumors in the cervical region that should be considered as differentials include mammary gland neoplasia, lymphosarcoma, fibrosarcoma, Zymbal's gland tumor, and peripheral nerve sheath tumor.

5.6.2.4 Other Conditions of the Esophagus
Acquired or congenital megaesophagus can occur in rats with typical esophageal dilatation and microscopic evidence of myofiber and neuronal cell degeneration (Figure 5.25A). Regurgitation with necrotizing bronchopneumonia has been reported as a corollary in a rat.

5.6.3 Gastric Conditions
Gastric erosion and ulceration of the nonglandular and glandular stomach may occur spontaneously in rats (Figure 5.25B). Affected animals may appear pale if bleeding is

significant, although this may be difficult to appreciate in pigmented animals. Animals may bleed out into the stomach or lower intestinal tract and die acutely following sudden and severe shock, and it may be difficult for the pathologist to pinpoint the actual site of bleeding on the mucosa. Predisposing factors typically involve management problems such as prolonged transportation during hot weather without access to water, exposure to adverse environmental temperatures or lack of access to food and water for 24 hours, particularly in younger animals.

5.6.3.1 Bacterial Conditions of the Stomach
Although rats are experimentally susceptible to gastric infection with a range of *Helicobacter* species, and infections do occur commonly in colonies of laboratory rats, spontaneous bacterial gastritis is not reported in pet rats.

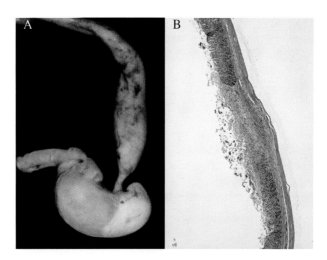

Figure 5.25 A: Megaesophagus in rat. B: Gastric ulcers are common in stressed rats and may result in sudden death if bleeding is prolonged.

Mild lymphoplasmacytic gastritis has been reported in wild rats with natural infections of *Helicobacter heilmanii*.

5.6.3.2 Gastric Neoplasia

Most spontaneous gastric tumors reported in rats have been found in aging laboratory animals and there are few, if any, reports of spontaneously occurring gastric tumors in pet rats. Older pet animals are not usually submitted for a post-mortem evaluation, and it is likely that tumors occur spontaneously with similar incidence in older pet rats but are undiagnosed.

Gastric tumors are uncommon and may involve the nonglandular or glandular stomach, or the stroma. Squamous cell carcinoma may occur within the nonglandular stomach and various adenomas, adenocarcinomas, and neuroendocrine cell tumors (carcinoids) with local invasion may be seen in the glandular stomach. Gastrointestinal stromal tumors, leiomyomas, and leiomyosarcomas may be seen with characteristics as described for other species. Histiocytic sarcoma, lymphosarcoma, and mesothelioma can involve the gastric wall and often locally extensive mucosal ulceration is present overlying areas of histiocytic or lymphocytic neoplastic cell infiltrates.

5.6.3.3 Other Gastric Conditions

Generalized **mucosal atrophy** with cystic dilatation of glands is a common finding in aging rats, particularly at the junction between the glandular and nonglandular stomach. The gastric muscularis, mucosa, and associated blood vessels may be mineralized in animals with severe, chronic renal disease.

Ectopic islands of **exocrine pancreas** or **liver** cells are occasionally seen within the submucosa or subserosa of the stomach or small intestine, and are interpreted as incidental.

Gastric impaction and death following buprenorphine-induced pica have been reported in rats. The incidence is higher in rats housed on sawdust or hardwood chip bedding immediately following surgery. High dose or prolonged therapy with nonsteroidal anti-inflammatory drugs may lead to gastric or intestinal ulceration with perforation (Figure 5.26A).

5.6.4 Enteric Conditions

Adult immunocompetent animals are generally quite resistant to diarrhea; however, there are several bacterial and viral agents that may induce diarrhea in young or debilitated animals.

5.6.4.1 Enterococcosis

Enterococcus species have been isolated in several outbreaks of neonatal diarrhea of suckling rats. Affected pups fail to grow and thrive, and are dehydrated with liquid yellow feces. Pups surviving the acute phase of the disease continue to nurse but are small compared with unaffected pups. Histologically, there is massive blanketing of the small intestinal villi by Gram-positive cocci but villi are otherwise of normal length and appearance, suggesting malabsorption as the basis for the diarrhea observed (Figure 5.27A). Adult animals are either unaffected or exhibit transient soft feces. Bacteria may be cultured readily from tissues. Enterococci are part of the normal flora of rodents but are found only within the lumen and do not adhere to the surface epithelium. Affected cages should be handled last to minimize transmission to unaffected breeding animals. Coinfection with enteric viruses may exacerbate the disease in affected animals.

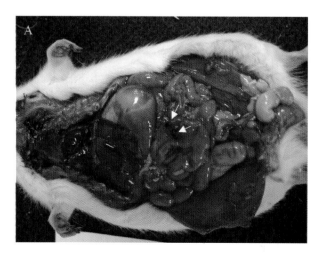
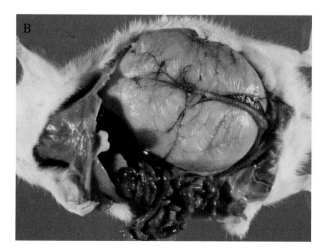

Figure 5.26 A: Iatrogenic nonsteroidal anti-inflammatory drug-induced cecal perforation (arrow) in a male rat with secondary peritonitis. B: Intra-abdominal lipoma in an adult rat.

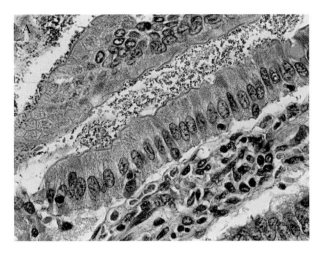
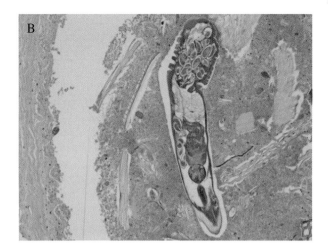

Figure 5.27 A: *Enterococcus* sp. infection in a rat pup presenting with diarrhea. Gram positive coccoid bacteria are seen blanketing the intestinal epithelial surface. B: Section of an adult, gravid, female *Syphacia* spp. pinworm in the intestine of a rat.

5.6.4.2 Salmonellosis

Salmonella enterica serovars Enteritidis and Typhimurium may be carried as an inapparent infection by pet or feeder rats or may induce soft stools, diarrhea, and sudden death in infected animals. In a number of cases, these bacteria have been demonstrated to have resistance to multiple antimicrobials. Infections may be acquired by rats during mixing of rodents from different sources in large distribution centers. Both live and frozen animals may transmit the disease, making routine hand washing essential after touching or holding rats. The bacteria are transmitted by a fecal-oral route and human infections have been reported following handling of contaminated rats. Treatment is not recommended for animals shedding bacteria and many feeder rodent breeding operations irradiate packages of frozen animals before sale to minimize the spread of disease.

5.6.4.3 Tyzzer's Disease

Tyzzer's disease may occur in rats as sporadic cases or outbreaks. Infections are usually subclinical in immunocompetent animals, but concomitant stressors, such as poor hygiene, overcrowding, concomitant disease or poor nutrition may induce outright disease. The disease is caused by *Clostridium piliforme*, a Gram-negative, spore-forming, anaerobic rod-shaped bacillus. Affected animals may present off feed with a ruffled hair coat. Diarrhea may or not be present and some animals may die peracutely with no premonitory signs. A classic triad of lesions is seen grossly in rats, including acute multifocal hepatic necrosis, dilatation and subserosal hemorrhage of the distal small intestine, and grey, circumscribed myocardial lesions. Microscopically, coagulation necrosis is present in affected tissues and bacteria are visualized with a Warthin-Starry or Steiner stain as "bundles of sticks" around the periphery of lesions. Serology can be used to monitor

exposure, but false positives are common. *C. piliforme* cannot be cultured by traditional means but requires embryonated hen's eggs or co-culture with other cell lines. Fecal PCR assays may be used to determine whether an animal is shedding spores into the environment. Spores are resistant to desiccation and may persist for years. There is no effective treatment for the disease, and colonies have to be rederived to eliminate the infection. *C. piliforme*-related disease occurs in many species, including immunosuppressed humans exposed to feces of feral rats. Feral animals should always be excluded from breeding colonies to minimize disease transmission.

5.6.4.4 Viral Enteritis

Rotaviruses are nonenveloped, double-stranded RNA viruses associated with enteritis outbreaks in all species. Rats are infected with type B rotaviruses, whereas most human infections are caused by type A rotaviruses. Infection of breeding colonies may result in mild, transient diarrhea in suckling rats with runting, poor hair coat, and perianal soiling. Villus atrophy with enterocyte syncytia at the villus tips and enterocyte vacuolation may be seen microscopically. Most serologic assays are based on type A viruses found in mice and do not cross-react with type B antigens. Virus isolation, EM, or PCR may be conducted on fecal samples to confirm infection. There are sporadic reports of type B rotavirus enteric infections in humans that cross-infect rat pups, suggesting that rat rotavirus may be transmitted to human caregivers. The virus may persist in the environment, and application of an appropriate virucidal detergent or decontaminating solution is necessary to ensure elimination.

Astroviruses, non-enveloped single stranded RNA viruses, have been isolated recently from the feces of wild brown rats in China. Astroviruses are a common cause of viral diarrhea in humans but infected animals were asymptomatic. Sequence analyses of viruses isolated from rats indicate phylogenetic similarity to the human viruses, but zoonotic potential is unknown. Astroviruses are not surveyed routinely in pet or laboratory rats and the prevalence of infection in these populations is undetermined.

Hepatitis E virus is a non-enveloped single strand RNA virus in the genus Hepevirus. Viruses have been isolated from asymptomatic wild rats; however, the sequence is distinct from hepatitis E viral sequences isolated from infected humans.

5.6.4.5 Parasitic Enteric Conditions

Several enteric parasites may infect rats; however, most are nonpathogenic and detection at necropsy is incidental. Pinworms (oxyurids) are detected with high frequency in feral and pet rats of all ages both in-life and at necropsy. The life cycle is direct and simple and animals are infected by ingesting embryonated eggs. There are three species seen in rats, *Syphacia muris*, *S. obvelata*, and *Aspiculuris tetraptera*, which can be differentiated by length of worm, shape of egg, and differing prepatent periods. Co-infection with multiple species is possible. *Syphacia* spp. lay eggs around the anus, which may generally be detected by perianal application of cellophane tape with subsequent microscopic examination, whereas eggs of *Aspiculuris* sp. can be detected only by fecal flotation, histopathology or PCR. Mild pruritus and rectal prolapse are anecdotally reported in heavily infested animals. Cross-sections of adult worms and larvae are seen readily in the cecal and colonic lumena with minimal mucosal reaction in infected animals (Figure 5.27B). The parasites are not zoonotic, but infections are difficult to eliminate from conventional colonies as eggs resist desiccation, they persist in the environment for long periods, and the eggs are very light, resulting in ready air-borne dispersion under conventional open-topped caging conditions.

Rodentolepis nana and *Hymenolepis diminuta* are cestodes seen incidentally in pet and feral rats. *R. nana* has a direct life cycle, but *H. diminuta* requires an insect intermediate host. Whereas humans can be infected with both tapeworms, the human *R. nana* strain appears to be host-specific, suggesting that infections are not transmitted by pet rodents. *Rodentolepis* adult worms are approximately the size of an intestinal villus, whereas *H. diminuta* is much larger and is found within the intestinal lumen. Adult tapeworms are found in the small intestine or biliary and pancreatic ducts, and generally induce minimal reaction.

Rats are the intermediate host for the cat tapeworm *Taenia taeniaformis* and often manifest the larval form, *Cysticercus fasciolaris*, as one or several opaque, white

cysts on the liver capsule. The cyst contains a single coiled larva, which may be up to 20 cm long. Most infections in pet and wild rats are asymptomatic, however, there are several reports of poorly differentiated, metastatic hepatic sarcomas arising in association with chronic inflammation induced by the strobilicercus.

Echinococcosis multilocularis infection has been reported in wild rats. Cestode infections are transmitted by fecal contamination of rodent food by other rodents, cats, and arthropod vectors.

Overgrowth of certain opportunistic enteric protozoa, such as *Giardia muris* and *Spironucleus muris*, may occur in young animals with intercurrent enteric disease.

5.6.4.6 Enteric Neoplasia

Spontaneous neoplasia of the small intestine is rare in rats. Adenomas, adenocarcinoma, squamous cell carcinoma, lipoma (Figure 5.26B), and lymphosarcoma have been described in the rat intestine and colon. Colonic adenocarcinoma in association with *Campylobacter*-like chronic inflammation has been described in laboratory but not pet rats. Mesothelioma is seen sporadically (Figure 5.28).

5.6.4.7 Other Enteric Conditions

Spontaneous and fatal adynamic ileus occurs sporadically in rats after intraperitoneal administration of specific agents, such as chloral hydrate or chloral hydrate-containing mixtures. Animals present off feed with a distended abdomen correlated grossly with a massively distended ileum. The mucosa is intact histologically and there are no microscopic lesions. This condition should be differentiated from fatal megacolon (**aganglionosis of the colon**), a polygenic congenital condition occurring in

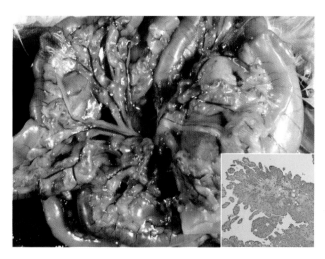

Figure 5.28 Mesothelioma in the abdominal cavity of a rat. Inset: Microscopically, classic papillary structures covered with epithelioid cells are seen.

rats with pigmentation abnormalities, including white spotting of the fur, white facial or body stripes or in animals with different colored eyes. Colonic aganglionosis may have an early or delayed onset, and adult animals present off feed with marked abdominal distension and with a history of either constipation or diarrhea. Defects in neural crest melanocyte migration are responsible for the white pigmentation irregularities and aganglionosis in colonic smooth muscle. Histologically, there is a complete lack of nerves within the colonic smooth muscle of affected rats.

5.6.5 Pancreatic Conditions

Exocrine pancreatic tumors are uncommonly reported in pet rats. Atrophy of the exocrine pancreas with loss of acinar cell zymogen granules is a common nonspecific finding in animals experiencing inanition.

5.6.6 Hepatobiliary Conditions

Hepatocellular perinuclear rarefaction may be marked in rats after feeding, and atrophy of hepatic cords appears rapidly after periods of fasting or inanition of 12 hours or longer (Figure 5.29). Bile ductule hyperplasia, characterized as multiple profiles of bile ducts lined by low cuboidal epithelium within the portal triads, with or without mild periportal lymphoplasmacytic infiltrates, may be seen as a nonspecific change during any condition inducing mild hepatic inflammation or irritation, and is a common incidental finding in geriatric rats. Random, multifocal microgranulomas, consisting of several neutrophils and monocytes surrounding 1 or 2 degenerating hepatocytes, are observed commonly in conventionally housed rats and generally represent nonspecific portal bacterial distribution from the gut. Islands of extramed-

ullary hematopoiesis and myelopoiesis may be seen in the livers of adult animals in cases in which there is an extra demand for their production. Clusters of hematopoietic cells may be seen within periportal areas or within sinusoids. Yellow-brown lipofuscin pigment accumulation may be seen in hepatocytes of aging rats and represents lysosomal digestion residues, as in other species. Rarely, exocrine pancreatic cell metaplasia may occur within the hepatic parenchyma.

5.6.6.1 Bacterial Hepatitis

Hepatic abscessation and necrosis may occur from disseminated infections with *C. kutscheri*, *S. aureus*, *C. piliforme*, and other bacteria. Multifocal miliary to discrete abscesses may be seen on the liver surface and throughout the parenchyma. In terms of possible differential diagnoses for acute multifocal hepatic necrosis, spontaneous liver disease is unusual in rats, although inadvertent intoxication from household chemicals may occur. Animals should always be supervised when allowed to exercise.

Several *Helicobacter* species are commonly isolated from laboratory rats, including *H. bilis*, *H. typhlonius*, *H. hepaticus*, and *H. rodentium*. Spontaneous enteric or hepatic disease caused by *Helicobacter* spp. is not reported in immunocompetent animals.

5.6.6.2 Viral Hepatitis

Hepatitis E antibodies are common in wild rats in North America and Europe; however, the specific isolates obtained from rats are not homologous with human isolates, and the disease cannot be transmitted to nonhuman primates, suggesting that rats are not a reservoir for human hepatitis E infections. Hepatitis E antibodies have not been reported in pet rats. The disease is subclinical in

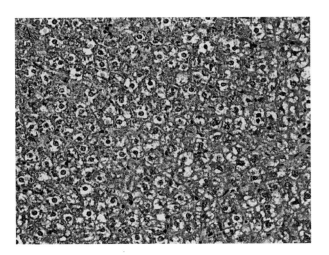
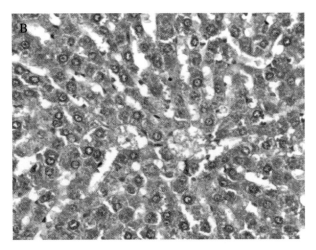

Figure 5.29 Significant glycogen accumulation occurs in rats after a meal, conferring perinuclear rarefaction and a moth-eaten appearance to liver sections (A). A 12h fast induces atrophy of hepatic cords (B). Given that pet rats fed ad lib will consume 20 or more small meals each day, this feature can be useful for determining whether inanition is present.

wild and laboratory rats and no clinical, gross or histologic lesions are reported in experimentally infected animals.

5.6.6.3 Hepatobiliary Neoplasia

Spontaneous liver tumors are uncommon in pet rats but are common in laboratory rats intentionally exposed to various toxicants. Hepatomas, hepatocellular carcinoma, and cholangiocarcinomas may occur with characteristics as described for other companion animal species. The liver is frequently involved in spontaneous cases of lymphosarcoma and histiocytic sarcoma, with periportal and sinusoidal aggregations of neoplastic cells (see Section 5.10.2).

5.6.6.4 Other Hepatobiliary Conditions

Long Evans cinnamon rats have a defect in the copper-transporting ATPase gene, resulting in **copper accumulation**. Jaundice may be detected in some animals, and the disease may manifest earlier in females. Affected rats develop spontaneous hepatitis and cholangiofibrosis as young adults, which can become chronic, resulting in hepatocellular carcinoma or cholangiocarcinoma development later in life. Hepatic copper concentrations in affected animals are over 50-fold greater than levels seen in normal LE rats. Grossly, there may be irregular lobar to diffuse fibrosis and macronodular hepatic regeneration. In early disease, there is single cell necrosis of hepatocytes, macro- and microvesiculation of hepatocytes, dissecting fibrosis, islands of hepatocellular regeneration, and lymphoplasmacytic infiltrates. Copper accumulation is readily detected with a rhodamine stain.

5.7 Cardiovascular Conditions

Degenerative changes are common in the heart and vasculature of aging rats, however, proliferative lesions are rare. Rats are resistant to the development of atherosclerosis and the condition does not occur spontaneously.

5.7.1 Cardiomyopathy

Degenerative cardiomyopathy is a common incidental finding at necropsy in rats and may be seen histologically in some stocks and strains, such as Sprague–Dawley, as early as 12 weeks of age. The extent of the condition is often not appreciated ante-mortem. Lesions are typically more severe in males than in females and are more common in the left and right ventricular free walls and apex. Changes include patchy to locally extensive myofiber fragmentation, vacuolation, and degeneration with interstitial mononuclear cell infiltrates, loss of cross striations, and infiltration by fibroblasts with collagen deposition (Figure 5.30A). Mineralization of necrotic fibers can occur and cartilage and osseous metaplasia also may be seen. Dietary restriction significantly reduces the incidence of this condition. There is no correlation between cardiac troponin I levels and the total area of myocardial degeneration in rats.

5.7.2 Cardiovascular Neoplasia

Spontaneous cardiac and vascular tumors are rare in rats, with an estimated frequency less than 0.3%. Schwannomas, either endocardial or intramural, are the most common tumor reported within the hearts of rats, and are seen predominantly in the left ventricle, but also in endocardial locations. The tumors consist of dense

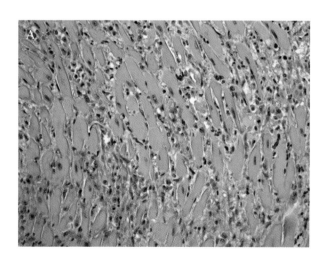
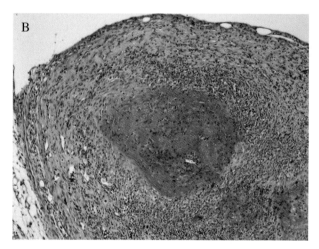

Figure 5.30 A: Cardiomyocyte degeneration and fibrosis are common incidental findings in aged rats. Pulmonary changes or hepatic congestion may be seen when the condition is clinical. B: Mesenteric polyarteritis in an aged rat. There is marked fibrinoid degeneration and inflammation of the vascular medial tunic and subtotal lumenal occlusion.

sheets of infiltrating pleomorphic spindle cells with palisading nuclei and occasional whorl formation within a moderate fibrovascular stroma. Mitoses are plentiful and cells are usually immunopositive for S-100.

Hemangioma, hemangiosarcoma, and hemangiopericytoma are all described in aged rats but these are uncommon masses. They should be differentiated from histiocytic sarcomas, which also may present as firm, raised, red, solitary cutaneous masses.

5.7.3 Other Cardiovascular Conditions

Left ventricular **cardiomyofiber mineralization** may occur in rats with chronic renal disease. Fibrosis is not a characteristic of this condition.

Interstitial fatty infiltrates can be seen in older obese animals. **Left atrial thrombosis** can occur in older rats and may be associated with deteriorating cardiac function secondary to degeneration or to valvular disease.

Idiopathic arteritis (polyarteritis nodosa) is seen incidentally at necropsy in aging rats, particularly in males. Grossly, tortuous, dilated, and thickened vessels may be seen anywhere, but are most common in the mesenteric, pancreatic, and peritesticular arteries. The lesion is degenerative and involves all arterial layers, characterized by initial medial fibrinoid necrosis with mixed leukocytic infiltrates, subsequent fibrosis, and perivascular inflammation (Figure 5.30B).

Myocarditis and endocarditis are seen sporadically as a sequela to bacteremia (Figure 5.31).

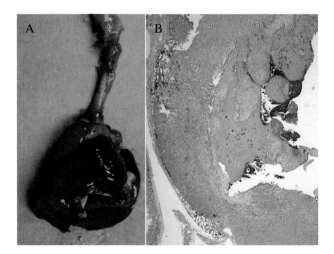

Figure 5.31 A: Valvular and mural septic endocarditis in an 8-month-old rat. *Pasteurella pneumotropica* was cultured from the heart. B: Dense basophilic colonies of bacteria are embedded within the fibrinosuppurative exudate adherent to the endocardium. There is marked suppurative inflammation and necrosis of the ventricular free wall.

5.8 Genitourinary Conditions

The rat kidney is unipapillate and mild proteinuria (up to 10 mg per day) is common. Young, intact, sexually mature male rats synthesize major urinary proteins (MUPs; previously known as alpha$_2\mu$ globulin) in the liver as precursor molecules and renal tubular epithelial cells excrete these proteins into the urine. Aggregates of the protein appears as hyaline droplets in the proximal renal tubular epithelial cells. These proteins are also synthesized by other tissues, including mammary, preputial, and salivary glands, and nasal and respiratory epithelia. MUPs are members of the lipocalin family and they may serve as pheromones or for other forms of olfactory communication when excreted in the urine. Synthesis and excretion of the urinary form of the protein is highly influenced by testosterone. Male rats excrete 120-fold more MUPs than female or castrated male rats, and production is minimal in aged rats.

The kidneys of rats continue to grow throughout their lives; however, there is no change in the number of nephrons; growth occurs by increasing tubular length and glomerular size.

5.8.1 Urinary Tract Conditions

5.8.1.1 Chronic Renal Disease

Chronic degenerative renal disease (chronic progressive nephropathy or CPN) is very common in all strains and breeds of rats, although wild rats may be less susceptible to developing chronic progressive nephropathy. The condition is much more common in males than females.

Presenting Clinical Signs Signs of renal disease may be nonspecific. Animals may present with anorexia, depression, dehydration, hunched posture, and may have a history of polyuria and polydipsia. Urine staining or scalding of the perineal area may be apparent. As the disease progresses, there may be a significant increase in daily water consumption of up to 70%, and the cage will appear wet.

Pathology Grossly, there is mild pallor and enlargement of the kidneys in early stages of the disease. As the disease progresses, the cortical surfaces become pitted and granular. Early microscopic changes can be seen in some strains of rats at 7–8 weeks of age and consist of tubular degeneration and regeneration, characterized by tubular epithelial cell basophilia and hyperplasia with basement membrane thickening, followed by tubular dilatation and epithelial attenuation with accumulation of hyaline casts. Glomerular changes are variable, some become atrophied while others become enlarged with thickening of the

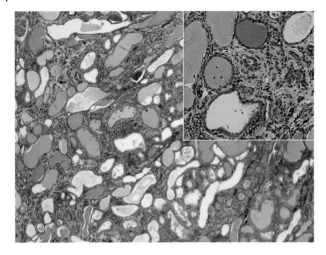

Figure 5.32 Chronic renal failure in an aged male rat. There is marked tubular dilatation, degeneration, and regeneration, and scattered glomerular tufts are sclerosed. Tubules are filled with eosinophilic acellular casts. Inset: Mild to moderate interstitial lymphoplasmacytic infiltrates and interstitial fibrosis are seen.

mesangial tuft and synechiae formation between the glomerulus and Bowman's capsule. Interstitial fibrosis and lymphoplasmacytic infiltrates occur as the disease progresses (Figure 5.32). Progressive renal deterioration and inability to adequately control calcium and phosphorus excretion may result in secondary hyperparathyroidism with mineralization of soft tissues throughout the body. Fibrous osteodystrophy and osteosclerosis are seen at times in rats with secondary hyperparathyroidism.

Laboratory Diagnostics Tubular loss of albumen with albuminuria is the earliest biomarker of renal disease in rats. There is a concomitant decrease in serum albumen and an increase in serum cholesterol. In urine samples obtained by free flow or cystocentesis, reduction in urine specific gravity is readily detected as the condition progresses.

Disease and Colony Management The progression of chronic progressive nephropathy in rats can be significantly retarded by maintaining dietary protein levels at 14% and by restricting the overall diet to just meet the daily needs.

5.8.1.2 Urolithiasis

Urolithiasis is common in pet rats and likely related to diet. Uroliths may be large and numerous and induce urinary bladder irritation with subsequent cystitis and hematuria or urethral blockage with anuria and subsequent urinary bladder rupture (Figure 5.33). Uroliths also may be found in the renal pelvis resulting in secondary nodular hyperplasia of the renal pelvis, mixed leukocytic infiltrates, mineralization and hemorrhage. In severe cases, obstructive nephropathy may occur. Most uroliths in rats are composed of ammonium magnesium phosphate (struvite), although some may be composed of calcium oxalate, depending on the diet. Risk factors for urolith development include concurrent bacterial cystitis, diet, dehydration, and bladder threadworm infestation. Concurrent infection with *Corynebacterium renale* has been reported in some rats with urolithiasis. Dietary deficiencies in vitamin A may predispose rats to urolithiasis and cystitis. Excessive dietary calcium levels and certain toxic contaminants, such as melamine, may also predispose rats to urolithiasis.

5.8.1.3 Cystitis, Pyelonephritis, and Nephritis

Bacterial cystitis occurs in older rats, and is more common in males, possibly because of concurrent prostatitis in some animals. Infections of the urinary tract may be

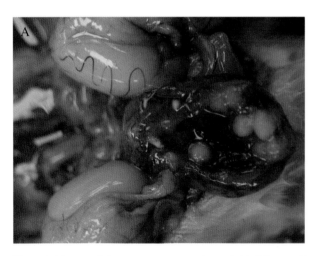

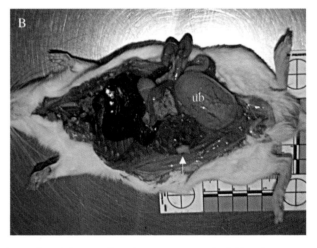

Figure 5.33 A: Urolithiasis in a mature male rat. B: Uroliths may block the urethra with secondary obstructive uropathy (ub) and hydronephrosis (arrow), as depicted in this animal.

due to hematogenous spread or ascending bacterial colonization. Animals can present with hematuria, a history of excessive grooming of the perineal area, urine staining or scalding, tenesmus, and hunched posture. The urinary bladder can be markedly dilated if there is concurrent obstruction. Microscopically, there may be erosion or ulceration of the urinary bladder epithelium with edema, hemorrhage, and marked suppurative infiltrates. Pyelonephritis and uni- or bilateral nephritis are common sequelae (Figure 5.34). A range of bacteria may be isolated from urine or tissue samples, including *C. renale*, *E. coli*, *Klebsiella* spp., *Proteus* sp., *S. aureus* or *Pseudomonas aeruginosa*. Differential diagnoses for apparent hematuria in rats include urolithiasis, bladder threadworm infection, urinary tract tumors, uterine tumors, prostatitis, fighting injuries, and trauma.

5.8.1.4 Urinary Bladder and Renal Masses

Spontaneous tumors of the urinary bladder are rare in rats but may be induced by chronic irritation and inflammation secondary to chronic urolithiasis. Papillomas and transitional or squamous cell carcinomas can occur.

Renal tumors may be seen on occasion but may not be diagnosed ante-mortem as they tend to occur in aged animals with concurrent conditions or diseases. Tumor types include renal adenomas, carcinomas, renal mesenchymal tumors, renal tubule carcinomas, and nephroblastomas. Nephroblastomas occur in young animals, whereas renal mesenchymal tumors are seen only in older rats. Metastases are rare for all renal and urinary bladder tumors.

The kidney may be involved secondarily in cases of lymphosarcoma and histiocytic sarcoma, and aggregates of neoplastic cells are seen often in perivascular and interstitial locations, although neoplastic cells may be generalized with end stage disease. In rats of both sexes with the latter tumor, there may be dense accumulations of hyaline proteins in the apical cytoplasm of renal tubular epithelial cells within the P2 segment. Accumulations are approximately proportional to the degree of tumor burden in the body. In mice, these hyaline droplets have been found to contain several antigens to monocyte-expressed proteins, including lysozyme and Mac-2.

5.8.1.5 Other Renal Conditions

Unilateral congenital renal agenesis, **congenital hydronephrosis**, and **congenital renal cysts** are seen sporadically. Hepatic or biliary cysts may also be present when renal cysts are detected.

Renal infarction secondary to thrombosis and bacteremia or septicemia occurs sporadically in rats. Lesions are generally wedge-shaped and may be swollen and hemorrhagic (acute) or collapsed and fibrotic (chronic), depending on the age of the lesion. Old infarction lesions can be an incidental finding at necropsy, often indicative of a historical event from which the animal recovered spontaneously.

Renal tubular mineralization (nephrocalcinosis) occurs commonly in female rats of certain strains and breeds and is characterized histologically as focal mineralization of renal tubules, usually at the corticomedullary junction. Elevated dietary phosphorus levels are linked to this condition, and nephrocalcinosis is common in female rats fed diets with calcium:phosphorus ratios less than 1.2:1. Mineral deposition occurs up to 12 weeks of age and is irreversible, underlining the critical importance of offering a high quality balanced diet to young, growing animals.

A proteinaceous plug admixed with sloughed epithelial cells and spermatozoa may be seen in the urethra of male

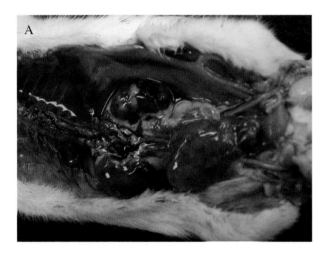
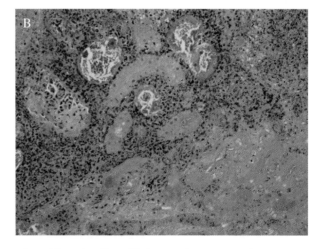

Figure 5.34 A: Unilateral suppurative nephritis in a male rat. *E. coli* was cultured from the affected kidney. B: There is marked regionally extensive liquefactive necrosis of the affected kidney with numerous dense bacterial colonies within the interstitium and tubular lumena.

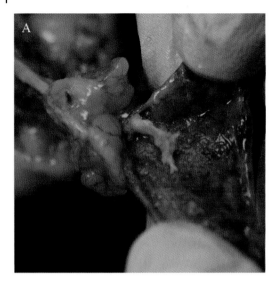 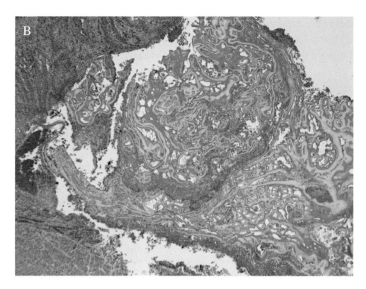

Figure 5.35 A: The urethra of this male rat is partially obstructed with a firm yellow concretion. B: Microscopically, the concretion consisted of lamellated, partially mineralized amorphous protein. The surrounding urethral epithelium is eroded, in places, from mechanical trauma and there are moderate neutrophilic infiltrates within and around the concretion.

rats at post-mortem. These are common, incidental findings in many rodent species. Post-mortem lesions, such as a distended urinary bladder that cannot be expressed readily at necropsy, a ruptured urinary bladder, hydroureter, or hydronephrosis must be present concurrently to diagnose pathologic urethral obstruction (Figure 5.35).

Bladder threadworm infection (*Trichosomoides crassicauda*) is common in wild rats and conventional breeding colonies. Infections are usually subclinical, although animals may present with hematuria when heavy worm burdens are present. Ingested eggs hatch into larvae within the intestine and undergo pulmonary migration, eventually migrating through the bloodstream to the urinary bladder. The adult female (up to 1 cm long) embeds within the urinary bladder epithelium, whereas the male worm (up to 3.5 mm long) parasitizes the female's uterus (Figure 5.36). Ova are thick-walled, light brown, ovoid and bioperculated, and are shed into the bladder lumen and excreted with urine. Minimal, nonsuppurative, local inflammation is seen typically in the urinary bladder submucosa, although more extensive inflammation can occur. Mild, focal, pulmonary hemorrhage or granulomatous inflammation may be seen in animals with recent larval migration. Rarely, parasites may be found in the kidney or within the distal urinary outflow tract. Ante-mortem diagnosis is made by evaluating urinary sediment for eggs. The environment must be disinfected thoroughly when attempting to eradicate the parasite.

Leptospirosis is an important zoonotic disease, and humans are susceptible to a number of serovars carried by rats. *Leptospira interrogans* serogroup icterohaemorrhagiae or copenhageni may be carried subclinically by pet or wild rats, and exposure to infected urine can induce leptospirosis (Weil's disease) in humans. Typical cases involve sewer or construction workers exposed to fresh feral rat urine. The organism does not survive drying. Several recent human cases have occurred when rats of unknown background have been adopted as pets, an increasingly common scenario with the rise of various pet rat rescue societies. No renal lesions are reported in infected animals. Prevalence rates of 40% or greater can be seen in wild rat populations and feral animals must be excluded from breeding colonies to minimize disease transmission. Clients, veterinarians, clinic workers, and

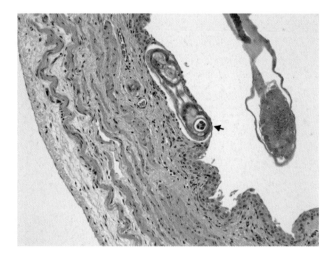

Figure 5.36 Bladder threadworms (*Trichosomoides crassicauda*) in the urinary bladder of a young rat. One female nematode is free within the lumen of the urinary bladder while another gravid female (arrow indicates an egg) lies within the superficial urothelium. There is minimal associated inflammation.

pathologists should always wash hands carefully after handling rats or their urine or tissues. *Leptospira* organisms may be cultured from urine and subsequently serotyped or visualized in urine samples of infected rats via dark-field microscopy.

A number of **hantaviruses** may induce serious systemic and respiratory diseases in humans, but they are not carried by pet rodents. The virus is highly prevalent and carried subclinically by specific strains of wild mice and rats (including *Rattus rattus* and *Rattus norvegicus*, black and brown rats, respectively) and shed in the urine, saliva, and droppings. Between rodents, the disease is transmitted via bite wounds from infected animals. Humans are infected when they ingest or inhale fresh or dried material containing virus, for example, when cleaning outdoor sheds or garages in areas where the virus is prevalent in wild rodent populations. Feral rodents must be excluded from human habitations and rodent breeding colonies to minimize disease transmission.

5.8.2 Reproductive Tract Conditions

Accessory sex glands in male rats consist of a multilobed prostate, paired seminal vesicles and coagulating glands (anterior prostate glands), paired bulbourethral glands, and paired periurethral glands. Male rats also have preputial glands whereas female rats have clitoral glands, both of which are flattened, paired, pale tan structures found subcutaneously on the ventrocaudal abdomen, anterior to the urogenital papilla. While not accessory sex glands, infections, hyperplasia, cysts, and tumors may arise in these specialized sebaceous glands.

Microscopic evaluation of vaginal smears is used routinely for staging the rat estrous cycle. At 9–12 months of age, fertility in female rats decreases, with concomitant decreases in litter size. Cystic endometrial hyperplasia and adenomyosis (presence of endometrial glands within the myometrium) are not uncommon in aged female rats and are usually an incidental finding on microscopic examination of uterine tissues.

Mycoplasma pulmonis can induce urogenital tract infections, and suppurative endometritis, salpingitis, and oophoritis have been reported in affected animals. Females may be infected during self- or mutual grooming.

Prostatitis occurs with moderate frequency in older male rats. This may contribute to bacterial cystitis and pyelonephritis. Acute to chronic necrosis with edema and suppurative to mixed inflammatory cell infiltrates may be seen. Inflammation may also be seen in other accessory sex glands in chronic infections. Common bacterial isolates include *S. aureus* and *E. coli*.

5.8.3 Reproductive Masses

Vaginal and endometrial stromal polyps are relatively common in aged female rats and may be associated with vaginal and uterine prolapses (Figure 5.37). Nonclinical polyps, which are not hormonally sensitive, are generally single and pedunculated, and are considered an incidental finding at necropsy. Histologically, they consist of benign, poorly cellular, fibrous masses in which entrapped well differentiated endometrial glands may be present. Polypoid masses occasionally may be infarcted with secondary inflammation. Spontaneous uterine tumors are seen rarely. While most are estrogen receptor positive, progesterone receptor expression is highly variable. In female Wistar rats, there is an inverse relationship between mammary and uterine masses, likely related to opposing effects of prolactin levels on these tissues. Granulosa cell tumors are the most commonly observed ovarian tumor, but the incidence is also very low.

An ovarian yolk sac carcinoma was diagnosed in a 1.4-year-old Long Evans rat presenting in poor body condition with dysnea, abdominal distension and jaundice. Miliary firm, yellow masses were noted throughout the abdomen and were adherent the peritoneum as well as the omentum and visceral serosa (Figure 5.38). The ovaries were enlarged and diffusely infiltrated. Both nests and cords as well as papillary projections of vacuolated stellate cells were noted, as well as an abundant PAS positive acellular matrix. This is a rare germ cell tumor and differential diagnoses include other ovarian tumors, as well as mesothelioma.

Interstitial cell or Leydig tumors are the most common tumor of the testis with an incidence up to 100% in certain strains of rats. Tumors are benign and bilateral, and

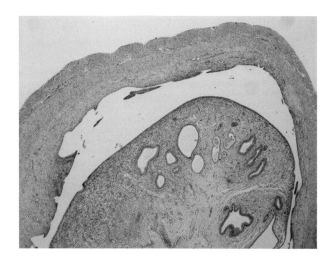

Figure 5.37 Endometrial stromal polyp from the uterus of an aged female rat. Entrapped and cystic endometrial glands are present in the mass. Polyps are generally incidental findings at necropsy.

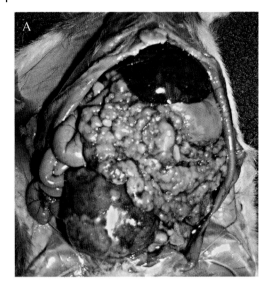
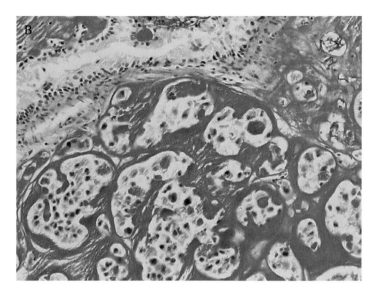

Figure 5.38 A: Ovarian yolk sac carcinoma in a Long Evans rat. Miliary firm yellow masses are present throughout the abdomen. The animal presented with abdominal distension and dyspnea. B: Nests of stellate neoplastic germ cells are embedded in a dense eosinophilic acellular matrix. *Source:* A and B: Courtesy of T. Cooper.

may induce hypercalcemia and hypercalciuria. Tumors are embedded within the testes, which may be enlarged, and, on cut section, these tumors bulge and are yellow-tan and multilobulated, sometimes with cystic, hemorrhagic or mineralized areas. Normal testicular tissue may be effaced entirely. Tumor cells have abundant pale eosinophilic cytoplasm with clear cell boundaries and a central round nucleus (Figure 5.39). The surrounding tissue may be compressed with a mild mixed inflammatory cell infiltrate.

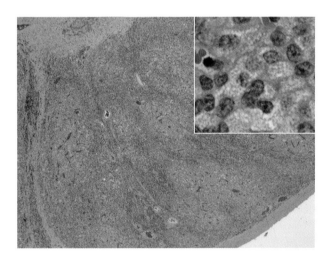

Figure 5.39 Interstitial cell tumor from the testicle of a male rat. Tumors are firm, bilateral, and often multilobulated, and are composed of bland interstitial cells with abundant, pale eosinophilic granular cytoplasm (inset). These are common benign tumors of intact male rats.

5.8.4 Other Reproductive Conditions

Uterine prolapse occurs sporadically in older rats and may be induced by straining secondary to uterine masses or cystitis (Figure 5.40A).

Peritesticular hemorrhage may occur in young adult rats infected with specific strains of parvovirus (see Section 5.10.1).

5.9 Nervous System Conditions

Primary neurologic conditions of rats must be differentiated from other common causes of weakness, paresis, head tilt, and ataxia, such as inanition, heat stress, infection, renal disease, otitis media (Figure 5.41), and trauma. Neuropil vacuolation and neuronal darkening are common artefacts of brain handling and fixation, and pathologists should be cautious about overinterpreting potential lesions.

Lipofuscin pigment accumulation is common in the neurons, astrocytes, and oligodendrocytes of aging rats, and such accumulation is interpreted as incidental. Decreases in cerebellar Purkinje cell numbers are found on occasion in older animals. Mild to moderate segmental demyelination and Wallerian degeneration of peripheral nerves (polyradiculoneuropathy) can be seen in older rats, particularly at the level of the lumbar spinal cord, affecting the sciatic nerve along its length. Affected nerves demonstrate segmental areas of swelling and fragmentation with mononuclear cell infiltrates and scattered digestion chambers. The condition is more

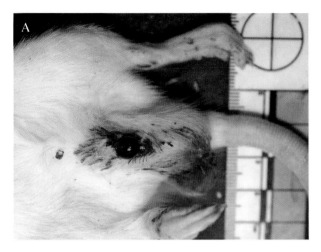
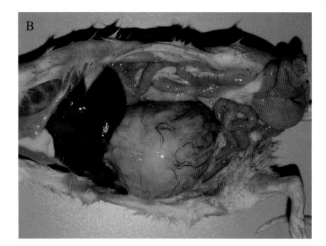

Figure 5.40 A: Vaginal prolapse in an aged female rat. B: Periuterine abscess in a severely debilitated female feeder-breeder colony rat. *Bacteroides* spp. was cultured from the abscess.

common in male rats and may be correlated clinically with posterior paresis or paralysis.

5.9.1 Cerebrospinal Masses

The most common mass seen in the brain of rats is the pituitary adenoma (see Section 5.3). Other spontaneous intracerebral tumors are highly uncommon. Of those described, astrocytoma, granular cell tumor, glial tumors, and meningioma are the most common. Neoplasia of the spinal cord is even less common, with too few cases reported to describe common tumor types. Secondary tumor infiltration of the spinal cord and peripheral nerves, for example, by lymphosarcoma or histiocytic sarcoma, is moderately common, and can account for ante-mortem paresis or paralysis in aging animals.

5.9.2 Other Conditions of the Brain and Spinal Cord

Congenital hydrocephalus is reported anecdotally in rats, but most affected pups die soon after birth. Acquired hydrocephalus is most common secondary to pituitary adenoma. Ataxia and subtle granular cerebellar degeneration have been reported in rats fed a thiamine-deficient diet.

Seizures are described anecdotally in pet rats. Differential diagnoses to consider include head trauma, neoplasia, intoxication, abscessation, and end stage systemic infectious disease, for example, that caused by *Streptococcus pneumoniae* (Figure 5.42).

Cerebellar hypoplasia of infant rats and acute, multifocal cerebral hemorrhage and subsequent death may

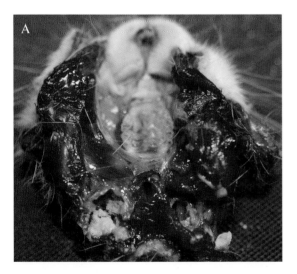
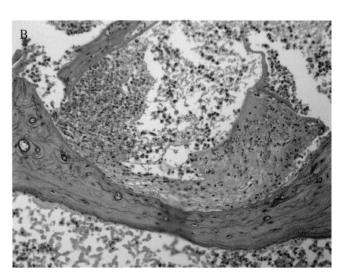

Figure 5.41 A: Bilateral suppurative to caseous otitis media from a rat infected with *Mycoplasma pulmonis*. Otitis media is a common cause of head tilt in a rat. B: Marked otitis interna and media in a rat found dead, caused by an acute *Streptococcus pneumoniae* infection. A marked fibrinosuppurative exudate can be seen filling the lumen and the membranous inner ear lining is markedly edematous.

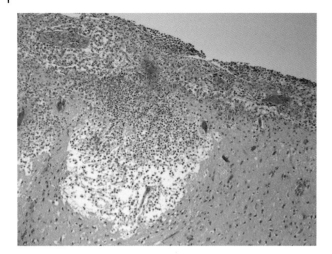

Figure 5.42 Fibrinosuppurative meningoencephalitis in an 8-month-old male Dumbo rat with *S. pneumoniae* septicemia. One animal in the family group had died 2 weeks previously and this animal was noted to be seizuring before it died. There is marked meningeal expansion secondary to inflammation with extension of the infection into the subtending parenchyma.

occur in young adult rats infected with Kilham's rat virus, a specific strain of parvovirus (see Section 5.10).

Both **granulomatous meningoencephalitis** and **encephalomyelitis** have been seen with spontaneous cases of central *Frenkelia* sp. and *Mucor*-like (fungal) infections.

Bilateral symmetrical **idiopathic necrotizing encephalitis** has been reported in asymptomatic adult Sprague–Dawley rats of both sexes. Sometimes these lesions were noted grossly at post mortem as a focus of red discoloration. Affected areas demonstrated white matter rarefaction and neuronal and glial cell necrosis with minimal inflammation. No etiology for this lesion has been determined.

Rats may be infected subclinically with several different **murine theiloviruses**, which are cardioviruses in the picornavirus family. No clinical or microscopic findings are noted, and detection occurs by serology.

5.10 Hematopoietic and Lymphoid Conditions

The erythrocyte half-life in rats is between 45 to 67 days and bone marrow remains active throughout life. The cellularity of marrow is approximately 80% in young animals and reduces to approximately 65% in 2-year-old animals. Infectious disease, inanition, and other sources of systemic stress can markedly affect the cellularity and the ratio of the lineages represented in bone marrow sections. Extramedullary hematopoiesis (erythroid, myeloid, and megakaryocyte) occurs throughout life, but is not as prominent in the rat spleen as in the mouse (Figure 5.43A). Splenic red pulp hyperplasia and granulopoiesis may be significant in response to infection. Accessory splenic tissue may be seen within the omentum or attached to the serosa of other viscera.

Leukocyte values show diurnal variation with higher white blood cell counts obtained during the day and subtle differences in white cell counts found depending on the blood collection site.

The thymus continues to develop after birth in the rat and reaches maximal size at sexual maturity, thereafter undergoing involution. Islands of ectopic thymic tissue may be found in the cervical area of some animals.

Peyer's patch size, location and number may vary among different strains and breeds of rats. Approximately 50% of the rat's lymphoid cells can be

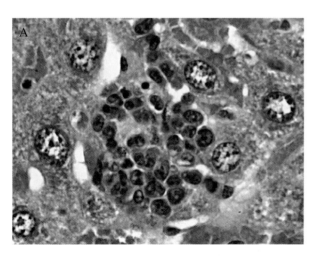

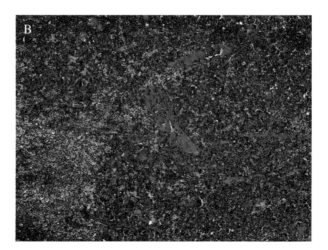

Figure 5.43 A: Extramedullary myelopoiesis is seen sporadically in rats and is most common in the liver. B: Massive thymic hemorrhage in a rat found dead acutely after transportation. No other lesions were noted to account for the sudden death.

found in mucosa-associated lymphoid tissue. Significant development of peripheral lymphoid tissue occurs postnatally, reaching functional maturation around 6–7 weeks of age. The appearance and size of lymphoid aggregates in various tissues as well as the peripheral lymph nodes are highly correlated to the degree of antigenic stimulation. For example, large periarteriolar lymphoid aggregates are common and generally considered incidental in companion rats without other signs of pulmonary disease, whereas they are rare to nonexistent in laboratory rats held under conditions of strict environmental hygiene.

5.10.1 Infectious Hematopoietic and Lymphoid Conditions

At least six rat parvoviruses have been identified to date, including Kilham's rat virus (KRV), H-1, rat parvovirus-1, and three different rat minute viruses. Infection of rats is largely asymptomatic; however, several outbreaks of disease, characterized by multi-organ hemorrhagic diathesis, have been documented in laboratory rats infected with the KRV strain. Peritesticular and intracerebral hemorrhage classic lesions of infection; however, the viruses are pantropic and lesions can be seen in multiple organs and cell types. Lymphoid tissue necrosis is common with infection. Large, eosinophilic intranuclear inclusion bodies can be seen in infected cells. Definitive characterization of infection is done by PCR assay.

5.10.2 Hematopoietic and Lymphoid Neoplasia

Hematopoietic and lymphoid neoplasia (Figure 5.44A) are generally uncommon in aging rats. The exception is large granular lymphocytic leukemia, which occurs with high incidence in F344 rats. These tumors are not seen widely in other strains and breeds. The disease is characterized by marked hepatosplenomegaly and very high white cell counts. Neoplastic round cells are small and pleomorphic with large nuclei and they contain reddish granules within the cytoplasm that are visible with Wright's stains on smears. Leukemia is common in advanced disease.

Lymphoblastic lymphoma (Figure 5.44B) and histiocytic sarcoma are the other major lymphohematopoietic tumors seen in rats. Lymphoblastic lymphomas may be B or T cell in origin and can be identified via immunohistochemistry. Epitheliotropic T cell lymphoma is rarely seen.

Histiocytic sarcomas may be seen in any tissue, but the liver, lung, spleen, lymph nodes, and subcutaneous tissues predominate as tumor sites. Tumors are pale and firm but may contain necrotic or hemorrhagic areas. They are characterized microscopically by large, infiltrative pleiomorphic mononuclear cells with abundant cytoplasm and indistinct cell borders. Nuclei are vesicular and multinucleated giant cells and mitoses are usually abundant (Figure 5.45). A variable fibrous matrix may be present. Hyaline droplets may be seen in the renal tubular epithelial cells of rats with histiocytic sarcoma. The droplets are positively labeled by lysozyme and are thought to be produced by neoplastic histiocytes.

Hemangiosarcoma is rarely described in rats. A multinodular pulmonary hemangiosarcoma involving 75% of the lung tissue has been described in an adult pet rat. Microscopically, neoplastic cells formed irregular, blood-filled channels that were surrounded by invading lymphoplasmacytic and histiocytic infiltrates. Immunologic markers for vWF, CD31, and VEGF were used to support the diagnosis. Mast cell tumors are rare in rats.

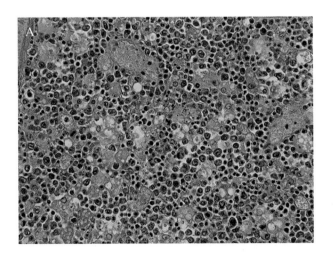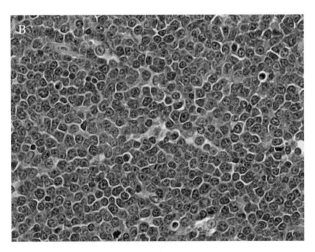

Figure 5.44 A: Splenic lymphoma in an aging rat. Neoplastic cells are pleomorphic and there is a high mitotic index. B: Thymic lymphoma in a rat, characterized by small neoplastic lymphocytes with scant basophilic cytoplasm and scattered mitoses.

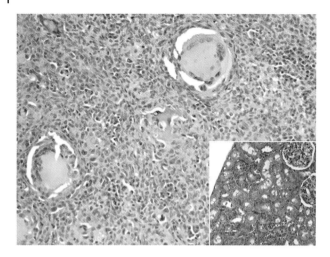

Figure 5.45 Histiocytic sarcoma in a mesenteric lymph node of a rat. Neoplastic mononuclear cells have indistinct cytoplasmic borders and several multinucleated giant cells are present. Inset: Hyaline droplets are present in the renal tubular epithelial cells from this animal, consistent with lysozyme secretion from neoplastic histiocytes.

5.10.3 Other Hematopoietic and Lymphoid Conditions

There are anecdotal reports from several countries of **heritable bleeding disorders** (hemophilia) in blue-coated rats, however, the clinical syndrome and associated etiopathogenesis have not been investigated.

Acute thymic hemorrhage and death are seen sporadically in rats, generally following transportation or some other management stressor (Figure 5.43B).

Lymphoid atrophy and **ectasia**, characterized by cystic dilatation of lymphoid sinuses, are common in aged rats and may be accompanied by vascular sinus ectasia. There may be moderate hemosiderin accumulation within macrophages found in lymph nodes and the splenic red pulp, interpreted as an incidental finding.

5.11 Ophthalmic Conditions

Rats have several lacrimal glands, including the Harderian gland, a large merocrine gland that almost encircles the globe, which is attached to the third eyelid by its duct. There is sexual dimorphism in lacrimal gland size, related to androgen production. Lipid and porphyrin-containing ocular secretions are predominantly produced by the Harderian gland, which are visualized microscopically as yellow brown proteinaceous globules within the center of acini. Any infectious or noninfectious stimulus that heightens parasympathetic stimulation may lead to increased Harderian gland secretion of porphyrin-containing tears.

The rat's eye is large for its size, spherical in shape, and continues to grow with age. The eye and optic nerve are otherwise similar morphologically and microscopically to other mammals, although the distribution and types of photoreceptors in the retina vary between species.

Unlike hamsters, exophthalmos is uncommon in rats and spontaneous occurrence is often related to a retrobulbar tumor. Microphthamos and anophthalmos are very uncommon congenital conditions in rats.

5.11.1 Conditions of the Lacrimal Glands and Ducts

There is normally marked anisokaryosis and anisocytosis of the exorbital lacrimal gland (Figure 5.46A).

Chromodacryorrhea is a nonspecific indication of systemic stress (Figure 5.45B). Management changes, poor nutrition, *M. pulmonis* infections, and infection with SDAV and subsequent Harderian gland inflammation (see Section 5.4.1.1) are examples of conditions that may induce this condition.

Inexpert blood sampling from the orbital venous plexus may result in periocular hemorrhage and lacrimal gland inflammation.

5.11.2 Conditions of the Eyelid and Conjunctiva

Conjunctivitis is moderately common in pet rats and may arise secondarily to infection with *M. pulmonis*, *P. pneumotropica*, *C. kutscheri*, *S. aureus*, and *Streptococcus* spp (Figure 5.47A).

Periocular dermatitis is common in hairless varieties of rats. Amelanotic melanomas have been reported on the palpebrae of albino rats.

5.11.3 Conditions of the Cornea and Anterior Chamber

Hyalinization or mineralization of the corneal stroma is a common and incidental lesion in aging animals. Single to multifocal punctate idiopathic corneal opacities are moderately common in some strains of rats.

Corneal ulcers and hypopyon may be seen in rats anesthetized with injectable drug combinations that are not supplemented concurrently with oxygen (Figure 5.47B). Lesions may be seen in rats anesthetized with inhalant agents without concurrent use of eye lubricant, as rats do not completely close their eyes during anesthesia. In the most severe cases, there is marked stromal edema, neovascularization, mixed leukocytic infiltration, and mineralization.

Punctate uni- or bilateral corneal opacities are common in some rat strains and correlated histologically to focal to multifocal mineral deposits. They are interpreted as an incidental finding in pet rats.

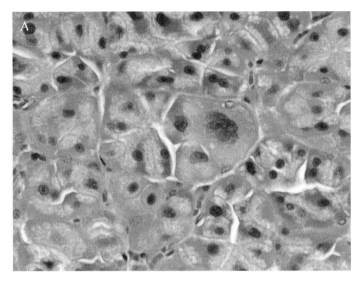 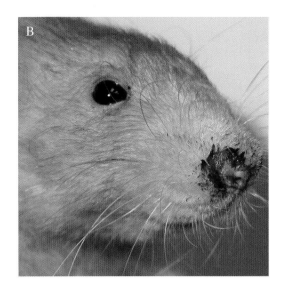

Figure 5.46 A: The normal exorbital lacrimal gland demonstrates moderate anisocytosis and anisokaryosis. This is more pronounced in male rats. B: Excessive oculonasal porphyrin discharge (chromodacryorrhea) is seen in rats that have experienced significant stressors or in animals suffering from intercurrent disease, such as respiratory disease. *Source* B: Courtesy of The Links Road Animal and Bird Clinic.

Keratitis and ulceration may occur secondarily to SDAV infection or self-trauma in animals with severe bacterial conjunctivitis.

5.11.4 Uveal and Lenticular Conditions

While uncommon, ocular melanomas have been reported in both pigmented and albino rats. Those occurring in albino animals are amelanotic melanomas. Tumors often arise from the iris or ciliary body and may induce exophthalmos as they enlarge.

Iris colobomas are reported in rats but are uncommon conditions. Uni- or bilateral cataracts are common in aging rats and may be heritable or acquired. Glaucoma is reported infrequently.

5.11.5 Retinal Conditions

Retinal degeneration is a common finding in many strains and breeds of rats and may be congenital in nature or acquired (Figure 5.48A). In affected animals, there is often marked loss of the outer nuclear layer and

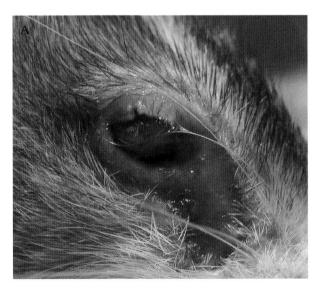 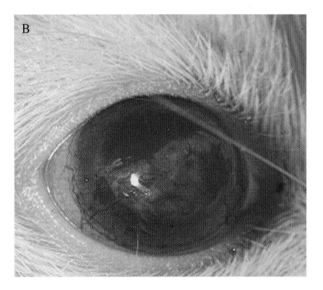

Figure 5.47 A: Keratitis and conjunctivitis following fighting in a pet rat. Courtesy of The Links Road Animal and Bird Clinic. B: Corneal ulceration with scarring and neovascularization following anesthesia with ketamine/zylazine in a young adult, male rat. These lesions can be avoided by providing supplemental oxygen during anesthesia. *Source:* Turner (2005). Reprinted with permission from AALAS.

A

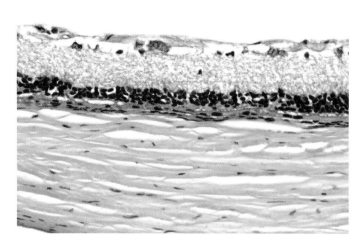

B

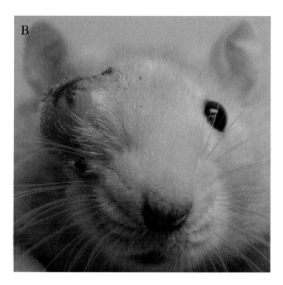

Figure 5.48 A: Marked retinal degeneration in an albino rat. There is a complete loss of retinal nuclear layers. B: Retrobulbar abscess in a pet rat. *Source* B: Courtesy of The Links Road Animal and Bird Clinic.

degeneration of both segments of the photoreceptor layer. In albino animals, exposure to bright light has been demonstrated to accelerate the degenerative process. Age-related loss of retinal neurons is common.

Retinal folding and colobomas of the optic disk are reported as incidental findings. Ophthalmic masses are uncommon in rats. Retrobulbar abscesses are seen sporadically (Figure 5.48B).

Bibliography

Introduction

Greaves, J.H. (1981) Wavy: a new recessive rexoid mutant in the Norway rat. *Journal of Heredity*, **72**(4), 291–292.

Harkness, J.E., Turner, P.V., VandeWoude, S., and Wheler, C.L. (2010) *Harkness and Wagner's Biology and Medicine of Rabbits and Rodents*, 5th edn. Wiley-Blackwell, Ames, IA.

Hayssen, V. (1997) Effects of the nonagouti coat-color allele on behavior of deer mice (*Peromyscus maniculatus*), a comparison with Norway rats (*Rattus norvegicus*). *Journal of Comparative Psychology.* **111**(4), 419–423.

Keeler, C.E. (1947) Coat color, physique, and temperament; materials for the synthesis of hereditary behavior trends in the lower mammals and man. *Journal of Heredity*, **38**(9), 271–277.

Kuramoto, T., Hirano, R., Kuwamura, M., and Serikawa, T. (2010) Identification of the rat Rex mutation as a 7-bp deletion at splicing acceptor site of the Krt71 gene. *Journal of Veterinary Medical Science.* **72**(7), 909–912.

Kuramoto, T., Yokoe, M., Yagasaki, K., *et al.* (2010) Genetic analyses of fancy rat-derived mutations. *Experimental Animals.* **59**(2), 147–55.

Fiedler, L.A. (1990) Rodents as a food source, in *Proceedings of the Fourteenth Vertebrate Pest Conference.* Paper 30. http://digitalcommons.unl.edu/vpc14/30 (accessed Aug. 25, 2015).

Kwit, N., Nelson, C., and Kugeler, K., *et al.* (2015) Human plague — United States, 2015. *Morbidity and Mortality Weekly Reports.* **64**,: 1–2.

Matthews, I. (1898) *Full Revelations of a Professional Rat-Catcher after 25 Years' Experience.* A Project Gutenberg eBook: www.gutenberg.org

Panteleyev, A.A. and Christiano, A.M. (2001) The Charles River "hairless" rat mutation is distinct from the hairless mouse alleles. *Comparative Medicine.* **51**(1), 49–55.

Priestley, G.C. (1966) Rates and duration of hair growth in the albino rat. *Journal of Anatomy*, **100**(1), 147–157.

Voisey, J. and van Daal, A. (2002) Agouti: from mouse to man, from skin to fat. *Pigment Cell Research*, **15**(1), 10–18.

Alopecia

Inalöz, H.S., Deveci, E., Inalöz, S.S., Unal, B., Eralp, A., and Can, I. (2002) The effects of tamoxifen on rat skin. *European Journal of Gynaecology and Oncology*, **23**(1), 50–52.

McElwee, K.J. and Hoffmann, R. (2002) Alopecia areata – animal models. *Clinical and Experimental Dermatology*, **27**(5), 410–417.

Morgan, A.F. and Simms, H.D. (1939) Greying of fur and other disturbances in several species due to vitamin deficiency. *Journal of Nutrition*, **16**, 233–250.

Bacterial Dermatitis

Fox, J.G., Niemi, S.M., Murphy, J.C., and Quimby, F.W. (1977) Ulcerative dermatitis in the rat. *Laboratory Animal Science.* **27**(5 Pt 1), 671–678.

Nakamura, Y., Oscherwitz, J., Cease, K.B., *et al.* (2013) Staphylococcus δ-toxin induces allergic skin disease by activating mast cells. *Nature*, **503**(7476), 397–401.

Wagner, J.E., Owens, D.R., LaRegina, M.C., and Vogler, G.A. (1977) Self trauma and *Staphylococcus aureus* in ulcerative dermatitis of rats. *Journal of the American Veterinary Medical Association.* **171**(9), 839–841.

Dermatophytoses

Chermette, R., Ferreiro, L., and Guillot, J. (2008) Dermatophytoses in animals. *Mycopathologia*, **166**, 385–405.

Lane, R.F. (2003) Diagnostic testing for fungal diseases. *Veterinary Clinics of North America: Exotic Animal Practice*, **6**, 301–314.

Lopez-Martinez, R., Mier, T., and Quirarte, M. (1984) Dermatophytes isolated from laboratory animals. *Mycopathologia*, **88**:111–3.

Papini, R., Gazzano, A., and Mancianti, F. (1997) Survey of dermatophytes isolated from the coats of laboratory animals in Italy. *Laboratory Animal Science.* **47**(1), 757–7.

Pollock, C. (2003) Fungal diseases of laboratory rodents. *Veterinary Clinics of North America: Exotic Animal Practice*, **6**(2), 401–413.

Parasitic Dermatitis

Baumstark, J., Beck, W., and Hofmann, H. (2007) Outbreak of tropical rat mite (*Ornithonyssus bacoti*) dermatitis in a home for disabled persons. *Dermatology*, **215**(1), 66–68.

Beck, W. and Pfister, K. (2004) Mites as newly emerging disease pathogens in rodents and human beings. *Veterinary Dermatology*, **15**(Suppl 1), 35.

Beck, W. (2008) Occurrence of a house-infesting tropical rat mite (*Ornithonyssus bacoti*) on murides and human beings. *Travel Medicine and Infectious Disease*, **6**(4), 245–249.

Bond, R., Riddle, A., Mottram, L., Beugnet, F., and Stevenson, R. (2007) Survey of flea infestation in dogs and cats in the United Kingdom during (2005. *Veterinary Record*, **160**(15), 503–506.

Chung, S.L., Hwang, S.J., Kwon, S.B., *et al.* (1998) Outbreak of rat mite dermatitis in medical students. *International Journal of Dermatology*, **37**(8), 591–594.

Civen, R., and Ngo, V. (2008) Murine typhus: an unrecognized suburban vectorborne disease. *Clinical Infectious Diseases*, **46**(6), 913–918.

Cole, J.S., Sabol-Jones, M., Karolewski, B., and Byford, T. (2005) *Ornithonyssus bacoti* infestation and elimination from a mouse colony. *Contemporary Topics in Laboratory Animal Science.* **44**(5), 27–30.

Durbin, P.W., Williams, M.H., Jeung, N., and Arnold, J.S. (1966) Development of spontaneous mammary tumors over the life-span of the female Charles River (Sprague–Dawley) rat: the influence of ovariectomy, thyroidectomy, and adrenalectomy-ovariectomy. *Cancer Research*, **26**(3), 400–411.

Engel, P.M., Welzel, J., Maass, M., Schramm, U., and Wolff, H.H. (1998) Tropical rat mite dermatitis: case report and review. *Clinical Infectious Diseases.* **27**(6), 1465–1469.

Eremeeva, M.E., Warashina, W.R., Sturgeon, M.M., *et al.* (2008) *Rickettsia typhi* and *R. felis* in rat fleas (*Xenopsylla cheopis*), Oahu, Hawaii. *Emerging Infectious Diseases*, **14**(10), 1613–1615.

Fisher, M., Beck, W., and Hutchson, M.J. (2007) Efficacy and safety of selamectin (Stronghold®/Revolution™) used off-label in exotic pets. *International Journal of Applied Research in Veterinary Medicine*, **5**(3), 87–96.

Hill, P.B., Lo, A., Eden, C.A.N., *et al.* (2006) Survey of the prevalence, diagnosis and treatment of dermatological conditions in small animals in general practice. *Veterinary Record*, **158**, 533–539.

Kondo, S., Taylor, A., and Chun, S. (1998) Elimination of an infestation of rat fur mites (*Radfordia ensifera*) from a colony of Long Evans rats, using the micro-dot technique for topical administration of 1% ivermectin. *Contemporary Topics in Laboratory Animal Science.* **37**(1), 58–61.

Pizzi, R., Meredith, A., Thoday, K.L., and Walker, A. (2004) *Ornithonyssus bacoti* infestation on pets in the UK. *Veterinary Record*, **154**(18), 576.

Schwan, T.G., Thompson, D., and Nelson, B.C. (1985) Fleas on roof rats in six areas of Los Angeles County, California: their potential role in the transmission of plague and murine typhus to humans. *American Journal of Tropical Medicine and Hygiene*, **34**(2), 372–379.

Visser, M., Rehbein, S., and Wiedemann, C. (2001) Species of flea (*Siphonoptera*) infesting pets and hedgehogs in Germany. *Journal of Veterinary Medicine B: Infectious Diseases and Veterinary Public Health.* **48**(3), 197–202.

Zingg, B.C., Brown, R.N., Lane, R.S., and LeFebvre, R.B. (1993) Genetic diversity among *Borrelia burgdorferi* isolates from wood rats and kangaroo rats in California. *Journal of Clinical Microbiology*, **31**(12), 3109–3114.

Mastitis

Hong, C.C., and Ediger, R.D. (1978) Chronic necrotizing mastitis in rats caused by *Pasteurella pneumotropica*. *Laboratory Animal Science.* **28**(3), 317–320.

Kunstýr, I., Ernst, H., and Lenz, W. (1995) Granulomatous dermatitis and mastitis in two SPF rats associated with a slowly growing *Staphylococcus aureus*–a case report. *Laboratory Animals.* **29**(2), 177–179.

Cutaneous Masses and Neoplasia

Barsoum, N.J., Gough, A.W., Sturgess, J.M., and de la Iglesia, F.A. (1984) Morphologic features and incidence of spontaneous hyperplastic and neoplastic mammary gland lesions in Wistar rats. *Toxicologic Pathology.* **12**(1), 26–38.

Becker, C., Kurth, A., Hessler, F., *et al.* (2009) Cowpox virus infection in pet rat owners: not always immediately recognized. *Deutsches Ärzteblatt International*, **106**(19), 329–334.

Campe, H., Zimmermann, P., Glos, K., *et al..* (2009) Cowpox virus transmission from pet rats to humans, Germany. *Emerging Infectious Diseases*, **15**(5), 777–780.

Capel-Edwards, M. (1970) Foot-and-mouth disease in the brown rat. *Journal of Comparative Pathology.* **80**, 543–548.

Esfandiari, A., Loya, T., and Lee, J.L. (2002) Skin tumors in aging Long Evans rats. *Journal of National Medical Association.* **94**(6), 506–510.

Evans, M.G., Cartwright, M.E., Sahota, P.S., and Clifford, C.B. (1997) Proliferative lesions of the skin and adnexa of rats. In: *Guides for Toxicologic Pathology.* STP/ARP/AFIP, Washington, DC. Available at: http://www.toxpath.org/ssdnc/SkinProliferativeRat.pdf (accessed November 22, 2011).

Harleman, J.H., Hargreaves, A., Andersson, H., and Kirk, S. (2012) A review of the incidence and coincidence of uterine and mammary tumors in Wistar and Sprague–Dawley rats based on the RITA database and the role of prolactin. *Toxicologic Pathology.* **40**(6), 926–930.

Hotchkiss, C.E. (1995) Effect of surgical removal of subcutaneous tumors on survival of rats. *Journal of the American Veterinary Medical Association.* **206**(10), 1575–1579.

Kalthoff, D., König, P., Meyer, H., Beer, M., and Hoffmann, B. (2011) Experimental cowpox virus infection in rats. *Veterinary Microbiology.* **153**(3–4), 382–385.

Maiboroda, A.D. (1982) Experimental infection of Norwegian rats (*Rattus norvegicus*) with ratpox virus. *Acta Virology*, **26**(4), 288–291.

Marennikova, S.S. (1979) Field and experimental studies of poxvirus infections in rodents. *Bulletin of the WHO*, **57**(3), 461–464.

Marennikova, S.S., Shelukhina, E.M., and Fimina, V.A. (1978) Pox infection in white rats. *Laboratory Animals (UK).* **12**(1), 33–36.

Martina, B.E., van Doornum, G., Dorrestein, G.M., *et al.* (2006) Cowpox virus transmission from rats to monkeys, the Netherlands. *Emerging Infectious Diseases*, **12**(6), 1005–1007.

Morehead, J., and Barthold, S.W. (1997) Hemangiopericytoma in a rat. *Contemporary Topics in Laboratory Animal Science.* **36**(5), 71–72.

Nakazawa, M., Tawaratani, T., Uchimoto, H., *et al.* (2001) Spontaneous neoplastic lesions in aged Sprague–Dawley rats. *Experimental Animals.* **50**(2), 99–103.

Ninove, L., Domart, Y., Vervel, C., *et al.* (2009) Cowpox virus transmission from pet rats to humans, France. *Emerging Infectious Diseases*, **15**(5), 781–784.

Okada, M., Takeuchi, J., Sobue, M., *et al.*(1981) Characteristics of 106 spontaneous mammary tumours appearing in Sprague–Dawley female rats. *British Journal of Cancer.* **43**(5), 689–695.

Pires, M.A., Seixas, F., Pires, I., and Queiroga, F. (2003) Mammary neoplasia with lung metastasis in a rat (*Rattus norvegicus*). *Veterinary Record*, **153**(25), 783–784.

Prats, M., Fondevila, D., Rabanal, R.M., Marco, A., Domingo, M., and Ferrer, L. (1994) Epidermotropic cutaneous lymphoma (mycosis fungoides) in an SD rat. *Veterinary Pathology.* **31**, 396–398.

Reznik, G., and Reznik-Schüller, H. (1980) Pathology of the clitoral and prepucial glands in aging F344 rats. *Laboratory Animal Science.* **30**(5), 845–850.

Russo, J., Gusterson, B.A., Rogers, A.E., Russo, I.H., Wellings, S.R., and van Zwieten, M.J. (1990) Comparative study of human and rat mammary tumorigenesis. *Laboratory Investigations*, **62**(3), 244–278.

Russo, J., and Russo, I.H. (2000) Atlas and histologic classification of tumors of the rat mammary gland. *Journal of Mammary Gland Biology and Neoplasia*, **5**(2), 187–200.

Schulz, E., Gottschling, M., Wibbelt, G., Stockfleth, E., and Nindl, I. (2009) Isolation and genomic characterization of the first Norway rat (*Rattus norvegicus*) papillomavirus and its phylogenetic position within Pipapillomavirus, primarily infecting rodents. *Journal of General Virology*, **90**(Pt 11), 2609–2614.

Sommer, M.M. (1997) Spontaneous skin neoplasms in Long-Evans rats. *Toxicologic Pathology.* **25**(5), 506–510.

Tantawi, H.H., Zaghloul, T.M., and Zakaria, M. (1983) Poxvirus infection in a rat (*Rattus norvegicus*) in Kuwait. *International Journal of Zoonoses.* **10**(1), 28–32.

Welsch, C.W., and Nagasawa, H. (1977) Prolactin and murine mammary tumorigenesis: a review. *Cancer Research*, **37**(4), 951–963.

Yoshitomi, K., Elwell, M.R., and Boorman, G.A. (1995) Pathology and incidence of amelanotic melanomas of the skin in F-344/N rats. *Toxicologic Pathology.* **23**(1), 16–25.

Zwicker, G.M., Eyster, R.C., Sells, D.M., and Gass, J.H. (1995) Spontaneous vascular neoplasms in aged Sprague–Dawley rats. *Toxicologic Pathology.* **23**(4), 518–526.

Other

Crippa, L., Gobbi, A., Ceruti, R.M., *et al.* (2000) Ringtail in suckling Munich Wistar Fromter rats: a histopathologic study. *Comparative Medicine*, **50**(5), 536–9.

Kitagaki, M., Suwa, T., Yanagi, M., and Shiratori, K. (2003) Auricular chondritis in young ear-tagged Crj:CD(SD) IGS rats. *Laboratory Animals (UK)*, **37**(3), 249–253.

McEwen, B.J., and Barsoum, N.J. (1990) Auricular chondritis in Wistar rats. *Laboratory Animals (UK)*. **24**(3), 280–283.

Morrow, D.T., Robinette, L.R., Saubert, C.W. IVth, and Van Hoosier, G.L. Jr. (1977) Poditis in the rat as a complication of experiments in exercise physiology. *Laboratory Animal Science*. **27**(5 Pt 1), 679–681.

Owens, N.C., Ootsuka, Y., Kanosue, K., and McAllen, R.M. (2002) Thermoregulatory control of sympathetic fibres supplying the rat's tail. *Journal of Physiology*, **543**(Pt 3), 849–858.

Prieur, D.J., Young, D.M., and Counts, D.F. (1984) Auricular chondritis in fawn-hooded rats. A spontaneous disorder resembling that induced by immunization with type II collagen. *American Journal of Pathology*. **116**(1), 69–76.

Totton, M. (1958) Ringtail in new-born Norway rats; a study of the effect of environmental temperature and humidity on incidence. *Journal of Hygiene (Lond)*. **56**(2), 190–196.

Tynes, V.V. (2013) Behavioral dermatopathies in small mammals. *Veterinary Clinics of North America: Exotic Animal Practice*, **16**, 801–820.

General

Harkness, J.E., Turner, P.V., VandeWoude, S., and Wheler, C.L. (2010) *Harkness and Wagner's Biology and Medicine of Rabbits and Rodents*, 5th edn. Wiley-Blackwell, Ames, IA.

Hoppmann, E., and Wilson Barron, H. (2007) Rodent dermatology. *Journal of Exotic Pet Medicine*, **16**(4), 238–255.

Diabetes Mellitus

Colella, R.M., Bonner-Weir, S., Braunstein, L.P., Schwalke, M., and Weir, G.C. (1985) Pancreatic islets of variable size--insulin secretion and glucose utilization. *Life Science*. **37**(11), 1059–1065.

Collins, B.R. (2008) Endocrine diseases of rodents. *Veterinary Clinics of North America: Exotic Animal Practice*, **11**, 153–162.

Wright, J., Yates, A., Sharma, H., and Thibert, P. (1985) Histopathological lesions in the pancreas of the BB Wistar rat as a function of age and duration of diabetes. *Journal of Comparative Pathology*. **95**(1), 7–14.

Endocrine Masses and Neoplasia

Adissu, H.A., and Turner, P.V. Insulinoma and squamous cell carcinoma with peripheral polyneuropathy in an aged Sprague–Dawley rat. *Journal of the American Association of Laboratory Animal Science*.**49**(6), 856–859.

Allen Durrand, A.M., Fisher, M., and Adams, M. (1964) Histology in rats as influenced by age and diet. I. Renal and cardiovascular systems. *Archives of Pathology*. **77**, 268–277.

Almaden, Y., Felsenfeld, A.J., Rodriguez, M., *et al.* (2003) Proliferation in hyperplastic human and normal rat parathyroid glands: role of phosphate, calcitriol, and gender. *Kidney International*, **64**(6), 2311–2317.

Attia, M.A. (1985) Neoplastic and nonneoplastic lesions in aging female rats with special reference to the functional morphology of the hyperplastic and neoplastic changes in the pituitary gland. *Archives of Toxicology*, **57**(2), 77–83.

Barsoum, N.J., Moore, J.D., Gough, A.W., Sturgess, J.M., and De La Iglesia, F.A. (1985) Morphofunctional investigations on spontaneous pituitary tumors in Wistar rats. *Toxicologic Pathology*. **13**(3), 200–8.

Berkvens, J.M., van Nesselrooy, J.H.J., and Kroes, R. (1980) Spontaneous tumours in the pituitary gland of old Wistar rats. A morphological and immunocytochemical study. *Journal of Pathology*. **130**, 179–191.

Brown, W.R., Gough, A., Hamlin, M.H. II, Hottendorf, G.H., and Patterson, D.R. (1995) Proliferative lesions of the adrenal glands in rats. E-4, in *Guides for Toxicologic Pathology*. STP/ARP/AFIP, Washington, DC.

Greenacre, C.B. (2004) Spontaneous tumors of small mammals. *Veterinary Clinics of North America: Exotic Animal Practice*, 7(3), 627–651.

Halloran, B., Udén, P., Duh, Q.Y., Kikuchi, S., Wieder, T., Cao, J., and Clark, O. (2002) Parathyroid gland volume increases with postmaturational aging in the rat. *American Journal of Physiology: Endocrinology and Metabolism*, **282**(3), E557–E563.

Kaspareit-Rittinghausen, J., Wiese, K., Deerberg, F., and Nitsche, B. (1990) Incidence and morphology of spontaneous thyroid tumours in different strains of rats. *Journal of Comparative Pathology*. **102**(4), 421–432.

Lindsay, S., Nichols, C.W. Jr, and Chaikoll, I.L. (1968) Naturally occurring thyroid carcinoma in a rat. *Archives of Pathology*. **86**, 353–364.

Nakazawa, M., Tawaratani, T., Uchimoto, H., *et al.* (2001) Spontaneous neoplastic lesions in aged Sprague–Dawley rats. *Experimental Animals*. **50**(2), 99–103.

Pace, V. and Perentes, E. (2001) Mixed pituitary adenoma-gangliocytoma in a female albino rat. *Acta Neuropathology* **101**(3), 277–280.

Pickering, C.E. and Pickering, R.G. (1984) The effect of repeated reproduction on the incidence of pituitary tumours in Wistar rats. *Laboratory Animals (UK).* **18**(4), 371–378.

Reznik, G., Ward, J.M., and Reznik-Schüller, H. (1980) Ganglioneuromas in the adrenal medulla of F344 rats. *Veterinary Pathology.* **17**(5), 614–621.

Son, W.C., Bell, D., Taylor, I., and Mowat, V. (2010) Profile of early occurring spontaneous tumors in Han Wistar rats. *Toxicologic Pathology.* **38**(2), 292–296.

Spencer, A.J., Andreu, M., and Greaves, P. (1986) Neoplasia and hyperplasia of pancreatic endocrine tissue in the rat: an immunocytochemical study. *Veterinary Pathology.* **23**, 11–15.

Stromberg, P.C., Wilson, F., and Capen, C.C. (1983) Immunocytochemical demonstration of insulin in spontaneous pancreatic islet cell tumors of Fisher rats. *Veterinary Pathology.* **20**, 291–297.

Thorson, L. (2014) Thyroid diseases in rodent species. *Veterinary Clinics of North America: Exotic Animal Practice,* **17**, 51–67.

Trouillas, J., Girod, C., Claustrat, B., Curé, M., and Dubois, M.P. (1982) Spontaneous pituitary tumors in the Wistar/Furth/Ico rat strain. An animal model of human prolactin adenoma. *American Journal of Pathology.* **109**(1), 57–70.

van Nesselrooij, J.H., Kuper, C.F., and Bosland, M.C. (1992) Correlations between presence of spontaneous lesions of the pituitary (adenohypophysis) and plasma prolactin concentration in aged Wistar rats. *Veterinary Pathology.* **29**(4), 288–300.

General

Dillberger, J.E. (1994) Age-related pancreatic islet changes in Sprague–Dawley rats. *Toxicologic Pathology.* **22**(1), 48–55.

Frith, C.H., Botts, S., Jokinen, M.P., *et al.* (2000) Non-proliferative lesions of the endocrine system in rats. E-1, in *Guides for Toxicologic Pathology.* STP/ARP/AFIP, Washington, DC.

Goodman, D.G., Ward, J.M., Squire, R.A., *et al.* (1980) Neoplastic and nonneoplastic lesions in aging Osborne-Mendel rats. *Toxicology and Applied Pharmacology,* **55**(3), 433–447.

Han, E.S., Evans, T.R., Lee, S., and Nelson, J.F. (2001) Food restriction differentially affects pituitary hormone mRNAs throughout the adult life span of male F344 rats. *Nutrition,* **131**(6), 1687–1693.

Han, E.S., Levin, N., Bengani, N., Roberts, J.L., Suh, Y., Karelus, K., and Nelson, J.F. (1995) Hyperadrenocorticism and food restriction-induced life extension in the rat: evidence for divergent regulation of pituitary proopiomelanocortin RNA and adrenocorticotropic hormone biosynthesis. *Gerontology A: Biol Science. Med Science.* **50**(5), B288–B294.

MacKenzie, W.F., and Garner, F.M. (1973) Comparison of neoplasms in six sources of rats. *National Cancer Institute* **50**, 1243–1257.

Masoro, E.J. (1988) Food restriction in rodents: An evaluation of its role in the study of aging. *Gerontology,* **43**(3), B59–B64.

Molon-Noblot, S., Keenan, K.P., Coleman, J.B., Hoe, C.M., and Laroque, P. (2001) The effects of ad libitum overfeeding and moderate and marked dietary restriction on age-related spontaneous pancreatic islet pathology in Sprague–Dawley rats. *Toxicologic Pathology.* **29**, 353–362.

Solleveld, H.A., Haseman, J.K., and McConnell, E.E. (1984) Natural history of body weight gain, survival, and neoplasia in the F344 rat. *Journal of the National Cancer Institute,* **72**(4), 929–940.

Takemori, K., Kimura, T., Shirasaka, N., *et al.* (2011) Food restriction improves glucose and lipid metabolism through Sirt1 expression: a study using a new rat model with obesity and severe hypertension. *Life Sciences.* **88**(25–26), 1088–1094.

Wright, J.R. Jr, Senhauser, D.A., Yates, A.J., Sharma, H.M., and Thibert, P. (1983) Spontaneous thyroiditis in BB Wistar diabetic rats. *Veterinary Pathology.* **20**(5), 522–530.

Mycoplasmosis

Davidson, M.K., Lindsey, J.R., Brown, M.B., Schoeb, T.R., and Cassell, G.H. (1981) Comparison of methods for detection of *Mycoplasma pulmonis* in experimentally and naturally infected rats. *Journal of Clinical Microbiology,* **14**(6), 646–655.

Ferreira, J.B., Yamaguti, M., Marques, L.M., Oliveira, R.C., Neto, R.L., Buzinhani, M., and Timenetsky, J. (2008) Detection of *Mycoplasma pulmonis* in laboratory rats and technicians. *Zoonoses and Public Health.* **55**(5), 229–234.

Pitcher, D.G. and Nicholas, R.A. (2005) *Mycoplasma* host specificity: fact or fiction? *Veterinary Journal,* **170**(3), 300–306.

Razin, S., Yogev, D., and Naot, Y. (1998) Molecular biology and pathogenicity of mycoplasmas. *Microbiology and Molecular Biology Reviews,* **62**(4), 1094–1156.

Reyes, L., Shelton, M., Riggs, M., and Brown, M.B. (2004) Rat strains differ in susceptibility to maternal and fetal infection with *Mycoplasma pulmonis. American Journal of Reproductive Immunology,* **51**(3), 211–9.

Reyes, L., Steiner, D.A., Hutchison, J., Crenshaw, B., and Brown, M.B. (2000) *Mycoplasma pulmonis* genital disease: effect of rat strain on pregnancy outcome. *Comparative Medicine,* **50**(6), 622–627.

Schoeb, T.R., Davidson, M.K., and Lindsey, J.R. (1982) Intracage ammonia promotes growth of *Mycoplasma pulmonis* in the respiratory tract of rats. *Infection and Immunity,* **38**(1), 212–217.

Whittlestone, P., Lemcke, R.M., and Olds, R.J. (1972) Respiratory disease in a colony of rats. II. Isolation of *Mycoplasma pulmonis* from the natural disease, and the experimental disease induced with a cloned culture of this organism. *Journal of Hygiene (Lond)*, **70**(3), 387–407.

Filobacterium rodentium or Cilia-Associated Respiratory Bacillus

Cundiff, D.D., Besch-Williford, C.L., Hook, R.R. Jr, Franklin, C.L., and Riley, L.K. (1995) Characterization of cilia-associated respiratory bacillus in rabbits and analysis of the 16S rRNA gene sequence. *Laboratory Animal Science.* **45**(1), 22–26.

Cundiff, D.D., Riley, L.K., Franklin, C.L., Hook, R.R. Jr, and Besch-Williford, C. (1995) Failure of a soiled bedding sentinel system to detect cilia-associated respiratory bacillus infection in rats. *Laboratory Animal Science.* **45**(2), 219–221.

Franklin, C.L., Pletz, J.D., Riley, L.K. *et al.* (1999) Detection of cilia-associated respiratory (CAR) bacillus in nasal-swab specimens from infected rats by use of polymerase chain reaction. *Laboratory Animal Science.* **49**(1), 114–117.

Ike F, Sakamoto M, Ohkuma M, Kajita A, Matsushita S, KokuboT. (2016). Filobacterium rodentium gen. nov., sp. nov., a member of Filobacteriaceae fam. nov. within the phylum Bacteroidetes, and includes microaerobic filamentous bacterium isolated from rodent respiratory disease specimens. International Journal of Systematic and Evolutionary Microbiology, **66**(1):150–157.

Kawano, A., Nenoi, M., Matsushita, S., Matsumoto, T., and Mita, K. (2000) Sequence of 16S rRNA gene of rat-origin cilia-associated respiratory (CAR) bacillus SMR strain. *Journal of Veterinary Medical Science.* **62**(7), 797–800.

Matsushita, S. (1986) Spontaneous respiratory disease associated with cilia-associated respiratory (CAR) bacillus in a rat. *Nihon Juigaku Zasshi.* **48**(2), 437–440.

Medina, L.V., Fortman, J.D., Bunte, R.M., and Bennett, B.T. (1994) Respiratory disease in a rat colony: identification of CAR bacillus without other respiratory pathogens by standard diagnostic screening methods. *Laboratory Animal Science.* **44**(5), 521–525.

Schoeb, T.R., Davidson, M.K., and Davis, J.K. (1997) Pathogenicity of cilia-associated respiratory (CAR) bacillus isolates for F344, LEW, and SD rats. *Veterinary Pathology.* **34**(4), 263–270.

Streptococcal Respiratory Infections

Baer, H., and Preiser, A. (1969) Type 3 diplococcus pneumonia in laboratory rats. *Canadian Journal of Comparative Medicine*, **33**(2), 113–7.

Borkowski, G.L., and Griffith, J.W. (1990) Diagnostic exercise: pneumonia and pleuritis in a rat. *Laboratory Animal Science.* **40**(3), 323–325.

Chiavolini, D., Pozzi, G., and Ricci, S. (2008) Animal models of *Streptococcus pneumoniae* disease. *Clinical Microbiology Review*, **21**(4), 666–685.

Corning, B.F., Murphy, J.C., and Fox, J.G. (1991). Group G streptococcal lymphadenitis in rats. *Journal of Clinical Microbiology*, **29**(12), 2720–2723.

Ford, T.M. (1965) An outbreak of pneumonia in laboratory rats associated with *Diplococcus pneumoniae* type 8. *Laboratory Animal Care.* **15**, 448–451.

Hardie, J.M. and Whiley, R.A. (1997) Classification and overview of the genera *Streptococcus* and *Enterococcus*. *Society of Applied Bacteriology Symposium Series*, **26**, 1S–11S.

Mirick, G.S., Richter, C.P., Schaub, I.G., *et al.* (1950) An epizootic due to pneumococcus type II in laboratory rats. *American Journal of Hygiene.* **52**, 48–53.

Shuster, K.A., Hish, G.A., Selles, L.A., *et al.* (2013) Naturally occurring disseminated group B *Streptococcus* infections in postnatal rats. *Comparative Medicine*, **63**(1), 55–61.

Van der Linden, M., Al-Lahham, A., Nicklas, W., and Reinert, R.R. (2009) Molecular characterization of pneumococcal isolates from pets and laboratory animals. *PLoS ONE.* **4**(12), e8286.

Other Bacterial Infections

Amao, H., Akimoto, T., Komukai, Y., *et al.* (2002) Detection of *Corynebacterium kutscheri* from the oral cavity of rats. *Experimental Animals.* **51**(1), 99–102.

Amao, H., Komukai, Y., Akimoto, T., *et al.* (1995) Natural and subclinical *Corynebacterium kutscheri* infection in rats. *Laboratory Animal Science.* **45**(1), 11–14.

Bemis, D.A., Shek, W.R., and Clifford, C.B. (2003) *Bordetella bronchiseptica* infection of rats and mice. *Comparative Medicine*, **53**(1), 11–20.

Ford, T.M. and Joiner, G.N. (1968) Pneumonia in a rat associated with *Corynebacterium pseudotuberculosis*. A case report and literature survey. *Laboratory Animal Care.* **18**(2), 220–223.

Holmes, N.E. and Korman, T.M. (2007) *Corynebacterium kutscheri* infection of skin and soft tissue following rat bite. *Journal of Clinical Microbiology*, **45**(10), 3468–3469.

Jackson, N.N., Wall, H.G., Miller, C.A., and Rogul, M. (1980) Naturally acquired infections of *Klebsiella pneumoniae* in Wistar rats. *Laboratory Animals (UK)*, **14**(4), 357–361.

McEwen, S.A. and Percy, D.H. (1985) Diagnostic exercise: pneumonia in a rat. *Laboratory Animal Science.* **35**(5), 485–487.

Wang, R.F., Campbell, W., Cao, W.W., *et al.* (1996) Detection of *Pasteurella pneumotropica* in laboratory mice and rats by polymerase chain reaction. *Laboratory Animal Science.* **46**(1), 81–85.

Fungal Infections

Albers, T.M., Simon, M.A., and Clifford, C.B. (2009) Histopathology of naturally transmitted "rat respiratory virus": progression of lesions and proposed diagnostic criteria. *Veterinary Pathology.* **46**(5), 992–999.

Chabé, M., Aliouat-Denis, C.M., Delhaes, L., *et al.* (2011) *Pneumocystis*: from a doubtful unique entity to a group of highly diversified fungal species. *FEMS Yeast Research,* **11**(1), 2–17.

Chang, S.C., Hsuan, S.L., Lin, C.C., *et al.* (2013) Probable *Blastomyces dermatitidis* infection in a young rat. *Veterinary Pathology.* **50**(2), 343–346.

Icenhour, C.R., Rebholz, S.L., Collins, M.S., and Cushion, M.T. (2001) Widespread occurrence of *Pneumocystis carinii* in commercial rat colonies detected using targeted PCR and oral swabs. *Journal of Clinical Microbiology,* **39**(10), 3437–3441.

Livingston, R.S., Besch-Williford, C.L., Myles, M.H., *et al.* (2011) *Pneumocystis carinii* infection causes lung lesions historically attributed to rat respiratory virus. *Comparative Medicine,* **61**(1), 45–59.

Weisbroth, S.H., Geistfeld, J., Weisbroth, S.P., *et al.* (1999) Latent *Pneumocystis carinii* infection in commercial rat colonies: comparison of inductive immunosuppressants plus histopathology, PCR, and serology as detection methods. *Journal of Clinical Microbiology,* **37**(5), 1441–1446.

Viral Respiratory Diseases

Burek, J.D., Zurcher, C., Van Nunen, M.C., and Hollander, C.F. (1977) A naturally occurring epizootic caused by Sendai virus in breeding and aging rodent colonies. II. Infection in the rat. *Laboratory Animal Science.* **27**(6), 963–971.

Everitt, J.I. and Richter, C.B. (1990) Infectious diseases of the upper respiratory tract: implications for toxicology studies. *Environmental Health Perspectives,* **85**, 239–247.

Giddens, W.E., Van Hoosier, G.L., and Garlinghouse, L.E. (1987) Experimental Sendai virus infection in laboratory rats II. Pathology and immunohistochemistry. *Laboratory Animal Science.* **37**, 442–448.

Kashuba, C., Hsu, C., Krogstad, A., and Franklin, C. (2005) Small mammal virology. *Veterinary Clinics of North America: Exotic Animal Practice,* **8**(1), 107–22.

Parker, J.C., Cross, S.S., and Rowe, W.P. (1970) Rat coronavirus (RCV): a prevalent, naturally occurring pneumotropic virus of rats. *Arch Gesammelte Virusforschung,* **31**(3), 293–302.

Pulmonary Masses and Neoplasia

Chen, H.C., Liang, C.T., Hong, C.C., Huang, Y.J., and Pan, I.J. (1996) Spontaneous pulmonary squamous cell carcinoma in an aging CD rat. *Veterinary Pathology.* **33**(2), 228–30.

Goodman, D.G., Ward, J.M., Squire, R.A., *et al.* (1980) Neoplastic and nonneoplastic lesions in aging Osborne-Mendel rats. *Toxicology and Applied Pharmacology,* **55**(3), 433–447.

Greenacre, C.B. (2004) Spontaneous tumors of small mammals. *Veterinary Clinics of North America: Exotic Animal Practice,* **7**(3), 627–651.

Prejean, J.D., Peckham, J.C., Casey, A.E., *et al.* (1973) Spontaneous tumors in Sprague–Dawley rats and Swiss mice. *Cancer Research,* **33**(11), 2768–2773.

General

Cowie, R.H. (2013) Biology, systematics, life cycle, and distribution of *Angiostrongylus cantonensis*, the cause of rat lungworm disease. *Hawaii Journal of Medicine and Public Health.* **72**(6 Suppl 2), 6–9.

Kling, M.A. (2011) A review of respiratory system anatomy, physiology, and disease in the mouse, rat, hamster, and gerbil. *Veterinary Clinics of North America: Exotic Animal Practice,* **14**(2), 287–337.

Martins, Y.C., Tanowitz, H.B., and Kazacos, K.R. (2015) Central nervous system manifestations of *Angiostrongylus cantonensis* infection. *Acta Tropica,* **141**(Pt A), 46–53.

Renne, R.A., Dungworth, D.L., Keenan, C.M., Morgan, K.T., Hahn, F.F., and Schwartz, L.W. (2003) Non-proliferative lesions of the respiratory tract in rats. R-1, in *Guides for Toxicologic Pathology,* STP/ARP/AFIP, Washington, DC.

Reznik, G.K. (1990) Comparative anatomy, physiology, and function of the upper respiratory tract. *Environmental Health Perspectives,* **85**, 171–176.

Thiengo, S.C., Simões Rde, O., Fernandez, M.A., and Maldonado, A. Jr. (2013) *Angiostrongylus cantonensis* and rat lungworm disease in Brazil. *Hawaii Journal of Medicine and Public Health,* **72**(6 Suppl 2), 18–22.

York, E.M., Creecy, J.P., Lord, W.D., and Caire, W. (2015) Geographic range expansion for rat lungworm in North America. *Emerging Infectious Diseases,* **21**(7), 1234–1236.

Musculoskeletal Conditions

Feinstein, R.E. and Eld, K. (1989) Naturally occurring erysipelas in rats. *Laboratory Animals (UK).* **23**, 256–260.

Jackson, T.A., Chrisp, C.E., Dysko, R.C., and Carlson, B.M. (1997) Spontaneous hypertrophic osteopathy in a Wistar rat. *Contemporary Topics in Laboratory Animal Science.* **36**(5), 68–70.

Katerji, S., Vanmuylder, N., Svoboda, M., Rooze, M., and Louryan, S. (2009) Expression of Msx1 and Dlx1 during Dumbo rat head development: Correlation with morphological features. *Genetics and Molecular Biology,* **32**(2), 399–404.

Kato, M. and Onodera, T. (1984) Spontaneous osteochondrosis in rats. *Laboratory Animals (UK)*, **18**(2), 179–187.

Kato, M. and Onodera, T. (1987) Early changes of osteochondrosis in medial femoral condyles from rats. *Veterinary Pathology.* **24**(1), 80–86.

Schaid, D.J., Kunz, H.W., and Gill, T.J. 3rd. (1982) Genic interaction causing embryonic mortality in the rat: epistasis between the Tal and GRC genes. *Genetics*, **100**(4), 615–632.

van Steenis, G. and Kroes, R. (1971) Changes in the nervous system and musculature of old rats. *Veterinary Pathology.* **8**(4), 320–332.

Yamasaki, K. and Houshuyama, S. (1994) Proliferative bone lesions in Sprague Dawley rats. *Laboratory Animal Science*, **44**(2), 177–179.

Neoplasia

Brockus, C.W., Rakich, P.M., King, C.S., and Broderson, J.R. (1999) Rhabdomyosarcoma associated with incisor malocclusion in a laboratory rat. *Contemporary Topics in Laboratory Animal Science.* **38**(6), 42–43.

Nagamine, C.M., Jackson, C.N., Beck, K.A., *et al.* (2005) Acute paraplegia in a young adult long-Evans rat resulting from T-cell lymphoma. *Contemporary Topics in Laboratory Animal Science.* **44**(6), 53–56.

Ruben, Z., Rohrbacher, E., and Miller, J.E. (1986) Spontaneous osteogenic sarcoma in the rat. *Journal of Comparative Pathology.* **96**(1), 89–94.

Oral Conditions

Adissu, H.A. and Turner, P.V. (2010) Insulinoma and squamous cell carcinoma with peripheral polyneuropathy in an aged Sprague–Dawley rat. *Journal of the American Association of Laboratory Animal Science*, **49**(6), 856–859.

Capello, V. (2008) Diagnosis and treatment of dental disease in pet rodents. *Journal of Exotic Pet Medicine*, **17**(2), 114–123.

Horn, C.C., Kimball, B.A., Wang, H., *et al.* (2013) Why can't rodents vomit? A comparative behavioral, anatomical, and physiological study. *PLoS One*, **8**(4), e60537.

Legendre, L.F. (2003) Oral disorders of exotic rodents. *Veterinary Clinics of North America: Exotic Animal Practice*, **6**(3), 601–628.

Long, P.H., Leininger, J.R., Nold, J.B., and Lieuallen, W.G. (1993) Proliferative lesions of bone, cartilage, tooth, and synovium in rats. MST-2, in, *Guides for Toxicologic Pathology.* STP/ARP/AFIP, Washington, DC.

Whitely, L.O., Anver, M.R., Botts, S., and Jokinen, M.P. (1996) Proliferative lesions of the intestine, salivary glands, oral cavity, and esophagus in rats, GI-1/2/4, in *Guides for Toxicologic Pathology.* STP/ARP/AFIP, Washington, DC.

Salivary Gland and Esophageal Conditions

Banerjee, P., Ali, Z., and Fowler, D.R. (2011) Rat bite fever, a fatal case of *Streptobacillus moniliformis* infection in a 14-month-old boy. *Journal of Forensic Science.* **56**(2), 531–533.

Centers for Disease Control. (2003) Fatal rat-bite fever – Florida and Washington. *Morbidity and Mortality Weekly Reports*, **53**(51 & 52), 1198–1202.

Cunningham, B.B., Paller, A.S., and Katz, B.Z. (1998) Rat bite fever in a pet lover. *Journal of the American Academy of Dermatology*, **38**(2 Pt 2), 330–332.

Elliott, S.P. (2007) Rat bite fever and *Streptobacillus moniliformis*. *Clinical Microbiology Reviews*, **20**(1), 13–22.

Gresik, E.W. (1980) Postnatal developmental changes in submandibular glands of rats and mice. *Journal of Histochemistry and Cytochemistry*, **28**(8), 860–870.

Hagelskjaer, L., Sørensen, I., and Randers, E. (1998) *Streptobacillus moniliformis* infection: 2 cases and a literature review. *Scandinavian Journal of Infectious Diseases*, **30**(3), 309–311.

Halter, S.A., Wetherall, N., and Holscher M. (1983) Adenocarcinoma of the parotid gland in nude rats. *Laboratory Animal Science.* **33**, 287–289.

Harkness, J.E., and Ferguson, F.G. (1979) Idiopathic megaesophagus in a rat (*Rattus norvegicus*). *Laboratory Animal Science.* **29**(4), 495–498.

Hayashimoto, N., Yoshida, H., Goto, K., and Takakura, A. (2008) Isolation of *Streptobacillus moniliformis* from a pet rat. *Journal of Veterinary Medical Science.* **70**(5), 493–495.

Hosokawa, S., Imai, T., Hayakawa, K., Fukuta, T., and Sagami, F. (2000) Parotid gland papillary cystadenocarcinoma in a Fischer 344 rat. *Contemporary Topics in Laboratory Animal Science.* **39**(3), 31–33.

Meier, H. (1960) Spontaneous cytomegalic inclusion body disease involving lacrimal glands of caesarian-derived (so-called) pathogen-free rats. *Nature*, **188**, 506–507.

Mudd, B.D., and White, S.C. (1975) Sexual dimorphism in the rat submandibular gland. *Journal of Dental Research*, **54**(1), 193.

Percy, D.H., Hayes, M.A., Kocal, T.E., and Wojcinski, Z.W. (1988) Depletion of salivary gland epidermal growth factor by sialodacryoadenitis virus infection in the Wistar rat. *Veterinary Pathology.* **25**:183–192.

Percy, D.H., Wojcinski, Z.W., and Schunk, M.K. (1989) Sequential changes in the harderian and exorbital lacrimal glands in Wistar rats infected with sialodacryoadenitis virus. *Veterinary Pathology.* **26**(3), 238–245.

Ruben, Z., Rohrbacher, E., and Miller, J.E. (1983) Esophageal impaction in BHE rats. *Laboratory Animal Science.* **33**, 63–65.

Tsunenari, I., Yamate, J., and Sakuma, S. (1997) Poorly differentiated carcinoma of the parotid gland in a six-week-old Sprague–Dawley rat. *Toxicologic Pathology.* **25**, 225–228.

Ward, J.M., Lock, A., Collins, M.J. Jr, Gonda, M.A., and Reynolds, C.W. (1984) Papovaviral sialoadenitis in athymic nude rats. *Laboratory Animals (UK)*, **18**(1), 84–89.

Wullenweber, M. (1995) *Streptobacillus moniliformis*–a zoonotic pathogen. Taxonomic considerations, host species, diagnosis, therapy, geographical distribution. *Laboratory Animals (UK)*, **29**(1), 1–15.

Gastric Conditions

Bosgraaf, C.A., Suchy, H., Harrison, C., and Toth, L.A. (2004) What's your diagnosis? Dyspnea and porphyria in rats. *Laboratory Animals (NY)*, **33**(3), 21–23.

Frantz, J.D., Betton, G., Cartwright, M.E., *et al.* (1991) Proliferative lesions of the nonglandular and glandular stomach in rats, *GI-3, in Guides for Toxicologic Pathology*. STP/ARP/AFIP, Washington, DC.

Fujimoto, H., Shibutani, M., Kuroiwa, K., *et al.* (2006) A case report of a spontaneous gastrointestinal stromal tumor (GIST) occurring in a F344 rat. *Toxicologic Pathology.* **34**(2), 164–167.

Giusti, A.M., Crippa, L., Bellini, O., Luini, M., and Scanziani, E. (1998) Gastric spiral bacteria in wild rats from Italy. *Journal of Wildlife Diseases*, **34**(1), 168–172.

Majka, J.A. and Sher, S. (1989) Spontaneous gastric carcinoid tumor in an aged Sprague–Dawley rat. *Veterinary Pathology.* **26**(1), 88–90.

Shibuya, K., Tajima, M., and Yamate, J. (1993) Multicystic peritoneal mesothelioma in a Fischer-344 rat. *Toxicologic Pathology.* **21**(1), 87–90.

Tanigawa, H., Onodera, H., and Maekawa, A. (1987) Spontaneous mesotheliomas in Fischer rats–a histological and electron microscopic study. *Toxicologic Pathology.* **15**(2), 157–163.

Enteric Conditions

Centers for Disease Control. (2005) Outbreak of multidrug-resistant *Salmonella* Typhimurium associated with rodents purchased at retail pet stores – United States, December 2003–October 2004. *Morbidity and Mortality Weekly Reports*, **54**(17), 429–433.

Chu, D.K., Chin, A.W., Smith, G.J., *et al.* (2010) Detection of novel astroviruses in urban brown rats and previously known astroviruses in humans. *Journal of General Virology*, **91**(Pt 10), 2457–2462.

Dubois, A., Weise, V.K., and Kopin, I.J. (1973) Postoperative ileus in the rat: physiopathology, etiology and treatment. *Annals of Surgery*, **178**(6), 781–786.

Easterbrook, J.D., Kaplan, J.B., Glass, G.E., Watson, J., and Klein, S.L. (2008) A survey of rodent-borne pathogens carried by wild-caught Norway rats: a potential threat to laboratory rodent colonies. *Laboratory Animals (UK)*, **42**(1), 92–98.

Eiden, J., Vonderfecht, S., and Yolken, R.H. (1985) Evidence that a novel rotavirus-like agent of rats can cause gastroenteritis in man. *Lancet*, **2**(8445), 8–11.

Etheridge, M.E., Yolken, R.H., and Vonderfecht, S.L. (1988) *Enterococcus hirae* implicated as a cause of diarrhea in suckling rats. *Journal of Clinical Microbiology*, **26**(9), 1741–1744.

Fleischman, R.W., McCracken, D., and Forbes, W. (1977) Adynamic ileus in the rat induced by chloral hydrate. *Laboratory Animal Science.* **27**(2), 238–243.

Franklin, C.L., Motzel, S.L., Besch-Williford, C.L., Hook, R.R. Jr, and Riley, L.K. (1994) Tyzzer's infection: host specificity of *Clostridium piliforme* isolates. *Laboratory Animal Science.* **44**(6), 568–572.

Gades, N.M., Mandrell, T.D., and Rogers, W.P. (1999) Diarrhea in neonatal rats. *Contemporary Topics in Laboratory Animal Science.* **38**(6), 44–46.

Hanes, M.A., and Stribling, L.J. (1995) Fibrosarcomas in two rats arising from hepatic cysts of *Cysticercus fasciolaris*. *Veterinary Pathology.* **32**(4), 441–444.

Hill, W.A., Randolph, M.M., and Mandrell, T.D. (2009) Sensitivity of perianal tape impressions to diagnose pinworm (*Syphacia* spp.) infections in rats (*Rattus norvegicus*) and mice (*Mus musculus*). *Journal of the American Association of Laboratory Animal Science.* **48**(4), 378–380.

Hoover, D., Bendele, S.A, Wightman, S.R., Thompson, C.Z., and Hoyt, J.A. (1985) Streptococcal enteropathy in infant rats. *Laboratory Animal Science.* **35**(6), 635–41.

Huber, A.C., Yolken, R.H., Mader, L.C., Strandberg, J.D., and Vonderfecht, S.L. (1989) Pathology of infectious diarrhea of infant rats (IDIR) induced by an antigenically distinct rotavirus. *Veterinary Pathology.* **26**(5), 376–385.

Irizarry-Rovira, A.R., Wolf, A., and Bolek, M. (2007) *Taenia taeniaeformis*-induced metastatic hepatic sarcoma in a pet rat (*Rattus norvegicus*). *Journal of Exotic Pet Medicine*, **16**(1), 45–48.

Johne, R., Heckel, G., Plenge-Bönig, A. *et al.* (2010) Novel hepatitis E virus genotype in Norway rats, Germany. *Emerging Infectious Diseases*, **16**(9), 1452–1425.

Jonas, A.M., Percy, D.H., and Craft, J. (1970) Tyzzer's disease in the rat. Its possible relationship with megaloileitis. *Archives of Pathology.* **90**(6), 516–521.

Macnish, M.G., Morgan, U.M., Behnke, J.M., and Thompson, R.C. (2002) Failure to infect laboratory rodent hosts with human isolates of *Rodentolepis* (= *Hymenolepis*) *nana*. *Journal of Helminthology*, **76**(1), 37–43.

Mahesh Kumar, J., Reddy, P.L., Aparna, V., *et al.* (2006) *Strobilocercus faScience. olaris* infection with hepatic sarcoma and gastroenteropathy in a Wistar colony. *Veterinary Parasitology*, **141**(3–4), 362–367.

Public Health Agency of Canada. Public Advisory: Illness linked to frozen rodents used as pet food. Sept 30, (2010. http://www.phac-aspc.gc.ca/alert-alerte/salmonella/advisory-avis_20100930-eng.php

Reavill, D. (2014) Pathology of the exotic companion mammal gastrointestinal system. *Veterinary Clinics of North America: Exotic Animal Practice*, **17**:145–164.

Rowlatt, U., and Roe, F.J. (1967) Epithelial tumors of the rat pancreas. *Journal of National Cancer Institute*, **39**(1), 17–32.

Silverman, J., and Muir, W.W. 3rd. (1993) A review of laboratory animal anesthesia with chloral hydrate and chloralose. *Laboratory Animal Science.* **43**(3), 210–216.

Smith, K.J., Skelton, H.G., Hilyard, E.J., *et al.* (1996) *Bacillus piliformis* infection (Tyzzer's disease) in a patient infected with HIV-1: confirmation with 16S ribosomal RNA sequence analysis. *Journal of the American Academy of Dermatology*, **34**(2 Pt 2), 343–348.

Stedham, M.A., and Bucci, T.J. (1970) Spontaneous Tyzzer's disease in a rat. *Laboratory Animal Care*, **20**(4 Pt 1), 743–6.

Swanson, S.J., Snider, C., Braden, C.R., *et al.* (2007) Multidrug-resistant *Salmonella enterica* serotype Typhimurium associated with pet rodents. *New England Journal of Medicine*, **356**(1), 21–28.

Taffs, L.F. (1976) Pinworm infections in laboratory rodents: a review. *Laboratory Animals (UK)*, **10**(1), 1–13.

Vandenberghe, J., Verheyen, A., Lauwers, S., and Geboes, K. (1985) Spontaneous adenocarcinoma of the ascending colon in Wistar rats: the intracytoplasmic presence of a *Campylobacter*-like bacterium. *Journal of Comparative Pathology.* **95**(1), 45–55.

Vonderfecht, S.L., Huber, A.C., Eiden, J., Mader, L.C., and Yolken, R.H. (1984) Infectious diarrhea of infant rats produced by a rotavirus-like agent. *Journal of Virology*, **52**(1), 94–98.

Exocrine Pancreas Conditions

Hansen, J.F., Ross, P.E., Makovec, G.T., Eustis, S.L., and Sigler, R.E. (1995) Proliferative and other selected lesions of the exocrine pancreas in rats, *in Guides for Toxicologic Pathology*. STP/ARP, AFIP, Washington, DC.

Hepatobiliary Conditions

Goodman, D.G., Maronpot, R.R., Newberne, P.M., Popp, J.A., and Squire, R.A. (1994) Proliferative and other selected lesions of the liver in rats. GI-5. In: *Guides for Toxicologic Pathology*. STP/ARP/AFIP, Washington, DC.

Institute of Laboratory Animal Resources (1980) *Histologic Typing of Liver Tumors of the Rat*. National Research Council, National Academy of Science, Washington, D.C.

Li, Y., Togashi, Y., Sato, S., *et al.* (1991) Spontaneous hepatic copper accumulation in Long-Evans Cinnamon rats with hereditary hepatitis. A model of Wilson's disease. *Journal of Clinical Investigations*, **87**(5), 1858–1861.

Livingston, R.S., and Riley, L.K. (2003) Diagnostic testing of mouse and rat colonies for infectious agents. *Laboratory Animals (UK)*, **32**, 44–51.

Purcell, R.H., Engle, R.E., Rood, M.P. *et al.* (2011) Hepatitis E virus in rats, Los Angeles, California, USA. *Emerging Infectious Diseases*, **17**(12), 2216–2222.

Riley, L.K., Franklin, C.L., Hook, R.R. Jr, and Besch-Williford, C. (1996) Identification of murine helicobacters by PCR and restriction enzyme analyses. *Journal of Clinical Microbiology*, **34**, 942–946.

Schilsky, M.L., Quintana, N., Volenberg, I., Kabishcher, V., and Sternlieb, I. (1998) Spontaneous cholangiofibrosis in Long-Evans Cinnamon rats: a rodent model for Wilson's disease. *Laboratory Animal Science.* **48**(2), 156–161.

Turner, P.V., Albassam, M.A., and Walker, R.M. (2001) The effects of overnight fasting, feeding, or sucrose supplementation prior to necropsy in rats. *Contemporary Topics in Laboratory Animal Science.* **40**(4), 38–42.

Whary, M.T., and Fox, J.G. (2004) Natural and experimental *Helicobacter* infections. *Comparative Medicine*, **54**(2), 128–58.

Wu, J., Forbes, J.R., Chen, H.S., and Cox, D.W. (1994) The LEC rat has a deletion in the copper transporting ATPase gene homologous to the Wilson disease gene. *Nature: Genetics*, **7**(4), 541–545.

Yamaguchi, Y., Heiny, M.E., Shimizu, N., Aoki, T., and Gitlin, J.D. (1994) Expression of the Wilson disease gene is deficient in the Long-Evans Cinnamon rat. *Biochemistry Journal*, **301** (Pt 1), 1–4.

General Gastrointestinal References

Johnson-Delaney, C.A. (2006) Anatomy and physiology of the rabbit and rodent gastrointestinal system. *AEMV Proceedings*, pp 9–17.

Kararli, T.T. (1995) Comparison of the gastrointestinal anatomy, physiology, and biochemistry of humans and commonly used laboratory animals. *Biopharmaceutical and Drug Disposition*, **16**(5), 351–380.

Moolenbeek, C. and Ruitenberg, E.J. (1981) The "Swiss roll": a simple technique for histological studies of the rodent intestine. *Laboratory Animals (UK)*, **15**(1), 57–59.

Morotomi, M., Watanabe, T., Suegara, N., Kawai, Y., and Mutai, M. (1975) Distribution of indigenous bacteria in the digestive tract of conventional and gnotobiotic rats. *Infection and Immunity*, **11**(5), 962–968.

Suegara, N., Morotomi, M., Watanabe, T., Kawai, Y., and Mutai, M. (1975) Behavior of microflora in the rat stomach: adhesion of lactobacilli to the keratinized epithelial cells of the rat stomach in vitro. *Infection and Immunity*, **12**(1), 173–179.

Cardiovascular Conditions

Alison, R.H., Elwell, M.R., Jokinen, M.P., Dittrich, K.L., and Boorman, G.A. (1987) Morphology and classification of 96 primary cardiac neoplasms in Fischer 344 rats. *Veterinary Pathology.* **24**(6), 488–494.

Chanut, F., Kimbrough, C., Hailey, R. *et al.* (2013) Spontaneous cardiomyopathy in young Sprague–Dawley rats: evaluation of biological and environmental variability. *Toxicologic Pathology.* **41**(8), 1126–1136.

Heatley, J.L. (2009) Cardiovascular anatomy, physiology, and disease of rodents and small exotic mammals. *Veterinary Clinics of North America: Exotic Animal Practice*, **12**, 99–113.

Katsuta, O., Doi, T., Okazaki, Y., Wako, Y., and Tsuchitani, M. (1999) Case report: spontaneous hemangiosarcoma in the pancreas of a Fischer rat. *Toxicologic Pathology.* **27**(4), 463–7.

Keenan, K.P., Soper, K.A., Hertzog, P.R., *et al.* (1995) Diet, overfeeding, and moderate dietary restriction in control Sprague–Dawley rats: II. Effects on age-related proliferative and degenerative lesions. *Toxicologic Pathology.* **23**(3), 287–302.

Morehead, J., and Barthold, S.W. (1997) Hemangiopericytoma in a rat. *Contemporary Topics in Laboratory Animal Science.* **36**(5), 71–72.

Novilla, M.N., Sandusky, G.E., Hoover, D.M., Ray, S.E., and Wightman, K.A. (1991) A retrospective survey of endocardial proliferative lesions in rats. *Veterinary Pathology.* **28**(2), 156–165.

Robertson, J.L., Garman, R.H., and Fowler, E.H. (1981) Spontaneous cardiac tumors in eight rats. *Veterinary Pathology.* **18**, 30–37.

Rosenbaum, M.D., Feirer, M.R., Fox, K., and Kendall, L. (2010) Solitary foot mass on a Sprague–Dawley rat. Cutaneous histiocytic sarcoma. *Laboratory Animals (NY)*, **39**(2), 36–39.

Ruben, Z., Arceo, R.J., Bishop, S.P., *et al.* (2000) Nonproliferative lesions of the heart and vasculature in rats. CV-1, in *Guides for Toxicologic Pathology.* STP/ARP/AFIP, Washington, DC.

Teredesai, A., and Wöhrmann, T. (2005) Endocardial schwannomas in the Wistar rat. *Journal of Veterinary Medicine A: Physiol Pathol Clinical Medicine*, **52**(8), 403–406.

Zwicker, G.M., Eyster, R.C., Sells, D.M., and Gass, J.H. (1995) Spontaneous vascular neoplasms in aged Sprague–Dawley rats. *Toxicologic Pathology.* **23**(4), 518–526.

Chronic Renal Disease

Goldstein, R.S., Tarloff, J.B., and Hook, J.B. (1988) Age-related nephropathy in laboratory rats. *FASEB Journal*, **2**(7), 2241–2251.

Hard, G.C., and Khan, K.N. (2004) A contemporary overview of chronic progressive nephropathy in the laboratory rat, and its significance for human risk assessment. *Toxicologic Pathology.* **32**(2), 171–180.

Itakura, C., Iida, M., and Goto, M. (1977) Renal secondary hyperparathyroidism in aged Sprague–Dawley rats. *Veterinary Pathology.* **14**(5), 463–469.

Keenan, K.P., Soper, K.A., Hertzog, P.R., *et al.* (1995) Diet, overfeeding, and moderate dietary restriction in control Sprague–Dawley rats: II. Effects on age-related proliferative and degenerative lesions. *Toxicologic Pathology.* **23**(3), 287–302.

Peter, C.P., Burek, J.D., and van Zwieten, M.J. (1986) Spontaneous nephropathies in rats. *Toxicologic Pathology.* **14**(1), 91–100.

Rao, G.N. (2002) Diet and kidney diseases in rats. *Toxicologic Pathology.* **30**(6), 651–656.

Seely, J.C. and Frazier, K.S. (2015) Regulatory forum opinion piece: Dispelling confusing terminology: Recognition and interpretation of selected rodent renal tubule lesions. *Toxicologic Pathology.* **43**, 457–463.

Seely, J.C. and Hard, G.C. (2008) Chronic progressive nephropathy in the rat: Review of pathology and relationship to renal tumorigenesis. *Journal of Toxicologic Pathology.* **21**, 199–205.

Urolithiasis and Cystitis

Magnussen, G. and Ramsay, C-H. (1971) Urolithiasis in the rat. *Laboratory Animals (UK).* **5**, 153–162.

Munday, J.S., McKinnon, H., Aberdein, D., *et al.* (2009) Cystitis, pyelonephritis, and urolithiasis in rats accidentally fed a diet deficient in vitamin A. *Journal of the American Association of Laboratory Animal Science.* **48**(6), 790–794.

Olson, M.E., Nickel, J.C., and Costerton, J.W. (1989) Infection-induced struvite urolithiasis in rats. *American Journal of Pathology.* **135**(3), 581–583.

Osanai, T., Miyoshi, I., Hiramune, T., and Kasai, N. (1994) Spontaneous urinary calculus in young LEW rats caused by Corynebacterium renale. *Journal of Urology*, **152**(3), 1002–1004.

Osanai, T., Ohyama, T., Kikuchi, N., Takahashi, T., Kasai, N., and Hiramune, T. (1996) Distribution of *Corynebacterium renale* among apparently healthy rats. *Veterinary Microbiology*, **52**(3–4), 313–315.

Peterson, C.A., Baker, D.H., and Erdman, J.W. Jr. (1996) Diet-induced nephrocalcinosis in female rats is irreversible and is induced primarily before the completion of adolescence. *Journal of Nutrition*, **126**(1), 259–265.

Ritskes-Hoitinga, J., and Beynen, A.C. (1992) Nephrocalcinosis in the rat: a literature review. *Progress in Food Nutrition Science.* **16**(1), 85–124.

Ritskes-Hoitinga, J., Mathot, J.N., Danse, L.H., and Beynen, A.C. (1991) Commercial rodent diets and nephrocalcinosis in weanling female rats. *Laboratory Animals (UK)*, **25**(2), 126–132.

Takahashi, T., Tsuji, M., Kikuchi, N., *et al.* (1995) Assignment of the bacterial agent of urinary calculus in young rats by the comparative sequence analysis of the 16S rRNA genes of corynebacteria. *Journal of Veterinary Medical Science.* **57**(3), 515–517.

Other Renal Conditions

Bettini, G., Mandrioli, L., and Morini, M. (2003) Bile duct dysplasia and congenital hepatic fibrosis associated with polycystic kidney (Caroli syndrome) in a rat. *Veterinary Pathology.* **40**(6), 693–694.

Bowman, M.R., Paré, J.A., and Pinckney, R.D. (2004) *Trichosomoides crassicauda* infection in a pet hooded rat. *Veterinary Record*, **154**(12), 374–375.

Carter, M.E., and Cordes, D.O. (1980) Leptospirosis and other infections of *Rattus rattus* and *Rattus norvegicus*. *New Zealand Veterinary Journal*, **28**(3), 45–50.

Childs, J.E., Glass, G.E., Korch, G.W., and LeDuc, J.W. (1989) Effects of hantaviral infection on survival, growth and fertility in wild rat (*Rattus norvegicus*) populations of Baltimore, Maryland. *Journal of Wildlife Diseases*, **25**(4), 469–476.

Gaudie, C.M., Featherstone, C.A., Phillips, W.S., *et al.* (2008) Human *Leptospira interrogans* serogroup *icterohaemorrhagiae* infection (Weil's disease) acquired from pet rats. *Veterinary Record*, **163**(20), 599–601.

Jansen, A., and Schneider, T. (2011) Weil's disease in a rat owner. *Lancet Infectious Diseases*, **11**(2), 152.

LeDuc, J.W., Smith, G.A., and Johnson, K.M. (1984) Hantaan-like viruses from domestic rats captured in the United States. *American Journal of Tropical Medicine and Hygiene*, **33**(5), 992–998.

Lejnieks, D.V. (2007) Urethral plug in a rat (*Rattus norvegicus*). *Journal of Exotic Pet Medicine*, **16**(3), 183–185.

O'Donoghue, P.N., and Wilson, M.S. (1977) Hydronephrosis in male rats. *Laboratory Animals (UK)*, **11**(3), 193–194.

Rand, M.S. (1994) Hantavirus: an overview and update. *Laboratory Animal Science.* **44**(4), 301–304.

Solleveld, H.A. and Boorman, G.A. (1986) Spontaneous renal lesions in five rat strains. *Toxicologic Pathology.* **14**(2), 168–174.

Strugnell, B.W., Featherstone, C., Gent, M., *et al.* (2009) Weil's disease associated with the adoption of a feral rat. *Veterinary Record*, **164**(6), 186.

Yanagihara, R. (1990) Hantavirus infection in the United States: epizootiology and epidemiology. *Review of Infectious Diseases*, **12**(3), 449–457.

Zeier, M., Handermann, M., Bahr, U., *et al.* (2005) New ecological aspects of hantavirus infection: a change of a paradigm and a challenge of prevention – a review. *Virus Genes*, **30**(2), 157–180.

Renal and Reproductive Masses

Attia, M.A. (1985) Neoplastic and nonneoplastic lesions in aging female rats with special reference to the functional morphology of the hyperplastic and neoplastic changes in the pituitary gland. *Archives of Toxicology*, **57**(2), 77–83.

Cohen, S.M. (2002) Comparative pathology of proliferative lesions of the urinary bladder. *Toxicologic Pathology.* **30**(6), 663–671.

Cook, J.C., Klinefelter, G.R., Hardisty, J.F., Sharpe, R.M., and Foster, P.M. (1999) Rodent Leydig cell tumorigenesis: a review of the physiology, pathology, mechanisms, and relevance to humans. *Critical Reviews in Toxicology*, **29**(2), 169–261.

Cooper, T.K., Dumpala, P.R., and Whitcomb, T.L. (2014) Diagnostic exercise: aScience, tes, abdominal masses, and diffuse peritoneal nodules in a rat. *Veterinary Pathology.* **51**(3), 659–662.

Davis, B. (2012) Endometrial stromal polyps in rodents: Biology, etiology, and relevance to disease in women. *Toxicologic Pathology.* **40**, 419–424.

de Rijk, E.P., Ravesloot, W.T., Wijnands, Y., and van Esch, E. (2003) A fast histochemical staining method to identify hyaline droplets in the rat kidney. *Toxicologic Pathology.* **31**(4), 462–464.

Dontas, I.A., and Khaldi, L. (2006) Urolithiasis and transitional cell carcinoma of the bladder in a Wistar rat. *Journal of the American Association of Laboratory Animal Science.* **45**(4), 64–67.

Frazier, K.S., Seely, J.C., Hard, G.C., *et al.* (2012) Proliferative and nonproliferative lesions of the rat and mouse urinary system. *Toxicologic Pathology.* **40**(4 Suppl), 14S–86S.

Greenacre, C.B. (2004) Spontaneous tumors of small mammals. *Veterinary Clinics of North America: Exotic Animal Practice*, **7**, 627–651.

Hard, G.C. and Grasso, P. (1976) Nephroblastoma in the rat: histology of a spontaneous tumor, identity with respect to renal mesenchymal neoplasms, and a review of previously recorded cases. *Journal of the National Cancer Institute*, **57**(2), 323–329.

Hard, G.C. and Snowden, R.T. (1991) Hyaline droplet accumulation in rodent kidney proximal tubules: an association with histiocytic sarcoma. *Toxicologic Pathology.* **19**(2), 88–97.

Harleman, J.H., Hargreaves, A., Andersson, H., and Kirk, S. (2012) A review of the incidence and coincidence of uterine and mammary tumors in Wistar and Sprague–

Dawley rats based on the RITA database and the role of prolactin. *Toxicologic Pathology*. **40**(6), 926–930.

Kudo, K., Hoshiya, T., Nakazawa, T., Saito, T., *et al.* (2012) Spontaneous renal tumors suspected of being familial in Sprague–Dawley rats. *Journal of Toxicologic Pathology*. **25**(4), 277–280.

Morton, D., Mirsky, M.A., Meier, W.A., and Thulin, J.D. (1994) Vaginal stromal polyps in aging rats. *Veterinary Pathology*. **31**(2), 287–289.

Qureshi, S.R., Perentes, E., Ettlin, R.A., Kolopp, M., Prentice, D.E., and Frankfurter, A. (1991) Morphologic and immunohistochemical characterization of Leydig cell tumor variants in Wistar rats. *Toxicologic Pathology*. **19**(3), 280–286.

Reznik, G., and Ward, J.M. (1981) Morphology of hyperplastic and neoplastic lesions in the clitoral and preputial gland of the F344 rat. *Veterinary Pathology*. **18**(2), 228–238.

Seely, J.C. (2004) Renal mesenchymal tumor vs nephroblastoma: Revisited. *Journal of Toxicologic Pathology*, **17**, 131–136.

Troyer, H., Sowers, J.R., and Babich, E. (1982) Leydig cell tumor induced hypercalcemia in the Fischer rat: morphometric and histochemical evidence for a humoral factor that activates osteoclasts. *American Journal of Pathology*. **108**(3), 284–290.

Wakui, S., Muto, T., Kobayashi, Y. *et al.* (2008) Sertoli-Leydig cell tumor of the testis in a Sprague–Dawley rat. *Journal of the American Association of Laboratory Animal Science*. **47**(6), 67–70.

Ward, J.M. and Sheldon, W. (1993) Expression of mononuclear phagocyte antigens in histiocytic sarcoma of mice. *Veterinary Pathology*. **30**(6), 560–565.

Willson, C.J., Herbert, R.A., and Cline, J.M. (2015) Hormone receptor expression in spontaneous uterine adenocarcinoma in Fischer 344 rats. *Toxicologic Pathology*. **43**(6), 865–871.

Other Reproductive Conditions

Cohen, B.J., Anver, M.R., Ringler, D.H., and Adelman, R.C. (1978) Age-associated pathological changes in male rats. *Federation Proceedings*, **37**(14), 2848–2850.

Cora, M.C., Kooistra, L., and Travlos, G. (2015) Vaginal cytology of the laboratory rat and mouse: Review and criteria for the staging of the estrous cycle using stained vaginal smears. *Toxicologic Pathology*. **43**(6), 776–793.

General Urinary Tract References

Corman, B., Pratz, J., and Poujeol, P. (1985) Changes in anatomy, glomerular filtration, and solute excretion in aging rat kidney. *American Journal of Physiology*, **248**(3 Pt 2), R282–R287.

Fisher, P.G. (2006a) Exotic mammal renal disease: Causes and clinical presentation. *Veterinary Clinics of North America: Exotic Animal Practice*, **9**, 33–67.

Fisher, P.G. (2006b) Exotic mammal renal disease: Diagnosis and treatment. *Veterinary Clinics of North America: Exotic Animal Practice*, **9**, 69–96.

Gómez-Baena, G., Armstrong, S.D., Phelan, M.M., Hurst, J.L., and Beynon, R.J. (2014) The major urinary protein system in the rat. *Biochemical Society Transactions*, **42**(4), 886–892.

Kulkarni, A.B., Gubits, R.M., and Feigelson, P. (1985) Developmental and hormonal regulation of alpha 2u-globulin gene transcription. *Proceeding of the National Academy of Sciences. USA*, **82**(9), 2579–2582.

Montagna, W. and Noback, C.R. (1946) The histology of the preputial gland of the rat. *Anatomical Record*, **96**, 41–54.

Cerebrospinal Masses

Kaspareit-Rittinghausen, J., and Deerberg, F. (1989) Spontaneous tumours of the spinal cord in laboratory rats. *Journal of Comparative Pathology*. **100**(2), 209–215.

Krinke, G., Naylor, D.C., Schmid, S., Fröhlich, E., and Schnider, K. (1985) The incidence of naturally-occurring primary brain tumours in the laboratory rat. *Journal of Comparative Pathology*. **95**(2), 175–192.

Krinke, G.J., Kaufmann, W., Mahrous, A.T., and Schaetti, P. (2000) Morphologic characterization of spontaneous nervous system tumors in mice and rats. *Toxicologic Pathology*. **28**(1), 178–192.

Maekawa, A., Onodera, H., Furuta, K., *et al.* (1989) Teratoma of the pituitary gland in a young male rat. *Journal of Comparative Pathology*. **100**(3), 349–352.

Newman, A.J., and Mawdesley-Thomas, L.E. (1974) Spontaneous tumours of the central nervous system of laboratory rats. *Journal of Comparative Pathology*. **84**(1), 39–50.

Other Neurologic Conditions

Collins, G.H., and Converse, W.K. (1970) Cerebellar degeneration in thiamine-deficient rats. *American Journal of Pathology*. **58**(2), 219–233.

De Jonghe, S., Abbott, D., Vinken, P., *et al.* (2015) Bilateral symmetrical idiopathic necrotizing encephalopathy: A new syndrome in Sprague–Dawley rats. *Toxicologic Pathology*. **43**(8), 1141–1148.

Drake, M.T., Riley, L.K., and Livingston, R.S. (2008) Differential susceptibility of SD and CD rats to a novel rat theilovirus. *Comparative Medicine*, **58**(5), 458–464.

Eldadah, A.H., Nathanson, N., Smith, K.O., *et al.* (1967) Viral hemorrhagic encephalopathy of rats. *Science*. **156**(3773), 392–394.

Hayden, D.W., King, N.W., and Murthy, A.S. (1976) Spontaneous *Frenkelia* infection in a laboratory-reared rat. *Veterinary Pathology*. **13**(5), 337–342.

Moody, K.D., Griffith, J.W., and Lang, C.M. (1986) Fungal meningoencephalitis in a laboratory rat. *Journal of the American Veterinary Medical Association*. **189**(9), 1152–1153.

Ohsawa, K., Watanabe, Y., Miyata, H., and Sato, H. (2003) Genetic analysis of a Theiler-like virus isolated from rats. *Comparative Medicine*, **53**(2), 191–196.

Rodrigues, D.M., Martins, S.S., Gilioli, R., Guaraldo, A.M., and Gatti, M.S. (2005) Theiler's murine encephalomyelitis virus in nonbarrier rat colonies. *Comparative Medicine*. **55**, 459–464.

General Nervous System

Jortner, B.S. (2006) The return of the dark neuron. A histological artifact complicating contemporary neurotoxicologic evaluation. *Neurotoxicology*, **27**(4), 628–634.

Krinke, G. (1983) Spinal radiculoneuropathy in aging rats. Demyelination secondary to neuronal dwindling. *Acta Neuropathologica*. **59**, 63–69.

Krinke, G., Suter, J., and Hess, R. (1981) Radicular myelinopathy in aging rats. *Veterinary Pathology*. **18**(3), 335–341.

Meredith, A.L., and Ricardson, J. (2015) Neurological diseases of rabbits and rodents. *Journal of Exotic Pet Medicine*, **24**, 21–33.

van Steenis, G., and Kroes, R. (1971) Changes in the nervous system and musculature of old rats. *Veterinary Pathology*. **8**(4), 320–332.

Infectious Hematopoietic and Lymphoid Conditions

Coleman, G.L., Jacoby, R.O., Bhatt, P.N., Smith, A.L., and Jonas, A.M. (1983) Naturally occurring lethal parvovirus infection of juvenile and young-adult rats. *Veterinary Pathology*. **20**(1), 49–56.

Fritz, T.E., Tolle, D.V., and Flynn, R.J. (1968) Hemorrhagic diathesis in laboratory rodents. *Proceedings of the Society for Experimental Biology and Medicine*, **128**(1), 228–234.

Gaertner, D.J., Jacoby, R.O., Johnson, E.A., *et al.* (1993) Characterization of acute rat parvovirus infection by in situ hybridization. *Virus Research*, **28**(1), 1–18.

Jacoby, R.O., Ball-Goodrich, L.J., Besselsen, D.G., *et al.* (1996) Rodent parvovirus infections. *Laboratory Animal Science*. **46**(4), 370–380.

Kashuba, C., Hsu, C., Krogstad, A., and Franklin, C. (2005) Small mammal virology. *Veterinary Clinics of North America: Exotic Animal Practice*, **8**(1), 107–122.

Salzman, L.A., and Jori, L.A. (1970) Characterization of the Kilham rat virus. *Journal of Virology*, **5**(2), 114–122.

Wan, C.H., Bauer, B.A., Pintel, D.J., and Riley, L.K. (2006) Detection of rat parvovirus type 1 and rat minute virus type 1 by polymerase chain reaction. *Laboratory Animals (UK)*, **40**(1), 63–69.

Wan, C.H., Söderlund-Venermo, M., Pintel, D.J., and Riley, L.K. (2002) Molecular characterization of three newly recognized rat parvoviruses. *Journal of General Virology*, **83**(Pt 8), 2075–2083.

Hematopoietic and Lymphoid Neoplasia

Barsoum, N.J., Hanna, W., Gough, A.W., Smith, G.S., Sturgess, J.M., and de la Iglesia, F.A. (1984) Histiocytic sarcoma in Wistar rats. A light microscopic, immunohistochemical, and ultrastructural study. *Archives of Pathology and Laboratory Medicine*, **108**(10), 802–807.

Baselmans, A.H., Kuijpers, M.H., and van Dijk, J.E. (1996) Brief communication: Histopathology of a spontaneously developing mast cell sarcoma in a Wistar rat. *Toxicologic Pathology*. **24**(3), 365–369.

de Rijk, E.P., Ravesloot, W.T., Wijnands, Y., and van Esch, E. (2003) A fast histochemical staining method to identify hyaline droplets in the rat kidney. *Toxicologic Pathology*. **31**(4), 462–464.

Frith, C.H. (1988) Morphologic classification and incidence of hematopoietic neoplasms in the Sprague–Dawley rat. *Toxicologic Pathology*. **16**(4), 451–457.

Frith, C.H., Ward, J.M., and Chandra, M. (1993) The morphology, immunohistochemistry, and incidence of hematopoietic neoplasms in mice and rats. *Toxicologic Pathology*. **21**(2), 206–218.

Hard, G.C. and Snowden, R.T. (1991) Hyaline droplet accumulation in rodent kidney proximal tubules: an association with histiocytic sarcoma. *Toxicologic Pathology*. **19**(2), 88–97.

Hayashi, S., Nonoyama, T., and Miyajima, H. (1989) Spontaneous nonthymic T cell lymphomas in young Wistar rats. *Veterinary Pathology*. **26**(4), 326–332.

Kaspareit-Rittinghausen, J., Deerberg, F., and Sommer, R. (1989) Atypical epithelial thymomas in rats. *Laboratory Animals (UK)*, **23**(4), 337–339.

Matsushima, K., Yamaka, S., Edamoto, H., Yamaguchi, Y., Nagatani, M., and Tamura, K. (2010) Spontaneous malignant T-cell lymphoma in a young adult Crl:CD (SD) rat. *Journal of Toxicologic Pathology*. **23**, 49–52.

Naylor, D.C., Krinke, G.J., and Ruefenacht, H.J. (1988) Primary tumours of the thymus in the rat. *Journal of Comparative Pathology*. **99**(2), 187–203.

Smith, G.R., Nemeth, N.M., Howerth, E.W., Butler, A.M., and Gottdenker, N.L. (2014) Spontaneous pulmonary hemangiosarcoma in a Norway rat (*Rattus norvegicus*). *Journal of Exotic Pet Medicine*, **23**, 101–106.

Son, W.C., Bell, D., Taylor, I., and Mowat, V. (2010) Profile of early occurring spontaneous tumors in Han Wistar rats. *Toxicologic Pathology.* **38**(2), 292–296.

Squire, R.A., Brinkhous, K.M., Peiper, S.C., Firminger, H.I., Mann, R.B., and Strandberg, J.D. (1981) Histiocytic sarcoma with a granuloma-like component occurring in a large colony of Sprague–Dawley rats. *American Journal of Pathology.* **105**(1), 21–30.

Ward, J.M., and Reynolds, C.W. (1983) Large granular lymphocyte leukemia. A heterogeneous lymphocytic leukemia in F344 rats. *American Journal of Pathology.* **111**(1), 1–10.

General Hematopoietic Conditions

Cesta, M.F. (2006) Normal structure, function, and histology of mucosa-associated lymphoid tissue. *Toxicologic Pathology.* **34**(5), 599–608.

Cesta, M.F. (2006) Normal structure, function, and histology of the spleen. *Toxicologic Pathology.* **34**(5), 455–465.

Lindstrom, N.M., Moore, D.M., Zimmerman, K., and Smith, S.A. (2015) Hematologic assessment in pet rats, mice, hamsters, and gerbils. *Veterinary Clinics of North America: Exotic Animal Practice*, **18**, 21–32.

Parker, G.A., Picut, C.A., Swanson, C., and Toot, J.D. (2015) Histologic Features of Postnatal Development of Immune System Organs in the Sprague–Dawley Rat. *Toxicologic Pathology.* **43**(6), 794–815.

Pearse, G. (2006) Normal structure, function and histology of the thymus. *Toxicologic Pathology.* **34**(5), 504–514.

Pilny, A.A. (2008) Clinical hematology of rodent species. *Veterinary Clinics of North America: Exotic Animal Practice*, **11**(3), 523–533.

Travlos, G.S. (2006) Normal structure, function, and histology of the bone marrow. *Toxicologic Pathology.* **34**(5), 548–565.

Ward, J.M., Erexson, C.R., Faucette, L.J., Foley, J.F., Dijkstra, C., and Cattoretti, G. (2006) Immunohistochemical markers for the rodent immune system. *Toxicologic Pathology.* **34**(5), 616–630.

Willard-Mack, C.L. (2006) Normal structure, function, and histology of lymph nodes. *Toxicologic Pathology.* **34**(5), 409–424.

Conditions of the Cornea and Anterior Chamber

Bellhorn, R.W., Korte, G.E., and Abrutyn, D. (1988) Spontaneous corneal degeneration in the rat. *Laboratory Animal Science.* **38**(1), 46–50.

Turner, P.V., and Albassam, M.A. (2005) Susceptibility of rats to corneal lesions following anesthesia. *Comparative Medicine*, **55**(2), 182–189.

Conditions of the Uveal Tract and Retina

Hubert, M.F., Gillet, J.P., and Durand-Cavagna, G. (1994) Spontaneous retinal changes in Sprague Dawley rats. *Laboratory Animal Science.* **44**(6), 561–567.

Kuwahara, T., and Funahashi, M. (1976) Light damage in the developing rat retina. *Archives of Ophthalmology*, **94**, 1369–1374.

Lin, W.L., and Essner, E. (1988) Retinal dystrophy in Wistar-Furth rats. *Experimental Eye Research.*, **46**(1), 1–12.

Magnusson, G., Majeed, S., and Offer, J.M. (1978) Intraocular melanoma in the rat. *Laboratory Animals (UK)*, **12**(4), 249–252.

Manning, W.S. Jr, Greenlee, P.G., and Norton, J.N. (2004) Ocular melanoma in a Long Evans rat. *Contemporary Topics in Laboratory Animal Science.* **43**(1), 44–46.

Ninomiya, H., Kuno, H., and Inagaki, S. (2005) Vascular changes associated with chorioretinal and optic nerve colobomas in rats (Crj: CD(SD), IGS). *Veterinary Ophthalmology*, **8**(5), 319–323.

Schardein, J.L., Lucas, J.A., and Fitzgerald, J.E. (1975) Retinal dystrophy in Sprague–Dawley rats. *Laboratory Animal Science.* **25**(3), 323–326.

Yoshitomi, K. and Boorman, G.A. (1991) Spontaneous amelanotic melanomas of the uveal tract in F344 rats. *Veterinary Pathology.* **28**(5), 403–409.

Yoshitomi, K. and Boorman, G.A. (1993) Palpebral amelanotic melanomas in F344 rats. *Veterinary Pathology.* **30**(3), 280–286.

General Ophthalmic Conditions

Beaumont, S.L. (2002) Ocular disorders of pet mice and rats. *Veterinary Clinics of North America: Exotic Animal Practice*, **5**(2), 311–324.

Kern, T.J. (1997) Rabbit and rodent ophthalmology. *Seminars in Avian and Exotic Pet Medicine*, **6**(3), 138–145.

Williams, D. (2007) Rabbit and rodent ophthalmology. *European Journal of Comparative Animal Practice*, **17**(3), 242–252.

6

Hamsters

6.1 Introduction

The most common species of pet hamster is the golden Syrian hamster (*Mesocrictus auratus*), although there are many other species. Long-haired hamsters, also called "teddy bear" hamsters, are also Syrian hamsters. Other species of hamsters seen occasionally as pets include Siberian hamsters (*Phodopus sungorus*), Dungarian hamsters (*Phodopus campbelli*), and Chinese hamsters (*Cricetulus griseus*). Most information available about hamster health relates to the Syrian hamster and this is the species that will be emphasized throughout this chapter. Readers are cautioned to avoid making sweeping generalizations about hamster conditions and diseases, as other hamsters are of different genera and have different disease susceptibilities. Much of the information about neoplastic diseases of Syrian hamsters comes from long-term carcinogenicity studies in toxicology, which can be extrapolated to companion hamsters.

Hamsters have prominent stores of brown adipose tissue beneath and between the scapulae, in the axillary areas, and around the thymus, thyroid and adrenal glands, kidneys, and ureters. Hamsters are permissive hibernators and under conditions of reduced food availability combined with low ambient temperatures, may display reduced heart and respiration rates with very shallow breaths and become motionless (i.e., achieve a state of estivation). The pathologist should ensure that the animal is truly dead before commencing post-mortem examination.

6.2 Integument Conditions

Both male and female Syrian hamsters have bilateral flank sebaceous glands, but glands in the male are more darkly pigmented and larger with black bristly hairs. In dwarf hamsters, the scent glands are single, raised, sometimes hairless structures on the ventrum near the umbilicus, and can be are associated with a greasy or waxy yellow secretion. When the male is sexually stimulated, he will lick the scent glands until the area is wet and the fur may become matted with secretions. These scent glands are used for marking territory, are involved in the mating ritual, and convert testosterone to dihydroxytestosterone.

6.2.1 Alopecia

Roughened hair coats and patchy to generalized hair loss are commonly seen in older hamsters in response to a number of conditions, including chronic renal disease, amyloidosis, endocrine disorders such as hyperadrenocorticism and hypothyroidism, epitheliotropic lymphoma, acariasis, dermatophytosis, and fighting. Alopecia is also associated with feeding low-protein diets (<16%) and feeding pelleted rodent chow is recommended instead of seed mixes to prevent hamsters from selectively consuming preferred high fat seeds. Mechanical facial hair loss can occur with constant rubbing on exercise wheels, feeders, drinkers or rough bedding.

Allergic dermatitis is poorly characterized in hamsters and can present as generalized hair loss, swollen feet, and periocular and periauricular seborrhoea. Allergens may include bedding and dietary components, but hamsters can develop allergies to various household products and perfumes.

6.2.2 External Parasites

6.2.2.1 Acariasis

Mite infestations are relatively common in hamsters but mites themselves are of low pathogenicity. Clinical disease is typically seen in aged hamsters, those with intercurrent disease, immunocompromise or poor nutrition. Young hamsters acquire mites from their dam during suckling. The two most common species of mites seen include *Demodex criceti*, a short broad mite found in the superficial keratin and epidermal pits, and *D. aurati*, a long, slender mite that is generally located in hair follicles and ducts of sebaceous glands.

Presenting Clinical Signs In cases of demodectic mange, lesions include nonpruritic patchy alopecia with erythema or seborrhea, dry scaling skin, and miliary pustules or

Pathology of Small Mammal Pets, First Edition. Patricia V. Turner, Marina L. Brash and Dale A. Smith.
© 2018 John Wiley & Sons, Inc. Published 2018 by John Wiley & Sons, Inc.

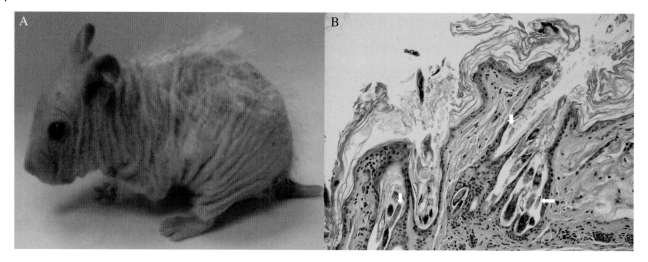

Figure 6.1 A: Hamster with severe demodectic mange. Mite infestations are relatively common but clinical disease is seen typically in aged hamsters, those with intercurrent disease, immunocompromised animals and animals with poor nutrition. There is generalized nonpruritic alopecia with seborrhea. B: The epidermis is thrown into folds with moderate superficial and follicular hyperkeratosis, mild epidermal hyperplasia, minimal dermal inflammation, and numerous mites (arrows) within the surface keratin and dilated follicle lumena, which is atypical. The two most common species of mites found in hamsters are *D. criceti*, a short broad mite found predominantly in the superficial keratin and epidermal pits, and *D. aurati*, a long, slender mite that is located in hair follicles and ducts of sebaceous glands. *Source:* A: Courtesy of The Links Road Animal and Bird Clinic.

hemorrhages over the neck, back, rump, and less often, forelimbs (Figure 6.1). Notoedric mange may occur in hamsters and is caused by the highly contagious burrowing ear mite, *N. notoedres*. Clinical signs of infestation include pruritus, hyperemia, crusting, erosions, and hyperpigmentation, generally involving the ears, face, legs, tail, and perigenital skin. *N. cati*, the cat mange mite, has been associated with skin lesions in hamsters, as has *Sarcoptes scabiei*. The latter causes facial hair loss and severe pruritus and can be transferred to other animals and humans.

Tropical rat mite (*Ornithonyssus bacoti*) and nasal mite (*Spleorodens clethrionomys*) infestations can occur in hamsters. *O. bacoti* has a nonselective host range and can cause debilitation and anemia in animals with heavy infestations. A pet hamster boarded for a short time at a local pet store resulted in bites on the skin of human family members subsequent to its return home, although the hamster had no clinical signs. *O. bacoti* mites were later identified on the hamster and family members.

Pathology Histologically, in cases of demodicosis, superficial and follicular hyperkeratosis is seen with serocellular crusts, epidermal hyperplasia, minimal dermal inflammation, and scant mites within the surface keratin and dilated follicle lumens.

Laboratory Diagnostics Mites can be demonstrated in deep skin scrapings or skin biopsies and in skin samples that have undergone potassium hydroxide digestion. Digested skin sample results are more reliable than histology for mite detection. Male hamsters often yield more fruitful

results upon examination as they usually carry a larger *Demodex* burden than do females.

Differential Diagnoses Differential diagnoses for demodicosis include various endocrine disorders, such as hyperadrenocorticism and hypothyroidism, epitheliotropic lymphoma, dermatophytosis, bacterial dermatitis, and trauma from fighting.

Disease/Colony Management *S. scabiei* and *O. bacoti* are both zoonotic conditions that may cause pruritus in people. *O. bacoti* is a vector that can transmit rickettsial and bacterial diseases, such as *Coxiella burnetii*, *Borrelia burgdorferi*, and *Yersinia* spp. to humans.

6.2.2.2 Fleas
Ctenocephalides spp. (i.e., cat and dog fleas) can occasionally be identified on hamsters housed with dogs and cats. Clinical signs of infestation include a dull hair coat, severe pruritus, patchy alopecia, and erythema. Diagnosis is based on seeing fleas or flea excreta on hamsters.

6.2.3 Subcutaneous Abscesses and Bacterial Dermatitis

Cellulitis and abscesses are commonly seen anywhere on the body secondary to bite wounds from fighting or from cannibalization of flank glands by pen mates. Cheek pouches may also become impacted with food with secondary bacterial infection and fistulation, necessitating major debridement or surgical removal.

Diagnostic investigation of the flank glands is warranted if the hamster shows changes in behavior or if the glands are erythematous, edematous, painful, or present with unusual discharge, surface crusting, and ulceration. Bacterial adenitis may underlie the change in the glands but neoplasia should also be considered (see Section 6.7.2.4).

Abscesses with secondary fistulation can develop from dental caries and periodontitis, and may extend to involve surrounding tissues, including the retroorbital space, Harderian glands, and brain, with embolic showering of the lungs and kidneys. Contributing factors include suboptimal management, inappropriate diet, and poorly maintained cages with rough edges. Bacterial agents cultured from cutaneous abscesses of hamsters include *Staphylococcus aureus*, *Pasteurella pneumotropica*, and *Streptococcus pyogenes*. *Klebsiella pneumoniae* has been associated with a cluster of facial abscesses (Figure 6.2) and multifocal embolic hepatitis and pneumonia.

Multiple cases have been reported of bacterial pseudomycetomas presenting as dermal and subcutaneous masses on the distal limbs of both dwarf and Siberian hamsters (Figure 6.3). Histologically, pseudomycetomas consist of basophilic coccoid bacteria surrounded by eosinophilic rims of Splendore-Hoeppli material embedded in pyogranulomatous inflammation. Culture was consistent with *Staphylococcus epidermidis*. Because bacterial pseudomycetomas respond poorly to antibiotic therapy, surgical removal should be considered; however, abscesses may recur if excision is incomplete. Hepatic pyogranulomas were also seen but did not contain bacteria.

Spontaneous mycobacterial infections are infrequent in hamsters. *Mycobacterium chelonae* was isolated from a hamster with chronic pododermatitis and ulcerative cheilitis. On post-mortem examination, enlarged draining lymph nodes were noted; however, visceral organs were not grossly affected. Microscopically, systemic mycobacteriosis was confirmed in the enlarged lymph

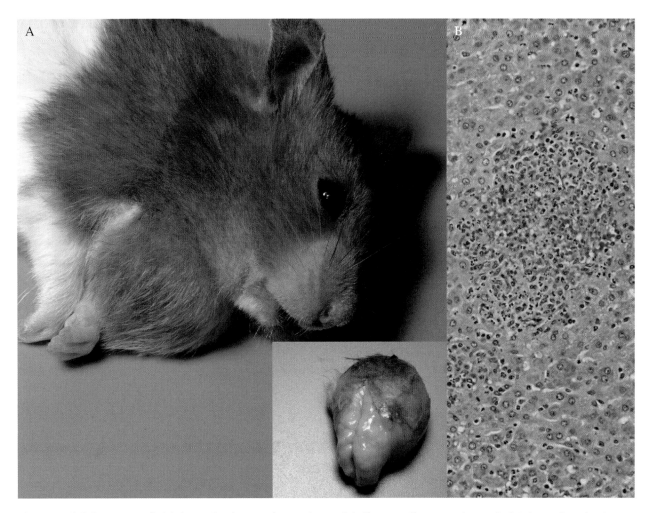

Figure 6.2 A: Subcutaneous facial abscess in a hamster from a cluster of similar cases. *K. pneumoniae* was isolated on culture. Inset: Dissected and opened abscess. B: Most of the affected hamsters also had embolic suppurative hepatitis, as demonstrated in this photomicrograph and pneumonia.

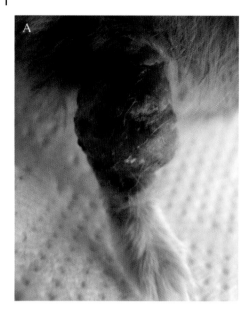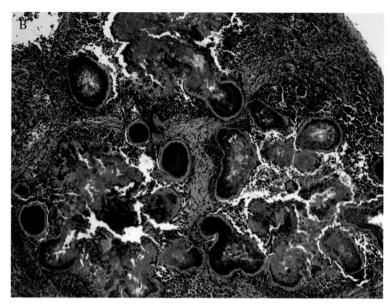

Figure 6.3 A: Bacterial pseudomycetoma on distal leg of a Siberian hamster. B: Microscopically, pseudomycetomas contain characteristic granules composed of basophilic coccoid bacteria rimmed with eosinophilic Splendore-Hoeppli material embedded in pyogranulomatous inflammation. Gram stains confirmed Gram-positive cocci morphologically resembling *Staphylococcus* spp. *Source:* A and B: Courtesy of D. Eshar.

nodes, and liver, spleen and lung contained granulomatous foci with multinucleated giant cells bearing low numbers of acid-fast bacteria. *M. chelonae* is an atypical fast-growing mycobacterial specie found in soil, water, and dust, and is considered mildly pathogenic. Major risk factors for infection are trauma and immunosuppression. Human infection is uncommon and thought to be primarily contracted from the environment, but could result from contact with infected pets.

Granulomatous inflammation with necrosis and ulceration of the foot and upper leg can occur if bedding material penetrates the footpad and migrates. Footpad erosions and ulcers can develop secondary to urine scald if the cage is not maintained appropriately or if cage components, such as exercise wheels, and flooring, are poorly maintained.

6.2.4 Mastitis

Mastitis is uncommon in hamsters, but may occur under conditions of poor environmental hygiene. Clinical signs of mastitis include swollen, painful, warm or hot mammary glands, reduced appetite, hunched posture, refusal to nurse, and cannibalism of the pups. Milk should be expressed and cultured. β-hemolytic *Streptococcus* spp., *P. pneumotropica*, *S. aureus*, and *E. coli* have been isolated from mastitis cases in hamsters.

6.2.5 Bacterial Otitis

Bacterial otitis can be associated with suppurative oculonasal discharge, conjunctivitis, matting of hair on the forelegs, dyspnea, head tilt, and pneumonia. Possible etiologic agents include *Streptococcus* spp., *Pasteurella* spp., *Klebsiella pneumoniae*, *Bordetella* spp. and *S. aureus*.

6.2.6 Dermatophytosis

Dermatophytosis (ringworm) is uncommon in hamsters and infections can be asymptomatic or clinical, presenting as patchy, dry, circular crusted skin lesions. Microscopically, there is hyperkeratosis, epithelial hyperplasia, suppurative to granulomatous perifolliculitis and furunculosis, with arthrospores surrounding the hair shafts and fungal hyphae within the hairs. Differential diagnoses include endocrine disorders such as hyperadrenocorticism and hypothyroidism, epitheliotropic lymphoma, bacterial dermatitis, and trauma from fighting.

Histochemical stains, such as periodic acid Schiff (PAS) or Gomori's methenamine silver (GMS), are useful for demonstrating fungal hyphae and arthrospores. Skin scrapings and hair plucked from lesion margins can be cultured using fungal media and examined microscopically following KOH digestion. Ultraviolet fluorescence of the lesions is not a useful test as *Trichophyton mentagrophytes* is the most common etiologic agent isolated from hamsters and it does not fluoresce.

Hamsters housed in solid plastic cages are more likely to develop ringworm because of reduced ventilation, which may allow the bedding to become damp, encouraging fungal growth. Infected hamsters serve as a potential source of infection for other animals and humans. Transmission of the fungal arthrospores is by direct contact of infected animals or fomites so hand washing and disinfection of equipment before each use and between cages or rooms are advised. All organic materials should be discarded as they can be contaminated with fungal spores. If animals are suspected or known to be infected, the handler should wear gloves.

6.2.7 Cutaneous Masses and Neoplasia

Neoplasia is very common in older hamsters and often multiple tumors are present at postmortem examination. In general, cutaneous masses are moderately common, ranking second to endocrine tumors. Flank glands, testicles, and cheek pouches filled with food can all be mistaken for tumors.

6.2.7.1 Melanoma and Melanocytoma

Melanocytoma, a benign circular blue nevus, is occasionally seen in hamsters. Histologically, these masses are small and composed of nests of pigmented cells located close to the basal lamina of the epithelium.

Melanomas are commonly seen in hamsters, with a higher incidence in males. In one survey, all the skin tumors reported were heavily pigmented nodular melanomas of the tail or flank and almost 50% had metastasized to lymph nodes and lungs (Figure 6.4).

6.2.7.2 Epitheliotropic Lymphoma

Epitheliotropic lymphoma is another common skin tumor of hamsters that is not associated with virus infection and is similar to mycosis fungoides in humans. This tumor is seen most often in adult hamsters and affected animals initially present with focal alopecia and flaking skin with progression to generalized exfoliative dermatitis, alopecia, and development of multiple firm cutaneous reddened nodules or plaques, some of which may be ulcerated (Figure 6.5). Pruritus may or may not be present. The condition progresses rapidly and in one series of cases, the mean survival time was less than 10 weeks. Lethargy, anorexia and weight loss develop later in the course of the disease, in conjunction with generalized skin lesions.

At post-mortem, systemic involvement was noted in one hamster with neoplastic masses present in axillary lymph nodes and the liver. Histologically, aggregates of neoplastic lymphocytes are seen within the dermis with extension into the underlying panniculus and involvement of hair follicles and other adnexal structures. Neoplastic lymphocytes infiltrate the overlying epidermis either singly or in small clusters forming Pautrier's microabscesses. Neoplastic lymphocytes generally are of medium size with oval, often bean-shaped nuclei and moderate amounts of cytoplasm. Positive cytoplasmic immunohistochemistry labeling for CD3 antigen, a pan T-cell marker, can be used to confirm the cell origin.

6.2.7.3 Trichoepithelioma

Trichoepitheliomas in hamsters are commonly associated with polyoma virus infection (see Section 6.6.4.15) and are found in young hamsters 3 months to 1 year of age. These present as irregular exophytic masses often involving the face and feet (Figure 6.6A), but they can arise anywhere on body. Trichoepitheliomas are benign and do not metastasize, but can lead to debilitation, depending upon the location, size, and number. Although

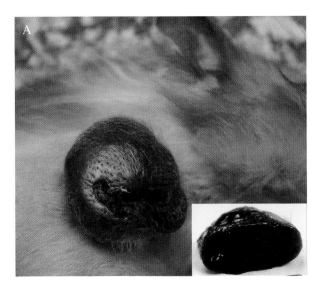
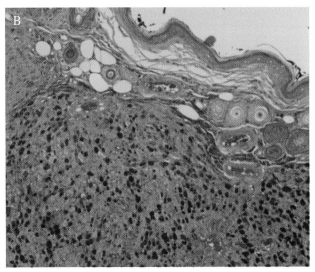

Figure 6.4 A: Heavily pigmented cutaneous melanoma on shoulder of a Syrian hamster. Inset bottom: The cut surface of the mass demonstrates diffuse pigmentation. B: Although grossly, the mass appeared diffusely pigmented, microscopically, the mass is seen to be composed of both poorly pigmented and heavily pigmented melanocytes. The mass was excised without further incident. *Source:* A: Courtesy of The Links Road Animal and Bird Clinic.

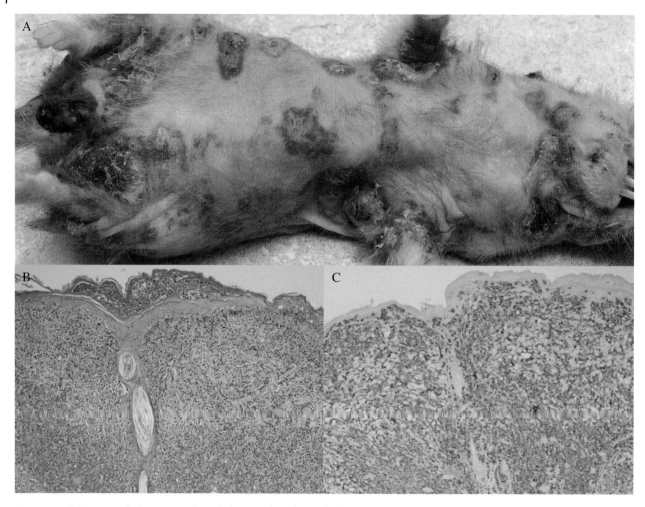

Figure 6.5 A: Ventrum of a hamster with epitheliotropic lymphoma displaying the characteristic alopecia and wide-spread, raised, reddened and ulcerated cutaneous plaques with crusting. B: Histologically, aggregates of neoplastic lymphocytes are seen within the dermis and extending to involve hair follicles. Neoplastic lymphocytes infiltrate the overlying thickened epidermis in small clusters forming Pautier microabscesses. There is superficial hyperkeratosis and serocellular crusting. C: There is positive immunohistochemical labeling (alkaline phosphatase red) for CD3 antigen, a pan T-cell marker, confirming the cell origin. *Source:* A: Courtesy of The Links Road Animal and Bird Clinic.

cells may contain hamster polyomavirus, virus transmission occurs through shedding the urine. Histologically, the dermis contains a multiloculated basal cell tumor with abrupt central keratinization and lamellated keratin filling the central cystic cavities (Figure 6.6B).

6.2.7.4 Flank Gland Neoplasia
Neoplasms seen in the sebaceous flank glands of hamsters include adenoma, adenocarcinoma, squamous cell carcinoma, and melanoma.

6.2.7.5 Other Skin Neoplasms
Other skin-associated neoplasms found in hamsters include papillomas, squamous cell carcinomas, sebaceous adenomas (Figure 6.7), fibromas, plasmacytomas, mast cell tumor, apocrine adenocarcinoma, extraskeletal osteosarcomas, and undifferentiated soft tissue sarcomas (Figure 6.8).

A myxoma was reported on the right flank of a mature hamster. The mass was well encapsulated, gelatinous, shiny, and slightly opaque with central focal hemorrhage. Histologically, the mass had an outer fibrous capsule surrounding very loosely woven spindle cells with abundant pale blue-staining extracellular mucinous ground substance consistent with a myxoma.

A myofibroblastic sarcoma was reported in a 1.5-year-old female Djungarian hamster. The animal presented with a large, slow-growing, subcutaneous mass involving the right shoulder that interfered with ambulation. A short time later, the hamster died and at necropsy, a large, irregular, pale gray mass was noted to be infiltrating the right thoracic wall. Histologically, the mass was highly cellular, and composed of spindle to stellate cells and multinucleated giant cells arranged in bundles intermingled with fine collagen fibres. More than 90% of the neoplastic cells were positive

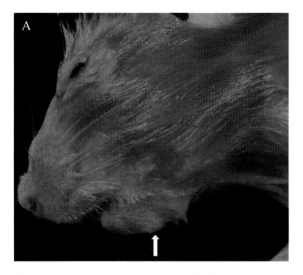

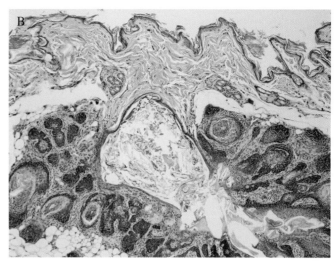

Figure 6.6 A: Small exophytic trichoepithelioma (arrow) on the chin of a 10-month-old Syrian hamster. Numerous cutaneous nodules were seen elsewhere on the body, including the ventral abdomen, back, limbs, and eyelids. The thoracic cavity contained abundant chylous effusion and there was a large thymic mass at the base of the heart. B: Trichoepitheliomas are multiloculated basal cell tumors displaying characteristic features of abrupt central keratinization and lamellated keratin filling the central cystic cavities. This hamster also had lymphosarcoma involving the thymus, lungs, and perirenal lymph nodes. The thymic tumor was positively immunolabelled for hamster polyomavirus (HaPV). There is an association between trichoepitheliomas and HaPV infection in hamsters. *Source:* A and B: Courtesy of A. Beck.

for vimentin and the remainder of the cells were positive for smooth muscle actin (SMA); neurofilament labeling was negative. Myofibroblastic sarcomas are microscopically similar to fibrosarcomas but differ in SMA positivity.

6.2.7.6 Mammary Neoplasia

Mammary tumors, including adenoma, tubulopapillary adenocarcinoma, and complex carcinoma are seen in aging female hamsters. Carcinomas may be locally infiltrative, but there is usually no evidence of invasion of lymphatics or blood vessels. Most of these tumors

express androgen receptors and almost half are positive for estrogen receptor alpha.

6.3 Endocrine Conditions

Pathologists are often rewarded for close examination of endocrine tissues of aging hamsters at postmortem, as disorders or tumors of these tissues are very common, with one or multiple tissues affected by a single or different disease processes.

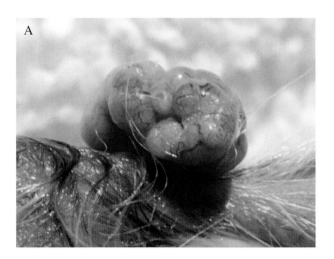

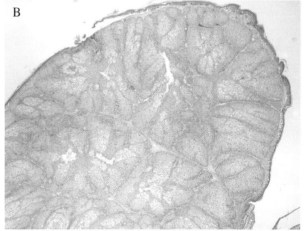

Figure 6.7 A: Small, multinodular pedunculated sebaceous adenoma on the distal hind limb of a 1.5-year-old hamster. B: The sebaceous adenoma is composed of multiple lobules of well differentiated sebaceous cells rimmed peripherally by basal reserve cells not associated with ducts. *Source:* A: Courtesy of The Links Road Animal and Bird Clinic.

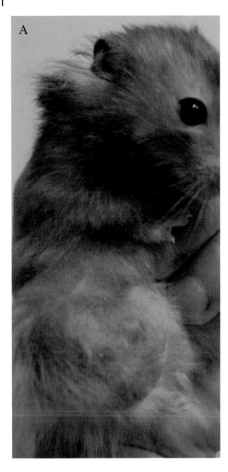
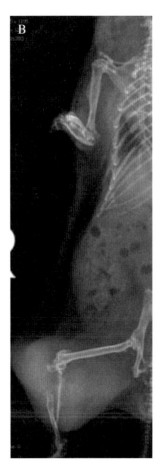
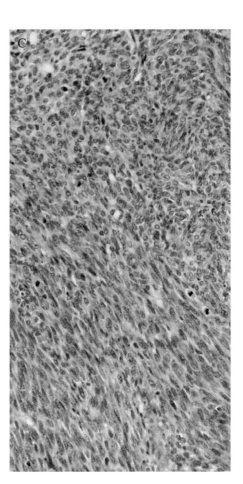

Figure 6.8 A: Rapidly growing soft tissue tumor encompassing most of the right hind leg of a 1-year old hamster compromising its ability to ambulate. B: Radiograph demonstrating soft tissue mass and lysis of the tibia. C: Microscopically, the soft tissue sarcoma is composed of interlacing bands of densely packed spindle cells displaying moderate anisokaryosis and up to 6 mitoses/400x field with no evidence of further cellular differentiation. *Source:* A and B: Courtesy of The Links Road Animal and Bird Clinic.

6.3.1 Adrenal Gland Conditions

The adrenal glands of male hamsters are up to several times larger than those of females due to an expanded zona reticularis.

6.3.1.1 Adrenocortical Amyloidosis

The adrenal gland is one of many tissues to be affected by amyloid deposition in hamsters. Deposition is age-related with some animals being affected as early as 5 months of age, although the condition is more commonly seen in animals 12 months of age and older. Rate of amyloid deposition may be augmented by ongoing chronic inflammatory processes. Amyloid is deposited initially in the zona fasciculata and zona reticularis with subsequent widespread deposition throughout the adrenal cortex. Amyloid protein appears as amorphous, homogenous eosinophilic material and may be identified using a Congo red stain, looking for apple green birefringence of amyloid fibrils under a polarized light. Loss or

necrosis of the adrenal cortex may be seen in conjunction with amyloid deposition, as well as vascular dilatation, cavitation, and marked congestion or hemorrhage. Concurrent mineralization is uncommon.

6.3.1.2 Adrenal Gland Pigmentation

Adrenocortical pigmentation seen commonly in animals greater than eight months of age. Varying amounts of brown-black, coarse granular, intracellular pigment is found primarily within the zona fasciculata and zona reticularis. The pigment is partially PAS and Oil Red O positive, mildly positive for iron, but acid-fast negative. The pathogenesis underlying pigment deposition is uncertain.

6.3.1.3 Hyperadrenocorticism

Hyperadrenocorticism or Cushing's disease is seen infrequently in both males and females and can result from adrenocortical hyperplasia or neoplasia or the condition may arise secondary to excess ACTH production from a pituitary tumor or from glucocorticoid treatments. Hyperadrenocorticism

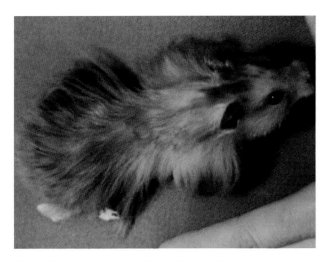

Figure 6.9 Hamster with Cushing's disease. Note the characteristic bilaterally symmetrical alopecia. *Source:* Courtesy of C. Wheler.

was associated with a pituitary chromophobe adenoma in one hamster and at necropsy the pituitary gland was enlarged to 3 mm by 2 mm with a cystic dilated cleft, causing compression of the overlying brainstem.

Presenting Clinical Signs The clinical signs in hamsters are similar to those reported in other species with hyperadrenocorticism, and include bilaterally symmetrical alopecia without pruritus, hyperpigmentation, comedone formation, thinning of the skin, polyphagia, polydipsia, and polyuria (Figure 6.9). Behavioral changes may also occur.

Differential Diagnoses Differential diagnoses include dermatophytosis, epitheliotropic lymphoma, demodecosis, bacterial dermatitis, diabetes mellitus, nephrosclerosis, and hypothyroidism.

Laboratory Diagnostics The diagnosis is primarily based on the clinical signs. Results for ACTH stimulation and dexamethasone suppression tests have been described in laboratory hamsters but may not be feasible for a pet hamster because of the need for repeated testing, the quantities of blood required, and the stress to the animal from repeated handling and anesthesia for blood collection. A urine cortisol:creatinine ratio can be used but requires that reference ranges be developed. Elevated serum cortisol or alkaline phosphatase levels may be useful but hamsters secrete both cortisol and corticosterone, which may confound interpretation of tests. Ultrasound and survey radiography may demonstrate enlargement of the adrenal gland.

6.3.1.4 Adrenocortical Hyperplasia and Neoplasia

Adrenocortical hyperplasia is an age-related change seen in hamsters that are older than 12 months of age, and more commonly, in hamsters 18–36 months of age. Hyperplastic foci are usually composed of two different cell types, including cortical cells and spindle type cells. In ferrets, spindle cell proliferation is reported in adrenocortical tumors and identified as smooth muscle. Further studies are needed in hamsters to determine if the cell types are similar.

Adrenocortical neoplasia is common and more often reported in males. Bilateral involvement of the glands is usual but there is not always equal involvement. Both adenomas and adenocarcinomas are seen and carcinomas are locally invasive with rare metastases. Similar to adrenocortical hyperplasia, two cell types; cortical cells and spindle cells, are identified in both adrenal cortical adenomas and adenocarcinomas.

Pheochromocytomas are in frequently seen in hamsters. Cells of these tumors are arranged in cords or nodules and are well demarcated from the surrounding normal medulla. These tumors have only been identified as incidental findings at necropsy and it is unknown if they are functional.

Lymphosarcomas involving the adrenal glands are uncommon.

6.3.2 Conditions of the Thyroid Gland

6.3.2.1 Thyroid Gland Amyloidosis

Deposition of amyloid in the thyroid gland is an age-related change and part of a generalized amyloid deposition condition that may be seen in hamsters. Amyloid deposits occur predominantly in hamsters greater than 17 months of age and range from mild to marked perifollicular deposition with atrophy and loss of normal follicles over time.

6.3.2.2 Follicular Cysts

Follicular cysts are seen in hamsters aged 11–29 months and the colloid-containing cysts are quite variable in size and shape. The clinical significance is unknown and these are usually an incidental finding upon microscopic examination of tissues.

6.3.2.3 Hypothyroidism

Thyroxine-responsive hypothyroidism has been reported anecdotally in hamsters. Clinical signs include alopecia, hyperpigmentation and thickening of skin, listlessness, and lack of tolerance to the cold. No pathologic correlates have been reported.

6.3.2.4 Thyroid Gland Neoplasia

Thyroid gland neoplasia is not commonly identified at necropsy. An incidence of 1.5% to 2.6% was reported in one hamster colony. Both solid and follicular papillary thyroid adenomas are seen with the solid adenomas confined mostly to the mid portion of the gland and follicular papillary adenomas located within the mid to lower portion of the gland (Figure 6.10). Thyroid glands

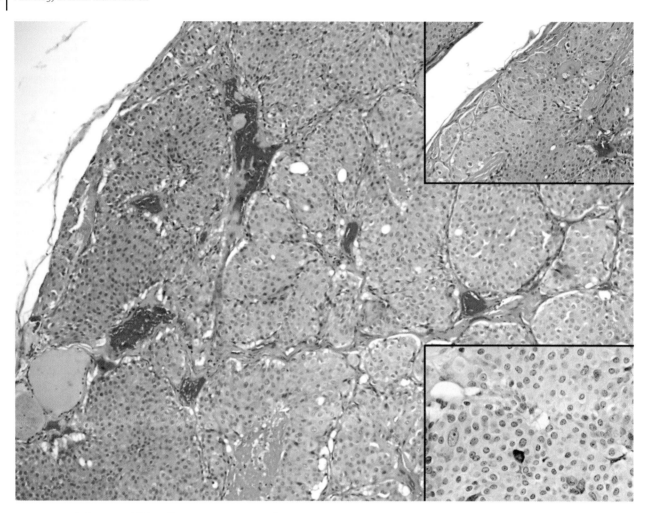

Figure 6.10 A: A 2-year-old dwarf hamster was presented in acute respiratory distress with inspiratory stridor and inflated cheek pouches. A 0.5 x 1cm mass was identified in the tissues of the anterior neck at post-mortem. Histologically, the mass is composed of nodules of polygonal cells with round to oval nuclei, prominent nucleoli and abundant cytoplasm with distinct borders, rare mitotic figures and separated by fine vascularized fibrous septa and occasional structures resembling colloid-containing thyroid follicles. The C-cell carcinoma was likely causing compression of the upper trachea which would explain the presenting clinical signs of inspiratory stridor. Inset upper: Small nests of neoplastic cells are penetrating the surrounding fibrous capsule. Inset lower: Variable positive immunohistochemistry labelling for calcitonin are noted within several tumor cells confirming the identify as thyroid gland C-cells. No specific immunohistochemistry labelling was present for thyroglobulin or thyroid transcription.

carcinomas tend to be solid in nature. A single case of melanoma originating in skin with metastasis to thyroid gland has been reported in a hamster.

Both multifocal C-cell hyperplasia and foci of ectopic C-cell hyperplasia can occasionally be seen within laryngotracheal tissues near the thyroid glands.

6.3.3 Conditions of the Parathyroid Gland

6.3.3.1 Parathyroid Gland Hyperplasia and Neoplasia
Parathyroid gland hyperplasia and adenomas are infrequent but in one study were second only to adrenal gland proliferative lesions in hamsters older than 18 months old. Differentiation of hyperplastic from adenomatous lesions is challenging, and criteria include anaplasia,

identification of a circumscribed capsule, and compression of surrounding parenchyma. Parathyroid cysts are rare and may be mistaken for thyroid follicular cysts. In other species, these cysts are often associated with hyperparathyroidism, but this relationship has not been established in hamsters. The cysts are lined by ciliated epithelium and are thought to arise from remnants of the pharyngeal pouches.

6.3.4 Conditions of the Pituitary Gland

Pituitary gland cysts can be seen in older animals and in one report, females were affected more frequently than males. Cysts are usually small but can be multiple, filled with homogenous eosinophilic material with a lining epithelium that is often ciliated. Other age-related changes include glandular degeneration and mineralization.

A functional pituitary chromophobe adenoma was reported as the cause of hyperadrenocorticism in a 1.5-year-old female hamster. Some 25% of aged hamsters with adenomas and adenocarcinomas of the pars distalis also had cerebral lateral ventricular dilation in one long-term study. Pituitary gland hyperplasia was reported in a 14-month-old male in one case study. Hyperplasia of the pars distalis was reported more often in aged females than males in multiple long-term studies.

6.3.5 Conditions of the Endocrine Pancreas

6.3.5.1 Diabetes Mellitus

Diabetes mellitus occurs in Chinese hamsters (*Cricetulus griseus*) as a spontaneous disease, and is autosomal recessive in some sublines, but has a polygenic mode of inheritance in others. Diabetes mellitus can also be induced experimentally in Syrian hamsters following intraperitoneal inoculation of hamsters with encephalomyocarditis virus (EMC)-D (diabetogenic variant).

Presenting Clinical Signs   Clinically, diabetes can be clinically identified in hamsters by three months of age based on signs of hyperphagia, hyperglycemia and glucosuria, polydipsia, and polyuria. Animals are not typically overweight, are occasionally ketouric, and may have concurrent urinary bladder infection. Diabetes mellitus has been linked with the increased risk of developing early onset atherosclerosis in hamsters.

Pathology   Early in the course of the disease, there is incomplete β-cell degranulation and hypertrophy, and α-cells are located at the margins of the islets. As the condition develops, β-cell degranulation becomes intensified and β-cells become vacuolated. Overall; however, islet size and appearance are variable, although ketotic hamsters have islets that are reduced in size, with reduced numbers of β cells and more pronounced degranulation and vacuolar changes with fibrosis within islets. There is no difference in the appearance or function of the exocrine pancreas between normal and diabetic hamsters.

Renal glomerulopathy is also seen with mesangial thickening and increased cellularity, and cystic dilatation of capillaries and a reduction of capillary loops resulting from capillary fusion. Glomerular lipidosis may be present.

In hamsters infected with EMC-D, there is marked subcapsular and interlobular edema of the pancreas. Initially, there is acute generalized necrosis of acinar cells with edema and moderate to marked mixed inflammatory cell infiltrates progressing to fibroplasia and ductular hyperplasia. The islets are not affected at first, but by day 7, islets are reduced in size with a reduction in insulin content, based on the results of immunoperoxidase staining.

Differential Diagnoses   Differential diagnoses for diabetes mellitus in hamsters include hyperadrenocorticism, renal amyloidosis, and nephrosclerosis.

Laboratory Diagnostics   Diagnosis of the condition is based on clinical signs, persistent glycosuria, and elevated blood glucose levels.

Disease/Colony Management   The onset of clinical signs can be delayed by restricting food intake and feeding low fat diets.

In minimally biosecure research facilities and pet distribution centers, the possibility exists for transfer of EMC-D from other small rodents to hamsters.

6.4 Respiratory Conditions

6.4.1 Conditions of the Nasal Cavity

6.4.1.1 Rhinitis

Rhinitis is not commonly seen in isolation in hamsters and is more often found together with pneumonia and conjunctivitis. Etiologic agents include *Streptococcus* spp., *S. pneumoniae*, *Pasteurella* spp., *Klebsiella pneumonia*, and *Bordetella* spp. Animals may have oculonasal discharge and can develop otitis media and interna. With bacteria such as *Pasteurella* spp. and *Streptococcus* spp., abscesses can form elsewhere in the body, especially in the uterus. Drafts and fine sawdust from bedding can also cause oculonasal irritation, as can cigarette smoke and aerosolized products, such as furniture polish, hair spray, and perfumes. Anecdotally, allergies to food and bedding may present as rhinitis together with generalized alopecia and sore feet.

Microscopically, rhinitis can range from a focal suppurative condition to generalized inflammation of the nasal mucosa with large numbers of infiltrating neutrophils and macrophages to necrotizing rhinitis with mucosal ulceration and fibrin, neutrophils, and necrotic cellular debris on the ulcerated surface and within the nasal passages.

6.4.1.2 Nasal Polyps

Nasal polyps are found sporadically and are variable in size, ranging from a small nodule of hyperplastic epithelium jutting into the nasal cavity to larger, obstructive, exophytic mucosal nodules lined by nasal epithelium with dilated and cystic nasal glands filled with inflammatory cells. Mixed leukocytic infiltrates may also be present in the surrounding connective tissue and within the nasal epithelium.

6.4.2 Conditions of the Trachea

Inflammation of the trachea is usually mild with mixed leukocytic infiltrates within the lamina propria and submucosa, sometimes involving the submucosal glands, which may be distended and lined by attenuated epithelium. Cystic dilatation of tracheal and laryngeal glands is a common incidental finding in adult hamsters. In these cases, cysts are lined by flattened epithelium and filled with eosinophilic PAS-positive, acellular material with occasional inflammatory cells. Rarely, amyloid is deposited in the tracheal connective tissue.

Tracheal neoplasia is rare and primary tumors are not reported. Metastatic tumors affecting the trachea include lymphosarcoma with neoplastic cells infiltrating the tracheal mucosa and submucosa, and metastases from an adrenocortical adenocarcinoma in the lymphatic vessels surrounding the trachea.

6.4.3 Pulmonary Conditions

6.4.3.1 Bacterial Pneumonia

Pneumonia is common in pet hamsters and is generally secondary to bacterial infection, although there are several murine respiratory viruses that infect hamsters that may act as co-factors in disease initiation and progression. Suppurative bronchopneumonia is typically associated with concurrent suppurative rhinitis and conjunctivitis, and presents clinically as dyspnea, ocular discharge, matting of the fur on the forelegs, otitis media and interna, and encephalitis. Etiologic agents include *Streptococcus* spp., *S. pneumoniae*, *Pasteurella* spp., *P. pneumotropica*, *Klebsiella pneumoniae*, cilia-associated respiratory bacillus (CARB), and *Bordetella* spp. *Mycoplasma pulmonis* has been rarely isolated from hamsters with no associated lesions, thus, the pathogenicity in hamsters is questionable. There is a single case report of *Corynebacterium paulometabulum*-associated acute edematous pneumonia in a 1-year-old hamster.

Streptococcus agalactiae and *S. pneumoniae* infections are associated with acute pleuropneumonia and septicemia and may be transmitted from humans to hamsters. Streptococcal pneumonias are relatively uncommon in hamsters and are associated with stress. Hamsters are infected via aerosol and clinical signs include depression, anorexia, oculonasal discharge, dehydration, dyspnea, and weight loss. The course of disease is short, approximately 3 days or less, and diagnosis is based on clinical signs, necropsy findings, and bacterial culture. Bacteria can usually be recovered from the lung, spleen, and liver of affected hamsters.

Pasteurella pneumotropica can cause acute and chronic bacterial pneumonia in hamsters and hamsters may also be subclinically infected. In addition, affected hamsters may have cutaneous abscesses, conjunctivitis, and otitis

interna. Clinical signs associated with bronchopneumonia include dyspnea, nasal exudate, and weight loss. At necropsy, there are multifocal areas of pulmonary consolidation. *Pasteurella* spp. may be transmitted from human caregivers, such as children, to hamsters.

Experimentally, hamsters are very susceptible to CARB infection with a mouse origin isolate. Transmission is by direct contact with infected animals and interspecies transmission is possible; however, the organism is usually less virulent in the heterologous host. There is increased opportunity to disseminate infections among different rodent species as a consequence of mixing small mammals in distribution centers destined for the pet retail market. In hamsters, experimental infection with CARB produced multifocal to coalescing pyogranulomatous bronchopneumonia with bronchiectasis and enlargement of mediastinal and bronchial lymph nodes. Diagnosis is based on the identification of filamentous bacteria intercalating between cilia using a Warthin-Starry stain.

Hamsters can carry other opportunistic organisms subclinically in their respiratory tract, including *Pasteurella multocida*, *S. pneumoniae*, *Staphylococcus aureus*, *Klebsiella pneumoniae*, *Bordetella* spp. and *Salmonella* spp. The most effective control measure is elimination of carrier animals from breeding colonies, and isolation and quarantine of new animals before introduction into the colony.

6.4.3.2 Viral Pneumonias

Sendai virus is an RNA virus of the family Paramyxoviridae, genus Paramyxovirus, species parainfluenza type 1. Mice, rats, hamsters, and guinea pigs are natural hosts. Historically, a high percentage of conventional hamster breeding colonies have been seropositive for Sendai virus with no associated clinical disease. The virus is highly contagious and is transmitted by aerosol and contact with respiratory secretions. Infection can be demonstrated by the development of antibodies to Sendai virus only a few weeks after introduction to the contaminated colony. During experimental studies, neonatal hamsters were shown to be susceptible to infection following nasal instillation of the virus and increased mortality was observed due to pneumonia. In adult animals, no clinical signs are noted after intranasal challenge. In another study, groups of hamsters were treated with an immunosuppressant and then challenged with aerosolized Sendai virus. At necropsy, the lungs were extensively consolidated and all animals died within 7–9 days of severe hemorrhagic pneumonia. With damage to the nasal and tracheal mucosa, animals may be predisposed to a secondary bacterial pneumonia. Diagnosis is by serologic assay, including ELISA and IFA. Virus can be recovered from respiratory tissues. Continued breeding and the availability of young, naïve animals allows for the persistence of this virus in a small mammal breeding facility. Closing the facility to new introductions and temporarily discontinuing breeding for at least 8 weeks will break the cycle of reinfection and virus propagation. Rodent vermin should be excluded from breeding colonies to minimize disease transmission.

Pneumonia virus of mice (PVM) is an RNA virus of the family Paramyxoviridae, genus *Pneumovirus*. Mice, rats, and hamsters can be infected, although infection in hamsters is subclinical. The virus is transmitted horizontally by aerosol and by contact with respiratory secretions. Experimentally, following intranasal instillation of the virus, hamsters become lethargic, develop sneezing and dyspnea, and may die within 1 to 2 weeks post infection. At necropsy, lung involvement is extensive with consolidation, edema, and purple discoloration and nasal turbinates may be swollen and erythematous. Histologically rhinitis and an interstitial pneumonia are seen, with alveolar septal thickening by mixed mononuclear cell infiltrates and a serocellular alveolar exudate. Healthy hamsters placed in close contact with intranasally challenged hamsters may exhibit clinical signs and at necropsy had mild pulmonary involvement. Diagnosis is best achieved by serology.

Simian Virus 5 (SV5) is an RNA virus of the family Paramyxoviridae, genus *Paramyxovirus*, and is classified as a parainfluenza type 5 virus. Seroconversion to SV5 is common in hamsters but infection is generally subclinical.

6.4.3.3 Pulmonary Neoplasia

Primary neoplasia, such as adenocarcinoma, is infrequently seen in hamsters. Metastatic tumors including lymphosarcoma, adrenocortical adenocarcinoma, and melanoma are more likely to occur.

6.4.3.4 Other Pulmonary Conditions

In cases of **pulmonary histiocytosis**, thickened alveolar septa are lined by hypertrophic and hyperplastic pneumocytes and alveoli contain numerous macrophages with abundant foamy cytoplasm and long, slender, needle-shaped crystals resembling cholesterol clefts. The lesions may develop as a result of inhalation of foreign material, possibly containing lipid, but are also likely idiopathic aging lesions.

Pulmonary granulomas were reported as incidental findings in a study involving a group of Chinese hamsters. At necropsy, lungs contained multifocal to coalescing 1–2 mm, gray subpleural nodules. Microscopically, the nodules consisted of alveolar aggregates of lipid-filled macrophages with focal fibrosis, some mixed inflammatory cells, lymphoid nodules, and occasional cholesterol clefts. The etiology of the pulmonary lesions was not determined but a viral etiology was suspected. Animals were housed in different types of cages and had different bedding material so inhaled bedding material was discounted as a possible etiology of the lesions. The description of these lesions is similar to pulmonary adenomatosis.

6.5 Musculoskeletal Conditions

Hamsters are solitary animals and fighting will occur when hamsters are mixed together. Adult females are particularly aggressive and only allow cohabitation with a male during breeding. Injuries from bite wounds are common and can result in fracture or loss of limbs, traumatic skin and muscle injuries, and abscessation. Old healed fractures may be seen at postmortem as a result of traumatic running wheel injuries, inappropriate diets or inadvertent falls during restraint.

6.5.1 Myodystrophy

Myodystrophy has been described in inbred strains of Syrian hamsters. Some of these strains of hamsters with muscular dystrophy also have cardiomyopathy (see Section 6.7.2).

6.5.1.1 Presenting Clinical Signs

Historical reports suggest that clinical signs associated with skeletal myopathy are manifested in older animals in contrast with cardiac lesions, which occur when hamsters are quite young. Most affected hamsters will die from cardiac failure before showing any loss of function associated with skeletal myopathy. More recent investigations have demonstrated gait abnormalities in 3- and 9-month-old myodystrophic hamsters. The significance of these findings may not translate to pet hamsters, although given that hamsters are very active and are usually provided with exercise wheels, lameness may be seen with this condition.

6.5.1.2 Pathology

The first change reported in the skeletal muscle is a perinuclear halo with irregular borders and fine granular material that gradually enlarges and becomes more eosinophilic. As the disease progresses, this halo fuses to form a clear zone around rows of nuclei. The supraspinatus (shoulder) muscle is most affected. In hamsters less than one month of age, centrally located nuclei and nuclear rowing are normal, thus myofiber necrosis is the only lesion seen. After seven months of age, a few centrally located nuclei, rare nuclear rowing, and myofiber basophilia and nuclear changes are considered pathognomonic for muscular dystrophy. Muscle fiber necrosis, inflammation, and fibrosis can be seen in aged animals; however, the lesions are focal and may reflect aging changes or healed bite wounds incurred from fighting.

In a case of polymyopathy in an 8-month-old Syrian golden hamster, the animal presented for necropsy because the hind legs were stretched backwards preventing the animal from walking. Several muscles, including those of the hind limbs and the neck, were also markedly swollen, causing the overlying skin to be stretched very tightly. There was no evidence of weakness. Histologically, there was marked variation in size of myofiber bundles, with splitting and fragmentation of swollen or atrophic myofibers, hypereosinophilia, loss of cross striations, and vacuolation. Centrally located nuclei or pyknotic nuclei were common. There was evidence of regeneration with sarcoplasmic basophilia and enlarged nuclei arranged in rows. Neutrophils or a mixture of mononuclear cells including macrophages and plasma cells were clustered around necrotic myofibers and there was a mild increase in connective tissue. The etiology was not determined and a hereditary muscular dystrophy was considered.

6.5.2 Osteoarthritis

Osteoarthritis is seen in aged animals and affects the femorotibial joint (stifle joint) most commonly. Physical exercise at an early age in hamsters is beneficial as it contributes to cartilage maturation but may be associated with an increased incidence of osteoarthritis at a later age.

6.5.3 Osteoporosis

Hamsters may develop osteoporosis as a result of poorly balanced diets, such as all seed diets. Bone fractures are more likely to occur secondary to increased bone fragility so careful restraint and provision of safe housing and surroundings are needed to prevent entrapment or other trauma.

6.5.4 Fibrous Osteodystrophy

Fibrous osteodystrophy can occur in hamsters, likely due to secondary hyperparathyroidism resulting from chronic renal failure with retention of phosphorus and development of hypocalcemia. Chronic renal disease may also impair formation of 1, 25-dihydroxyvitamin D_3, reducing calcium absorption from the intestine and contributing to hypocalcemia. Reduced bone density and fractures may be evident in survey radiographs. Histologically, features of fibrous osteodystrophy include increased bone resorption with prominent osteoclast activity, fibroplasia, and increased osteoblast activity producing woven bone.

6.5.5 Injection-induced Myonecrosis

Skeletal muscle necrosis has been associated with intramuscular injections of ketamine and xylazine in the caudal thigh muscle. Early lesions of myonecrosis with hemorrhage and edema are replaced by suppurative myositis and cellulitis of the intermuscular connective tissue continuous with overlying epithelial ulceration. If left untreated, the necrotic muscle will slough. In chronic lesions, fibrous replacement of muscle tissue may be seen with variable mineralization and areas of myofiber regeneration.

Similar lesions and more extensive lesions involving nervous tissue can be induced by the injection of many types of irritants. The injection of bacteria contaminated substances must also be considered but would be expected to produce more inflammation with evidence of bacterial colonization. Other routes of injection, such as subcutaneous or intraperitoneal, are preferable in small rodents because of their very small muscle mass.

6.5.6 Neoplasia

Muscle and bony neoplasms are rarely noted in hamsters with rare reports of osteochondroma and osteosarcoma.

6.6 Gastrointestinal Conditions

Hamsters have cheek pouches, which are evaginations of the lateral buccal wall that extend beneath the skin dorsolaterally over the shoulders. These are considered immunologically privileged sites as tumors can be transplanted into this site and grow without rejection. The skin covering the lateral and dorsal neck and shoulders is loose to accommodate expansion of the cheek pouches.

The hamster stomach has two distinct compartments separated by a muscular sphincter; the nonglandular stomach or forestomach, which has a squamous mucosa similar to the esophagus (Figure 6.11), a high pH, and contains fermentative microorganisms, and the glandular

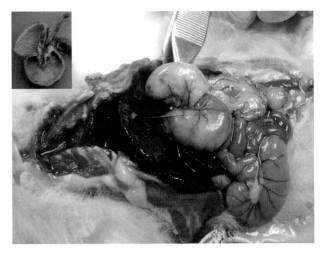

Figure 6.11 The hamster stomach has two distinct compartments separated by a muscular sphincter, the nonglandular stomach or forestomach, and the glandular or true stomach. Inset: Fixed stomach emptied of contents. *Source:* Courtesy of M. Ritter.

or true stomach. Because of the anatomy of the stomach and esophageal sphincter, a hamster cannot regurgitate. Hamsters are coprophagic, like other rodents, consuming feces directly from the anus several times per day.

Hamsters carry a number of bacteria in their mouth as either normal commensals or opportunistic agents, which may cause disease in human caregivers. For example, *Acinetobacter anitratus* is considered a normal commensal agent of low virulence and is carried in the oral cavity of hamsters. A pet hamster bit the distal finger of an otherwise healthy 8-year-old boy and 24 hours later, the area around the bite was reddened, swollen and tender. Eventually, tenosynovitis and osteomyelitis of the distal phalanx were diagnosed and *A. anitratus* was isolated from the wound. The hamster died shortly afterwards and *A. anitratus* was recovered from oral swabs of the animal. *Acinetobacter* spp. are considered to be commensals and of low virulence but do have an association with osteomyelitis in humans following animal bites. Other potential oral bacteria include *Corynebacterium* spp., *Pasteurella* spp., and *Yersinia* spp. Because hamsters are prone to biting when disturbed at rest, they are not generally considered good pets for very small children. Hands should be washed well after handling hamsters and bites should be carefully cleaned.

6.6.1 Conditions of the Cheek Pouch

Cheek pouches are used for carrying and storing food (Figure 6.12) but can become impacted with various substances, including feed and bedding material. Rupture can occur with spillage of contents into the surrounding sub-

cutaneous tissues and subsequent development of a foreign body inflammatory reaction and cellulitis. Cheek pouches can evert spontaneously and may become lacerated, requiring surgical intervention.

Tumors of cheek pouch and oral cavity are infrequently reported in aged hamsters and include osteosarcoma and squamous cell carcinoma. A spontaneous fibroma was reported in the right cheek pouch of a 1.5-year-old pet female Syrian hamster. The 2.5 x 3.0 cm ulcerated fluctuant mass initially presented as a white papule that was lanced and drained but regrew within two months. The mass was surgically removed because it interfered with chewing. Microscopically, the well-demarcated, partially encapsulated submucosal mass was composed of loosely arranged interdigitating bundles of spindle to stellate cells separated by amorphous mucopolysaccharide ground substance.

6.6.2 Conditions of the Oral Cavity

Similar to other rodents, hamsters have continuously growing incisors and malocclusion is common. Clinical signs include anorexia, weight loss, emaciation, ptyalism, and visual abnormalities of incisors. Overgrowth of incisors can be an underlying cause of cheek pouch impaction. Associated lesions include gingival hyperplasia, bone loss, and osteosclerosis with subsequent abscessation extending to include the Harderian gland and brain, with eventual vascular dissemination to lungs and kidneys.

6.6.2.1 Hamster Parvovirus Infection

Marked tooth discoloration, malformed or missing incisors, a pot-bellied appearance, and domed calvaria are reported in suckling and weanling Syrian hamsters

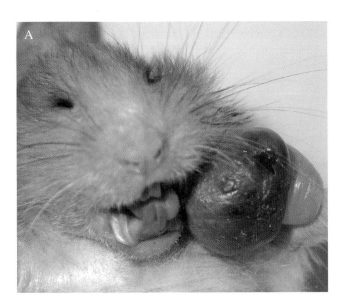
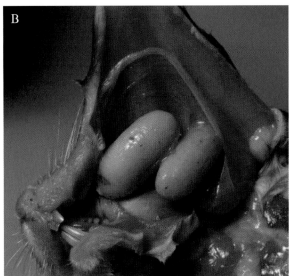

Figure 6.12 A: Large partially cystic cheek pouch mass protruding from mouth. The etiology was undetermined. B: The hamster cheek pouches are very large, extend caudally over the shoulders and are used for carrying and storing food and other materials, as depicted. Food-filled cheek pouches can be mistaken for tumors or other masses. *Source:* A: Courtesy of The Links Road Animal and Bird Clinic.

infected with hamster parvovirus (HaPV). Morbidity and mortality approached 100% in experimentally infected pups. HaPV has high homology with MPV-3 (a mouse parvovirus), suggesting that the mouse is likely the natural host with interspecies transmission to hamsters. Histologic lesions following infection in hamsters include incisor enamel hypoplasia, periodontitis, and suppuration of the dental pulp with hemorrhage and mineralization. Other lesions may include multifocal cerebral mineralization and testicular atrophy with necrosis and mineralization of the seminiferous tubules epithelium, and perivasculitis of the pampiniform plexus. Suckling hamsters inoculated with HaPV died with hemorrhagic lesions in the kidneys, gastrointestinal tract, testicles/uterus and brain, and histologic lesions of vascular thrombosis with evidence of intranuclear parvovirus inclusions in endothelial cells.

An outbreak of high mortality and malformation and absence of incisors has also been described in young hamster pups that seroconverted to Toolan's H-1 virus, a parvovirus of rats.

There is increased opportunity to disseminate infections among and between small mammal species when they are mixed and held in distribution centers for retail pet markets. The entry of wild mice and rats into small mammal breeding and holding centers is also facilitated by suboptimal rodent control programs, which may allow for interspecies transmission of various disease agents, including parvovirus.

6.6.2.2 Salivary Gland Cytomegalovirus-like Infection

One report describes naturally occurring cytomegalovirus-like inclusions predominantly in the acini and only rarely concurrently in the ducts of the serous portion of the submaxillary glands in a large percentage of mature hamsters. Mucous cells of the submaxillary glands were less frequently affected.

6.6.2.3 Oral Neoplasia

Oral squamous cell papilloma and molar odontomas are seen infrequently in aged hamsters. Salivary gland adenomas, adenocarcinomas, and mixed sarcomas are also rare.

6.6.3 Gastric Conditions

6.6.3.1 Helicobacter-induced Gastritis

Chronic antral gastritis and intestinal metaplasia are seen in hamsters naturally infected with *Helicobacter aurati* and a second novel *Helicobacter* sp. Histologically, lesions are most intense in the distal gastric antrum near the pyloroduodenal junction, presenting as multifocal to diffuse lymphoplasmacytic mucosal infiltrates, with

fewer neutrophils and eosinophils, and scattered deep mucosal lymphoid nodules. Mucosal epithelial hyperplasia and dysplasia are noted with numerous goblet cells within the gastric antral pits. An invasive gastric adenocarcinoma at the pyloric-duodenal junction was seen in an aged female hamster from the same colony of hasmters naturally infected with multiple *Helicobacter* spp. including *H. aurati*. The only ante-mortem sign was weight loss. Experimentally, *H. pylori* has been reported to readily colonize the hamster stomach, although the implications for cross-transfer between pets and their human caregivers is unknown.

6.6.3.2 Gastric Candidiasis and Cryptosporidiosis

Candida spp., other yeasts, and bacteria are commonly seen in the stomach of hamsters and without indication of mucosal invasion are an incidental finding. Opportunistic overgrowth of yeast, bacteria, and protozoa, such as *Cryptosporidia* sp. may occur in animals suffering from other conditions and infections, and the pathologist should look elsewhere for a primary disease. Because of the ability of *Cryptosporidia* to transfer among a broad range of host species, they must be considered a potential human health hazard.

6.6.3.3 Gastric Ulceration

Acute ulceration of the forestomach or the glandular stomach may occur in hamsters and result in sudden death. Management causes, such as lack of access to food or water, recent shipping or poor handling practices may lead to acute hemorrhage and exsanguination. Necropsy findings include dark gastric content with or without mucosal petechiation.

6.6.3.4 Gastric Neoplasia

Gastric squamous papillomas of the forestomach are seen sporadically and appear as raised, irregular, roughened masses. Microscopically, these represent papillary outgrowths of parakeratotic squamous epithelium with accumulation of surface keratin, sometimes with focal ulceration and inflammation.

6.6.4 Intestinal Conditions

Diarrhea (wet tail) is a common and nonspecific clinical sign in pet hamsters and may be initiated by both infectious and noninfectious causes, such as management changes, transportation or social stress, and sudden dietary changes. Of cases involving infectious agents, bacterial causes predominate. Enteric adenovirus can be present in young, weanling hamsters with characteristic large amphophilic intranuclear inclusion bodies noted in enterocytes, but infection is not associated with clinical illness. Intestinal parasitism is very common in pet hamsters acquired from conventional sources and heavy, mixed burdens of pinworms, tapeworms, and protozoa may be present with few clinical signs.

Amyloid deposition within the lamina propria of the intestine and exocrine pancreas is uncommon in aging hamsters.

6.6.4.1 Intestinal Obstruction and Intussusception

Enteritis, luminal tumors, foreign bodies, post-anesthetic intestinal atony, pica, and heavy infestations of intestinal parasites, such as cestodes, have all been associated with intestinal obstruction and intussusception in hamsters. Hamsters appear to be more susceptible to colonic intussusceptions than small intestinal invaginations. Rectal prolapse may occur as sequela to straining due to rectal irritation from large parasite burdens or conditions causing diarrhea.

6.6.4.2 Proliferative Enteritis

Proliferative enteritis or transmissible ileal hyperplasia is caused by *Lawsonia intracellularis. L. intracellularis* infection causes similar diseases in rabbits, pigs, calves, and ferrets, however, there is strong evidence of host susceptibility to specific bacterial subspecies. Transmission is by the fecal-oral route; young post-weaned hamsters are highly susceptible. Underlying stress factors enhancing susceptibility to infection and disease include weaning, pups from first litters, dietary changes, suboptimal diets, overcrowding, transportation, intercurrent disease, surgery, and environmental changes.

Presenting Clinical Signs Clinical signs vary and include an acute onset of lethargy, unkempt hair coat, irritability, hunched posture, anorexia, profuse diarrhea, dehydration, weight loss, and high mortality within 24–48 hours. Subacute disease presents as diarrhea, weight loss, palpable intestinal thickening, variable mortality, and ileal obstruction, intussusception, peritonitis, impaction, and colonic and rectal prolapses as sequelae. Chronic disease may occur in asymptomatic carriers with palpable intestinal thickening or intestinal and intra-abdominal granulomas, abscesses and reactive lymph nodes.

Pathology At necropsy, affected hamsters are emaciated with soiling of the perineum and fecal staining and matting of the fur around the tail and ventral abdomen. In acute cases, the ileum may be dilated, hyperemic, and filled with blood-tinged fluid. The lower ileum may be segmentally thickened and edematous with serosal abscesses and fibrinous to fibrous adhesions to nearby organs. Generalized peritonitis can result from intestinal or abscess rupture with complete or partial obstruction of the ileum. The affected ileal serosa can have an exaggerated cerebriform pattern of folds and the subtending mucosa may be thickened and corrugated. Mesenteric lymph nodes and Peyer's patches can be enlarged, hemorrhagic, and edematous. Characteristically, crypt hyperplasia is present characterized by irregular, elongate, tortuous and branching crypts lined by hyperplastic, pseudostratified columnar epithelium and scant goblet cells. Hyperplastic crypts can extend laterally and penetrate the underlying muscularis. Ileal crypts frequently contain neutrophils, macrophages, and luminal cellular debris with formation of crypt and subserosa abscesses. Lamina proprial inflammation and necrosis is common with a mixed cellular infiltrate, fibrin deposition, and congestion.

Laboratory Diagnostics Abundant curved, rod-shaped bacteria typical of *Lawsonia intracellularis* are present in the apical cytoplasm of hyperplastic enterocytes with a Warthin-Starry silver stain. PCR of affected intestinal tissues is confirmatory.

Differential Diagnoses Differential diagnoses include Tyzzer's disease (*Clostridium piliforme* infection), salmonellosis, colibacillosis, and clostridial enterocolitis. Often outbreaks of enteritis occur from mixed infections from agents such as *Escherichia coli, Salmonella* spp., *Campylobacter jejuni, Helicobacter* spp., and protozoal organisms such as *Giardia* sp., *Entamoeba* sp., *Spironucleus muris*, tritrichomonads ands *Cryptosporidia* sp.

6.6.4.3 Colibacillosis

Escherichia coli has been isolated from hamsters with proliferative ileitis and may also directly induce enteritis in hamsters. Enteropathogenic *E. coli* can cause disease alone or may act in concert with other pathogens such as *L. intracellularis*.

At necropsy, the small intestine may be hyperemic with segmental dilatation of the small or large intestine and yellow or dark red fluid content. Histologically, villi are blunted and fused with attenuation of the epithelium or ulceration and fibrin and neutrophils may be present in the lamina propria, crypts, or lumen. Mesenteric lymph nodes may be reactive or contain neutrophilic infiltrates. Random, multifocal hepatic necrosis may be seen rarely.

6.6.4.4 Salmonellosis

Historically, salmonellosis is an important disease of pet and laboratory hamsters but is now uncommon in North America. When encountered, the infection may present as an outbreak with high mortality. *Salmonella* Typhimurium and *Salmonella* Enteritidis are isolated most commonly and both are zoonotic. Recently, human illness from a multidrug resistant strain of *S.* Typhimurium DT 120 was linked to rodent exposure, including hamsters. In one case, a young child developed salmonellosis nine days after the acquisition of a hamster that had died two days following purchase from a pet store. Around the same time, a commercial pet distributor experienced approximately 60% mortality in hamsters from which a similar multidrug resistant strain of *S.* Typhimurium was isolated. *S.* Typhimurium was recovered from samples taken from rodent feed, bedding, and transport cages. Interspecies transmission was likely facilitated through the use of contaminated transport cages. Salmonellosis typically has a fecal-oral route of transmission and clinical signs in hamsters can include depression, ruffled hair coat, anorexia, dyspnea, diarrhea, high mortality, and peracute death.

Acute necrohemorrhagic enterocolitis may occur following infection with some strains of *Salmonella*. Commonly, in cases of salmonellosis in hamsters lesions at necropsy include patchy pulmonary hemorrhage, erythematous mediastinal lymph nodes, and acute, multifocal, miliary hepatic necrosis with no obvious signs of enteritis. Histologic lesions include pulmonary congestion and hemorrhage with focal interstitial pneumonitis, lobular atelectasis, and rarely, pleuritis with septic thrombophlebitis. Multifocal hepatic necrosis is often present with varying degrees of inflammation and venous thromboses, multifocal splenic necrosis, septic renal glomerular emboli, and suppurative pericarditis. Acute enteritis with necrosis of Peyer's patches is seen less often. Bacterial organisms are readily cultured from lesions and blood filtering tissues.

6.6.4.5 Clostridial Enterotoxemia

Syrian hamsters are very sensitive to *Clostridium difficile* toxins and disruption of the normal intestinal flora or loss of mucosal barrier is likely a prerequisite for development of *C. difficile*-associated enterocolitis. Hamsters may carry *C. difficile* spores as part of their normal intestinal flora and these organisms have difficulty colonizing a host with robust intestinal flora. Narrow spectrum antibiotics including penicillins, cephalosporins, macrolide antibiotics, lincosamides, and glycopeptide antibiotics may induce *C. difficile* enterocolitis by altering beneficial intestinal flora, particularly when administered orally. *C. difficile* typhlitis has also developed following topical administration of a broad spectrum antibiotic that contained polymyxin B sulphate, neomycin sulphate, and bacitracin zinc. Dietary changes and transportation stress may also trigger the condition.

Two virulence factors for clostridial enterocolitis are toxins A, a potent enterotoxin, and B, a potent cytotoxin, and either toxin or both in combination can produce disease. The disease has a neural component and stimulation of primary sensory neurons leads to the release of substance P and subsequent mast cell degranulation.

Presenting Clinical Signs Clinical signs in hamsters include ataxia, lethargy, anorexia, rough hair coat, diarrhea, dehydration, weight loss, fecal staining of

perianal area, and sudden death. At necropsy, there is hyperemia of the distal ileum and colon with serosal hemorrhage and gaseous distension of the cecum. Cecal content is yellow to blood-tinged fluid and the colon can contain formed feces or fluid content.

Pathology Microscopically, within the cecum, ileum, and colon, there is diffuse mucosal necrosis with proprial congestion, hemorrhage, edema and fibrin exudation, and mixed submucosal inflammatory cell infiltrates. The lumen may contain necrotic cellular debris, and sloughed epithelial and inflammatory cells. *C. difficile* has also been associated with more chronic cecal mucosal pathology. In one report, in addition to the typical acute cecal lesions, thickened and firm ceca were noted. This was microscopically correlated with glandular proliferation and dilatation with increased glandular depth, mild tortuosity, and numerous mitoses.

Laboratory Diagnostics Diagnosis of *C. difficile* enterotoxemia is based on gross and histologic lesions, isolation of the organism by anaerobic culture of cecal content, and demonstration of toxin elaboration in cecal content by ELISA or tissue by PCR. Gram stains may demonstrate large numbers of Gram positive rods within the cecal lumen.

6.6.4.6 Tyzzer's Disease

Clostridium piliforme is an obligate intracellular, spore-forming, anaerobic, slender, rod-shaped bacterium with a fecal-oral route of transmission. Infective spores can remain viable in contaminated bedding, environment, and feed for extended periods of time, but the vegetative form is very fragile. Animals co-infected with enteropathogenic attaching and effacing *E. coli* may increase the susceptibility of animals to secondary infection with *C. piliforme* and may also exacerbate the enteric lesions.

Presenting Clinical Signs Clinical signs of infection include hunched posture, depression, lethargy, unkempt hair coat, diarrhea with perineal staining, dehydration, and sudden death or rapid progression to death. Likely, most infections are subclinical subclinical following ingestion of spores, with only sporadic episodes of clinical disease. Predisposing factors include poor sanitation, stressful events such as transportation, poor environmental conditions, overcrowding, intercurrent disease, inadequate nutrition, and young age.

Pathology At necropsy, a triad of lesions involving the heart, liver, and small or large intestine may be present but are not always seen. Lesions include hyperemia, hemorrhage, and edema of the ileum, cecum, and colon with fluid content, enlarged, congested mesenteric lymph nodes, and hepatomegaly with multiple small pale

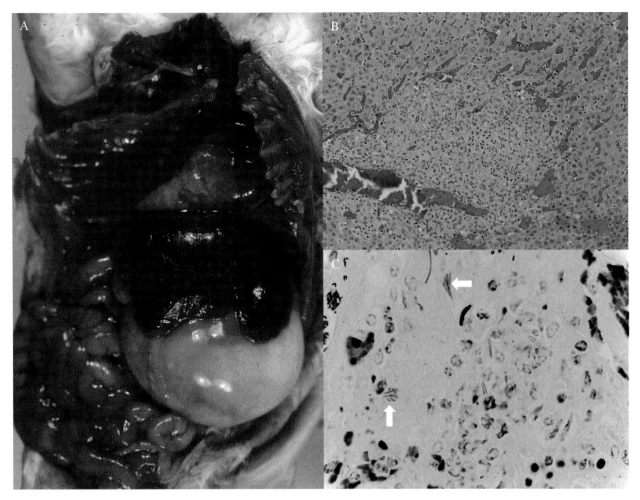

Figure 6.13 A: Tyzzer's disease in a hamster with characteristic acute, multifocal hepatic necrosis. A triad of lesions involving heart, liver and intestine may be present but is not compulsory. B: Liver from a 3-month-old hamster that died suddenly. There is acute, multifocal hepatic necrosis. C: This same hamster also had ulcerative typhlitis and bundles of *Clostridium piliforme* bacteria are seen within the cecal mucosa (arrows). Warthin-Starry.

necrotic foci (Figure 6.13). Microscopically, the intestinal mucosa is focally eroded with infiltration of the edematous lamina propria by a mixed neutrophilic and lymphocytic infiltrate. Typical intracellular bundles of bacilli ("pick-up sticks") can be visualized with a Warthin-Starry silver stain in nearby unaffected enterocytes bordering the lesion. Within the liver, there is multifocal necrosis with varying numbers of infiltrating leukocytes and intracellular bundles of bacteria seen at the periphery of lesions. Myocardial necrosis may be seen in some animals.

Laboratory Diagnostics Diagnosis is based on compatible lesions and the demonstration of characteristic bacteria with Warthin-Starry staining. PCR testing is available that targets 16 S ribosomal rRNA genomic sequences and the cecal wall and content are the preferred tissues for testing.

6.6.4.7 Campylobacteriosis
Campylobacter jejuni has been isolated from hamsters with diarrhea, proliferative ileitis, as well as from asymptomatic hamsters. Clinical signs included lethargy, ruffled fur, and diarrhea with staining of the tail and perineum. At necropsy, the ileum, cecum, and colon may be segmentally distended with fluid and the mucosa reddened and edematous. Histologically, the severity of the lesions is variable with shortening and distortion of small intestinal villi, epithelial hyperplasia and infiltrates of neutrophils within the lamina propria. *C. jejuni* is also a zoonotic agent and asymptomatic hamsters can shed the organisms in their feces for extended periods of time.

6.6.4.8 Helicobacter Typhocolitis
Spontaneous proliferative and dysplastic typhlocolitis occurs in aging Syrian hamsters naturally infected with

Helicobacter spp. At necropsy, the ileocecocolic junction may be thickened with a cobblestone appearance to the cecal mucosa. This correlates histologically to cecal mucosal thickening with focal erosions and mixed leukocytic lamina proprial infiltrates, gland abscesses, and submucosal herniation of glands.

6.6.4.9 Other Causes of Bacterial Enteritis

Yersinia pseudotuberculosis infections in hamsters are rare and not typically seen in well-managed breeding facilities. Organisms may be introduced through feed, water or bedding material contaminated from wild rodents or birds. Clinical signs include progressive emaciation, intermittent diarrhea, and eventual death. Nodular foci of caseous necrosis can be found in the intestines, mesenteric lymph nodes, liver, spleen, and lungs. Bacterial culture of affected tissues is diagnostic. Colony management includes removal of the affected hamsters, sanitation, repopulation with unaffected hamsters, and re-evaluation of biosecurity protocols. Inadequate rodent control programs facilitate the entry of wild mice and rats into large distribution and holding centers where various species of small mammals are assembled and allow for interspecies transmission of various diseases including yersiniosis.

Pasteurella pneumotropica is a zoonotic pathogen that can be found in the oropharynx and intestinal tract of rodents and was reported as the etiologic agent of peritonitis in a child on peritoneal dialysis. The child had recently acquired a pet hamster and the child and hamster were sleeping together at night. A pinhole was detected in the dialysis tubing and that same morning the child diagnosed with peritonitis. It is likely that the hamster either bit the tubing or licked the tubing at the site of the opening, thus introducing the bacterium. *P. pneumotropica* has been associated with outbreaks of enteritis in hamster breeding colonies with rectal prolapses occurring in severely affected animals. Diagnosis is based on bacterial culture.

6.6.4.10 Enteric Giardiasis

Giardia muris infections are common in in weanling hamsters with and without diarrhea, suggesting that infections may be subclinical except in the face of stress or chronic diseas. *Giardia* organisms have also been identified in cases of chronic gastritis associated with *Helicobacter aurati* infection. Histologically, there are moderate lymphoplasmacytic lamina proprial infiltrates with flattening of duodenal enterocytes. Abundant 7–13 by 5–10 μm pear- to crescent-shaped flagellated binucleate trophozoites may be seen along the brush border of villi and within crypts and intervillus spaces (Figure 6.14). Diagnosis includes identification of the organisms in histologic sections or observation of characteristic tumbling movement

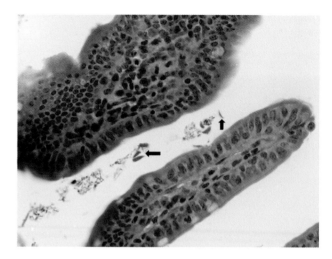

Figure 6.14 *Giardia muris* infections are common in hamsters and are seen in weanling animals with and without diarrhea, suggesting infections may be clinical or subclinical. Histologically, lymphoplasmacytic lamina proprial infiltrates are present with flattening of duodenal enterocytes. 7-13 μm x 5-10 μm pear- to crescent-shaped flagellated trophozoites (arrows) may be seen along the brush border of villi and within crypts and intervillus spaces.

on wet mount small intestinal preparations. ELISA or PCR can be used to confirm infection.

6.6.4.11 Cryptosporidiosis

Cryptosporidial infections often occur concurrently with bacterial disease in hamsters. *Cryptosporidia* spp. were initially considered to be host-specific; however, interspecies transmission studies have demonstrated this to be incorrect and cattle isolates of *Cryptosporidia* have been successfully transferred to many species of animals and birds, including hamsters. Because of this ability to transfer among a broad range of host species, *Cryptosporidia* have to be considered to be a potential human health hazard. Diagnosis is based on the identification of numerous small, round, 1 to 3 μm basophilic organisms within the microvilli of enterocytes in hematoxylin and eosin-stained histologic sections or by the identification of oocysts from feces using either saturated sugar or salt flotation solutions.

6.6.4.12 Spironucleosis

Spironucleus muris is a flagellated protozoan found deep within small intestinal crypts and is likely a normal commensal organism, although overgrowth may occur with intercurrent enteric disease. Trophozoites are torpedo-shaped and are approximately 9 by 3 μm without the flagella (Figure 6.15). Diagnosis is based on identification of trophozoites in intestinal crypts in hematoxylin and eosin, periodic acid Schiff (PAS), or Gomori's methenamine silver-stained sections or by the characteristic fast, forward linear movements of the protozoa on wet mount

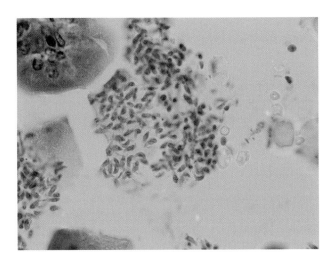

Figure 6.15 *Spironucleus muris* is a commensal flagellated protozoan normally found in small intestinal crypts of hamsters, although overgrowth may occur with intercurrent enteric disease. This hamster had been treated with a broad-spectrum antibiotic for suspected nephritis. Trophozoites are torpedo-shaped and are approximately 9 μm x 3 μm without the flagella.

small intestinal preparations. *S. muris* can be transmitted from hamsters to mice and the organism can cause clinical disease in young, immunosuppressed or inbred mice.

Other protozoa are commonly seen in sections of hamster colon, including *Tritrichomonas muris* and *Entamoeba muris*, and these are considered to be non-pathogenic.

6.6.4.13 Oxyuriasis

Hamsters can be infected with different types of pinworms including the hamster pinworm, *Syphacia mesocriceti*, as well as other murine pinworms, including *S. obvelata* and *S. muris*. Concomitant infections of golden hamsters with multiple pinworm species can occur, although none of these infestations poses a zoonotic risk for human handlers.

Pinworm infections are usually subclinical even with a high worm burden. Adults are 1–4 mm in length and are located in the lumen of the cecum and colon, closely associated with the mucosal surface, where they may induce mild catarrhal inflammation. Infestations can be diagnosed by identification of characteristic ova on fecal flotations or in histologic sections of large intestine, or from observation of eggs or larvae in impression smears made from cellophane tape applied to the hamster perianal region. Transmission occurs by ingestion of embryonated ova from feces, feed or water contaminated with feces, by ingestion of ova from the perianal skin or via retrograde migration of larval forms.

6.6.4.14 Cestodiasis

Two species of tapeworms infect hamsters, *Rodentolepis nana* and *Hymenolepis diminuta*. Infections are typically subclinical but when the worm burden is high, catarrhal

enteritis, weight loss, and death can result. *Rodentolepis nana* adults are small (20–30 mm long by 1 mm wide) and are found in the small intestine. Following ingestion of the ova-bearing proglottids, the oncospheres or hexacanth larvae (16–25 by 24–30 μm) within the eggs are released into the small intestine and penetrate the villi, forming cysticercoid larvae (16–25 by 24–30 μm) in the lamina propria. After 4–5 days, the cysticercoids leave the villi, evert their scolices and attach to the intestinal mucosa further down the small intestine and develop into adults. (See Section 7.6.4.7 in Chapter 7, for a fuller description of the life cycle of *R. nana*.)

Hymenolepis diminuta is found in the upper small intestine and is visible to the unaided eye (20–60 cm long by 0.4 mm wide). Heavy infestations of *H. diminuta* can lead to intestinal obstruction, impaction, intussusception, rectal prolapse, and death. Other signs of infestation include constipation, catarrhal enteritis, retarded growth, and emaciation. *H. diminuta* has an indirect life cycle and gravid proglottids are passed in the feces of the infected definitive host (rodents, including hamsters) and ova are ingested by an intermediate host (various arthropod adult or larval forms). Oncospheres are released from the eggs to develop into cysticercoid larvae in the host intestine, where they can persist. Following ingestion of the intermediate host, cysticeroid larvae are released, the scolices evert, and the parasite attaches to the mucosa, maturing to an adult. Diagnosis is primarily based on identifying the cestodes in the intestinal lumen at necropsy or by microscopic identification of adult or larval forms in tissue section (Figure 6.16). Adult cestodes are dorsoventrally flattened with calcareous corpuscles (mineralized concretions) embedded in the parenchyma and no body cavity. Proglottid segments containing both female and male reproductive organs and eggs are found caudal to the scolices. Because intact gravid proglottid segments are shed into the feces, fecal flotation for identification of ova is not reliable.

6.6.4.15 Intestinal Hyperplasia and Neoplasia

Cystadenomatous cecal polyps are infrequently associated with chronic proliferative colitis in adult hamsters. Intestinal adenomas are seen sporadically and appear as exophytic mucosal masses with a narrow connecting fibrovascular stalk. The thickened epithelium is arranged in folds with hyperplastic epithelial cells, increased basophilia and increased mucus production.

Intestinal adenocarcinoma was reported in a group of unthrifty weanling hamsters with diarrhea. Most had mild thickening of the jejunal mucosa and terminal ileum and a few hamsters also had similar lesions involving the colon. Histologically, the early lesions consisted of jejunal and ileal crypt hyperplasia progressing to carcinoma *in situ*. More extensive lesions were identified in the ileum close to the ileocecal orifice with large nodules of

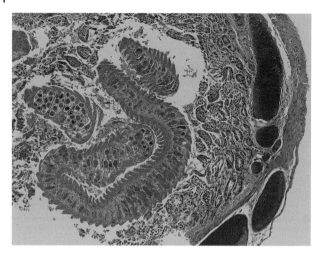

Figure 6.16 *Hymenolepis diminuta* is found in the upper small intestine and because of its large size, is visible to the unaided eye (20-60cm x 0.4mm). Heavy infestations of *H. diminuta* can lead to intestinal obstruction, impaction, intussusception, rectal prolapse, and death. Other signs of infestation include constipation, catarrhal enteritis, delayed growth, and emaciation. Histologic features of adult cestodes in the intestinal lumen include segmentation, dorsoventral flattening, parenchymatous body cavity, calcareous corpuscles (mineralized concretions) embedded in the parenchyma, and an anterior scolex.

proliferative neoplastic mucosa projecting into the lumen resulting in partial to complete luminal obstruction. Colonic adenocarcinomas were focal and invasive but with no involvement of regional lymph nodes. It is unknown whether these animals were co-infected with bacteria such as *Helicobacter* spp. or *L. intracellularis*, which might have contributed to pre-existing chronic inflammation.

Hamster polyomavirus (HaPV) (see Section 6.2.7.3, for more information about hamster polyoma virus) is a naturally occurring highly transmissible virus that causes multisystemic disease. The virus persists in the kidney and is shed in the urine, and possibly, feces. Infective virus-containing trichoepitheliomas develop in hamsters from enzootically infected colonies or when adult hamsters are infected with HaPV. When the virus is introduced into a naïve colony of hamsters, up to 80% of young hamsters will develop **multicentric lymphosarcoma** within a time span of 1 to 7 months. The lymphoid tumors do not contain infective HaPV virions, but do contain HaPV DNA. Once HaPV becomes enzootic within a colony the incidence of lymphosarcoma will decrease substantially. Clinical signs include lethargy, respiratory distress, nervous signs, reduced feed consumption, weight loss, patchy alopecia, and palpable abdominal masses. At necropsy, there is hepatosplenomegaly, enlargement of mesenteric lymph nodes, and various fibrinous visceral adhesions may be present. Histologically, dense aggregates of neoplastic lymphocytes with round to irregular vesicular nuclei and small to moderate amounts of cytoplasm infiltrate parenchymal organs and the intestines with marked effacement of normal architecture and development of large neoplastic lymphoid nodules with necrotic centres. Neoplastic involvement of other organs, including kidney and thymus, may occur. Diagnostic testing includes PCR using formalin-fixed, paraffin-embedded tissues to demonstrate HaPV DNA.

6.6.5 Conditions of the Liver and Gall Bladder

6.6.5.1 *Helicobacter*-Associated Hepatitis

Helicobacter bilis infections in hamsters may induce chronic hepatitis with fibrosis characterized by variable chronic periportal lymphohistiocytic- and neutrophil-rich infiltrates, with portal and perivenular fibrosis, bile ductile proliferation, and subsequent distortion of the lobular architecture with formation of hyperplastic or dyplastic hepatic nodules, foci of hepatic necrosis, vascular ectasia, and hemorrhage. It is difficult to positively identify organisms in tissue sections, even with Warthin-Starry staining and PCR identification is recommended. *H. bilis* may be zoonotic and has been identified in the bile and gallbladder from human cases of cholecystitis and in the bile from human cases of gallbladder and biliary tract neoplasia.

Chronic cholangiofibrosis with concurrent centrilobular pancreatitis has been reported in young Syrian hamsters infected with *Helicobacter cholecystus*. Histologic lesions of the liver are as described above. Mild pancreatic lesions range from mild periductular neutrophilic and lymphocytic aggregates to more extensive periductular inflammation with extension into pancreatic ducts and surrounding pancreatic tissue. *H. cholecystus* may enter the common bile duct from the intestinal tract and may play a role in the development of hepatic and pancreatic lesions either by initiating or intensifying the hepatic and pancreatic lesions. *Helicobacter* spp. may be identified by PCR from fecal samples or tissue.

6.6.5.2 Hepatic and Biliary Cysts

Hepatic and biliary cysts are a common incidental finding in older animals at postmortem. Polycystic disease is considered congenital in nature and thought to be caused by failure of intralobular and interlobular ducts to fuse or failure of redundant bile ducts to disappear. Clinical signs are rarely reported, although abdominal distension and dyspnea may occur if cysts are very numerous or large. At post-mortem, cysts are thin-walled, filled with clear colourless to amber fluid, and may be pedunculated or more deeply embedded in hepatic parenchyma (Figure 6.17). Cysts may be found on occasion in other organs, including epididymis, ovary, adrenal gland, seminal vesicles, renal pelvis, endometrium, pancreas, and esophagus. Males are more likely to have multiple cysts involving more than one

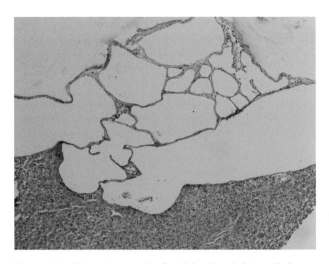

Figure 6.17 Photomicrograph of multiloculated, thin-walled, fluid-filled hepatobiliary cysts separated by slender bands of connective tissue lined by flattened epithelial cells.

tissue. Livers may be atrophied with variable amounts of fibrosis, fatty degeneration, lymphocytic aggregates, and biliary hyperplasia.

6.6.5.3 Hepatic Amyloidosis
Hepatic amyloidosis may be seen in aging hamsters. At necropsy, affected livers are swollen with an accentuated lobular pattern. Histologically, the eosinophilic, homogeneous proteinaceous material is initially deposited in and around portal areas and within vessel walls in the lobule centres and into the perisinusoidal Space of Disse, with subsequent atrophy of the hepatocellular cords.

6.6.5.4 Neoplasia of the Liver and Gall Bladder
Hepatic tumors are infrequently reported and include hepatocellular adenomas, carcinomas, cholangiomas, cholangiocarcinomas, hemangiosarcomas and hemangioendotheliomas. Adenomas of the gallbladder are rarely reported in hamster mortality surveys.

6.6.6 Conditions of the Exocrine Pancreas

6.6.6.1 Pancreatitis
Interstitial pancreatitis is one of the lesions seen with encephalomyocarditis (EMC) virus infection, to which hamsters are highly susceptible. When experimentally infected with EMC virus D (diabetogenic variant), infected animals developed marked weight loss, lethargy, and ruffled hair coats and males showed early elevated blood glucose levels. At necropsy, the pancreas has marked subcapsular and interlobular edema. Histologically, focal necrosis and neuronal loss has been reported in the hippocampal pyramidal layer and cerebellar granular layer. Myocardial lesions may include focal myocardial necrosis with mineralization and occasionally mild inflammatory

cell infiltrates. In the pancreas, there is often acute generalized necrosis of acinar cells with edema and moderate to marked mixed inflammatory cell infiltration progressing to fibroplasia and ductular hyperplasia. Small rodents are suspected to be carriers or reservoir hosts of EMCV and there is a potential risk of spread of EMC virus to other rodents, including hamsters, in large rodent distribution centers.

Centrilobular pancreatitis may be seen concurrently with cholangiofibrosis associated with *Helicobacter cholecystus* infection in young hamsters.

6.6.6.2 Pancreatic Neoplasia
Neoplasia of the exocrine pancreas is rare. Acinar adenomas are seen rarely and are composed of nodules of well-differentiated pancreatic acinar cells with supporting fibrous stroma. Ductular adenomas and papilloma of the common duct may be seen in combination with islet cell adenomas.

6.7 Cardiovascular Conditions

Anecdotally, cardiovascular disease is commonly reported in pet hamsters but the pathology is poorly documented such that the true prevalence of heart disease is unknown.

6.7.1 Congenital Abnormalities

Bicuspid aortic valves are a common finding in Syrian hamsters and may be associated with variations in coronary artery origin and morphology. The abnormal coronary arteries and aortic valves are not associated with disease unless ectopic coronary arteries originate at an acute angle such that blood flow is altered with resultant alterations to the coronary artery wall, including intimal thickening, inflammation, and disorganization of the elastic fibers of the tunica media.

An aortic coronary ostium is a rare anomaly in hamsters and can be located in the left or right aortic sinus or in the ventral aortic sinus of the biscuspid valve. This anomaly is usually not clinically significant. Cartilaginous foci may also be present sporadically within the interventricular septae and are thought to arise in response to mechanical stimulation.

6.7.2 Cardiomyopathy

Cardiomyopathy is common in Syrian hamsters with or without myodystrophy. The defect results from an autosomal recessive mutation in the δ-sarcoglycan gene found on chromosome 9 of hamsters. The disease presents with variable severity and progression and includes both hypertrophic and dilated forms.

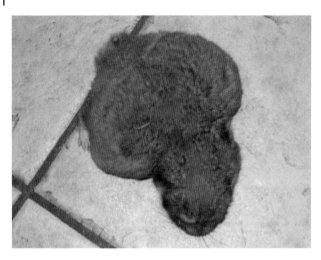

Figure 6.18 The abdomen of this hamster is severely distended with ascitic fluid. Differential diagnoses include cardiomyopathy, atrial thrombosis, chronic renal disease, and neoplasia. *Source: Courtesy of The Links Road Animal and Bird Clinic.*

6.7.2.1 Presenting Clinical Signs

Clinical signs include increased respiratory rate, cyanosis, reduced activity, anorexia, cold extremities, and ascites (Figure 6.18). Once clinical signs are observed, death is usually imminent.

6.7.2.2 Pathology

At necropsy, lesions include subcutaneous edema, hydrothorax, hydropericardium, and ascites. The heart is enlarged with biventricular dilatation or hypertrophy. The liver may also be enlarged and congested, while the spleen, lungs, and other organs may be congested. With cardiomyopathy, there are successive phases of focal vacuolation of myofibers or repeated myolysis followed by repair and proliferation of connective tissue and occasional mineralization. The heart responds with hypertrophy or dilation resulting in further dilatation, myofiber necrosis, and eventual cardiac failure.

6.7.2.3 Differential Diagnoses

Differential diagnoses include atrial thrombosis and chronic renal disease, including renal amyloidosis, nephrosclerosis, and glomerulonephrosis.

6.7.3 Atrial Thrombosis

Atrial thrombosis is seen commonly in aging hamsters with up to 45% prevalence in some colonies. Androgens are protective and administration of testosterone to neutered male and female hamsters markedly reduces the incidence of the condition.

6.7.3.1 Presenting Clinical Signs

Clinical signs are similar to those of cardiomyopathy and include tachypnea, tachycardia, cyanosis, generalized subcutaneous edema, hydrothorax, hydropericardium and ascites (Figure 6.19).

6.7.3.2 Pathology

The left atrium is involved most often and large firm thrombi are present, filling and distending the atrial lumen. Hearts may be enlarged with thickened valves, most frequently the mitral valve followed by the tricuspid and then aortic valves. Blood-tinged fluid may be present in the pleural and abdominal cavities. Histologically, atrial thrombi are laminated, and may be partially organized and undergoing incorporation into the underlying endocardium. Valvular lesions consist of deposits of mucinous ground substance with a mild increase in fibroelastic tissue. Myocardial degeneration may be a sequela, with nuclear hypertrophy, myofiber vacuolation and atrophy, loss of myofibers, and increased interstitial fibrous tissue. Focal coronary artery tunica media degeneration and calcification and plaque formation are also seen. Multifocal areas of hemorrhage and necrosis may be present in various organs.

It is thought that the atrial thrombosis arises from poor blood circulation secondary to myocardial dysfunction, with a terminal consumptive coagulopathy. In the hematologic profile of affected animals, there is a reduction in platelets, although the red and white blood cell values are within normal ranges. Factors II, VII, VIII, X, and plasminogen are reduced while fibrinogen-fibrin split products are increased, and prothrombin, thrombin, and partial thromboplastin times may be prolonged. Atrial thrombosis can develop secondary to renal amyloidosis as a consequence of urinary loss of the small molecular weight protein, antithrombin III.

6.7.3.3 Differential Diagnoses

Differential diagnoses include cardiomyopathy and chronic renal disease including renal amyloidosis, nephrosclerosis, and glomerulonephrosis.

6.7.4 Vasculopathy

Vascular calcification is seen in aging hamsters and involves the aorta, cardiac, renal, and gastric arteries. Typically, the arterial tunica media is involved but sometimes the lesion extends through the full thickness of the artery (Figure 6.20). Focal and mild hyaline arteriosclerosis of the spleen, testis, and glomeruli are occasionally identified in aged Chinese hamsters.

6.7.5 Myocarditis

Several infectious diseases may result in myocarditis in hamsters. Tyzzer's disease (see Section 6.6.4.6, for a more complete discussion), caused by infection with *Clostridium piliforme*, may result in multifocal myocardial necrosis and granulomas and intracellular bundles of bacilli are visible in the cardiomyofibers with a Warthin-

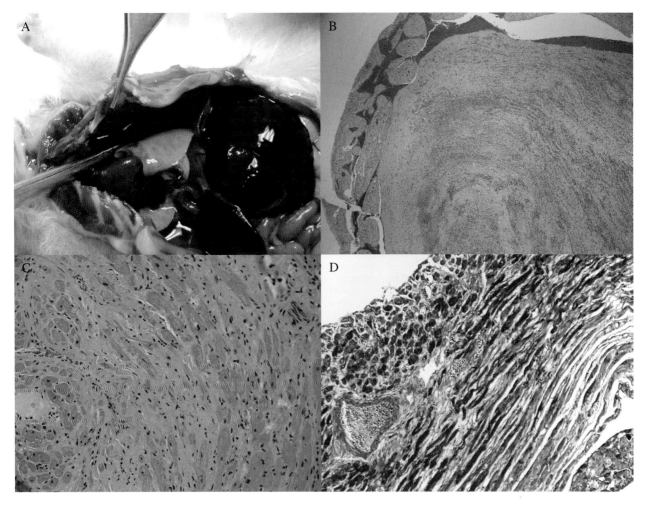

Figure 6.19 A: Gross findings with atrial thrombosis include hydrothorax and hydroperitoneum. The liver is enlarged and congested. B: The atrium contains a large lamellated thrombus. C. Myocardial degeneration may be seen as cardiomyofiber atrophy and loss with interstitial fibrosis. D: Myocardial atrophy with increased interstitial fibrous tissue, as demonstrated with a Masson's trichrome stain. *Source:* A: Courtesy of M. Ritter.

Starry stain. Salmonellosis due to *Salmonella* Enteritidis (see Section 6.6.4.4, for more details) may result in thrombophlebitis involving pulmonary veins and vessels, and suppurative pericarditis. Encephalomyocarditis virus infection (see Section 6.6.6.1, for more details) may induce small foci of myocardial necrosis with mineralization and occasionally mild inflammatory cell infiltrates.

6.7.6 Neoplasia

Primary neoplasia of the heart is not reported in hamsters, although metastatic lymphosarcoma is noted sporadically.

6.8 Genitourinary Conditions

Hamster kidneys are unipapillate and the papilla is long, extending well into each ureter. Urine has a high calcium carbonate content and is creamy white with a pH of 8.

6.8.1 Conditions of the Urinary Tract

Chronic renal disease and renal failure are common in aging hamsters. Clinical signs include reduced appetite or anorexia, poor body condition, ruffled fur, polyuria, polydipsia, ascites, hydrothorax, subcutaneous edema, and anasarca. Differential diagnoses include renal amyloidosis, nephrotic syndrome, arteriolar nephrosclerosis, and glomerulonephrosis.

6.8.1.1 Renal Amyloidosis
Amyloidosis is a common age-related condition of Syrian hamsters. There is a higher incidence, increased severity, and earlier onset of amyloidosis in females. In Syrian hamsters, the concentration of serum amyloid P (SAP), historically known as female protein, is under the control of acute phase inflammatory mediators (males) and sex steroids (females), such that female hamsters produce larger basal amounts of amyloid protein than do males, but males

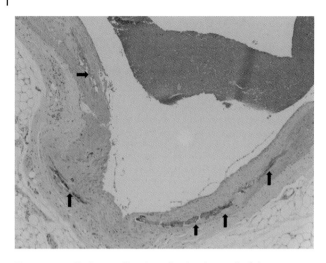

Figure 6.20 Tunica media mineralization (arrows) of the abdominal aorta was an incidental finding in a hamster with a highly vascularized uterine leiomyoma.

produce more SAP in response to chronic inflammation. Social stress induced by crowding increases the incidence of amyloidosis in both male and female Syrian hamsters.

Pathology At necropsy, kidneys are enlarged, irregular, and pale, with a granular capsular surface. Microscopically, eosinophilic, amorphous material is deposited in glomerular mesangial tufts and within basement membranes of tubules and glomeruli causing marked enlargement of glomeruli and alteration of normal architecture. Deposits may occur widely in other organs, including liver, adrenal glands, salivary glands, thyroid glands, parathyroid glands, spleen, meninges, trachea, lung, gall bladder, pancreas, urinary bladder, and rarely in the gastrointestinal tract.

Histologic confirmation of amyloidosis is with Congo red staining of affected renal tissues and identification of apple-green birefringence with polarized light or with thioflavine T labeling, which produces yellow-green fluorescent labeling when viewed under ultraviolet light.

Laboratory Diagnostics Chronic renal failure is the sequela to advanced renal amyloidosis. Any glomerular pathology, including glomerular amyloidosis, results in increased glomerular permeability with marked protein loss in the urine (proteinuria) and can progress to nephrotic syndrome, a clinical condition characterized by proteinuria, hypoalbuminemia, hypercholesterolemia, hyperlipemia, elevated creatinine and triglyceride levels, and generalized edema with anasarca, hydrothorax or ascites. The development of a hypercoaguable state secondary to the loss of low molecular weight proteins in the urine, such as antithrombin III, increases the risk for atrial thrombosis.

6.8.1.2 Chronic Progressive Glomerulopathy (Glomerulosclerosis)

There is lack of clarity regarding the etiopathogenesis of progressive renal disease in Syrian hamsters compared with what is known about progressive renal disease in other rodents. Non-amyloid glomerulonephropathy, without consistent arteriolar lesions, occurs sporadically in aging hamsters and the condition seems to develop more rapidly and is more severe in aging females. Glomerular abnormalities are present in young hamsters and progress with aging. At necropsy, kidneys are enlarged, pale white to tan, with an irregular granular appearance to the cortical surface (Figure 6.21).

In mildly affected kidneys, there is tubular atrophy and dilatation with luminal protein casts, and focal thickening of glomerular basement membranes and Bowman's capsules. In moderately affected kidneys, radiating linear- to wedge-shaped lesions extend from beneath the capsule to the medullary region and are characterized by atrophied and dilated tubules containing protein casts and thickened tubular basement membranes, as well as moderate interstitial fibrosis. There are segmental deposits of eosinophilic, PAS-positive and amyloid-negative protein within the glomerular capillary walls. In markedly affected kidneys, affected nephrons may have atrophied and dilated protein-filled tubules, interstitial fibrosis, and periarteriolar lymphoplasmacytic infiltrates.

6.8.1.3 Lymphocytic Choriomeningitis Virus (LCMV) Infection

Hamsters purchased from conventional sources are often carriers of LCMV, an arenavirus that infects a range of rodent species, as well as humans. Infections in hamsters are generally subclinical but viruria may persist for months, and renal lesions may develop over time. Following experimental subcutaneous inoculation, some hamsters develop interstitial nephritis with mild thickening of glomerular basement membranes and increased glomerular cellularity within four months. Renal vascular lesions, as described above, may also occur over time in some animals following exposure due to antigen-antibody complex deposition on glomerular basement membranes and arteriolar walls. Hamsters born to dams that were viremic during pregnancy are congenitally infected. LCMV infection has also been associated with pyometra and infertility in hamsters.

Infected animals can be detected using serologic techniques such as ELISA, indirect fluorescent antibody test and complement fixation. PCR testing and immunohistochemistry are useful for definitive diagnosis. Virus-contaminated urine from hamsters is a significant source of human infection and LCMV has been transmitted to human recipients following solid-organ transplants.

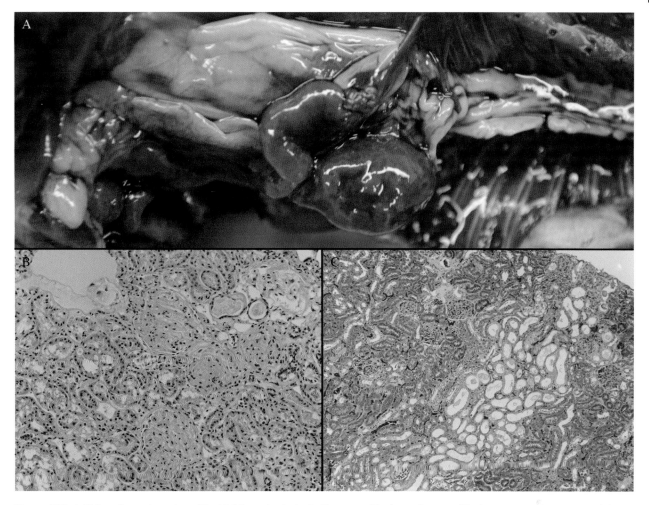

Figure 6.21 A: Kidney from a hamster with atrial thrombosis, hydrothorax, and hydroperitoneum. The lungs were edematous and the liver and spleen were enlarged and congested. Both kidneys had multiple, large, irregular depressions of the renal capsule. B: Microscopically, the kidney depicted in A contains enlarged renal glomeruli with generalized thickening of the mesangium, glomerular basement membranes, and Bowman's capsules. Tubules are dilated, lined by attenuated epithelium, and contain protein casts. Additional histochemical staining for amyloid (Congo red) was negative. C: Kidney from a hamster dying from non-renal related issues. Glomeruli are mildly enlarged with increased mesangial thickening, thickening of glomerular basement membranes, and periglomerular fibrosis. Segmentally, renal cortical tubules are dilated, lined by attenuated epithelium, and contain protein casts. Masson's trichrome.

6.8.1.4 Nephrocalcinosis

Nephrocalcinosis is seen sporadically in older animals with males affected almost twice as often as females. Lesions consist of focal mineralization of renal papillary tubular epithelium with accumulation of luminal mineral and dilatation of overlying tubules. The condition may extend to involve the inner medulla and cortex in more advanced cases.

6.8.1.5 Other Renal Conditions

Pyelitis and **pyelonephritis** occur sporadically in pet hamsters and are caused by various microorganisms, including *E. coli*, *Klebsiella* spp., and *S. aureus*. **Urolithiasis** is periodically seen in animals presenting with polyuria, polydipsia, dysuria, and hematuria.

Renal cortical cysts are infrequently identified and are part of generalized polycystic disease (see Section 6.6.5.2, for more details).

6.8.1.6 Renal Neoplasia

In colony mortality surveys, renal tumors are infrequently reported. Types of tumors noted include renal adenomas, which were multiple and most often cystic with a few demonstrating a tubular pattern. Nephroblastomas, embryonal tumors that develop from the renal blastema, were infrequent, only seen in females, and were invasive with renal vein thrombosis. Characteristic features of nephroblastomas include embryonal glomeruli and Bowman's spaces, vestigial tubules, and loose connective tissue stroma. Most tumors of the kidney represent metastases or local seeding, including adrenocortical carcinomas, various myelogenous tumors, multicentric lymphosarcoma (either spontaneous or associated with papovavirus infection), and melanomas. There is a single report of a clear cell renal carcinoma in the cranial pole of right kidney with metastasis to left kidney, liver, splenic hilus, peritoneal surface of diaphragm, and mesenteric and omental tissues. The tumor was poorly differentiated and composed of small cuboidal to spindle-shaped cells arranged in branching cords or interweaving clusters. Mitoses were numerous and intravascular tumor thrombi were frequent metastatic lesions. A unilateral renal adenocarcinoma was identified in a hamster reported to have died suddenly (Figure 6.22).

6.8.2 Conditions of the Female Genital Tract and Reproductive Problems

Hamsters are seasonal breeders with nonbreeding periods during the winter months. Female hamsters have a 4-day estrous cycle and following ovulation produce an abundant stringy white vaginal discharge with a distinctive odor that can be mistaken for pyometra. They have paired vaginal pouches that collect locally desquamated epithelial and inflammatory cells, decreasing the efficacy of vaginal cytology for estrus detection in this species. Females will not breed if sexually immature (<5 weeks of age), if older than 60 weeks of age or if overweight and hamsters that are older than 6–7 months of age at first breeding are more likely to be infertile. Some breeds of hamsters are more difficult to breed than others and have higher dietary protein requirements. Increased dietary protein during the breeding season may improve fertility in some colonies.

Pulmonary trophoblastic emboli are seen occasionally in pregnant hamsters and are considered an incidental finding. These cells can be greater than 400 μm in diameter with multiple nuclei. Hamsters have labyrinthine hemo-

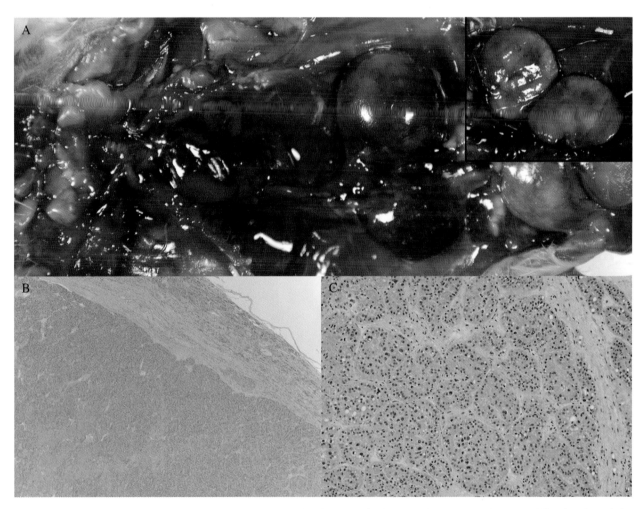

Figure 6.22 A: Unilaterally enlarged right kidney. Inset: Longitudinal section of enlarged kidney. The renal tissue is diffusely pale and the corticomedullary junction is blurred. B: Histologically, the renal adenocarcinoma is compressing the remaining atrophied renal parenchyma to the periphery. C: The adenocarcinoma is composed of disorganized solid and tubular structures lined by cuboidal to columnar epithelium with single vesicular nuclei displaying loss of polarity and marked anisokaryosis.

chorial placentation such that the maternal blood is in direct contact with the placental trophoblastic cells. Trophoblastic cells normally migrate beyond the blood vessels of the uterus into the mesometrial arteries where they induce vascular changes and remain until up to three weeks post partum.

Maternal infanticide and cannibalism are the most common causes of preweaning mortality and may account for over 95% of pup mortality. Factors such as cold temperatures, low maternal body weight, insufficient access to food and water, large litter sizes or litters with weak or sick pups, mastitis, handling of pups at an early age, an inadequate nest, and external noise can be risk factors. The dam and litter should be provided sufficient food and water and left undisturbed for at least one week following parturition to minimize cannibalism. Prenatal and perinatal pup mortality has been associated with maternal vitamin E deficiency. Increased postnatal mortality has been reported in hamster pups born to LCMV viremic mothers.

6.8.2.1 Cystic Ovaries

Cystic ovarian follicles can occur in older, intact female Syrian hamsters. Frequently, the condition is bilateral and the cysts may be very large. Clinical signs in affected animals include roughened hair coat, bilaterally symmetrical alopecia, distended abdomen, increased respiratory effort, reduced feed intake, and serosanguinous vaginal discharge. These are generally treated ante mortem by ovariohysterectomy. Ovarian bursal dilatations, cysts, and cystic rete ovarii are also reported in older intact female Syrian hamsters.

6.8.2.2 Pregnancy Toxemia

There are rare reports of pregnancy toxemia occurringin hamsters shipped just prior to parturition. The only clinical signs in hamsters that died were listlessness and roughened unkempt hair coats but the animals were otherwise in good body condition. Liver, kidneys, small intestine, and placenta were markedly congested and petechiated. Microscopically, there was marked renal congestion, and many glomerular capillaries contained fibrin thrombi, while proximal tubules were undergoing acute necrosis and some contained hyaline casts. There was marked necrosis of periportal hepatocytes and fibrinous thrombosis of portal vessels. Placentae were congested and numerous small vessels contained fibrin thrombi. The small intestinal lamina proprial vessels were also congested and contained fibrin thrombi. These lesions are similar to those described in guinea pigs with a circulatory form of pregnancy toxaemia and uteroplacental ischemia.

6.8.2.3 Other Uterine Conditions

Eimeria genitalia **sp.** *nova* has been noted incidentally in the vagina, uterus, and oviducts of hamsters. **Endometrial**

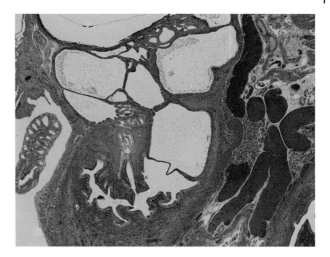

Figure 6.23 Cystic endometrial hyperplasia in a female mature hamster suffering from atrial thrombosis, hydrothorax, and hydroperitoneum. This was interpreted as an incidental finding.

cysts are seen sporadically and are considered to be part of the polycystic disease syndrome (see Hepatic Conditions: Polycystic Disease) (Figure 6.23). **Hydrometra** is seen with high frequency in some hamster colonies and may be heritable. **Pyometra** may be a sequela to respiratory infection with *Streptococcus* spp. or *Pasteurella pneumotropica*. LCMV infection has been associated with pyometra and infertility. **Ectopic pregnancies** are seen sporadically in hamster colonies and may have a familial basis.

6.8.2.4 Neoplasia

Vaginal bleeding is a common sign in hamsters with vaginal and uterine neoplasms (Figure 6.24). Uterine neoplasms include adenocarcinoma, leiomyomas, leiomyosarcomas, hemangioma, endometrial polyps, and metastatic mesothelioma. Leiomyosarcomas can be multiple and may metastasize to the lung. Cervical lymphosarcoma was noted in one hamster. A vaginal squamous papilloma has been described and characterized as an exophytic mass of keratinized vaginal epithelium. Foci of granular cells of unknown significance are reported often in the endometrium of aged Syrian hamsters.

In the ovaries, granulosa cell tumors, ovarian fibroma, and metastatic lymphosarcoma occur sporadically.

6.8.3 Conditions of the Male Genital Tract

Accessory sex glands in males include the ampullary gland, coagulating gland, prostate, and seminal vesicles. Secretions from these glands are not required to support the motility of sperm or the ability of the sperm to fertilize ova but are required for normal development of embryos.

Reduced fertility in males may be associated with aspermatogenesis, hypospermatogenesis, and testicular atrophy. Fibrinoid necrosis of testicular arteries is always

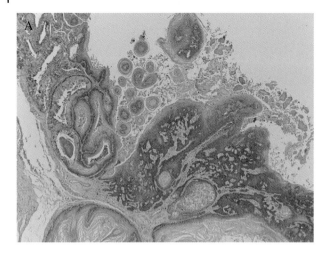
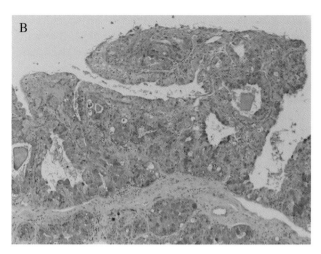

Figure 6.24 A: Hamster euthanized for generalized depression and vulvar bleeding. There was a mass in the vaginal wall and the vaginal lumen contained a blood clot. The exophytic vaginal mass is composed of papillary projections lined by squamous epithelium consistent with a vaginal squamous papilloma. B: This same hamster also had a 3 mm firm mass in the wall of the right uterine horn that was determined to be a uterine adenocarcinoma. The endometrium is thrown into folds by nests of neoplastic endometrial cells. Cells are also invading the myometrium.

associated with testicular atrophy. Congenital epididymal cysts are part of the polycystic disease syndrome reported in hamsters. Sperm granulomas are also reported in older hamsters and are characterized by necrotic centres with occasional mineralization and variable amounts of peripheral fibrosis and epididymitis.

Eimeria genitalia sp *nova* organisms have been identified in the epididymis and seminal vesicles of hamsters but the significance and prevalence are unknown.

Acute prostatitis is seen sporadically in aged males, with abundant macrophages and neutrophils filling the acinar lumena and attenuation of the lining epithelium. Prostatic calcification and cystic hypertrophy are also considered incidental age-related changes.

6.8.3.1 Neoplasia
Papillary cystic adenomas of bulbourethral glands have been reported infrequently in aged hamsters. There are otherwise very few cases of primary testicular tumors in hamsters. Generalized lymphosarcoma with secondary involvement of the testes has been reported.

6.9 Nervous System

6.9.1 Hydrocephalus

Hydrocephalus is a recessive trait and occurs sporadically in colonies of Syrian hamsters. Clinical signs are quite variable and less affected animals are able to breed and grow normally. Other pups may have domed skulls, lethargy, additional developmental abnormalities, such as motor deficits and delayed eye opening, and they may die

prior to weaning. The degree of hydrocephalus ranges from subtle to marked dilatations of the lateral ventricles with distortion or displacement of other cerebral structures. No infectious or toxic agents have been associated with the condition in hamsters and, in some cases, lesions may result from stenosis of the third ventricle.

6.9.2 Hereditary Cerebellar Atrophy

Hereditary cerebellar atrophy is an autosomal recessive trait and occurs sporadically in some hamster colonies. Homozygous offspring are smaller in size, can breed and care for offspring, and have a normal life span. Clinical signs become apparent around seven weeks of age and then slowly increase in severity to include moderate ataxia and a slight trembling of the head. Microscopically, a loss of Purkinje cells begins to occur at approximately 5 weeks of age and most Purkinje cells have disappeared by 18 months of age, with a 30% concurrent reduction in the density of the granular layer.

6.9.3 Spontaneous Hemorrhagic Necrosis (SHN) of Fetal Hamsters

In cases of spontaneous hemorrhagic necrosis, clinical signs include hemorrhage, visible grossly as a dark spot under the skull and sometimes in the posterior cranial fossa and as a line down the back in the region of the spinal cord, resulting in increased perinatal mortality. Affected offspring are born live but are quickly cannibalized by the dam. Microscopically, there is symmetrical subependymal vascular degeneration and hemorrhage, edema, and malacia of the parenchyma, which is most extensive in the forebrain and thalamus. The lesions increase in severity with increasing gestational age, and became progressively more widespread and severe in the more caudal regions with some involvement of the developing retina and inner ear. The spinal cord is affected last and damage is multifocal and random.

SHN has been reproduced in hamster pups by feeding the dams a diet low in vitamin E. Low-level dietary vitamin E supplementation reduced the incidence and severity of SHN and high levels of vitamin E supplementation eliminated the disease. There is variability in strain susceptibility to the disease, thus the best approach for disease prevention is to provide vitamin E supplementation during gestation and lactation, and to select strains of hamsters more resistant to disease. Vitamin E is very heat labile and so storage and length of feed retention are all important contributing factors.

6.9.4 Neoplasia of the Nervous System

Neoplasia of the nervous system is uncommon. Peripheral nerve sheath tumors, both benign and malignant, have been reported in aged animals. Malignant peripheral nerve sheath tumors may be identified by positive immunolabeling for S-100, vimentin, and neuron-specific enolase.

6.9.5 Other Conditions of the Nervous System

Excessive doses of dihydrostreptomycin and streptomycin may inhibit acetylcholine release in hamsters, causing a direct **neuromuscular blocking effect** with depression and ascending flaccid paralysis followed quickly by reduced respiration, coma, and death. The therapeutic safety margin for these antibiotics is low in hamsters and there are no specific histologic correlates because of the short clinical course of the toxicity.

Mineralization of the meninges and neuropil is considered to be an incidental postmortem finding, which may increase in frequency to affect approximately 50% of hamsters by 2 years of age. Foci of mineralization can be quite large, reaching a diameter of up to 500 μm. The etiology is undetermined and no correlation has been found with mineralization of other soft tissues. Increasing vacuolation of the neuropil is another age-related change of Syrian hamsters and the clinical significance is undetermined.

Heterotopic bone (Figure 6.25) is considered an incidental postmortem finding.

Lymphocytic choriomeningitis virus (LCMV; see Section 6.8.1.3, for more details) infection may induce mild nodular lymphoid infiltrates in the meninges in hamsters following inoculation of pups.

Experimental inoculation of hamsters with **encephalomyocarditis virus** (EMCV; see Section 6.6.6.1) resulted in marked weight loss, lethargy, and ruffled hair coat. Histologically, the hippocampal pyramidal layer

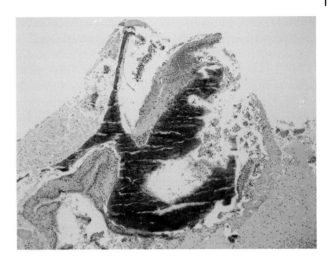

Figure 6.25 Heterotopic ossification in the cerebrum of an aged hamster, an incidental finding.

and cerebellar granular layer of the brain had focal necrosis and neuronal loss.

6.10 Hematopoietic and Lymphoid Conditions

Hamsters have neutrophils with ring-shaped lobulated nuclei and eosinophilic staining granules. The historical literature refers to these cells as heterophils but the cytoplasmic granules of these polymorphonuclear leukocytes contain the full complement of enzymes as per other mammals, suggesting that neutrophil is a more correct terminology.

6.10.1 Hematopoietic Conditions

6.10.1.1 Tularemia
Francisella tularensis is a Gram-negative, aerobic, pleomorphic, coccobacillary, facultative intracellular bacteria that multiplies within macrophages. Three subspecies are recognized and include the highly virulent *F. tularensis* spp. *tularensis* (Type A), the moderately virulent *F. tularensis* spp. *holarctica* (Type B), and *F. tularensis* spp. *Mediasiatica*, which is present in central Asia. *F. tularensis* has one of the largest host spectra of all bacteria, but principally causes disease in wild rodents and lagomorphs.

Syrian hamsters are an important source of infection for humans during outbreaks but are not considered a reservoir because they do not survive infection. Infection is direct and can occur by ingestion, inhalation, via bites or lacerations or introduced by blood-sucking arthropods, including mosquitoes, fleas, flies, and ticks. Tissues, blood, urine and feces of infected animals contain the organism. *F. tularensis* has been identified in hamsters dying shortly after arrival to pet stores and has also been transmitted to a child following a bite from an infected pet hamster that died shortly after purchase.

Presenting Clinical Signs In one outbreak of tularemia in 4- to 6-week-old hamsters in a closed hamster breeding colony the disease had a sudden onset, and within 48 hours, the hamsters were either moribund or found dead. The only clinical signs were reported 24 hours prior to death and included huddling and unkempt hair coats. The source of the infection was suspected to be fresh vegetables or bedding materials contaminated by urine or feces from infected wild rodents.

Pathology At necropsy, the lungs of affected hamsters demonstrated subpleural petechiation and ecchymoses. The liver, spleen, and lymph nodes were enlarged and the spleen was dotted with miliary white foci while the lymph nodes were mottled red and tan. Peyer's patches were enlarged and white. Microscopically, there was generalized necrosis of lymphoid tissue, and blood vessels and phagocytic cells contained numerous small Gram-negative bacteria.

Differential Diagnoses Differential diagnoses include salmonellosis, Tyzzer's disease, yersiniosis, pseudomoniasis, and other Gram-negative bacterial septicemias.

Laboratory Diagnostics Definitive diagnosis requires compatible gross and histologic lesions and a positive bacterial culture, but because this agent is a highly infectious zoonotic pathogen, culture should be carried out in level 2 or 3 biocontainment laboratory. *F. tularensis* grows slowly on most culture media and because of this slow growth, bacterial colonies can be overgrown by other faster proliferating organisms. Heart blood, liver, spleen, and bone marrow are the recommended tissues to culture. Organisms can be demonstrated in impression smears of the liver, spleen, bone marrow, kidney or lung or in histologic sections. Because of the zoonotic potential, post-mortem evaluations are recommended for pet hamsters dying unexpectedly. Human handlers should always wash their hands carefully after holding pet hamsters to minimize disease transmission.

6.10.2 Lymphoid Conditions

Splenic amyloidosis is common in aging hamsters with variable amyloid deposition, ranging from mild deposition in walls of the sinusoids to marked deposition with almost complete replacement of parenchyma.

Acute and chronic social subordination may suppress the humoral immune system in Syrian hamsters.

Cervical lymphadenopathy has been seen in one hamster colony and attributed to *S. aureus* infection.

Hamster polyomavirus (see Section 6.6.4.15) is a naturally occurring, highly transmissible virus that causes multisystemic disease, including lymphosarcoma, which is the most common neoplasm of hamsters. Typically, multiple lymph nodes are affected, in addition to the spleen. Spontaneous lymphosarcoma can occur but is considered rare.

Splenic hemangioma is rarely seen. Other tumors may metastasize to lymph nodes, including dermal melanoma and intestinal adenocarcinoma.

6.11 Ophthalmic Conditions

6.11.1 Conjunctivitis

Bacterial conjunctivitis in hamsters with or without associated rhinitis and pneumonia can be caused by various agents including *Streptococcus* spp., *Pasteurella* spp., *Klebsiella pneumoniae* and *Bordetella* spp. Animals may have oculonasal discharge, matting of hair on the forelegs, lethargy, hunched posture, a roughened hair coat, and be dull, depressed, and pyrexic. Affected animals can subsequently develop head tilt (otitis media) and ataxia. Abscesses can form in secondary sites, such as the uterus, in cases of *Pasteurella* spp. and *Streptococcus* spp. infections.

Keratitis and keratoconjunctivitis can occur secondary to irritation from exposure to drafts, cigarette smoke, dusty bedding or feed, aerosolized products such as furniture polish, hair products, perfume, excessive ammonia from urine-soaked bedding or an allergic reaction to bedding or feed. In cases of allergic conjunctivitis other clinical signs may be present, including generalized alopecia and sore feet.

Hamsters can develop entropion, which can result in corneal abrasion and secondary keratitis. This condition is likely hereditary so affected animals should not be used for breeding.

6.11.2 Conditions of the Globe and Lens

Facial or retrobulbar abscesses with swelling, exophthalmos, and secondary exposure keratitis may be a sequela to primary dental disease, including tooth root abscesses.

Ocular prolapse can be induced by excessive scruffing of the skin since the eyes have shallow orbits.

Buphthalmos has been reported in Djungarian hamsters. Hamsters had bilaterally enlarged eyes, poor vision, and dilated pupils with no light reflexes. Because of the small corneal surface, intraocular pressure could not be measured. On ophthalmic exam, the older hamsters had pale retinae and small optic nerves. Histologically, all affected eyes had uveal atrophy and reduced uveal pigmentation, and retinal atrophy with the most inner layer most severely affected. The etiology was not determined.

6.11.3   Ocular Neoplasia

Melanoma was identified in the right eyelid of a Syrian hamster and grew to be of sufficient size to compress the globe. At necropsy, the right submandibular lymph node was almost completely effaced by neoplastic melanocytes and multiple, subpleural pigmented nodules were present in the right diaphragmatic lung lobe. Intraocular melanoma was identified in a Chinese hamster with a week-long history of blepharospasm, mild ocular discharge, episcleral congestion, and hyphema. Following enucleation, a solid, sparsely pigmented melanoma was identified, composed of signet-ring cells infiltrating the iris, ciliary body, choroid, retina, and lens, obliterating the anterior and posterior chambers, and infiltrating the extraocular muscles.

6.11.4   Conditions of the Harderian Glands

Harderian gland inflammation can occur as a primary condition or subsequent to dental caries, periodontitis, and abscessation. Abscesses may extend into the brain or be disseminated to the lungs and kidneys.

Harderian gland tumors include adenomas, which display a papillary pattern composed of large cuboidal or columnar cells.

Bibliography

External Parasites

Beco, L., Petite, A., and Olivry, T. (2001) Comparison of subcutaneous ivermectin and oral moxidectin for the treatment of notoedric acariasis in hamsters. *Veterinary Record*, **149**(11), 324–327.

Fox, M.T., Baker, A.S., Farquhar, R., and Eve, E. (2004) First record of *Ornithonyssus bacoti* from a domestic pet in the United Kingdom. *Veterinary Record*, **154**(14), 437–438.

Harvey, C. (1995) Rabbit and rodent skin diseases. *Seminars in Avian and Exotic Pet Medicine*, **4**(4), 195–204.

Hoppmann, E. and Wilson Barron, H. (2007) Rodent dermatology. *Journal of Exotic Pet Medicine*, **16**(4), 238–255.

Meredith, A. (2010) Skin diseases of rodents. *In Practice*, **32**, 16–21.

Morrisey, J.K. (1996) Parasites of ferrets, rabbits, and rodents. *Seminars in Avian and Exotic Pet Medicine*, **2**, 106–114.

Owen, D. and Young, C. (1973) The occurrence of *Demodex aurati* and *Demodex criceti* in the Syrian hamster (*Mesocricetus auratus*) in the United Kingdom. *Veterinary Record*, **92**(11), 282–284.

Tani, K., Takeshi, I., Sonoda, K., Hayashiya, S., Hayashiya, M., and Taura, Y. (2001) Ivermectin treatment of demodicosis in 56 hamsters. *Journal of Veterinary Medical Science*, **63**(11), 1245–1247.

Welshman, M.D. (1973) Demodectic mange in hamsters. *Veterinary Record*, **92**(25), 684.

Subcutaneous Abscesses and Dermatitis

Endzweig, C.H., Strauss, E., Murphy, F., and Rao, B.K. (2001) A case of cutaneous *Mycobacterium chelonae abscessus* infection in a renal transplant patient. *Journal of Cutaneous Medical Surgery*, **5**(1), 28–32.

Eshar, D., Mayer, J., and Keating, J.H. (2010) Dermatitis in a Siberian hamster. *Laboratory Animals (NY)*, **39**(3), 71–73.

Grosset, C., Bellier, S., Lagrange, I., Moreau, S., Hedley, J., Hawkins, M., and Reyes-Gomez, E. (2014) Cutaneous botryomycosis in a Campbell's Russian dwarf hamster (*Phodopus campbelli*). *Journal of Exotic Pet Medicine*, **23**(4), 389–396.

Karbe, E. (1987) Disseminated mycobacteriosis in the golden hamster. *Journal of Veterinary Medicine*, **34**(5), 391–394.

Martorell, J., Gallifa, N., Fondevila, D., and Rabanal, R.M. (2006) Bacterial pseudomycetoma in dwarf hamster, *Phodopus sungorus*. *Veterinary Dermatology*, **17**, 449–452.

Pour, P., Althoff, J., Salmasi, S.Z., and Stepan, K. (1979) Spontaneous tumors and common diseases in three types of hamsters. *Journal of the National Cancer Institute*, **63**(3), 797–811.

Pour, P., Kmoch, N., Greiser, E., Mohr, U., Althoff, J., and Cardesa, A. (1976) Spontaneous tumors and common diseases in two colonies of Syrian hamsters. I. Incidence and sites. *Journal of the National Cancer Institute*, **56**(5), 931–935.

Wallace, R.J. Jr, Brown, B.A., and Onyi, G.O. (1992) Skin, soft tissue, and bone infections due to *Mycobacterium chelonae*: importance of prior corticosteroid therapy, frequency of disseminated infections, and resistance to oral antimicrobials other than clarithromycin. *Journal of Infectious Diseases*, **166**(2), 405–412.

Bacterial Otitis

Cooper, J.E. (1976) A survey of laboratory animal disease in Kenya. *Laboratory Animals (UK)*. **10**(1), 25–34.

Renshaw, H.W., Van Hoosier, G.L. Jr, and Amend, N.K. (1975) A survey of naturally occurring diseases of the Syrian hamster. *Laboratory Animals (UK)*. **9**(3), 179–191.

Dermatophytosis

Chitty, J., and Hendricks, A. (2007) Zoonotic skin disease in small animals. *In Practice*. **29**, 92–97.

Harkness, J.E., Turner, P.V., VandeWoude, S., and Wheler, C.L., (2010) *Harkness and Wagner's Biology and Medicine of Rabbits and Rodents*. 5th edn, Wiley-Blackwell. . Ames, IA, pp. 287–289.

Cutaneous Masses and Neoplasia

Beck, A.P., Compton, S.R., and Zeiss, C.J. (2014) Pathology in practice. HaPyV infection in a pet Syrian hamster. *Journal of the American Veterinary Medical Assoiation*, **244**(9), 1037–1039.

Foster, A.P., Brown, P.J., Jandrig, B., Grosch, A., Voronkova, T., Scherneck, S., and Ulrich, R. (2002) Polyomavirus infection in hamsters and trichoepitheliomas/cutaneous adnexal tumours. *Veterinary Record*, **151**(1), 13–17.

Greenacre, C.B. (2004) Spontaneous tumors of small mammals. *Veterinary Clinics of North America: Exotic Animal Practice*, **7**(3), 627–651.

Harvey, C. (1995) Rabbit and rodent skin diseases. *Seminars in Avian and Exotic Pet Medicine*, **4**(4), 195–204.

Harvey, R.G., Whitbread, T.J., Ferrer, L., and Cooper, J.E. (1992) Epidermotropic cutaneous T-cell lymphoma (mycosis fungoides) in Syrian hamsters (*Mesocricetus auratus*). A report of six cases and the demonstration of T-cell specificity. *Veterinary Dermatology*, **3**(1), 13–19.

Kondo, H., Onuma, M., Ito, H., Shibuya, H., and Sato, T. (2008) Spontaneous fibrosarcoma in a Djungarian hamster (*Phodopus sungorus*). *Comparative Medicine*, **58**(3), 294–296.

Kondo, H., Onuma, M., Shibuya, H., and Sato, T. (2008) Spontaneous tumors in domestic hamsters. *Veterinary Pathology*. **45**(5), 674–680.

Kondo, H., Onuma, M., Shibuya, H., and Sato, T. (2009) Morphological and immunohistochemical studies of spontaneous mammary tumors in Siberian hamsters (*Phodopus sungorus*). *Journal of Comparative Pathology*. **140**(2–3), 127–131.

Kondo, H., Takada, M., Shibuya, H., Shirai, W., Matsuo, K., and Sato, T. (2006) Cutaneous plasmacytoma in three golden hamsters (*Mesocrietus auratus*). *Journal of Veterinary Medicine, A Physiology and Pathology Clinical Medicine*, **53**(2), 74–76.

Madarme, H., Itoh, A., Hirose, M., and Ogihara, K. (2004) Spontaneous extraskeletal osteosarcomas of the subcutis in Djungarian hamsters (*Phodopus sungorus*), Report of two cases. *Journal of Veterinary Medicine*, **51**, 232–236.

Martorell, J., Martínez, and Soto, S. (2010) Complete ablation of vertical auditive conduct and ear pinna in a dwarf hamster (*Phodopus sungorus)* with an aural spontaneous squamous cell carcinoma. *Journal of Exotic Pet Medicine*, **19**(1), 96–100.

McKeon, G.P., Nagamine, C.M., Ruby, N.F., and Luong, R.H. (2011) Hematologic, serologic, and histologic profile of aged Siberian hamsters (*Phodopus sungorus*). *Journal of the American Association Laboratory Animal Science*, **50**(3), 308–316.

Meredith, A. (2010) Skin diseases of rodents. *In Practice*, **32**:16–21.

Pour, P., Althoff, J., Salmasi, S.Z., and Stepan, K. (1979) Spontaneous tumors and common diseases in three types of hamsters. *Journal of the National Cancer Institute*, **63**(3), 797–811.

Ridgway, R.L. (1977) Spontaneous myxoma in a pet hamster. *Veterinary Medicine Small Animal Clinics*, **72**(1), 75.

Saunders, G.K., and Scott, D.W. (1988) Cutaneous lymphoma resembling mycosis fungoides in the Syrian hamster (*Mesocricetus auratus*). *Laboratory Animal Science*, **38**(5), 616–617.

Urayama, F., Sato, T., Shibuya, H., Shirai, W., Matsutani, M., and Yamazaki, R. (2001) Apocrine adenocarcinoma in a golden hamster. *Journal of Veterinary Medical Science*, **63**(11), 1249–1252.

Adrenal Gland Conditions

Adamcak, A., Kaufman, A., and Quesenberry, K. (1998) Generalized alopecia in a Syrian (golden) hamster. *Laboratory Animals (NY)*. **27**(2), 19–20.

Bauck, L.B., Orr, J.P., and Lawrence, K.H. (1984) Hyperadrenocorticism in three teddy bear hamsters. *Canadian Veterinary Journal*, **25**(6), 247–250.

Deamond, S.F., Portnoy, L.G., Strandberg, J.D., and Bruce, S.A. (1990) Longevity and age-related pathology of LVG outbred golden Syrian hamsters (*Mesocricetus auratus*). *Experimental Gerontology*, **25**(5), 433–446.

Keeble, E. (2001) Endocrine diseases in small mammals. *In Practice*, **23**(10), 570–585.

Martinho, F. (2006) Suspected case of hyperadrenocorticism in a golden hamster (*Mesocricetus auratus*). *Veterinary Clinics of North Ameica: Exotic Animal Practice*, **9**(3), 717–721.

Newman, S.J., Bergman, P.J., Williams, B., Scase, T., and Craft, D. (2004) Characterization of spindle cell component of ferret (*Mustela putorius furo*) adrenal cortical neoplasms - correlation to clinical parameters and prognosis. *Veterinary Comparative Oncology*, **2**(3), 113–124.

Pour, P., Althoff, J., Salmasi, S.Z., and Stepan, K. (1979) Spontaneous tumors and common diseases in three types of hamsters. *Journal of the National Cancer Institute*, **63**(3), 797–811.

Schmidt, R.E., Eason, R.L., Hubbard, G.B., Young, J.T., and Eisenbrandt, D.L. (1983) *Pathology of Aging Syrian Hamsters*. CRC Press, Boca Raton, FL, pp. 141–175.

Thyroid Gland Conditions

Collins, B.R. (2008) Endocrine diseases of rodents. *Veterinary Clinics of North Ameica: Exotic Animal Practice*, **11**(1), 153–162.

Harkness, J.E., Turner, P.V., VandeWoude, S., and Wheler, C.L. (2010) *Harkness and Wagner's Biology and Medicine of Rabbits and Rodents*. 5th edn. Wiley-Blackwell. Ames, IA, pp. 220–228.

Keeble, E. (2001) Endocrine diseases in small mammals. *In Practice*, **23**(10), 570–585.

McInnes, E.F., Erhst, H., and Germain, P.G. (2013) Spontaneous nonneoplastic lesions in control Syrian hamsters in three 24-month long-term carcinogenicity studies. *Toxicologic Pathology*, **41**(1), 86–97.

Pour, P., Althoff, J., Salmasi, S.Z., and Stepan, K. (1979) Spontaneous tumors and common diseases in three types of hamsters. *Journal of the National Cancer Institute*, **63**(3), 797–811.

Sayers, I., and Smith, S. (2010) Mice, rats, hamsters and gerbils. In: *BSAVA Manual of Exotic Pets: A Foundation Manual (eds.* A. Meredith and C. Johnson-Delaney), BSAVA, Quedgeley.

Schmidt, R.E., Eason, R.L., Hubbard, G.B., Young, J.T., and Eisenbrandt, D.L. (1983) *Pathology of Aging Syrian Hamsters*. CRC Press, Boca Raton, FL, pp. 141–175.

Parathyroid Gland

Chen, H., Hayakawa, D., Emura, S., Ozawa, Y., Taguchi, H., Yano, R., and Shoumura, S. (2000) Occurrence of the parathyroid cyst in golden hamsters. *Annals of Anatomy*, **182**(6), 493–498.

Pour, P., Althoff, J., Salmasi, S.Z., and Stepan, K. (1979) Spontaneous tumors and common diseases in three types of hamsters. *Journal of the National Cancer Institute*, **63**(3), 797–811.

Schmidt, R.E., Eason, R.L., Hubbard, G.B., Young, J.T., and Eisenbrandt, D.L. (1983) *Pathology of Aging Syrian Hamsters*. CRC Press, Boca Raton, FL, pp. 141–175.

Conditions of the Pituitary Gland

Bauck, L.B., Orr, J.P., and Lawrence, K.H. (1984) Hyperadrenocorticism in three teddy bear hamsters. *Canadian Veterinary Journal*, **25**(6), 247–250.

Gerhauser, I., Wohlsein, P., Ernst, H., Germann, P.G., and Baumgärtner, W. (2013) Vacuolation and mineralisation as dominant age-related findings in hamster brains. *Experimental Toxicologic Pathology*, **65**(4), 375–381.

McInnes, E.F., Erhst, H., and Germain, P.G. (2013) Spontaneous nonneoplastic lesions in control Syrian hamsters in three 24-month long-term carcinogenicity studies. *Toxicologic Pathology*, **41**(1), 86–97.

Pour, P., Althoff, J., Salmasi, S.Z., and Stepan, K. (1979) Spontaneous tumors and common diseases in three types of hamsters. *Journal of the National Cancer Institute*, **63**(3), 797–811.

Schmidt, R.E., Eason, R.L., Hubbard, G.B., Young, J.T., and Eisenbrandt, D.L. (1983) *Pathology of Aging Syrian Hamsters*. CRC Press, Boca Raton, FL, pp. 141–175.

Conditions of the Endocrine Pancreas

Butler, L. (1967) The inheritance of diabetes in the Chinese hamster. *Diabetology*, **3**(2), 124–129.

Keeble, E. (2001) Endocrine diseases in small mammals. *In Practice*, **23**(10), 570–585.

Like, A.A., Gerritsen, G.C., Dulin, W.E., and Gaudreau, P. (1974) Studies in the diabetic Chinese hamster: light microscopy and autoradiography of pancreatic islets. *Diabetology*, **10** Suppl, 501–508.

Norimatsu, M., Doi, K., Itagaki, S., Honjo, K., and Mitsuoka, T. (1990) Glomerular lipidosis in a Syrian hamster of the APA strain. *Laboratory Animals (UK)*. **24**(1), 48–52.

Shigesato, M., Takeda, M., Hirasawa K., Itagaki, S., and Doi, K. (1995) Early development of encephalomyocarditis (EMC) virus-induced orchitis in Syrian hamsters. *Veterinary Pathology*, **32**(2), 184–186.

Shirai, T., Welsh, G.W., and Sims, E.A. (1974) Diabetes mellitus in the Chinese hamster. II. The evolution of renal glomerulopathy. *Diabetology*, **3**, 266–286.

Sugawara, Y., Hirasawa, K., Takeda, M., Han, J.S., and Doi, K. (1991) Acute infection of encephalomyocarditis (EMC) virus in Syrian hamsters. *Journal of Veterinary Medical Science*, **53**(3), 463–468.

Viral Pneumonias

Bauck, L. (1989) Ophthalmic conditions in pet rabbits and rodents. *Compendium of Continuing Education*, **11**(3), 258.

Benjamin, S.A., and Brooks, A.L. (1977) Spontaneous lesions in Chinese hamsters. *Veterinary Pathology*. **14**(5), 449–462.

Harkness, J.E., Turner, P.V., VandeWoude, S., and Wheler, C.L. (2010) *Harkness and Wagner's Biology and Medicine of Rabbits and Rodents*. 5th edn, Wiley-Blackwell Ames, pp. 220–228.

Renshaw, H.W., Van Hoosier, G.L. Jr, and Amend, N.K. (1975) A survey of naturally occurring diseases of the Syrian hamster. *Laboratory Animals (UK)*. **9**(3), 179–191.

Richardson, V.C.G. (2003) *Diseases of Small Domestic Rodents*. Blackwell, Oxford, pp. 133–175.

Sayers, I., and Smith, S. (2010) *BSAVA Manual of Exotic Pets: A Foundation Manual* (eds. A. Meredith and C. Johnson-Delaney). BSAVA, Quedgeley.

Schmidt, R.E., Eason, R.L., Hubbard, G.B., Young, J.T., and Eisenbrandt, D.L. (1983) *Pathology of Aging Syrian Hamsters*. CRC Press, Boca Raton, FL: pp: 21–45.

Pneumonia

Blandford, G., and Charlton, D. (1977) Studies of pulmonary and renal immunopathology after nonlethal primary sendai viral infection in normal and cyclophosphamide-treated hamsters. *American Review of Respiratory Diseases*, **115**(2), 305–314.

Brennan, P.C., Fritz, T.E., and Flynn, R.J. (1965) *Pasteurella pneumotropica*: cultural and biochemical characteristics, and its association with disease in laboratory animals. *Laboratory Animal Care.* **15**(5), 307–312.

Carthew, P., Sparrow, S., and Verstraete, A.P. (1978) Incidence of natural virus infections of laboratory animals 1976-1977. *Laboratory Animals (UK).* **12**(4), 245–246.

Castleman, W.L. (1983) Spontaneous pulmonary infections in animals affecting studies on comparative lung morphology and function. *American Review of Respiratory Diseases*, **128** (1–3), S83–S87.

Frisk, C.S. (1987) Bacterial and Mycotic Diseases. *Laboratory Hamsters* (eds. G.L. Van Hoosier and C.W. McPherson), Academic Press, Orlando, FL, pp. 112–134.

Gaertner, D.J., Boschert, K.R., and Schoeb, T.R. (1987) Muscle necrosis in Syrian hamsters resulting from intramuscular injections of ketamine and xylazine. *Laboratory Animal Science*, **37**(1), 80–83.

Nietfeld, J.C., Fickbohm, B.L., Rogers, D.G., Franklin, C.L., and Riley, L.K. (1999) Isolation of cilia-associated respiratory (CAR) bacillus from pigs and calves and experimental infection of gnotobiotic pigs and rodents. *Journal of Veterinary Diagnostic Investigation*, **11**(3), 252–258.

Parker, J.C., and Reynolds, R.K. (1968) Natural history of Sendai virus infection in mice. *American Journal of Epidemiology*, **88**(1), 112–125.

Percy, D.H., and Palmer, D.J. (1997) Pathogenesis of Sendai virus infection in the Syrian hamster. *Laboratory Animal Science*, **47**(2), 132–137.

Profeta, M.L., Lief, F.S., and Plotkin, S.A. (1969) Enzootic Sendai infection in laboratory hamsters. *American Journal of Epidemiology*, **89**(3), 316–324.

Renshaw, H.W., Van Hoosier, G.L. Jr, and Amend, N.K. (1975) A survey of naturally occurring diseases of the Syrian hamster. *Laboratory Animals (UK).* **9**(3), 179–191.

Tansey, G., Hoy, A.F., and Bivin, W.S. (1995) Acute pneumonia in a Syrian hamster: isolation of a *Corynebacterium* species. *Laboratory Animal Science*, **45**(4), 366–367.

Pulmonary Neoplasia

Mangkoewidjojo, S., and Kim, J.C.S. (1977) Malignant melanoma metastatic to the lung in a pet hamster. *Laboratory Animals (UK).* **11**(2), 125–127.

Schmidt, R.E., Eason, R.L., Hubbard, G.B., Young, J.T., and Eisenbrandt, D.L. (1983) *Pathology of Aging Syrian Hamsters*. CRC Press, Boca Raton, FL, pp. 21–45.

Neoplasia

Gaertner, D.J., Boschert, K.R., and Schoeb, T.R. (1987) Muscle necrosis in Syrian hamsters resulting from intramuscular injections of ketamine and xylazine. *Laboratory Animal Science*, **37**(1), 80–83.

Homburger, F. (1979) Myopathy of hamster dystrophy: history and morphologic aspects. *Annals of the New York Academy of Science*, **317**, 1–17.

Julkunen, P., Halmesmäki, E.P., Iivarinen, J., et al. (2010) Effects of growth and exercise on composition, structural maturation and appearance of osteoarthritis in articular cartilage of hamsters. *Journal of Anatomy*, **217**(3), 262–274.

Pour, P., Althoff, J., Salmasi, S.Z., and Stepan, K. (1979) Spontaneous tumors and common diseases in three types of hamsters. *Journal of the National Cancer Institute*, **63**(3), 797–811.

Renshaw, H.W., Van Hoosier, G.L. Jr, and Amend, N.K. (1975) A survey of naturally occurring diseases of the Syrian hamster. *Laboratory Animals (UK).* **9**(3), 179–191.

Schmidt, R.E., Eason, R.L., Hubbard, G.B., Young, J.T., and Eisenbrandt, D.L. (1983) *Pathology of Aging Syrian Hamsters*. CRC Press, Boca Raton, FL:. pp: 175–182.

Wijnands, M.V., and Woutersen, R.A. (1996) Polymyopathy in a Syrian golden hamster. *Laboratory Animals (UK).* **30**(1), 51–54.

Conditions of the Cheek Pouches and Oral Cavity

Besselsen, D.G., Gibson, S.V., Besch-Williford, C.L., et al. (1999) Natural and experimentally induced infection of Syrian hamsters with a newly recognized parvovirus. *Laboratory Animal Science*, **49**(3), 308–312.

Christie, R.D., Marcus, E.C., Wagner, A.M., and Besselsen, D.G. (2010) Experimental infection of mice with hamster parvovirus: evidence for interspecies transmission of mouse parvovirus 3. *Comparative Medicine*, **60**(2), 123–129.

Kondo, H., Onuma, M., Shibuya, H., and Sato, T. (2008) Spontaneous tumors in domestic hamsters. *Veterinary Pathology*, **45**(5), 674–680.

Lawrie, A.M., and Megahy, I.W. (1991) Tumours in Russian hamsters. *Veterinary Record*, **128**(17), 411–412.

Martorell, J., Fondevila, D., and Ramis, A. (2005) Spontaneous squamous cell carcinoma of the cheek pouch in two dwarf hamsters (*Phodopus sungorus*). *Veterinary Record*, **156**(20), 650–651.

Pour, P., Althoff, J., Salmasi, S.Z., and Stepan, K. (1979) Spontaneous tumors and common diseases in three types of hamsters. *Journal of the National Cancer Institute*, **63**(3), 797–811.

Pour, P., Kmoch, N., Greiser, E., Mohr, U., Althoff, J., and Cardesa, A. (1976) Spontaneous tumors and common diseases in two colonies of Syrian hamsters. I. Incidence and sites. *Journal of the National Cancer Institute*, **56**(5), 931–935.

West, W.L., Gaillard, E.T., and O'Connor, S.A. (2001) Fibroma (myxoma) molle in a hamster (*Mesocricetus auratus*). *Contemp Topics in Laboratory Animal Science*, **40**(6), 32–34.

Gastric Conditions

Lu, C., Zhang, L., Wang, R., et al. (2009) *Cryptosporidium* spp. in wild, laboratory and pet rodents in China: prevalence and molecular characterization. *Applied Environmental Microbiology*, **75**(24), 7692–7699.

Motzel, S.L., and Gibson, S.V. (1990) Tyzzer disease in hamsters and gerbils from a pet store supplier. *Journal of the American Veterinary Medical Association*, 19b7(9), 1176–1178.

Nambiar, P.R., Kirchain, S., and Fox, J.G. (2005) Gastritis-associated adenocarcinoma and intestinal metaplasia in a Syrian hamster naturally infected with *Helicobacter* species. *Veterinary Pathology*. **42**(3), 386–390.

Patterson, M.M., Schrenzel, M.D., Feng, Y., and Fox, J.G. (2000) Gastritis and intestinal metaplasia in Syrian hamsters infected with *Helicobacter aurati* and two other microaerobes. *Veterinary Pathology*, **37**(6), 589–596.

Pollock, W.B. (1975) Prolapse of invaginated colon through the anus in golden hamsters (*Mesocricetus auratus*). *Laboratory Animal Science*, **25**(3), 334–346.

Rainwater, K.A., Hawkins, M.G., Crabbs, T., and Malka, S. (2011) An anaplastic sarcoma of probable salivary origin in a Teddy-bear hamster (*Mesocricetus auratus*). *Journal of Exotic Pet Medicine*, **20**(2), 144–150.

Schmidt, R.E., Eason, R.L., Hubbard, G.B., Young, J.T., and Eisenbrandt, D.L. (1983) (eds.). *Pathology of Aging Syrian Hamsters*. CRC Press, Boca Raton, FL, pp 45–66.

Xiao, L. and Fayer, R. (2008) Molecular characterization of species and genotypes of *Cryptosporidium* and *Giardia* and assessment of zoonotic transmission. *International Journal of Parasitology*, **38**, 1239–1255.

Wagner, J.E. and Farrar, P.L. (1987) Husbandry and medicine of small rodents. *Veterinary Clinics of North America: Small Animal Practice*, **17**(5), 1061–1087.

Proliferative Enteritis

Fiskett, R.M. (2011) *Lawsonia intracellularis* infection in hamsters (*Mesocricetus auratus*). *Journal of Exotic Pet Medicine*, **20**(4), 277–283.

Jacoby, R.O. (1978) Transmissible ileal hyperplasia I. Histogenesis and immunohistochemistry. *American Journal of Pathology*. **91**, 433–451.

Jasni, S., McOrist, G., and Lawson, H.K. (1994) Experimentally induced proliferative enteritis in hamsters: an ultrastructural study. *Research in Veterinary Science*, **56**, 186–192.

Jasni, S., McOrist, G., and Lawson, H.K. (1994) Reproduction of proliferative enteritis in hamsters with a pure culture of porcine ileal symbiont intracellularis. *Veterinary Microbiology*, **41**:1–9.

Johnson, E.A. and Jacoby, R.O. (1978) Transmissible ileal hyperplasia II. Ultrastructure. *American Journal of Pathology*. **91**:451–468.

Vannucci, F.A., Pusterla, N., Mapes, S.M., and Gebhart, C. (2012) Evidence of host adaptation in *Lawsonia intracellularis* infections. *Veterinary Research*, **43**, 53.

Colibacillosis

Dillehay, D.L., Paul, K.S., Boosinger, T.R., and Fox, J.G. (1994) Enterocecocolitis associated with *Escherichia coli* and *Campylobacter*-like organisms in a hamster (*Mesocricetus auratus*) colony. *Laboratory Animal Science*, **44**(1), 12–16.

Frisk, C.S., Wagner, J.E., and Owens, D.R. (1978) Enteropathogenicity of *Escherichia coli* isolated from hamsters (*Mesocricetus auratus*) with hamster enteritis. *Infection and Immunity*, **20**(1), 319–320.

Frisk, C.S., Wagner, J.E., and Owens, D.R. (1981) Hamster (*Mesocricetus auratus*) enteritis caused by epithelial cell-invasive *Escherichia coli*. *Infection and Immunity*, **31**(3), 1232–1238.

Clostridial Enterotoxemia

Alworth, L., Simmons, J., Franklin, C., and Fish, R. (2009) Clostridial typhlitis associated with topical antibiotic therapy in a Syrian hamster. *Laboratory Animals (NY)*. **43**(3), 304–309.

Blankenship-Paris, T.L., Walton, B.J., Hayes, Y.O., and Chang, J. (1995) *Clostridium difficile* infection in hamsters fed an atherogenic diet. *Veterinary Pathology*. **32**(3), 269–273.

Hart, M., O'Connor, E., and Davis, M. (2010) Multiple peracute deaths in a colony of Syrian hamsters (*Mesocricetus auratus*). *Laboratory Animasl (NY)*. **39**(4), 99–102.

Hawkins, C.C., Buggy, B.P., Fekety, R., and Schaberg, D.R. (1984) Epidemiology of colitis induced by *Clostridium difficile* in hamsters: application of a bacteriophage and bacteriocin typing system. *Journal of Infectious Diseases*, **149**(5), 775–80.

Keel, M.K. and Songer, J.G. (2006) The comparative pathology of *Clostridium difficile*-associated disease. *Veterinary Pathology*, **43**(3), 225–240.

Kuehne, S.A., Cartman, S.T., Heap, J.T., Kelly, M.L., Cockayne, A., and Minton, N.P. (2010) The role of toxin A and toxin B in *Clostridium difficile* infection. *Nature.* **467**(7316), 711–3.

Lusk, R.H., Fekety, R., Silva, J., Browne, R.A., Ringler, D.H., and Abrams, G.D. (1978) Clindamycin-induced enterocolitis in hamsters. *Journal of Infectious Diseases*, **137**(4), 464–475.

Ryden, E.B., Lipman, N.S., Taylor, N.S., Rose, R., and Fox, J.G. (1991) *Clostridium difficile* typhlitis associated with cecal mucosal hyperplasia in Syrian hamsters. *Laboratory Animal Science.* **41**(6), 553–558.

Toshniwal, R., Silva, J. Jr, Fekety, R., and Kim, K.H. (1981) Studies on the epidemiology of colitis due to *Clostridium difficile* in hamsters. *Journal of Infect Diseases*, **143**(1), 51–54.

Wilson, K.H., Silva, J., and Fekety, F.R. (1981) Suppression of *Clostridium difficile* by normal hamster cecal flora and prevention of antibiotic-associated cecitis. *Infection and Immunity*, **34**(2), 626–628.

Tyzzer's Disease

Mahapatra, D., Fulton, H., Aboellail, T., Sprowls, R. and Naikare. H., (2007) *PCR evidence of co-infection of hamsters with Clostridium piliforme and enteropathogenic attaching and effacing E.coli.* Proceedings of the American Association Veterinary Laboratory Diagnostic Annual Conference, Reno, NV. Pg 168.

Motzel, S.L. and Gibson, S.V. (1990) Tyzzer disease in hamsters and gerbils from a pet store supplier. *Journal of the American Veterinary Medical Association*, **197**(9), 1176–1178.

Nakayama, M., Saegusa, J., Itoh, K., Kiuchi, Y., Tamura, T., Ueda, K., and Fujiwara, K. (1975) Transmissible enterocolitis in hamsters caused by Tyzzer's organism. *Japanese Journal of Experimental Medicine*, **45**(1), 33–41.

Takasaki, Y., Oghiso, Y., Sato, K., and Fujiwara, K. (1974) Tuzzer's disease in hamsters. *Japanese Journal of Experimental Medicine*, **44**(3), 267–270.

Zook, B.C., Huang, K., and Rhorer, R.G. (1977) Tyzzer's disease in Syrian hamsters. *Journal of the American Veterinary Medical Association*, **171**(9), 833–836.

Campylobacteriosis

Fox, J.G., Hering, A.M., Ackerman, J.I., and Taylor, N.S. (1983) The pet hamster as a potential reservoir of human campylobacteriosis. *Journal of Infectious Diseases*, **147**(4), 784.

Humphrey, C.D., Montag, D.M., and Pittman, F.E. (1985) Experimental infection of hamsters with *Campylobacter jejuni*. *Journal of Infectious Diseases*, **151**(3), 485–493.

Humphrey, C.D., Montag, D.M., and Pittman, F.E. (1986) Morphologic observations of experimental *Campylobacter jejuni* infection in the hamster intestinal tract. *American Journal of Pathology*. **122**(1), 152–159.

Lentsch, R.H., McLaughlin, R.M., Wagner, J.E., and Day, T.J. (1982) *Campylobacter fetus* subspecies *jejuni* isolated from Syrian hamsters with proliferative ileitis. *Laboratory Animal Science*, **32**(5), 511–514.

Other Enteric Conditions

Campos, A., Taylor, J.H., and Campbell, M. (2000) Hamster bite peritonitis: *Pasteurella pneumotropica* peritonitis in a dialysis patient. *Pediatric Nephrology*, **15**(1–2), 31–32.

Centers for Disease Control and Prevention. (2005) Outbreak of multidrug-resistant *Salmonella* typhimurium associated with rodents purchased at retail pet stores - United States, December 2003-October 2004. *Morbidity and Mortality Weekly Reports*,. **54**(17), 429–433.

Gadberry, J.L., Zipper, R., Tylor, J.A., and Wink, C. (1984) *Pasteurella pneumotropica* isolated from bone and joint infections. *Journal of Clinical Microbiology*, **19**(6), 926–927.

Gibson, S.V., Rottinghaus, A.A., Wagner, J.E., Srills, H.F. Jr, Stogsdill, P.L., and Kinden, D.A. (1990) Naturally acquired enteric adenovirus infection in Syrian hamsters (*Mesocricetus auratus*). *American Journal of Veterinary Research*, **51**(1), 143–147.

Innes, J.R., Wilson, C., and Ross, M.A. (1956) S*almonella enteritidis* infection causing septic pulmonary phlebothrombosis in hamsters. *Journal of Infectious Diseases*, **98**(2), 133–141.

Lesher, R.J., Jeszenka, E.V., and Swan, M.E. (1985) Enteritis caused by *Pasteurella pneumotropica* infection in hamsters. *Journal of Clinical Microbiology*, **22**(3), 448.

Martine, R., Martin, D., and Levy, C.S. (1988) Acinetobacter osteomyelitis from a hamster bite. *Pediatric Infectious Diseases*, **7**(5), 364–365.

Nambiar, P.R., Kirchain, S.M., Courmier, K., et al. (2006) Progressive proliferative and dysplastic typhlocolitis in aging Syrian hamsters naturally infected with *Helicobacter* spp.: a spontaneous model of inflammatory bowel disease. *Veterinary Pathology*, **43**(1), 2–14.

Intestinal Protozoa

Davis, A.J. and Jenkins, S.J. (1986) Cryptosporidiosis and proliferative ileitis in a hamster. *Veterinary Pathology*, **23**(5), 632–633.

Kunstýr, I. (1977) Infectious form of *Spironucleus* (*Hexamita*) *muris*: banded cysts. *Laboratory Animal (UK)*. **11**(3), 185–188.

O'Donoghue, P.J. (1985) *Cryptosporidium* infections in man, animals, birds and fish. *Australian Veterinary Journal*, **62**(8), 253–358.

Orr, J.P. (1988) *Cryptosporidium* infection associated with proliferative enteritis (wet tail) in Syrian hamsters. *Canadian Veterinary Journal*, **29**(10), 843–844.

Patterson, M.M., Schrenzel, M.D., Feng, Y., and Fox, J.G. (2000) Gastritis and intestinal metaplasia in Syrian hamsters infected with *Helicobacter aurati* and two other microaerobes. *Veterinary Pathology*. **37**(6), 589–596.

Rasmussen, K.R. and Healey, M.C. (1992) *Cryptosporidium parvum*: experimental infections in aged Syrian golden hamsters. *Journal of Infectious Diseases*, **165**(4), 769–772.

Schmidt, R.E. (1995) Protozoal diseases of rabbits and rodents. *Seminars in Avian and Exotic Pet Medicine*, **4**(3), 126–130.

Wilson Barron, H., Richley, L., Hernandex-Divers, S., and Ritchie, B. (2007) Etiology, pathology, and control of enterocolitis in a group of hamsters. *Proceedings of the Association of Exotic Mammal Veterinarians*, Providence, RI, pp. 123–126.

Intestinal Nematodes and Cestodes

Hasegawa, H., Sato, H., Iwakiri, E., Ikeda, Y., and Une, Y. (2008) Helminths collected from imported pet murids, with special reference to concomitant infection of the golden hamsters with three pinworm species of the genus *Syphacia* (Nematoda: oxyuridae). *Journal of Parasitology*, **94**(3), 752–754.

Macnish, M.G., Morgan, U.M., Behnke, J.M., and Thompson, R.C. (2002) Failure to infect laboratory rodent hosts with human isolates of *Rodentolepis* (*Hymenolepis*) *nana*. *Journal of Helminthology*, **76**(1), 37–43.

Intestinal Hyperplasia and Neoplasia

Beck, A.P., Compton, S.R., and Zeiss, C.J. (2014) Pathology in practice. HaPV infection in a pet Syrian hamster. *Journal of the American Veterinary Medical Associations*, **244** (9), 1037–1039.

Jonas, A.M., Tomita, Y., and Wyand, D.S. (1965) Enzootic intestinal adenocarcinoma in hamsters. *Journal of the American Veterinary Medical Associations*, **147**(10), 1102–1108.

Pour, P., Althoff, J., Salmasi, S.Z., and Stepan, K. (1979) Spontaneous tumors and common diseases in three types of hamsters. *Journal of the National Cancer Institute*, **63**(3), 797–811.

Scherneck, S., Ulrich, R., and Feunteun, J. (2001) The hamster polyomavirus - a brief review of recent knowledge. *Virus Genes*. **22**(1), 93–101.

Simmons, J.H., Riley, L.K., Franklin, C.L., and Besch-Williford, C.L. (2001) Hamster polyomavirus infection in a pet Syrian hamster (*Mesocricetus auratus*). *Veterinary Pathology*. **38**(4), 441–446.

Hepatic Conditions

Fox, J.G., Dewhirst, F.E., Shen, Z., et al. (1998) Hepatic *Helicobacter* species identified in bile and gallbladder tissue from Chileans with chronic cholecystitis. *Gastroenterology*, **114**(4), 755–763.

Fox, J.G., Shen, Z., Muthupalani, S., Rogers, A.R., Kirchain, S.M., and Dewhirst, F.E. (2009) Chronic hepatitis, hepatic dysplasia, fibrosis, and biliary hyperplasia in hamsters naturally infected with a novel Helicobacter classified in the *H. bilis* cluster. *Journal of Clinical Microbiology*, **47**(11), 3673–3681.

Franklin, C.L., Beckwith, C.S., Livingston, R.S., Riley, L.K., Gibson, S.V., Besch-Williford, C.L., and Hook, R.R. Jr. (1996) Isolation of a novel *Helicobacter* species, *Helicobacter cholecystus* sp. nov., from the gallbladders of Syrian hamsters with cholangiofibrosis and centrilobular pancreatitis. *Journal of Clinical Microbiology*, **34**(12), 2952–2958.

Gleiser, C.A., Van Hoosier, G.L., and Sheldon, W.G. (1970) A polycystic disease of hamsters in a closed colony. *Laboratory Animal Care*, **20**(5), 923–929.

Matsukura, N., Yokomuro, S., Yamada, S., Tajiri, T., Sundo, T., Hadama, T., Kamiya, S., Naito, Z., and Fox, J.G. (2002) Association between *Helicobacter bilis* in bile and biliary tract malignancies: *H. bilis* in bile from Japanese and Thai patients with benign and malignant diseases in the biliary tract. *Japanese Journal of Cancer Research*, **93**(7), 842–847.

McKeon, G.P., Nagamine, C.M., Ruby, N.F., and Luong, R.H. (2011) Hematologic, serologic, and histologic profile of aged Siberian hamsters (*Phodopus sungorus*). *Journal of the American Association Laboratory Animal Science*, **50**(3), 308–316.

Nambiar, P.R., Kirchain, S.M., Courmier, K., Xu, S., Taylor, N.S., Theve, E.J., Patterson, M.M., and Fox, J.G. (2006) Progressive proliferative and dysplastic typhlocolitis in aging Syrian hamsters naturally infected with *Helicobacter* spp.: a spontaneous model of inflammatory bowel disease. *Veterinary Pathology*, **43**(1), 2–14.

Pour, P., Althoff, J., Salmasi, S.Z., and Stepan, K. (1979) Spontaneous tumors and common diseases in three types of hamsters. *Journal of the National Cancer Institute*, **63**(3), 797–811.

Renshaw, H.W., Van Hoosier, G.L. Jr, and Amend, N.K. (1975) A survey of naturally occurring diseases of the Syrian hamster. *Laboratory Animals (UK)*, **9**(3), 179–191.

Schmidt, R.E., Eason, R.L., Hubbard, G.B., Young, J.T., and Eisenbrandt, D.L. (eds.). (1983) *Pathology of Aging Syrian Hamsters*. CRC Press, Boca Raton, FL, pp. 67–87.

Somvanshi, R., Iyer, P.K., Biswas, J.C., and Koul, G.L. (1987) Polycystic liver disease in golden hamsters. *Journal of Comparative Pathology*, **97**(5), 615–618.

Conditions of the Exocrine Pancreas

Doi, K. (2011) Experimental encephalomyocarditis virus infection in small laboratory rodents. *Journal of Comparative Pathology*, **144**, 25–40.

O'Leary, T.J., Costa, J., and Roth, J. (1982) Oncocytic nodules of the pancreas. *Laboratory Investigations*, **46**, 634.

Pour, P., Althoff, J., Salmasi, S.Z., and Stepan, K. (1979) Spontaneous tumors and common diseases in three types of hamsters. *Journal of the National Cancer Institute*, **63**(3), 797–811.

Schmidt, R.E., Eason, R.L., Hubbard, G.B., Young, J.T., and Eisenbrandt, D.L. (1983) *Pathology of Aging Syrian Hamsters*. CRC Press, Boca Raton, FL, pp. 67–87.

Shigesato, M., Takeda, M., Hirasawa, K., Itagaki, S., and Doi, K. (1995) Early development of encephalomyocarditis (EMC) virus-induced orchitis in Syrian hamsters. *Veterinary Pathology.* **32**(2), 184–186.

Sugawara, Y., Hirasawa, K., Takeda, M., Han, J.S., and Doi, K. (1991) Acute infection of encephalomyocarditis (EMC) virus in Syrian hamsters. *Journal of Veterinary Medical Science*, **53**(3), 463–468.

Pulmonary Conditions

Benjamin, S.A. and Brooks, A.L. (1977) Spontaneous lesions in Chinese hamsters. *Veterinary Pathology*, **14**(5), 449–462.

Doi, K., Yamamoto, T., Isegawa, N., Doi, C., and Mitsuoka, T. (1987) Age-related non-neoplastic lesions in the heart and kidneys of Syrian hamsters of the APA strain. *Laboratory Animal (UK)*, **21**(3), 241–248.

Durán, A.C., Fernández, B., Fernández, M.C., López-García, A., Arqué, J.M., and Sans-Coma, V. (2011) Ectopic origin of coronary arteries from the aorta in Syrian hamsters (*Mesocricetus auratus*). *Journal of Comparative Pathology*, **146**(2–3), 183–191.

Durán, A.C., Fernández-Gallego, T., Fernández, B., Fernández, M.C., Arqué, J.M., and Sans-Coma, V. (2005) Solitary coronary ostium in the aorta in Syrian hamsters. A morphological study of 130 cases. *Cardiovascular Pathology*, **14**(6), 303–311.

Durán, A.C., López, D., Guerrero, A., Mendoza, A., Arqué, J.M., and Sans-Coma, V. (2004) Formation of cartilaginous foci in the central fibrous body of the heart in Syrian hamsters (*Mesocricetus auratus*). *Journal of Anatomy*, **205**(3), 219–227.

Fernández, M.C., Durán, A.C., Real, R., López, D., Fernández, B., de Andrés, A.V., Arqué, J.M., Gallego, A., and Sans-Coma, V. (2000) Coronary artery anomalies and aortic valve morphology in the Syrian hamster. *Laboratory Animals (UK)*, **34**(2), 145–154.

Gertz, E.W. (1973) Cardiomyopathy. *American Journal of Pathology*, **70**(1), 151–154.

Goineau, S., Pape, D., Guillo, P., Ramée, M.P., and Bellissant, E. (2001) Hemodynamic and histomorphometric characteristics of dilated cardiomyopathy of Syrian hamsters (Bio TO-2 strain). *Canadian Journal of Physiology and Pharmacology*, **79**(4), 329–337.

Heatley, J.J. (2009) Cardiovascular anatomy, physiology, and disease of rodents and small exotic mammals. *Veterinary Clinics of North America: Exotic Animal Practice*, **12**(1), 99–113.

Innes, J.R., Wilson, C., and Ross, M.A. (1956) Epizootic *Salmonella enteritidis* infection causing septic pulmonary phlebothrombosis in hamsters. *Journal of Infectious Diseases*, **98**(2), 133–141.

López, D., Durán, A.C., Fernández, M.C., Guerrero, A., Arqué, J.M., and Sans-Coma, V. (2004) Formation of cartilage in aortic valves of Syrian hamsters. *Annals of Anatomy*, **186**(1), 75–82.

McMartin, D.N., and Dodds, W.J. (1982) Animal model of human disease: atrial thrombosis in aged Syrian hamsters. *American Journal of Pathology.* **107**(2), 277–279.

Motzel, S.L. and Gibson, S.V. (1990) Tyzzer disease in hamsters and gerbils from a pet store supplier. *Journal of the American Veterinary Medical Association*, **197**(9), 1176–1178.

Paterson, R.A., Layberry, R.A., and Nadkarni, B.B. (1972) Cardiac failure in the hamster: a biochemical and electron microscopic study. *Laboratory Investigations*, **26**(6), 755–766.

Pour, P., Althoff, J., Salmasi, S.Z., and Stepan, K. (1979) Spontaneous tumors and common diseases in three types of hamsters. *Journal of the National Cancer Institute*, **63**(3), 797–811.

Sakamoto, A., Ono, K., Abe, M., et al. (1997) Both hypertrophic and dilated cardiomyopathies are caused by mutation of the same gene, delta-sarcoglycan, in hamster: an animal model of disrupted dystrophin-associated glycoprotein complex. *Proceedings of the National Academy of Sciences*, **94**(25), 13873–13878.

Sans-Coma, V., Arqué, J.M., Durán, A.C., Cardo, M., and Fernández, B. (1991) Coronary artery anomalies and bicuspid aortic valves in the Syrian hamster. *Basic Research in Cardiology*, **86**(2), 148–153.

Schmidt, R.E. and Reavill, D.R. (2007) Cardiovascular disease in hamsters: review and retrospective study. *Journal of Exotic Pet Medicine*, **16**(1), 49–51.

Sichuk, G., Bettigole, R.E., Der, B.K., and Fortner, J.G. (1965) Influence of sex hormones on thrombosis of left atrium in Syrian (golden) hamsters. *American Journal of Physiology*, **208**, 465–470.

Sugawara, Y., Hirasawa, K., Takeda, M., Han, J.S., and Doi, K. (1991) Acute infection of encephalomyocarditis (EMC) virus in Syrian hamsters. *Journal of Veterinary Medical Science*, **53**(3), 463–468.

Wechsler, S.J. and Jones, J. (1984) Diagnostic IC exercise. *Laboratory Animal Science*, **34**(2), 137–139.

Zook, B.C., Huang, K., and Rhorer, R.G. (1977) Tyzzer's disease in Syrian hamsters. *Journal of the American Veterinary Medical Association*, **171**(9), 833–836.

Renal Amyloidosis

de Beer, M.C., de Beer, F.C., Beach, C.M., Gonnerman, W.A., Carreras, I., and Sipe, J.D. (1993) Syrian and Armenian hamsters differ in serum amyloid A gene expression. *Journal of Immunology*, **150**(12), 5361–5370.

Dowton, S.B., Woods, D.E., Mantzouranis, E.C., and Colten, H.R. (1985) Syrian hamster female protein: analysis of female protein primary structure and gene expression. *Science, 7*, **228**(4704), 1206–1208.

Gruys, E., Timmermans, H.J., and van Ederen, A.M. (1979) Deposition of amyloid in the liver of hamsters: an enzyme-histochemical and electron-microscopy study. *Laboratory Animals (UK)*, **13**(1), 1–9.

Llach, F. (1985) Hypercoagulability, renal vein thrombosis, and other thrombotic complications of nephrotic syndrome. *Kidney International*, **28**(3), 429–439.

Murphy, J.C., Fox, J.G., and Niemi, S.M. (1984) Nephrotic syndrome associated with renal amyloidosis in a colony of Syrian hamsters. *Journal of the American Veterinary Medical Association*, **185**(11), 1359–1362.

Oliveira, A.V., Roque-Barreira, M.C., Sartori, A., Campos-Neto, A., and Rossi, M.A. (1985) Mesangial proliferative glomerulonephritis associated with progressive amyloid deposition in hamsters experimentally infected with *Leishmania donovani. American Journal of Pathology*, **120**(2), 256–262.

Chronic Progressive Nephropathy (Glomerulosclerosis)

Doi, K., Yamamoto, T., Isegawa, N., Doi, C., and Mitsuoka, T. (1987) Age-related non-neoplastic lesions in the heart and kidneys of Syrian hamsters of the APA strain. *Laboratory Animals (UK)*, **21**(3), 241–248.

Fisher, P.G. (2006) Exotic mammal renal disease: causes and clinical presentation. *Veterinary Clinics of North America: Exotic Animal Practice*, **9**(1), 33–67.

Han, J-S., Norimatsu, M., Itagaki, S-I., and Doi, K. (1992) Early development of spontaneous glomerular lesion in Syrian hamsters of APA strain. *Journal of Veterinary Medical Science*, **54**(1), 149–151.

McInnes, E.F., Erhst, H., and Germain, P.G. (2013) Spontaneous nonneoplastic lesions in control Syrian hamsters in three 24-month long-term carcinogenicity studies. *Toxicologic Pathology*, **41**(1), 86–97. DOI:10.1177/0192623312448938

McKeon, G.P., Nagamine, C.M., Ruby, N.F., and Luong, R.H. (2011) Hematologic, serologic, and histologic profile of aged Siberian hamsters (*Phodopus sungorus*). *Journal of the American Association Laboratory Animal Science*, **50**(3), 308–316.

Schmidt, R.E., Eason, R.L., Hubbard, G.B., Young, J.T., and Eisenbrandt, D.L. (eds.). (1983) *Pathology of Aging Syrian Hamsters*. CRC Press, Boca Raton, FL, pp. 89–106.

Lymphocytic Choriomeningitis Virus (LCMV) Infection

Biggar, R.J., Woodall, J.P., Walter, P.D., and Haughie, G.E. (1975) Lymphocytic choriomeningitis outbreak associated with pet hamsters. Fifty-seven cases from New York State. *Journal of the American Medical Association*, **232**(5), 494–500.

Fischer, S.A., Graham, M.B., Kuehnert, M.J., et al. (2006) LCMV in Transplant Recipients Investigation Team. Transmission of lymphocytic choriomeningitis virus by organ transplantation. *New England Journal of Medicine*, **354**(21), 2235–2249.

Hotchin, J., Sikora, E., Kinch, W., Hinman, A., and Woodall, J. (1974) Lymphocytic choriomeningitis in a hamster colony causes infection of hospital personnel. *Science*, **185**(4157), 1173–1174.

Parker, J.C., Igel, H.J., Reynolds, R.K., Lewis, A.M. Jr, and Rowe, W.P. (1976) Lymphocytic choriomeningitis virus infection in fetal, newborn, and young adult Syrian hamsters (*Mesocricetus auratus*). *Infection and Immunity*, **13**(3), 967–981.

Skinner, H.H. and Knight, E.H. (1979) The potential role of Syrian hamsters and other small animals as reservoirs of lymphocytic choriomeningitis virus. *Journal of Small Animal Practice*, **20**(3), 145–161.

Thacker, W.L., Lewis, V.J., Shaddock, J.H., and Winkler, W.G. (1982) Infection of Syrian hamsters with lymphocytic choriomeningitis virus: comparison of detection methods. *American Journal of Veterinary Research*, **43**(8), 1500–1502.

Nephrocalcinosis

Pour, P., Althoff, J., Salmasi, S.Z., and Stepan, K. (1979) Spontaneous tumors and common diseases in three types of hamsters. *Journal of the National Cancer Institute*, **63**(3), 797–811.

Pour, P., Kmoch, N., Greiser, E., Mohr, U., Althoff, J., and Cardesa, A. (1976) Spontaneous tumors and common diseases in two colonies of Syrian hamsters. I. Incidence and sites. *Journal of the National Cancer Institute*, **56**(5), 931–935.

Schmidt, R.E., Eason, R.L., Hubbard, G.B., Young, J.T., and Eisenbrandt, D.L. (eds.). (1983) *Pathology of Aging Syrian Hamsters*. CRC Press, Boca Raton, FL, pp. 89–106.

Renal Neoplasia

Fisher, P.G. (2006) Exotic mammal renal disease: causes and clinical presentation. *Veterinary Clinics of North America: Exotic Animal Practice*, **9**(1), 33–67.

Kirkman, H. (1974) Autonomous derivatives of estrogen-induced renal carcinomas and spontaneous renal tumors in the Syrian hamster. *Cancer Research*, **34**(10), 2728–4274.

Pour, P., Althoff, J., Salmasi, S.Z., and Stepan, K. (1979) Spontaneous tumors and common diseases in three types of hamsters. *Journal of the National Cancer Institute*, **63**(3), 797–811.

Pour, P., Kmoch, N., Greiser, E., Mohr, U., Althoff, J., and Cardesa, A. (1976) Spontaneous tumors and common diseases in two colonies of Syrian hamsters. I. Incidence and sites. *Journal of the National Cancer Institute*, **56**(5), 931–935.

Rainwater, K.A., Hawkins, M.G., Crabbs, T., and Malka, S. (2011) An anaplastic sarcoma of probable salivary origin in a Teddy-bear hamster (*Mesocricetus auratus*). *Journal of Exotic Pet Medicine*, **20**(2), 144–150.

Conditions of the Female Genital Tract

Benjamin, S.A. and Brooks, A.L. (1977) Spontaneous lesions in Chinese hamsters. *Veterinary Pathology*, **14**(5), 449–462.

Buckley, P. and Caine, A. (1979) A high incidence of abdominal pregnancy in the Djungarian hamster (*Phodopus sungorus*). *Journal of Reproductive Fertility*, **56**(2), 679–682.

Burek, J.D., Goldberg, B., Hutchins, G., and Strandberg, J.D. (1979) The pregnant Syrian hamster as a model to study intravascular trophoblasts and associated maternal blood vessel changes. *Veterinary Pathology*, **16**(5), 553–566.

Gleiser, C.A., Van Hoosier, G.L., and Sheldon, W.G. (1970) A polycystic disease of hamsters in a closed colony. *Laboratory Animal Care*, **20**(5), 923–929.

Kamino, K., Tillman, T., Boschmann, E., and Mohr, U. (2001) Age-related incidence of spontaneous nonneoplastic lesions in a colony of Han:AURA hamsters. *Experimental Toxicologic Pathology*, **53**, 157–164.

Kondo, H., Kimoto, H., Shibuya, H., Shirai, W., Matsuo, K., and Sato, T. (2007) Spontaneous uterine leiomyosarcoma in a golden hamster (*Mesocrietus auratus*). *Journal of Veterinary Medicine, A Physiology and Pathology Clinical Medicine*, **54**(1), 27–9.

McInnes, E.F., Erhst, H., and Germain, P.G. (2013) Spontaneous nonneop2lastic lesions in control Syrian hamsters in three 24-month long-term carcinogenicity studies. *Toxicologic Pathology*, **41**(1), 86–97. DOI:10.1177/0192623312448938

Peters, L.J. (1982) Abdominal pregnancy in a golden hamster (*Mesocricetus auratus*). *Laboratory Animal Science*, **32**(4), 392–393.

Pour, P., Althoff, J., Salmasi, S.Z., and Stepan, K. (1979) Spontaneous tumors and common diseases in three types of hamsters. *Journal of the National Cancer Institute*, **63**(3), 797–811.

Richter, A.G., Lausen, N.C., and Lage, A.L. (1984) Pregnancy toxemia (eclampsia) in Syrian golden hamsters. *Journal of the American Veterinary Medical Association*, **185**(11), 1357–1358.

Schmidt, R.E., Eason, R.L., Hubbard, G.B., Young, J.T., and Eisenbrandt, D.L. (eds.). (1983) *Pathology of Aging Syrian Hamsters*. CRC Press, Boca Raton, FL, pp. 219–230.

Conditions of the Male Genital Tract

Gleiser, C.A., Van Hoosier, G.L., and Sheldon, W.G. (1970) A polycystic disease of hamsters in a closed colony. *Laboratory Animal Care*, **20**(5), 923–929.

Homburger, F. and Nixon, C.W. (1970) Cystic prostatic hypertrophy in 2 inbred lines of Syrian hamsters. *Proceedings of the Society of Experimental Biology and Medicine*, **134**(1), 284–286.

Pour, P., Althoff, J., Salmasi, S.Z., and Stepan, K. (1979) Spontaneous tumors and common diseases in three types of hamsters. *Journal of the National Cancer Institute*, **63**(3), 797–811.

Shigesato, M., Takeda, M., Hirasawa, K., Itagaki, S., and Doi, K. (1995) Early development of encephalomyocarditis (EMC) virus-induced orchitis in Syrian hamsters. *Veterinary Pathology*, **32**(2), 184–186.

Sugawara, Y., Hirasawa, K., Takeda, M., Han, J.S., and Doi, K. (1991) Acute infection of encephalomyocarditis (EMC) virus in Syrian hamsters. *Journal of Veterinary Medical Science*, **53**(3), 463–468.

Infertility and Perinatal Mortality

Chow, P.H. and O, W.S. (1989) Effects of male accessory sex glands on sperm transport, fertilization and embryonic loss in golden hamsters. *International Journal of Andrology*, **12**(2), 155–163.

Keeler, R.F. and Young, S. (1979) Role of vitamin E in the etiology of spontaneous hemorrhagic necrosis of the central nervous system of fetal hamsters. *Teratology*, **20**(1), 127–132.

Parker, J.C., Igel, H.J., Reynolds, R.K., Lewis, A.M. Jr, and Rowe, W.P. (1976) Lymphocytic choriomeningitis virus infection in fetal, newborn, and young adult Syrian hamsters (*Mesocricetus auratus*). *Infection and Immunity*, **13**(3), 967–981.

Renshaw, H.W., Van Hoosier, G.L. Jr, and Amend, N.K. (1975) A survey of naturally occurring diseases of the Syrian hamster. *Laboratory Animals (UK)*, **9**(3), 179–191.

Schneider, J.E. and Wade, G.N. (1989) Effects of maternal diet, body weight and body composition on infanticide in Syrian hamsters. *Physiology and Behavior*, **46**(5), 815–821.

Schneider, J.E. and Wade, G.N. (1991) Effects of ambient temperature and body fat content on maternal litter reduction in Syrian hamsters. *Physiology and Behavior*, **49**(1), 135–139.

Other Conditions of the Nervous System

Akita, K. and Arai, S. (2009) The ataxic Syrian hamster: an animal model homologous to the *PCD* mutant mouse? *Cerebellum*, **8**(3), 202–210.

Edwards, J.F., Gebhardt-Henrich, S., Fischer, K., Hauzenberger, A., Konar, M., and Steiger, A. (2006) Hereditary hydrocephalus in laboratory-reared golden hamsters (*Mesocricetus auratus*). *Veterinary Pathology*, **43**(4), 523–529.

Gerhauser, I., Wohlsein, P., Ernst, H., Germann, P.G., and Baumgärtner, W. (2013) Vacuolation and mineralisation as dominant age-related findings in hamster brains. *Experimental Toxicologic Pathology*, **65**(4), 375–381.

Keeler, R.F., and Young, S. (1978a) Hemorrhagic necrosis of the central nervous system of fetal hamsters: litter incidence and age-related pathological changes. *Teratology*, **17**(3), 293–301.

Keeler, R.F. and Young, S. (1978b) Multifactorial contributions to the etiology of spontaneous hemorrhagic necrosis of the central nervous system of fetal hamsters. *Teratology*, **17**(3), 285–291.

Keeler, R.F., Young, S., Spendlove, R.S., Douglas, D.R., and Stallknecht, G.F. (1975) Occurrence of spontaneous hemorrhagic necrosis of the central nervous system in fetal hamsters. *Teratology*, **11**(1), 21–30.

Keeler, R.F. and Young, S. (1979) Role of vitamin E in the etiology of spontaneous hemorrhagic necrosis of the central nervous system of fetal hamsters. *Teratology*, **20**(1), 127–132.

Margolis, G. and Kilham, L. (1976) Hemorrhagic necrosis of the central nervous system: a spontaneous disease of fetal hamsters. *Veterinary Pathology*, **13**(4), 250–263.

Parker, J.C., Igel, H.J., Reynolds, R.K., Lewis, A.M. Jr, and Rowe, W.P. (1976) Lymphocytic choriomeningitis virus infection in fetal, newborn, and young adult Syrian hamsters (*Mesocricetus auratus*). *Infection and Immunity*, **13**(3), 967–981.

Pour, P., Althoff, J., Salmasi, S.Z., and Stepan, K. (1979) Spontaneous tumors and common diseases in three types of hamsters. *Journal of the National Cancer Institute*, **63**(3), 797–811.

Shigesato, M., Takeda, M., Hirasawa, K., Itagaki, S., and Doi, K. (1995) Early development of encephalomyocarditis (EMC) virus-induced orchitis in Syrian hamsters. *Veterinary Pathology*, **32**(2), 184–186.

Sugawara, Y., Hirasawa, K., Takeda, M., Han, J.S., and Doi, K. (1991) Acute infection of encephalomyocarditis (EMC) virus in Syrian hamsters. *Journal of Veterinary Medical Science*, **53**(3), 463–468.

Schmidt, R.E., Eason, R.L., Hubbard, G.B., Young, J.T., and Eisenbrandt, D.L. (1983) *Pathology of Aging Syrian Hamsters*. CRC Press, Boca Raton, FL, 141–175.

Snyder, L.A., Linder, K.E., and Neel, J.A. (2007) Malignant peripheral nerve sheath tumor in a hamster. *Journal of the American Association of Laboratory Animal Science*, **46**(6), 55–57.

Wagner, J.E. and Farrar, P.L. (1987) Husbandry and medicine of small rodents. *Veterinary Clinics of North America: Small Animal Practice*, **17**(5), 1061–1087.

Wightman, S.R., Mann, P.C., and Wagner, J.E. (1980) Dihydrostreptomycin toxicity in the Mongolian gerbil, *Meriones unguiculatus*. *Laboratory Animal Science*, **30**(1), 71–75.

Yoon, C.H., and Slaney, J. (1972) Hydrocephalus: a new mutation in the Syrian golden hamster. *Journal of Heredity*, **63**(6), 344–346.

Lymphoid Conditions

Gyuranecz, M., Dénes, B., Dán, A., et al. (2010) Susceptibility of the common hamster (*Cricetus cricetus*) to *Francisella tularensis* and its effect on the epizootiology of tularemia in an area where both are endemic. *Journal of Wildlife Diseases*, **46**(4), 1316–1320.

Jasnow, A.M., Drazen, D.L., Huhman, K.L., Nelson, R.J., and Demas, G.E. (2001) Acute and chronic social defeat suppresses humoral immunity of male Syrian hamsters (*Mesocricetus auratus*). *Hormones and Behavior*, **40**(3), 428–433.

Pape, J., Gershman, K., Petersen, J., Ferguson, D.D., and Staples, J.E. (2005) Brief report: tularemia associated with a hamster bite. *Morbidity and Mortality Weekly Reports*, **53**, 1202–1203.

Pour, P., Althoff, J., Salmasi, S.Z., and Stepan, K. (1979) Spontaneous tumors and common diseases in three types of hamsters. *Journal of the National Cancer Institute*, **63**(3), 797–811.

Renshaw, H.W., Van Hoosier, G.L. Jr, and Amend, N.K. (1975) A survey of naturally occurring diseases of the Syrian hamster. *Laboratory Animals (UK)*. **9**(3), 179–191.

Ophthalmic System

Bauck, L. (1989) Ophthalmic conditions in pet rabbits and rodents. *Comparative Cont Education*, **11**(3), 258.

Ekesten, B. and Dubielzig, R.R. (1999) Spontaneous buphthalmos in the djungarian hamster (*Phodopus sungorus campbelli*). *Veterinary Ophthalmology*, **2**, 251–254.

Lima, L., Montiani-Ferreira, F., Sousa, R., and Langohr, I. (2011) Intraocular signet-ring melanoma in a hamster (*Cricetulus griseus*). *Veterinary Ophthalmology*, **14**(4), 1–6.

Mangkoewidjojo, S., and Kim, J.C.S. (1977) Malignant melanoma metastatic to the lung in a pet hamster. *Laboratory Animals*, **11**(2), 125–127.

Parker, J.C., Igel, H.J., Reynolds, R.K., Lewis, A.M. Jr, and Rowe, W.P. (1976) Lymphocytic choriomeningitis virus infection in fetal, newborn, and young adult Syrian hamsters (*Mesocricetus auratus*). *Infection and Immunity*, **13**(3), 967–981.

Pour, P., Althoff, J., Salmasi, S.Z., and Stepan, K. (1979) Spontaneous tumors and common diseases in three types of hamsters. *Journal of the National Cancer Institute*, **63**(3), 797–811.

Pour, P., Kmoch, N., Greiser, E., Mohr, U., Althoff, J., and Cardesa, A. (1976) Spontaneous tumors and common diseases in two colonies of Syrian hamsters. I. Incidence and sites. *Journal of the National Cancer Institute*, **56**(5), 931–935.

Renshaw, H.W., Van Hoosier, G.L. Jr, and Amend, N.K. (1975) A survey of naturally occurring diseases of the Syrian hamster. *Laboratory Animals (UK)*. **9**(3), 179–191.

7

Gerbils

7.1 Introduction

Gerbils belong to the family *Muridae* and the subfamily *Gerbillinae* and there are numerous genera and species. The most common species seen in clinical practice is the Mongolian gerbil *(Meriones unguiculatus)*, also known as the clawed jird, jird, sand rat, desert rat or antelope rat. Other species that may be seen in pet practice are the Libyan gerbil (*M. libycus*), the fat-tailed gerbil (*Pachyuromys duprasi*), and Shaw's jird (*M. shawii*). Species and even sub-strains of species may respond differently to drugs and exhibit different behaviors and resistance to disease and stress so broad generalizations should be made cautiously. Most of the information in the literature and in this chapter relates to Mongolian gerbils unless otherwise specified.

Gerbils are gentle, curious animals that live well as monogamous lifelong pairs or as trios (one male with two females), if raised as cage mates. They live naturally in hot, arid, desert-like conditions, and will dig, climb, hop, and burrow if provided with an appropriate environment. Like other rodents, gerbils have constantly growing incisors and are avid chewers. Their lifespan averages 3–4 years and they are crepuscular.

In stark contrast to other rodent species and despite their lengthy popularity as a children's pet, there is a relative paucity of information about naturally occurring diseases and conditions of pet gerbils.

7.2 Integument Conditions

In the wild, gerbils burrow, which affords protection from the heat at ground level. Relative humidity levels that exceed 50% or lack of access to a sand bath may result in greasy, unkempt hair coats. Harderian gland secretions are normally mixed with saliva and applied widely to the face and the fur. This behavior, which enhances the gerbil's ability to withstand cold and wet conditions, may be an evolutionary trait contributing to the survival of gerbils in the cold desert conditions of Mongolia and Northeast China. Gerbils also can accelerate evaporative heat loss by applying saliva to their fur.

Both sexes of gerbils have a marking gland on the mid-ventral abdomen, which is defined by a well-demarcated orange-tan area of alopecia (Figure 7.1). The gland is sebaceous and as males reach sexual maturity, the gland enlarges and has an oily secretion, which is used for territorial marking. Hyperplasia of the marking gland is infrequently reported.

7.2.1 Alopecia

Patchy hair loss is associated with multiple conditions, including mechanical abrasion from the cage, feeder, or furnishings or from vigorous burrowing. Hair chewing or barbering may be seen periodically and may indicate an inappropriate social environment or boredom. Marking glands on the ventral abdomen are sparsely covered with coarser hair and can be mistaken for areas of alopecia. Excessive estrogen or corticosterone plasma levels occurring secondary to ovarian cysts or hyperadrenocorticism, respectively, can result in bilaterally symmetrical alopecia.

7.2.2 Bacterial Dermatitis

Acute bacterial dermatitis in weanling gerbils is often associated with a beta-hemolytic *Staphylococcus aureus* infection. Infections may be enzootic within colonies, with up to 75% of animals subclinically infected. Outbreaks of dermatitis may occur following a significant stressor, such as transportation or other factors, such as suboptimal housing, mixing of unfamiliar animals, and fighting. Adverse environmental conditions, such as high ambient temperatures and relative humidity, may exacerbate the condition.

7.2.2.1 Presenting Clinical Signs
Affected animals may initially present with perinasal hyperemia leading to local alopecia and moist dermati-

Pathology of Small Mammal Pets, First Edition. Patricia V. Turner, Marina L. Brash and Dale A. Smith.
© 2018 John Wiley & Sons, Inc. Published 2018 by John Wiley & Sons, Inc.

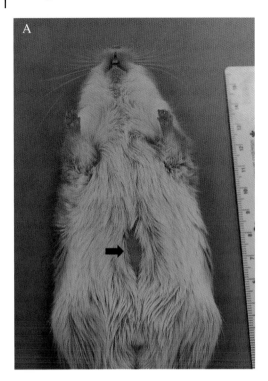

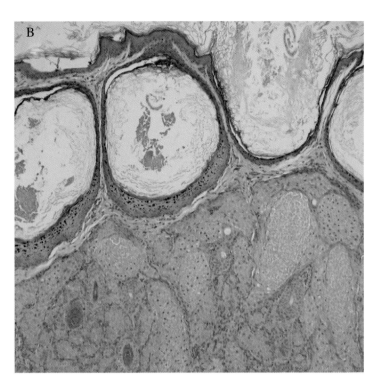

Figure 7.1 A: Normal gross appearance of a ventral abdominal marking gland (arrow). B: Normal histologic appearance of ventral abdominal marking gland. The gland is sebaceous and is composed of multiple lobules of acinar cells with abundant finely granular eosinophilic cytoplasm bearing characteristic large eosinophilic droplets.

tis. This inflammatory process may quickly progress to involve the feet, limbs, ventral and caudal abdomen, and tail (Figure 7.2). Some animals with chronic dermatitis will became stunted, emaciated, and eventually die.

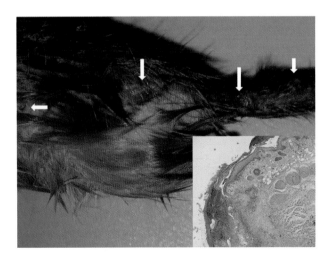

Figure 7.2 Skin punctures and lacerations of the lateral abdominal body wall, flank and tail (arrows) of gerbil following mixing of animals and associated aggression. Inset: Ulcerative, necrotizing, suppurative deep dermatitis and cellulitis of the tail. A mixture of *Staphylococcus* spp., including *S. xylosus*, *Streptococcus* spp., and *Proteus* spp. were isolated from the subcutaneous tissues.

7.2.2.2   Pathology
The skin is thickened, roughened, erythematous, and alopecic with brownish-yellow superficial exudation. Microscopically, lesions include acanthosis, hyperkeratosis, epidermal ulceration, suppurative dermatitis with epidermal microabscessation, dermal and follicular neutrophilic infiltration, and less frequently, suppurative panniculitis.

7.2.2.3   Differential Diagnoses
Nasal dermatitis (see below) and mechanical trauma should be considered.

7.2.2.4   Colony Management
The risk for introduction and spread of various pathogens is increased when pet stock from multiple sources are mixed in large distribution centers.

7.2.3   Dermatophytosis

Clinical dermatophytosis is rare in gerbils. Locally extensive, mildly pruritic areas of focal loss of hair or broken hair shafts and hyperkeratosis affecting the ears, head, back, and legs may be associated with *Trichophyton mentagrophytes* or *Microsporum gypseum* infections. Skin scrapings can be cultured using special fungal culture media and examined microscopically following KOH digestion for presence of hyphae and arthrospores.

Contaminated bedding, fomites from dust baths, and carrier animals are potential sources of infection. Infectious spores can also be transmitted between animals by caregivers. If animals are suspected or known to have dermatophytosis, the handler should wear gloves, as the condition is zoonotic.

7.2.4 Acariasis

Demodecosis in gerbils is caused by *Demodex meroni*. Clinical signs associated with infestation include a dry, unkempt haircoat with alopecia, focal ulcerative dermatitis with serocellular crusting, hyperkeratosis, and hyperemia. Histologic lesions include hyperkeratosis and focal epidermal ulceration. As in hamsters, clinical infection is seen in gerbils that are aged, immunocompromised, have poor nutrition or that are affected with chronic disease. Mites can be demonstrated in deep skin scrapings or tissue sections.

A forage mite, *Acarus farris*, frequently found in animal feed and bedding material, and reported to cause pruritic dermatitis in people, has also been associated with alopecia, hyperkeratosis, and skin erosions of the tail of gerbils. Immature mites (hypopi) have been seen on hair pluck samples. Hypersensitivity to the mite or its secretions could not be ruled out. Differential diagnoses include dermatophytosis and bacterial dermatitides.

Asymptomatic gerbils infested with avian mites, including *Ornithonyssus sylvarium* (northern fowl mite) and *Dermanyssus gallinae* (chicken mite) have been linked with human cases of avian mite-induced dermatitis.

Tropical rat mite (*Ornithonyssus bacoti*) infestations have been identified on Mongolian gerbils. The mites are considered to have a broad host range, including humans, with heavy infestations on gerbils resulting in agitation, pruritus, skin lesions, debilitation, and anemia.

7.2.5 Cutaneous Masses and Neoplasia

7.2.5.1 Ventral Marking Gland Tumors
Cutaneous neoplasms are moderately common in aging Mongolian gerbils of both sexes. Ventral sebaceous marking gland tumors are the most common neoplasms of the integument and occur more often in males. These may present as an adenoma, epithelioma, adenocarcinoma or squamous cell carcinoma (Figure 7.3). The latter neoplasm tends to be well-differentiated, locally invasive, and can metastasize to lung and regional lymph node. Ventral marking gland tumors can become ulcerated (Figure 7.4), secondarily infected, and may be subject to self trauma. Squamous papillomas of the skin with involvement and keratinization of the underlying sebaceous gland have also been seen.

7.2.5.2 Aural Cholesteatoma
Mongolian gerbils over two years of age may spontaneously develop aural cholesteatomas, an otherwise uncommon tumor in domestic animals. In the early stages of tumor development, there is accumulation of keratinized debris on the external surface of the tympanic membrane. Young gerbils tend to have minimal keratinization of the outer tympanic membrane surface but keratin accumulation increases with age. Keratinization and inflammation increase, resulting in displacement of tympanic membrane into the middle ear. The tympanic membrane becomes further displaced and contacts the temporal bone, resulting in resorption of bone and impingement on structures of the inner ear and associated nerves. Cholesteatomas are destructive and can also cause resorption of bone around the external auditory canal, with eventual intracranial extension. Animals present typically with a mass protruding from the external ear. Depending on the degree of invasiveness, a head tilt and dysphagia may be observed.

Microscopically, a cholesteatoma is composed of a keratin-containing cyst that is lined by keratinizing squamous epithelium. There may be variable amounts of mixed inflammatory cell infiltrates, cholesterol clefts, and abundant mixed bacterial populations, including *Pseudomonas* spp.

Sebaceous gland adenoma, squamous cell carcinoma and otitis media are potential differential diagnoses but the latter condition is not common in Mongolian gerbils. The Libyan gerbil (*M. libycus*) is reported to have a high incidence of otitis media.

7.2.5.3 Other Neoplasms
The following neoplasms are found:

Cutaneous melanotic and amelanotic melanomas are seen sporadically in gerbils. Masses may involve the pinna, foot, and perianal area.

A rapidly enlarging mass on the right mandible of an aged male Mongolian gerbil that was closely attached to the nearby skin and muscle was determined to be a primary cutaneous B cell lymphosarcoma using immunohistochemistry and flow cytometry.

Cytologic, histologic, immunohistochemical and electron microscopic features contributed to the identification of a poorly differentiated subcutaneous carcinoma in the axilla of a 3-year-old female gerbil.

Mammary adenocarcinoma and fibrosarcoma are rarely reported.

7.2.6 Other Integument Conditions

7.2.6.1 Degloving Injuries
Degloving injuries of the tail ("tail slip") can occur if gerbils are not restrained correctly and they are held by the distal third of the tail. The entire skin layer breaks away

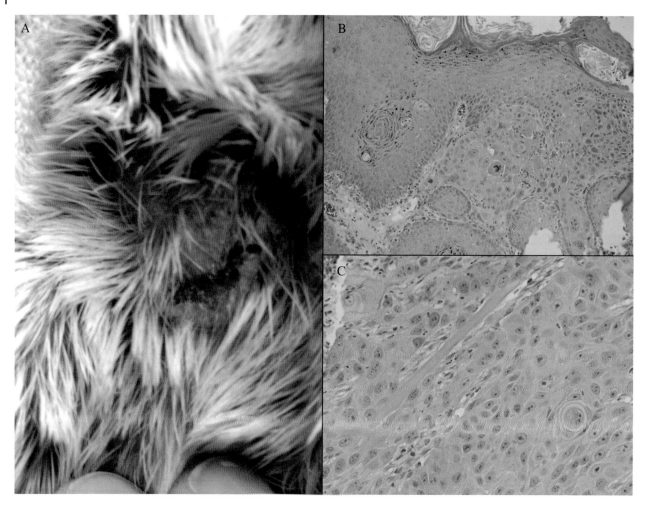

Figure 7.3 A: Squamous cell carcinoma of the ventral abdominal marking gland. B: Within the epidermis, is a cluster of dysplastic squamous epithelial cells and in the superficial dermis, in close proximity to the basal layer of epidermis, is a nest of neoplastic squamous epithelial cells with a centrally located cell displaying a large mitotic figure. C: Cords and sheets of neoplastic squamous cells have infiltrated into the subcutis and the underlying skeletal muscle obscuring the normal architecture. Within the center of the neoplastic cells is a small keratin pearl. *Source:* B and C: Courtesy of E. Brouwer.

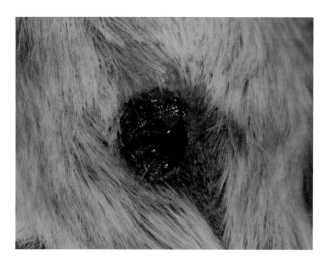

Figure 7.4 Enlarged and ulcerated ventral abdominal marking gland. *Source:* Courtesy of The Links Road Animal and Bird Clinic.

leaving the subcutaneous tissues of the distal portion of the tail exposed, which is then subject to dessication.

7.2.6.2 Nasal Dermatitis

Also known as sore nose or facial eczema, nasal dermatitis is an important condition of gerbils, with all age groups and both sexes being equally susceptible (Figure 7.5). Outbreaks have been reported in colonies during hot and humid weather when relative humidity levels exceed 60%. Stress from overcrowding, fighting or unsanitary cage conditions is also considered to be an initiating factor, resulting in increased Harderian gland porphyrin-containing secretions. Cutaneous irritation or self-trauma may occur as a consequence of accumulation of secretions around the eyes and external nares from hypersecretion or reduced self-grooming. Provision of regular access to a clean sand bath and switching to

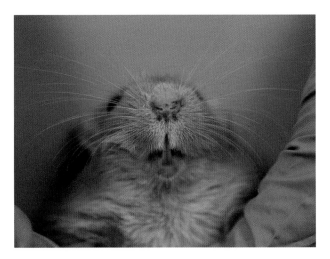

Figure 7.5 Nasal dermatitis (sore nose). This condition can occur with or without periocular dermatitis, conjunctivitis, and forepaw or ventral abdominal dermatitis. Sequelae include secondary bacterial infections with *Staphylococcus* spp.

bedding other than pine shavings may help to reduce the incidence of this condition.

Presenting Clinical Signs Initially, a red-brown crust that fluoresces under ultraviolet light develops below the external nares and alopecia of the underlying skin, extending later around the nostrils and over the upper and lower lip area, potentially to the proximal border of the vibrissae. Areas of alopecia can progress to develop a moist dermatitis with ulceration, pronounced red-brown crusting and secondary bacterial infections with *Staphylococcus* spp. Periocular dermatitis and protrusion of the nictitating membranes may be sequelae. Similar ulcerative and exudative dermatitis can develop on the paws and ventral abdomen.

Pathology Microscopically, there is acute, multifocal epidermal necrosis and ulceration with formation of micro-abscesses and microgranulomas. With longstanding dermatitis, there may be marked hyperkeratosis and acanthosis with irregular downgrowth of epidermal pegs and increased dermal melanin deposits. Concurrent adenomatous hyperplasia of the Harderian gland may be present with formation of lipid granulomas. Additionally, gerbils with periocular dermatitis may have non-suppurative conjunctivitis.

Differential Diagnoses Traumatic injuries secondary to overzealous burrowing and bacterial dermatitides should be considered. The classic location of the lesions combined with ultraviolet porphyrin fluorescence is a useful indicator.

Colony Management The condition may be prevented by improving the husbandry and management, including reducing relative humidity, enhancing sanitation, reducing overcrowding and other stressors, and provision of regular sand baths.

7.2.6.3 Unkempt Hair Coat

When relative humidity levels exceed 50%, the fur coat can become unkempt, greasy, and matted. Lack of proper ventilation, insufficient bedding changes, underlying disease, and inadequate nutrition should be considered. Oily haircoats can be prevented with the provision of sand baths several times weekly.

Fibers from synthetic nesting material may get wrapped around the limbs, resulting in ischemic necrosis.

7.3 Endocrine Conditions

7.3.1 Diabetes Mellitus

Obese gerbils are predisposed to developing hyperglycemia and glucose intolerance and are more prone to developing diabetes mellitus. Clinical signs include elevated blood glucose levels, polydipsia, polyuria, glycosuria, and urinary bladder infections. Pancreatic islet cell hyperplasia and pancreatic islet cell adenomas have been reported in Mongolian gerbils. In obese gerbils, it has been speculated that pancreatic islets hypertrophy and are able to maintain normal blood glucose levels despite the reduction in glucose tolerance.

7.3.2 Hyperadrenocorticism

Hyperadrenocorticism, associated with excess production of glucocorticoids by the adrenal gland or secondary to a functional pituitary tumor, is rarely seen in aged gerbils. Clinical signs include polyuria, polydipsia, polyphagia, and bilateral symmetrical alopecia of the flanks and lateral thighs. Differential diagnoses include diabetes and chronic interstitial nephritis. While the ACTH stimulation and dexamethasone suppression tests have been described for use in laboratory animals, the utility of these tests may not be feasible for a pet gerbil because of repeated testing, the quantities of blood required, and the stress to the animal from repeated handling and anesthesia. Thus, the diagnosis of this condition may be one of exclusion.

7.3.3 Endocrine Neoplasia

Disease surveys of Mongolian gerbils and other species of gerbils commonly report adrenal adenomas and adenocarcinomas; however, these conditions are only anecdotally reported in the clinical literature. One adrenal adenocarcinoma was found adherent to the renal vein, which contained tumor emboli. Pulmonary metastases were also noted in this animal. Another report detailing necropsy findings of healthy gerbils indicated identification of an adrenocortical adenocarcinoma and several adrenal cortical adenomas, but exclusively in females.

Some 8% of the female breeder gerbils in one study had nodules resembling pheochromocytomas, which compressed the remaining cortex against the surrounding capsule.

7.3.4 Other Endocrine Conditions

Amyloid deposition was reported in 16% of gerbils in one study, and the adrenal gland was occasionally affected. Many of the affected animals also had chronic renal disease, suggesting the amyloid deposition was secondary to chronic antigenic stimulation, such as is seen with persistent infections, inflammatory or neoplastic conditions in other species.

Rare cases of **thyroid atrophy** and **thyroiditis** have been reported in an aging colony of Mongolian gerbils. The clinical significance is unknown.

7.4 Respiratory Conditions

Respiratory disease is seen infrequently in gerbils and clinical signs include cyanosis, weight loss, inappetence, dyspnea, sneezing, and periocular and perinasal porphyrin staining. Upper respiratory infections may present primarily as conjunctivitis and sinusitis, and β-hemolytic *Streptococcus* spp. are often implicated. Irritation from dusty bedding or elevated levels of ammonia can cause similar clinical signs. Microscopic findings may include pulmonary hemorrhage, emphysema or pneumonia. Bacteria including *Klebsiella pneumoniae*, *Pasteurella pneumotropica*, *Streptococcus pneumoniae*, and *Mycoplasma pulmonis* have been associated with lower respiratory tract infections.

While gerbils can seroconvert to mouse viral respiratory pathogens, such as the paramyxoviruses, Sendai virus and pneumonia virus of mice, no clinical signs have been reported.

7.5 Musculoskeletal Conditions

Musculoskeletal conditions are noted with moderate frequency in pet gerbils. Other potential causes of paresis include stroke, weakness secondary to hypoglycemia, and neurologic disease.

7.5.1 Nutritional Osteodystrophy

Gerbils prefer sunflower seeds to pelleted rations; however, seeds are low in calcium and high in fat, such that diets composed primarily of sunflower seeds may predispose the gerbil to obesity, hypercholesterolemia, and secondary diseases including nutritional osteodystrophy. This condition can increase the incidence of pathological fractures. The histologic features of fibrous osteodystrophy include increased bone resorption with prominent osteoclast activity, fibroplasia, and increased osteoblast activity, leading to production of woven bone.

Limb fractures can occur from improper handling or exercise wheel entrapment. Solid exercise wheels are preferred to prevent limb or tail entrapment or sore hocks.

7.6 Gastrointestinal Conditions

Gerbil pups will start to eat solid food at approximately 14 days of age and should have food and water readily accessible at all times. Gerbils are unable to vomit because of their muscular cardia. Obesity and hypercholesterolemia are common in gerbils fed diets high in oily seeds.

7.6.1 Oral Conditions

7.6.1.1 Malocclusion
Gerbils, like other small rodents, have continuously growing incisors. If gerbils are not provided with the material to chew on, incisors will not be worn properly, resulting in overgrowth and possibly malocclusion.

7.6.1.2 Periodontal Disease
Gerbils can develop spontaneous periodontal disease as early as six months of age; however, periodontal lesions that are grossly identifiable do not appear before one year of age. Initial gingival changes include hyperplasia and edema, with deposition of soft plaque and brittle calculus. This is followed by resorption of the alveolar bone, with the formation of craters that are conducive to impaction with foreign material, such as hair and wood shavings. Exposure of interradicular tissues, excessive mobility of teeth, and subsequent loss of the third molar commonly occur in older animals.

7.6.1.3 Oral Neoplasia
Oral neoplasia is rare in gerbils with single reports of a locally invasive oral squamous cell carcinoma involving the lower incisor gingiva in a Libyan gerbil (*Meriones libycus*) and a fibromatous epulis in a Mongolian gerbil.

7.6.2 Salivary Gland Conditions

Sialoadenitis and amyloid deposition in the salivary gland are seen infrequently.

Salivary gland neoplasia is uncommon in gerbils. A large mass in the lower ventral neck of a 14-month-old male gerbil was diagnosed as an undifferentiated salivary gland sarcoma based on a lack of cellular differentiation, positive immunohistochemical labeling for vimentin and S-100, and an absence of labeling for cytokeratin.

7.6.3 Gastric Conditions

7.6.3.1 Gastric Bloat

Gastric dilatation with accumulation of gas is seen periodically in gerbils and the condition may occur following feeding of unsuitable or contaminated diets or secondary to ileus, inappetence or malocclusion. Clinical signs include bruxism, distension of the abdomen, respiratory distress, and cardiovascular impairment.

7.6.3.2 Gastric Yeast

Yeast organisms, suggestive of *Candida* spp. (Figure 7.6) have been identified in both the squamous and glandular portions of the gerbil stomach, and are considered incidental.

7.6.4 Enteric Conditions

7.6.4.1 Tyzzer's Disease

Gerbils of all ages are very susceptible to Tyzzer's disease, although the disease is more commonly manifested in younger animals. The condition is caused by *Clostridium piliforme*, a large, Gram-negative filamentous bacterium.

Presenting Clinical Signs Clinical signs in infected animals include depression, lethargy, dehydration, kyphosis, unkempt damp hair coat, moistening of the fur on the underside of the tail, and fecal staining of the perineum. Many animals will not demonstrate diarrhea; however, and gerbils may die suddenly with no premonitory signs. The bacterial spores are likely ubiquitous and predisposing factors include poor sanitation, stressful events, such as shipping, management changes,

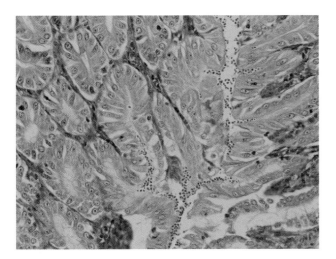

Figure 7.6 Yeast organisms, (suggestive of *Candida* spp.) are colonizing the mucosal surface and gastric pits of the glandular stomach. These are considered to an incidental finding in an otherwise healthy animal.

poor environmental conditions, overcrowding, concurrent disease, and inadequate nutrition.

Pathology The classic triad of lesions, consisting of hepatic, myocardial, and ileocecal necrosis, are often seen in infected gerbils. The most consistent lesion reported at necropsy is hepatomegaly with multiple small pale foci, sometimes with dark centers, on the capsular surface and extending into the parenchyma. Microscopically, acute multifocal hepatic necrosis is seen with necrotic foci surrounded by a rim of neutrophils and lymphocytes. With a Warthin-Starry stain, abundant bundles of long slender rod-shaped bacteria can be seen in the margins of necrotic areas. Intestinal lesions include acute edema, hemorrhage, congestion, necrosis, and mucosal ulceration of the ileum and cecum. Necrotic areas often contain neutrophilic infiltrates and intracellular bacteria. Myocarditis and pericarditis may be present, with *C. piliforme* organisms observed at the outer edges of necrotic foci.

Laboratory Diagnostics Diagnosis is based on compatible gross and microscopic lesions and the demonstration of the characteristic bacteria with a Warthin-Starry stain. PCR assays that target the 16S ribosomal rRNA sequence are available and the cecal wall and content are the preferred tissues for testing.

Differential Diagnoses There are many potential causes of diarrhea in gerbils, including dietary indiscretion, intestinal amyloidosis, cecal dysbiosis with overgrowth of *C. difficile*, and enteritis caused by other bacteria, such as *Salmonella* spp., *E. coli*, and *Citrobacter rodentium*.

Colony Management Tyzzer's disease is a heartbreaking condition in pet gerbils and breeding colonies, and is almost invariably fatal. Caging, equipment, and the general environment must be thoroughly cleaned and disinfected before they are used to house other gerbils or rodents. The spores persist for years within the environment and prevention by means of good management practices and cage hygiene is the best method of controlling the disease.

7.6.4.2 Salmonellosis

An outbreak of salmonellosis caused by *Salmonella* Typhimurium var Copenhagen, led to 90% mortality in a large group of 3 to 6-week-old gerbils shortly after shipping. Clinical signs included unkempt hair coat, lethargy, dehydration, moderate to marked diarrhea and fecal staining of the perineum, and peracute death of some animals. Affected gerbils had a leukocytosis with an absolute neutrophilia. At necropsy, findings included enlarged, congested livers, fibrinopurulent peritonitis with abscess formation, fluid- and gas-distended stomachs and intestines, and heavy infestations of

Rodentolepsis nana (small intestine) and *Entamoeba muris* (cecum). Microscopically, multifocal hepatic necrosis was seen, characterized by either small aggregates of predominantly mononuclear infiltrates or larger granulomas with caseous, partially calcified cores, which were surrounded by epithelioid macrophages, lymphocytes, neutrophils, and an outer fibrous capsule. Occasional intestinal crypt abscesses were seen. Predisposing factors for this outbreak included suspected contaminated feed combined with concurrent disease, the young age of the gerbils with associated recent weaning stress, and stressful events associated with shipping and a change in environment.

7.6.4.3 Enteric Dysbiosis and Clostridial Enterotoxemia

Gerbils are highly susceptible to developing intestinal dysbiosis when orally treated with narrow spectrum antibiotics, such as penicillins, cephalopsorins, and macrolides. These antibiotics suppress or kill normal bacterial flora and permit overgrowth of other pathogenic bacteria, such as *C. difficile*, resulting in enterocolitis and enterotoxemia. In one case, gerbils colonized by *Helicobacter* sp. were treated with triple-antibiotic wafers containing amoxicillin, metronidazole, and bismuth. After 7 days of treatment, two of five gerbils developed enterotoxemia and died suddenly with no premonitory signs.

Upon post-mortem examination, both gerbils had watery cecal content and colonic distension, and one animal had colonic mucosal hyperemia with patchy diphtheritic membrane formation. A necrohemorrhagic typhlocolitis was identified, characterized by diffuse exfoliation and necrosis of the superficial mucosa with lamina proprial hemorrhage, fibrin, edema, mats of degenerate and mature neutrophils, and small aggregates of Gram-positive bacilli. The intestinal lumen was filled with protein-rich exudate, necrotic epithelial cells, and short rod-shaped bacteria. The edematous submucosa and tunica muscularis contained perivascular aggregates of neutrophils and a sprinkling of macrophages and lymphocytes with a mild to moderate neutrophilic peritonitis. *C. difficile* toxins A and B were identified in the cecal contents of both animals by ELISA.

7.6.4.4 Citrobacter Infections

Citrobacter rodentium is a Gram-negative bacterial short rod related to *E. coli* and is a natural pathogen of small rodents. Colonic infections result in attaching and effacing mucosal lesions similar to those produced by enteropathogenic *E. coli*. Colony infections result in high morbidity and mortality with all ages affected, although young animals are more susceptible. In infected animals, clinical signs include an unkempt hair coat, emaciation, dehydration, bloody diarrhea, and perianal fecal stain-

ing. In the animals dying acutely, the colon and rectum are often thickened, with locally extensive mucosal ulceration. In animals that survive for longer periods, there is colonic goblet cell hyperplasia, distension of glands with debris, lamina proprial edema, dilatation of submucosal lymphatics, and sloughing of the superficial epithelium into the lumen. The bacterium can be difficult to isolate and may only be present in animals in the acute phase of the infection. Possible sources of contamination include feed, water, bedding, various fomites, or transfer by personnel.

7.6.4.5 Protozoal Infections

Gerbils are generally conventionally housed and have poorly defined flora. Various protozoal organisms, including *Tritrichomonas caviae*, *Giardia* spp., and *Entamoeba* sp. can be present in very large numbers in the cecum of normal and moribund animals (Figure 7.7). In general, even in very large numbers, these organisms are not associated with mucosal damage or inflammation, and are considered nonpathogenic.

None of these protozoa, including *Giardia*, are thought to pose a zoonotic threat to human caregivers except in very rare cases in which gerbils are infected with human strains. *Giardia duodenalis*, a human pathogen, can cause small intestinal villus atrophy, crypt hyperplasia, and increased mucus production in gerbils. Clusters of trophozoites collect at the tip and base of small intestinal villi leading to epithelial sloughing.

7.6.4.6 Nematode Infestations

Gerbils can be infested with several different species of pinworms, including the gerbil pinworm, *Dentostomella*

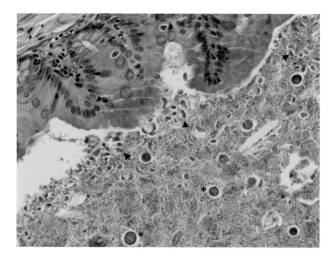

Figure 7.7 Photomicrograph of cecum from a healthy gerbil. Even large numbers of pyriform-shaped *Tritrichomonas* sp. (arrows) and *Entamoeba* sp. (*) trophozoites in the colon are considered to be nonpathogenic in conventionally housed gerbils and no mucosal reactivity is seen.

translucida, as well as other murine pinworms, including *Syphacia obvelata*, *S. muris*, and *Aspiculuris tetraptera*. Large numbers may be present, especially in animals with intercurrent enteric diseases, but infestations are almost always subclinical. In healthy animals, infestations are transient and self-limiting. Large small mammal pet distribution centers may provide the opportunity for interspecies transmission of pinworms.

The life cycle of *D. translucida* is direct with adult and juvenile pinworms located preferentially in the anterior third of the small intestine. In Mongolian gerbils, female pinworms range from 9.6–31 mm long and 0.38–1.0 mm wide, while males are 6.1–13.1 mm long and 0.37–0.53 mm wide. Animals with pinworm infestations may have focal lymphoplasmacytic or eosinophilic infiltrates within the small intestinal lamina propria. Diagnosis of *D. translucida* infection is by identification of adult or larval pinworms in the intestinal lumen at necropsy or by histology (Figure 7.8), by fecal flotation or by evaluating perineal cellophane tape impressions for eggs. Humans do not transmit *D. translucida*.

7.6.4.7 Cestode Infestations
Gerbils are susceptible to the rodent tapeworms, *Rodentolepis nana* and *R. diminuta*, but infestations do not persist in healthy, immunocompetent animals. Heavy infestations of *R. nana* can be seen in animals coinfected with other pathogens, such as *Salmonella* spp., and in animals debilitated by age or kept under conditions of poor hygiene. In these cases, the small intestines may be dilated and the lumina almost occluded with mucoid content and large numbers of tapeworms. Mucosal inflammation and necrosis may be evident with heavy infestations.

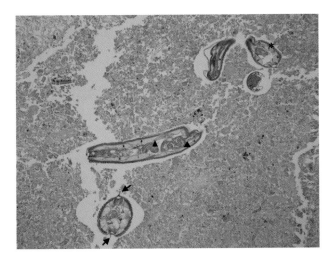

Figure 7.8 Cross- and longitudinal sections of pinworms from the small intestinal lumen. Identifying features include lateral alae (arrows), platymyarian musculature (*) and a digestive tract (triangles). Several species of pinworms can infect gerbils but typically are without clinical signs.

R. nana may undergo three life cycle routes. With a direct life cycle, ova-bearing proglottids are passed in the feces by one definitive host and are ingested by another. Because gerbils can be coprophagic, they can reinfect themselves. The second life cycle is an internal autoinfection cycle and the ova may hatch, releasing hexacanth larvae directly within the intestinal lumen. With the indirect life cycle, ova bearing proglottids are passed in the feces from a definitive host and taken up by an intermediate host, such as beetles, cockroaches or fleas, which are subsequently ingested by the next definitive host.

Historically, *R. nana* was believed to be zoonotic, but based on the results of recent studies, the subspecies of *R. nana* infective for humans has been determined to be genetically distinct from the subspecies that infects rodents. Infestations of *R. nana* can be spread between different species of rodents and have been detected for mouse-derived strains within immunosuppressed but not immunocompetent gerbils.

7.6.4.8 Gastroenteric Neoplasia
Gastric adenocarcinoma has been diagnosed in *P. duprasi*, another species of *Gerbillinae* and a duodenal adenocarcinoma was reported in a Mongolian gerbil. Cecal cystadenocarcinoma was reported in a 12-month-old male gerbil. This animal had an enlarged cecum with a smooth serosal surface and on cut surface, the wall was noted to be thickened and cystic. Histologically, the lamina propria, submucosa and muscle tunic contained multiple cysts lined by a single layer of enlarged epithelial cells with increased basophilia and bearing large eccentric nuclei containing one or two prominent nucleoli. Cecal carcinoma has been reported in two aged female gerbils.

7.6.5 Hepatic Conditions

7.6.5.1 Helicobacter Infection
Gerbils are susceptible to infection by both rodent and human species of *Helicobacter* and natural infections of *H. bilis* and *H. hepaticus* have been detected in gerbil research colonies. In one case, a single animal infected with *H. hepaticus* was anecdotally noted to have multifocal pale to white foci on the liver at necropsy, although this was not further evaluated microscopically. There may be zoonotic risks with maintaining *H. bilis*-infected rodents, as the bacterium has been isolated from bile and gall bladder tissue from human cases of cholecystitis as well as from the bile of some human patients with gall bladder and biliary tract neoplasia. Infections are readily detected by PCR analysis of feces.

7.6.5.2 Hepatic Lipidosis
A high fat diet may produce hepatic lipidosis and choleliths in gerbils. Obesity is common in gerbils and is

associated with the feeding of a predominantly seed-based ration, in particular, especially sunflower seeds.

7.6.5.3 Hepatic Amyloidosis

Hepatic amyloid deposition is moderately common in aging gerbils, with up to 8% prevalence in one survey of aged animals. Many of these animals also had chronic renal disease, suggesting that hepatic amyloid deposition was secondary to chronic antigenic stimulation and consistent with AA type amyloid derived from serum protein AA, an acute phase reactant protein produced by the liver.

7.6.5.4 Hepatobiliary Masses

Hepatic neoplasia is uncommon in gerbils but single reports of hepatic adenoma, hepatic lymphoangioma, and cholangiocarcinoma exist. Biliary cysts have been reported in aged gerbils.

7.6.6 Conditions of the Exocrine Pancreas

Interstitial pancreatitis is a prominent lesion associated with encephalomyocarditis (EMC) virus infection. Gerbils are highly susceptible to EMCV and when experimentally infected with a diabetogenic variant strain, mortality was noted to be higher in females. In severely affected gerbils, the peritoneal cavity contained abundant serous fluid, with marked subcapsular and interlobular pancreatic edema, and sporadic animals demonstrated foci of epicardial necrosis of the right ventricle. Histologically, there was marked interlobular edema and acute necrosis of exocrine pancreatic acinar cells with moderate to marked neutrophilic infiltrates and fewer lymphocytes. Islets were rarely involved. Foci of subendocardial necrosis with mineralization and nonsuppurative inflammation were present in some animals. Small rodents are suspected to be carriers or reservoir hosts of EMCV. The virus may spread between animals in breeding facilities and large pet rodent distribution centers.

Interstitial pancreatic amyloid deposition can be seen with low prevalence in aging gerbils.

Pancreatic fibrosarcoma has been reported in a Libyan gerbil.

7.7 Cardiovascular Conditions

Ventricular septal defect occurs with low prevalence in gerbils and other congenital heart defects are not reported.

Despite their propensity to develop hyperlipemia and hypercholesterolemia even while on low-fat diets, gerbils rarely develop atherosclerosis.

7.7.1 Cardiac Amyloidosis

Myocardial amyloidosis is uncommon in aging gerbils, occurring with less than 1% prevalence. Many affected animals also have concurrent chronic renal disease, suggesting that amyloid deposition is secondary to chronic antigenic stimulation.

7.7.2 Myocardial Degeneration and Fibrosis

Myocardial degeneration and fibrosis, and infrequently myocardial mineralization, are seen in gerbils greater than one year of age and the condition is more prevalent in males (Figure 7.9). The etiopathogenesis is not well understood.

7.7.3 Myocarditis and Pericarditis Complex

Tyzzer's disease, caused by infection with *Clostridium piliforme*, typically affects the heart, liver, and large intestine, but this triad of organ involvement is not essential. Necrotizing and pyogranulomatous myocarditis and granulomatous pericarditis can be seen exclusively in infected gerbils and the intracellular bundles of bacilli are sometimes visible in the myofibers at the outer margins of the lesions. A Warthin-Starry silver stain enhances bacterial visualization.

Gerbils experimentally infected intraperitoneally with encephalomyocarditis virus D (diabetogenic) variant developed white epicardial foci, correlating with myocardial necrosis with mineralization and nonsuppurative inflammation (see Section 7.6.6 for more details).

7.7.4 Hyperadrenocorticism and Cardiovascular Disease

In one study of 12-month-old virgin gerbils and breeding gerbils fed low fat diets, 30% of female breeders had grossly visible arteriosclerotic plaques and 65% of female breeders had histologic evidence of arterial degeneration with mild to marked deposition of plaques composed of mucopolysaccharide and calcium. Affected animals demonstrated fibrosis within the tunica intima and media with degeneration of the internal elastic membranes of the aorta, and mesenteric, renal and peripheral arteries. Histologically, 13% of these animals had multifocal myocardial necrosis or fibrosis. In comparison, none of the male breeders had gross evidence of arterial disease but approximately 25% had histologic evidence of aortic plaques and 60% had multifocal myocardial necrosis or fibrosis. Breeding animals had elevated levels of creatine kinase, triglycerides, free fatty acids, and corticosterone. These gerbils were also hyperlipemic, hypercholesterolemic and hyperglyemic with hepatic lipidosis and pancreatic islet hypertrophy. In addition, there was

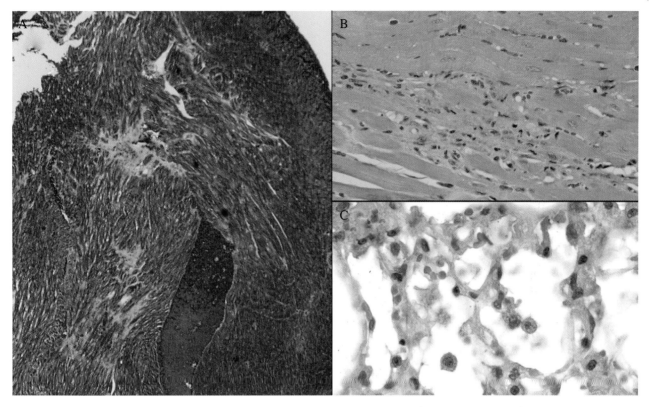

Figure 7.9 A: Focal myocardial degeneration and fibrosis are more commonly seen in gerbils greater than a year of age. Note the multiple pale blue foci of myocardial fibrosis within the left ventricular wall. Masson's trichrome. B: Small focus of myocardial fibrosis. With significant myocardial damage, heart failure can follow. C: Characteristic lesions of left-sided heart failure include pulmonary edema and congestion with alveoli containing low numbers of red blood cells and increased numbers of alveolar macrophages demonstrating erythrophagocytosis, resulting in cytoplasmic hemosiderin accumulation; commonly referred to as "heart failure" cells (arrows). A differential stain such as Perl's may be necessary to confirm the presence of small amounts of Iron.

marked thymic involution, adrenal gland hemorrhage and enlargement, and brown discoloration of the pancreas. Histologically, there was adrenocortical hyperplasia and changes in cortical lipid content with eight percent of the female breeders also having nodules resembling pheochromocytomas. The heart, kidney, and body weights of breeding animals were substantially heavier than for virgin gerbils and the breeders had larger depots of adipose tissue. Further details regarding the etiopathogenesis were not identified.

7.8 Genitourinary Conditions

Gerbils are well adapted to their natural desert environment as they require very little water to survive and produce small, dry, firm fecal pellets, and very concentrated urine. Their kidneys are unipapillate with a single long papilla that extends out into each ureter. The adrenal glands are large in proportion the gerbil's body weight and are thought to contribute to their unique ability to conserve water.

7.8.1 Genital Tract Conditions

Female gerbils, similar to other female mammals, possess a prostate gland, a small, paraurethral, hormonally-responsive gland (Figure 7.10). The gland is comparable to the ventral lobe of the postpubertal male prostate, with alveoli and ducts embedded in a vascularized fibromuscular stroma. The female prostate gland undergoes aging changes including secretory cell metaplasia and hyperplasia, with thickening of the smooth muscle and subepithelial collagen layers. Dysplastic and neoplastic epithelial changes can be seen in aged, multiparous females, whereas prostatitis is seen in both senile virgin and multiparous gerbils.

Pyometra and suppurative metritis can occur in female gerbils and must be differentiated from tumors of the reproductive tract as vulvar discharge or hemorrhage may be seen with both conditions. Gerbils in estrus may have a congested vulva, which must also be distinguished from vulvar staining by abnormal uterine or vaginal exudate. Cystic endometrial hyperplasia and myometrial mineralization are occasionally seen in aging females.

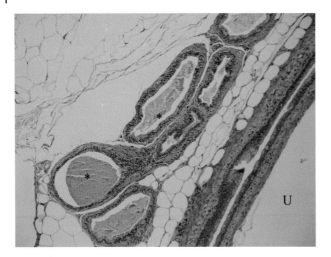

Figure 7.10 The paraurethrally-located prostate gland in a female gerbil. Anatomy is similar to the male prostate gland with alveoli and ducts embedded in vascularized fibromuscular stroma. Note the location of the urethra (U) and presence of alveolar eosinophilic microcalculi (*). Larger calculi that completely fill glandular lumena are also reported.

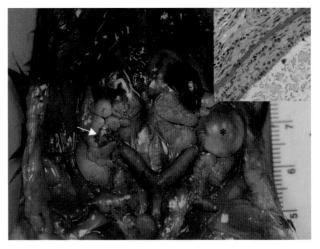

Figure 7.11 Thin-walled, serous fluid-filled unilateral paraovarian cyst in a retired breeding female (*). Note contralateral ovary with developing follicles embedded in adipose tissue (arrow). The uterine horns are thickened. Inset: Photomicrograph of a paraovarian cyst in a female gerbil. Note the cuboidal, ciliated epithelium lining the cyst lumen.

Orchitis, testicular mineralization, and prostatitis are infrequently seen in male gerbils of any age.

7.8.1.1 Cystic Ovaries

Female gerbils are prone to developing ovarian and parovarian cysts and the incidence and severity increases with age, with up to 50% of females older than 400 days of age affected in one study. Clinically affected gerbils may have bilaterally symmetrical, estrogen-induced alopecia and be inappetent, lethargic, and dyspneic with a distended abdomen. Ovulation can still occur in animals with cystic ovaries but litter sizes will be smaller and females eventually become infertile. Cysts may be uni- or bilateral and of variable size, ranging from <1 to >50 mm in diameter (i.e., up to 16% of the body weight). Cysts are thin-walled and filled with serous or serosanguinous fluid (Figure 7.11). Histologically, cyst walls are composed of delicate fibrovascular connective tissue lined by single to multiple layers of granulosa cells with multiple small clusters of lutenized thecal cells. In contrast, paraovarian cysts are lined by cuboidal, ciliated epithelium. Ovaries may simultaneously contain tumors and cysts.

7.8.1.2 Reproductive Tract Neoplasia

Ovarian tumors are frequently seen in female gerbils greater than two years of age and include granulosa, thecal, and luteal cell tumors, dysgerminomas, teratomas, and leiomyomas. Uterine leiomyomas, hemangiopericytomas, and adenocarcinomas are also seen sporadically. Gerbils with ovarian tumors may present with similar clinical signs as animals with ovarian cysts, including bilaterally symmetrical alopecia, inappetence, lethargy, dyspnea, and abdominal distension, as these tumors can be large and bilateral. Tumors may also result in vulvar discharge or hemorrhage, often associated with secondary bacterial infection.

Granulosa cell tumors are the most common ovarian tumor seen in aged female gerbils. Early tumors can be detected microscopically in nonbreeding females less than 2 years of age. Classically, granulosa cell tumors cause ovarian enlargement, and may be bilateral with a varied appearance ranging from solid to lobulated to cystic. Histologically, characteristic features include clusters and sheets of polygonal, pale staining, variably-sized granulosa cells with vacuolated cytoplasm within a fine fibrovascular stroma. Call-Exner bodies, pseudofollicles, and cystic or hemorrhagic areas may also be present but mitoses are rare. Invasion of the ovarian hilus, paraovarian fat, and ovarian fimbriae can be seen with metastases to the omentum and mesentery.

Dysgerminomas are encapsulated, solid, but soft tumors that are mottled red-yellow and may contain cysts enclosing dark red gelatinous to bloody material with scant stroma. Any remaining normal ovarian tissue may be found compressed within the outer capsule. Microscopically, dysgerminomas are composed of large cells with large nuclei rimmed by a fine nuclear membrane and containing inconsistent numbers of variably-sized nucleoli. They have rare mitoses but metastasis to mesenteric lymph nodes and the adrenal glands can occur.

Testicular teratoma, seminoma, and prostatic adenoma can all occur in male gerbils. Prostatic adenocarcinoma has been identified in a fat-tailed gerbil (*Pachyuromys duprasi*).

7.8.1.3 Perinatal Mortality

Small litters (less than three), insufficient nesting material, insufficient water, and excessive human handling of the young may all result in cannibalism or abandonment. Primary causes of postnatal mortality include maternal neglect, lactation failure due to mastitis or agalactia, and crushing or suffocation of pups in large litters. Adjustment of litter size and cross-fostering techniques can be applied successfully to gerbils.

Young gerbil pups will continue to nurse until 25 days of age but will begin to eat and drink at about 15 days of age so feeders and waterers need to be accessible or increased mortality may be experienced at weaning.

7.8.2 Urinary Tract Conditions

Mature, healthy male Mongolian gerbils may have a thickened Bowman's capsule affecting 2–3% of glomeruli in the superficial and juxtamedullary cortex. This lamina muscularis is composed of one to two layers of smooth muscle cells adjacent to the outer aspect of the basal lamina.

7.8.2.1 Chronic Renal Disease

Chronic renal disease and renal amyloidosis are commonly seen in aged gerbils (Figure 7.12). Affected animals may demonstrate a lymphoplasmacytic interstitial nephritis, tubular dilatation with eosinophilic proteinaceous or cellular luminal casts, atrophic tubular epithelium, glomerulonephropathy with mesangial thickening, distension of Bowman's spaces, and condensation of glomeruli with glomerulosclerosis, interstitial fibrosis and

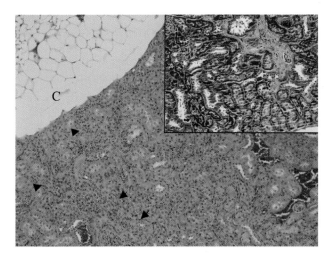

Figure 7.12 Photomicrograph of a kidney from retired female breeder with chronic renal fibrosis. The renal capsule (C) is pitted with cortical streaks of tubular atrophy, thickened tubular basement membranes, interstitial and periglomerular fibrosis (arrows). Inset: The cortical interstitial fibrosis is more obvious as is the tubular and glomerular atrophy. Masson's trichrome.

medullary mineralization. Renal amyloid deposits may be found within glomeruli or interstitial tissue.

Clinical signs of renal disease include weight loss, decreased feed intake, polyuria, polydipsia, and cystitis. Clinical chemistry changes in cases of renal disease are similar to those seen other mammals.

7.8.2.2 Lead Intoxication

Gerbils are active gnawers and burrowers and their risk of exposure to lead is high, if not housed in an appropriate environment. The risk of lead intoxication may be increased compared with other rodents because they accumulate four to six times more renal lead than do rats. In acute toxicity cases, large acid-fast intranuclear inclusions begin to accumulate in proximal convoluted tubular epithelium near the corticomedullary junction by week four, and by week six, the number of inclusions is markedly increased with shedding or attenuation of inner cortical tubular epithelium. Typically, the outer cortical proximal tubules, distal convoluted and medullary tubules, and glomeruli are unaffected.

With chronic lead exposure, gerbils become emaciated and lethargic with unkempt hair coats and some may show neurologic signs, including ataxia and seizures. At necropsy, livers are small, dark brown-black, and fibrotic, and may be adherent to the diaphragm. Kidneys are generally small, pale with pitted and adherent capsules. Microscopically, Kupffer cells and hepatocytes contain lipofuscin and infrequent intranuclear lead inclusions. Renal lesions include chronic nephropathy with tubular degeneration, interstitial fibrosis, blurring of the corticomedullary junction, and radiating streaks of degenerating tubules extending from the inner cortex to the capsular surface. Eosinophilic intranuclear lead inclusions may be present in numerous tubular epithelial cells. Concurrent hematologic abnormalities include a microcytic hypochromic anemia with marked erythrocytic basophilic stippling, marked anisocytosis and variably shaped erythrocytes.

7.8.2.3 Renal Neoplasia

Renal masses and neoplasias are infrequently diagnosed and include hemangiomas and hemangiosarcomas, Other renal vascular abnormalities include vascular hamartomas.

7.9 Nervous System Conditions

7.9.1 Epilepsy

Spontaneous epileptiform seizures in gerbils are typically observed first at 2 months of age and increase in frequency as the animals age. The seizures are variable in intensity and are triggered by increased stress-related stimulation such as handling or by environmental changes including moving cages and can be reduced if animals are habituated. The trait is inherited with variable penetrance so incidence in populations and strains of Mongolian gerbils can vary. Affected gerbils are deficient in the enzyme cerebral glutamine synthetase. Because of the heritable nature of this condition, it is likely that the gerbils raised for pets would be selected from seizure-resistant strains. There are no specific histologic lesions.

7.9.2 Other Neurologic Conditions

Meningitis and **suppurative encephalitis** of unknown etiology have been reported sporadically in preweaned gerbils.

In an outbreak of **Tyzzer's disease** in a colony of gerbils, neurologic signs such as rolling, ataxia, incoordination, and torticollis were noted. In addition to the classic hepatic, myocardial, and enteric lesions, acute purulent encephalitis and meningoencephalitis were noted with bacteria present only in the most severely affected brain tissues. See Section 7.6.4.1 for a further description of *C. piliforme* infection in gerbils.

A spontaneously occurring, predominantly solid and squamous **cranipharyngioma** was reported in a gerbil that presented clinically with emaciation, lethargy, and peripheral nervous signs. This tumor is thought to originate from the remnants of Rathke's pouch and is infrequently reported.

7.10 Hematopoietic and Lymphoid Conditions

The gerbil thymus is thoracic and is present into adulthood. Gerbil erythrocytes have a lifespan of approximately 10 days and normally have prominent basophilic stippling. Polychromasia and reticulocytosis are also common in adult gerbils. Sexual dimorphisms in gerbil erythrocyte parameters include higher packed red blood cell volumes, hemoglobin levels, total leukocyte, and lymphocyte counts in males. Neonatal gerbils have panleukocytosis, erythrocytic macrocytosis, and a reduced total erythrocyte count compared with adults.

Even when fed standard amounts of dietary fats, adult gerbils may have lipemia, which can result in apparent abnormally elevated hemoglobin levels. Hypercholesterolemia can be induced by adding 1% cholesterol to a standard rodent ration and a high fat diet will produce hepatic lipidosis and gallstones but not atherosclerosis.

Gerbils are similar to hamsters and guinea pigs in that they have neutrophils with eosinophilic staining granules, which have been termed heterophils. The cytoplasmic granules of polymorphonuclear leukocytes from these species contain the full complement of enzymes, suggesting that neutrophil is likely a more correct name for this cell type.

7.10.1 Amyloidosis

Spontaneous amyloid deposition is moderately common in aging gerbils, with deposition seen in the liver, spleen, lymph nodes, and other visceral organs. Concurrent chronic renal disease is common, suggesting that amyloid deposition occurs secondary to chronic antigenic stimulation (AA type).

7.10.2 Hematopoietic and Lymphoid Neoplasia

Hematopoietic tumors are infrequently seen in aging gerbils and lymphosarcomas are uncommon compared with other rodent species.

Histiocytic sarcoma of the spleen and liver was diagnosed in an aged pet gerbil. At necropsy, the spleen and liver were markedly enlarged and mottled yellow. Histologically, cohesive infiltrates of neoplastic histiocytes effaced the architecture of the spleen and liver. Neoplastic cells generally large, pleomorphic, predominantly ovoid, nuclei occasionally containing nucleoli with large amounts of pale eosinophilic vacuolated cytoplasm that often contained phagocytized red blood cells. The mitotic rate was high and similar populations of neoplastic histiocytic cells were present in the bone marrow, lung, adrenal gland, kidney, and lymph nodes.

Systemic mastocytosis with cutaneous involvement was reported in a young female gerbil that presented with emaciation, diarrhea, and a roughened hair coat. At necropsy, there was generalized enlargement of lymph nodes, with small gray nodules disseminated throughout the lung, thickening of the pyloric antrum, and dilatation of the glandular stomach, duodenum, and jejunum. The diagnosis was based on infiltrates of a homogeneous population of mast cells with amphophilic cytoplasm and metachromatic granules and round to oval central nuclei with fine chromatin and small nucleoli within bone marrow, lymph nodes, spleen, liver, gastrointestinal tract, lung, and numerous other tissues. Other red and white cell parameters were within normal ranges.

Other neoplasms identified in laboratory gerbils as part of disease surveillance studies include thymic lymphoepithelioma, splenic and renal hemangioma, and hepatic lymphangioma, characterized by accumulation of variably sized ducts devoid of lymphocytes lined by well-differentiated lymphatic endothelium.

7.11 Ophthalmic Conditions

The Harderian gland of gerbils and other rodents is red-brown and located ventromedially within the posterior orbit, and except for the hilus, is surrounded by

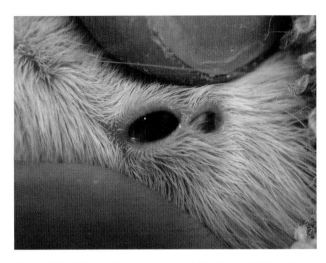

Figure 7.13 Unilateral segmental ankyloblepharon (failure of eyelids to completely separate). *Source:* Courtesy of The Links Road Animal and Bird Clinic.

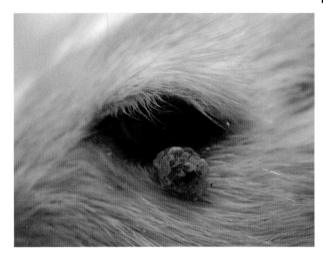

Figure 7.14 Papilloma on the eyelid of a gerbil. *Source:* Courtesy of The Links Road Animal and Bird Clinic.

orbital venous plexus. Secretions from the gland pass through the lacrimal canal and out the external nares, where they are mixed with saliva and applied to the pelage as part of normal daily grooming. Histologically, the gland is partitioned into ill-defined lobes composed of straight and coiled tubuloaveoli that drain into a single glandular branch connected to a single excretory duct. The glandular epithelial cells are tall and pyramidal with finely vacuolated eosinophilic cytoplasm. The Harderian gland produces a secretion containing protoporphyrins and melatonin, which fluoresces under ultraviolet light. This secretion may play a role in ocular lubrication, chemocommunication, and thermoregulation. Increased secretions of protoporphyrins may be produced in response to stress or as a result of reduced grooming. The oculonasal secretions can accumulate and owners may describe bleeding (chromodacryorrhea) from the nose or eyes. These secretions are irritating and with rubbing or scratching nasal and periocular dermatitis, blepharitis, and conjunctivitis may ensue. Management practices should always be reviewed when this sign is present.

Conjunctivitis and corneal ulcers can develop secondary to irritation from bedding particulates and volatile oils from softwood shavings. Softwood bedding should be kiln-dried before use to minimize this irritation. Facial swelling, exopthalmos and secondary exposure keratitis may be sequelae to primary dental disease, such as molar root abscesses. Unilateral segmental ankyloblepharon (failure of eyelids to completely separate) has been reported (Figure 7.13). Little information regarding eyelid tumors (Figure 7.14) is available for gerbils.

Since gerbil eyes have shallow orbits, ocular prolapse can be induced by excessive scruffing of the skin during restraint. Proptosis also occurs in aged gerbils. Corneal mineralization is a dystrophic aging change and foci can rarely become ulcerated. Reversible cataract formation is common in anesthetized rodents and these will usually resolve following recovery. Cataracts can also be associated with diabetes and are an age-related change.

Bibliography

General

Banks, R.E., Sharp, J.M., Doss, S.D., and Vanderford, D.A. (2010) *Exotic Small Mammal Care and Husbandry.* Wiley-Blackwell, Ames, IA, pp. 93–101.

Bihun, C. (2004) Basic anatomy, physiology, husbandry, and clinical techniques. in *Ferrets, Rabbits and Rodents: Clinical Medicine and Surgery* (eds. K.E. Quesenberry and J.W. Carpenter), 2nd edn. Saunders, St. Louis, MO, pp. 286–298.

Harkness, J.E., Turner, P.V., VandeWoude, S., and Wheler, C.L. (2010) *Harkness and Wagner's Biology and Medicine of Rabbits and Rodents.* 5th edn. Wiley-Blackwell, Ames, IA, pp. 74–83.

Keeble, E. (2002) Gerbils. In: *BSAVA Manual of Exotic Pets* (eds. A. Meredith and S. Redrobe), 4th edn. BSAVA, Quedgeley, pp. 34–46.

Laber-Laird, K., Swindle, M.M., and Flecknell, P.A. (eds.) (1996) *Handbook of Rodent and Rabbit Medicine.* Pergamon, Oxford, pp. 39–58.

Integument Conditions

Beck, W. (2008) Occurrence of a house-infesting tropical rat mite (*Ornithonyssus bacoti*) on murides and human beings. *Travel Medicine and Infectious Disease,* **6**(4), 245–249.

Benitz, K.F. and Kramer, A.W. Jr. (1965) Spontaneous tumors in the Mongolian gerbil. *Laboratory Animal Care*, **15**(5), 281–294.

Bingel, S.A. (1995) Pathologic findings in an aging Mongolian gerbil (*Meriones unguiculatus*) colony. *Laboratory Animal Science*, **45**(5), 597–600.

Bresnahan, J.F., Smith, G.D., Lentsch, R.H., Barnes, W.G., and Wagner, J.E. (1983) Nasal dermatitis in the Mongolian gerbil. *Laboratory Animal Science* **33**(3), 258–263.

Canny, C.J. and Gamble, C.S. (2003) Fungal diseases of rabbit. *Veterinary Clinics of North America: Exotic Animal Practice*, **6**(2), 429–433.

Cramlet, S.H., Toft, J.D., and Olsen, N.W. (1974) Malignant melanoma in a black gerbil (*Meriones unguiculatus*). *Laboratory Animal Science*, **24**(3), 545–547.

Deutschland, M., Denk, D., Skerritt, G., and Hetzel, U. (2011) Surgical excision and morphological evaluation of altered abdominal scent glands in Mongolian gerbils (*Meriones unguiculatus*). *Veterinary Record*, **169**(24), 636–641.

Donnelly, T.M. (1997) What's your diagnosis? Nasal lesions in gerbils. Nasal dermatitis ("Facial Eczema" or "Sore Nose"). *Laboratory Animals (NY,)* **26** (2), 17–18.

Farrar, P.L., Opsomer, M.J., Kocen, J.A., and Wagner, J.E. (1988) Experimental nasal dermatitis in the Mongolian gerbil: effect of bilateral harderian gland adenectomy on development of facial lesions. *Laboratory Animal Science*, **38**(1), 72–76.

Fenton, H., Forzán, M.J., Desmarchelier, M., et al. (2016) Poorly differentiated cutaneous carcinoma of non-sebaceous origin in a 3-year-old Mongolian gerbil (*Meriones unguiculatus*). *Canadian Veterinary Journal*, **57**(1), 80–83.

Fulghum, R.S. and Chole, R.A. (1985) Bacterial flora in spontaneously occurring aural cholesteatomas in Mongolian gerbils. *Infection and Immunity*, **50**(3), 678–81.

Henry, K.R., Chole, R.A., and McGinn, M.D. (1983) Age-related increase of spontaneous aural cholesteatoma in the Mongolian gerbil. *Archives of Otolaryngology*, **109**(1), 19–21.

Hoppmann, E., and Wilson Baron, H. (2007) Rodent dermatology. *Journal of Exotic Pet Medicine*, **16**(4), 238–255.

Jacklin, M.R. (1997) Dermatosis associated with *Acarus farris* in gerbils. *Journal of Small Animal Practice*, **38**(9), 410–411.

Keeble, E. (2002) Gerbils. In: *BSAVA Manual of Exotic Pets* (eds. A. Meredith and S. Redrobe), 4th edn. British Small Animal Veterinary Association, Quedgeley, pp. 34–46.

Lucky, A.W., Sayers, C., Argus, J.D., and Lucky. A. (2001) Avian mite bites acquired from a new source--pet gerbils: report of 2 cases and review of the literature. *Archives of Dermatology*, **137**(2), 167–170.

Meckley, P.E. and Zwicker, G.M. (1979) Naturally-occurring neoplasms in the Mongolian gerbil, *Meriones unguiculatus*. *Laboratory Animals*, **13**(3), 203–206.

McGinn, M.D., Chole, R.A., and Henry, K.R. (1984) Cholesteatoma induction. Consequences of external auditory canal ligation in gerbils, cats, hamsters, guinea pigs, mice and rats. *Acta Otolaryngology*, **97**(3–4), 297–304.

Peckham, J.C., Cole, J.R., Chapman, W.L., et al. (1974) Staphylococcal dermatitis in Mongolian gerbils. *Laboratory Animal Science*, **24**(1), 43.

Raflo, C.P., and Diamond, S.S. (1980) Metastatic squamous-cell carcinoma in a gerbil (*Meriones unguiculatus*). *Laboratory Animals*, **14**(3), 237–239.

Rowe, S.E., Simmons, J.L., Ringler, D.H., and Lay, D.M. (1974) Spontaneous neoplasms in aging Gerbillinae. A summary of forty-four neoplasms. *Veterinary Pathology*, **11**(1), 38–51.

Sayers, I., and Smith, S. (2010) Mice, rats, hamsters and gerbils. In: *BSAVA Manual of Exotic Pets* (eds. A. Meredith and S. Redrobe), 5th edn. BSAVA, Quedgeley.

Schwarzbrott, S.S., Wagner, J.E., and Frisk, C.S. (1974) Demodicosis in the Mongolian gerbil (*Meriones unguiculatus*), a case report. *Laboratory Animal Science*, **24**(4), 666–668.

Su, Y.C., Wang, M.H., and Wu, M.F. (2001) Cutaneous B cell lymphoma in a Mongolian gerbil (*Meriones unguiculatus*). *Contemporary Topics in Laboratory Animal Science*, **40**(5), 53–56.

Thiessen, D.D. and Kittrell, E.M. (1980) The Harderian gland and thermoregulation in the gerbil (*Meriones unguiculatus*). *Physiology and Behavior*, **24**(3), 417–424.

Thiessen, D.D. and Pendergrass, M. (1982) Harderian gland involvement in facial lesions in the Mongolian gerbil. *Journal of the American Veterinary Medical Association*, **181**(11), 1375–1377.

Thompson, T.A., Gardner, D., Fulghum, R.S., et al. (1981) Indigenous nasopharyngeal, auditory canal, and middle ear bacterial flora of gerbils: animal model for otitis media. *Infection and Immunity*, **32**(3), 1113–1118.

Vincent, A.L., Porter, D.D., and Ash, L.R. (1975) Spontaneous lesions and parasites of the Mongolian gerbil, *Meriones unguiculatus*. *Laboratory Animal Science*, **25**(6), 711–722.

Vincent, A.L., Rodrick, G.E., and Sodeman, W.A. Jr. (1979) The pathology of the Mongolian gerbil (*Meriones unguiculatus*): A review. *Laboratory Animal Science*, **29**(5), 645–651.

Endocrine Conditions

Benitz, K.F. and Kramer, A.W. Jr. (1965) Spontaneous tumors in the Mongolian gerbil. *Laboratory Animal Care*, **15**(5), 281–294.

Bingel, S.A. (1995) Pathologic findings in an aging Mongolian gerbil (*Meriones unguiculatus*) colony. *Laboratory Animal Science*, **45**(5), 597–600.

Boquist, L. (1972) Obesity and pancreatic islet hyperplasia in the Mongolian gerbil. *Diabetologia*, **8**(4), 274–282.

Keeble, E. (2001) Endocrine diseases of small mammals. *In Practice*, Nov/Dec, 570–585.

Keeble, E. (2002) Gerbils. In: *BSAVA Manual of Exotic Pets* (eds. A. Meredith and S. Redrobe), 4th edn. British Small Animal Veterinary Association, Quedgeley, pp. 34–46.

Laber-Laird, K., Swindle, M.M., and Flecknell, P.A (eds.). (1996) *Handbook of Rodent and Rabbit Medicine.* Pergamon, Oxford.

Rowe, S.E., Simmons, J.L., Ringler, D.H., and Lay, D.M. (1974) Spontaneous neoplasms in aging Gerbillinae. A summary of forty-four neoplasms. *Veterinary Pathology*, **11**(1), 38–51.

Sayers, I., and Smith, S. (2010) Mice, rats, hamsters and gerbils. In *BSAVA Manual of Exotic Pets.* (eds. A. Meredith and S. Redrobe), 5th edn. Quedgeley: British Small Animal Veterinary Association.

Troup, G.M., Smith, G.S., and Walford, R.L. (1969) Life span, chronologic disease patterns, and age-related changes in relative spleen weights for the Mongolian gerbil (*Meriones unguiculatus*). *Experimental Gerontology*, **4**(3), 139–143.

Wexler, B.C., Judd, J.T., Lutmer, R.F., and Saroff, J. (1971) Spontaneous arteriosclerosis in male and female gerbils (*Meriones unguiculatus*). *Atherosclerosis*, **14**(1), 107–119.

Respiratory Conditions

Johnson-Delaney, C.A. and Orosz, S.E. (2009) The respiratory system: Exotic companion mammals. *Proceedings of the Association of Exotic Mammal Veterinarians*, Milwaukee, WI, pp. 41–49.

Keeble, E. (2002) Gerbils. In: *BSAVA Manual of Exotic Pets.* (eds. A. Meredith and S. Redrobe), 4th edn. British Small Animal Veterinary Association, Quedgeley, pp. 34–46.

Kling, M.A. (2011) A review of respiratory system anatomy, physiology, and disease in the mouse, rat, hamster, and gerbil. *Veterinary Clinics of North America Exotic Animal Practice*, **14**(2), 287–290.

Troup, G.M., Smith, G.S., and Walford, R.L. (1969) Life span, chronologic disease patterns, and age-related changes in relative spleen weights for the Mongolian gerbil (*Meriones unguiculatus*). *Experimental Gerontology*, **4**(3), 139–143.

Musculoskeletal Conditions

Keeble, E. (2002) Gerbils. In: *BSAVA Manual of Exotic Pets.* (eds. A. Meredith and S. Redrobe), 4th edn. British

Small Animal Veterinary Association, Quedgeley, pp. 34–46.

Thompson, K. (2007) Bones and Joints. In: Jubb, Kennedy, and Maxie, MG (ed). *Palmer's Pathology of Domestic Animals.* 5th edn. Elsevier Saunders, Edinburgh, pp. 82–88.

Encephalomyocarditis Virus Infection

Doi, K. (2011) Experimental encephalomyocarditis virus infection in small laboratory rodents. *Journal of Comparative Pathology*, **144**, 25–40.

Matsukura, N., Doi, K., Mitsuoka, T., Tsuda, T., and Onodera, T. (1989) Experimental encephalomyocarditis virus infection in Mongolian gerbils (*Meriones unguiculatus*). *Veterinary Pathology*, **26**, 11–17.

Gastrointestinal Parasites

Araújo, N.S., Mundim, M.J., Gomes, M.A., et al. (2008) *Giardia duodenalis*: pathological alterations in gerbils, *Meriones unguiculatus*, infected with different dosages of trophozoites. *Experimental Parasitology*, **118**(4), 449–457.

Baker, D.G. (2007) *Flynn's Parasites of Laboratory Animals.* 2nd edn. Blackwell, Ames, IA, pp. 413–420.

Belosevic, M., Faubert, G.M., MacLean, J.D., Law, C., and Croll, N.A. (1983) *Giardia lamblia* infections in Mongolian gerbils: an animal model. *Journal of Infectious Diseases* **147**(2), 222–226.

Hasegawa, H., Sato, H., Iwakiri, E., Ikeda, Y., and Une, Y. (2008) Helminths collected from imported pet murids, with special reference to concomitant infection of the golden hamsters with three pinworm species of the genus *Syphacia* (*Nematoda: oxyuridae*). *Journal of Parasitology*, **94**(3), 752–754.

Johnson, S.S. and Conder, G.A. (1996) Infectivity of *Hymenolepis diminuta* for the Jird, *Meriones unguiculatus*, and utility of this model for anthelmintic studies. *Journal of Parasitology*, **82**(3), 492–495.

Lussier, G. and Loew, F.M. (1970) Case report. Natural *Hymenolepis nana* infection in Mongolian gerbils (*Meriones unguiculatus*). *Canadian Veterinary Journal*, **11**(5), 105–107.

Macnish, M.G., Morgan, U.M., Behnke, J.M., and Thompson, R.C. (2002) Failure to infect laboratory rodent hosts with human isolates of *Rodentolepis* (= *Hymenolepis*) *nana*. *Journal of Helminthology*, **76**(1), 37–43.

Majewska, A.C. (1994) Successful experimental infections of a human volunteer and Mongolian gerbils with *Giardia* of animal origin. *Transactions of the Royal Society of Tropical Medicine and Hygiene*, **88**(3), 360–362.

Pinto, R.M., Gomes, D.C. and Noronha, D. (2003) Evaluation of coinfection with pinworms (*Aspiculuris tetraptera, Dentostomella translucida*, and *Syphacia obvelata*) in gerbils and mice. *Contemporary Topics in Laboratory Animal Science*, **42**(4), 46–48.

Pritchett, K.R. and Johnston, N.A. (2002) A review of treatments for the eradication of pinworm infections from laboratory rodent colonies. *Contemporary Topics in Laboratory Animal Science*, **41**(2), 36–46.

Toft, J.D. and Ekstrom, M.E. (1980) Identification of metazoan parasites in tissue sections. The comparative pathology of zoo animals. *Proceedings of the Symposium of the National Zoologic Park, National Zoological Park.* (eds. R.G. Montali and G. Migaki). Smithsonian Institution, Washington, DC, pp. 369–78.

Vianna, G.J.C. and de Melo, A.L. (2007) Experimental infection and adaptation of *Rodentolepis nana* to the Mongolian jird, *Meriones unguiculatus*. *Journal of Helminthology*, **81**, 345–349.

Vincent, A.L., Porter, D.D., and Ash, L.R. (1975) Spontaneous lesions and parasites of the Mongolian gerbil, *Meriones unguiculatus*. *Laboratory Animal Science*, **25**(6), 711–722.

Hepatic Helicobacteriosis

Bergin, I.L., Taylor, N.S., Nambiar, P.R., and Fox, J.G. (2005) Eradication of enteric *Helicobacters* in Mongolian gerbils is complicated by the occurrence of *Clostridium difficile* enterotoxemia. *Comparative Medicine*, **55**(3), 265–268.

Fox, J.G., Dewhirst, F.E., Shen, Z., et al. (1998) Hepatic *Helicobacter* species identified in bile and gallbladder tissue from Chileans with chronic cholecystitis. *Gastroenterology*, **114**(4), 755–763.

Goto, K., Ohashi, H., Takakura, A., and Itoh, T. (2000) Current status of *Helicobacter* contamination of laboratory mice, rats, gerbils, and house musk shrews in Japan. *Current Microbiology*, **41**(3), 161–166.

Matsukura, N., Yokomuro, S., Yamada, S., et al. (2002) Association between *Helicobacter bilis* in bile and biliary tract malignancies: *H. bilis* in bile from Japanese and Thai patients with benign and malignant diseases in the biliary tract. *Japanese Journal of Cancer Research*, **93**(7), 842–847.

Other Gastrointestinal, Hepatic, and Pancreatic Conditions

Bergin, I.L., Taylor, N.T., and Fox, J.G. (2000) Antibiotic-associated *Clostridium difficile* colitis in Mongolian Gerbils (*Meriones unguiculatus*) treated with amoxicillin/metronidazole/bismuth wafers. *Proceedings of AALAS National Meeting.* San Diego, CA.

Bingel, S.A. (1995) Pathologic findings in an aging Mongolian gerbil (*Meriones unguiculatus*) colony. *Laboratory Animal Science*, **45**(5), 597–600.

Boquist, L. (1972) Obesity and pancreatic islet hyperplasia in the Mongolian gerbil. *Diabetology*, **8**(4), 274–282.

de la Puente-Redondo, V.A., Gutiérrez-Martín, C.B., Pérez-Martínez, C., et al. (1999) Epidemic infection caused by *Citrobacter rodentium* in a gerbil colony. *Veterinary Record*, **145**(14), 400–403.

Moskow, B.S., Wasserman, B.H., and Rennert, M.C. (1968) Spontaneous periodontal disease in the Mongolian gerbil. *Journal of Periodontal Research*, **3**(2), 69–83.

Motzel, S.L. and Gibson, S.V. (1990) Tyzzer disease in hamsters and gerbils from a pet store supplier. *Journal of the American Veterinary Medical Association*, **197**(9), 1176–1178.

Olson, G.A., Shields, R.P., and Gaskin, J.M. (1977) Salmonellosis in a gerbil colony. *Journal of the American Veterinary Medical Association*, **171**, 970–972.

Wagner, J.E. and Farrar, P.L. (1987) Husbandry and medicine of small rodents. *Veterinary Clinics of North America: Small Animal Practice*, **17**(5), 1061–1087.

Tyzzer's Disease

Veazey, R.S., Paulsen, D.B., Schaeffer, D.O. (1992) Encephalitis in gerbils due to naturally occurring infection with Bacillus piliformis (Tyzzer's Disease). *Laboratory Animal Science*, **42**(5), 516–518.

White, D.J. and Waldron, M.M. (1969) Naturally-occurring Tyzzer's disease in the gerbil. *Veterinary Record*, **85**, 111–114.

Gastrointestinal and Hepatic Neoplasia

Meckley, P.E. and Zwicker, G.M. (1979) Naturally-occurring neoplasms in the Mongolian gerbil, *Meriones unguiculatus*. *Laboratory Animals (UK)*, **13**(3), 203–206.

Rowe, S.E., Simmons, J.L., Ringler, D.H., and Lay, D.M. (1974) Spontaneous neoplasms in aging Gerbillinae. A summary of forty-four neoplasms. *Veterinary Pathology*, **11**(1), 38–51.

Vincent, A.L. and Ash, L.R. (1978) Further observations on spontaneous neoplasms in the Mongolian gerbil *Meriones unguiculatus*. *Laboratory Animal Science*, **28**(3), 297–300.

Cardiovascular Conditions

Bingel, S.A. (1995) Pathologic findings in an aging Mongolian gerbil (*Meriones unguiculatus*) colony. *Laboratory Animal Science*, **45**(5), 597–600.

Fox, J.G., Anderson, L.C., Loew, F.M., and Quimby, F.W. (2002) *Laboratory Animal Medicine*, 2nd edn. Academic Press, San Diego, CA, pp. 275–279.

Gordon, S. and Cekleniak, W.P. (1961) Serum lipoprotein pattern of the hypercholesterolemic gerbil. *American Journal of Physiology*, **201**, 27–28.

Hegsted, D.M. and Gallagher, A. (1967) Dietary fat and cholesterol and serum cholesterol in the gerbil. *Journal of Lipid Research*, **8**(3), 210–214.

Matsukura, N., Doi, K., Mitsuoka, T., Tsuda, T., and Onodera, T. (1989) Experimental encephalomyocarditis virus infection in Mongolian gerbils (*Meriones unguiculatus*). *Veterinary Pathology*, **26**, 11–17.

Veazey, R.S., Paulsen, D.B., and Schaeffer, D.O. (1992) Encephalitis in gerbils due to naturally occurring infection with Bacillus piliformis (Tyzzer's Disease). *Laboratory Animal Science*, **42**(5), 516–518.

Wexler, B.C., Judd, J.T., Lutmer, R.F., Saroff, J. (1971) Spontaneous arteriosclerosis in male and female gerbils (*Meriones unguiculatus*). *Atherosclerosis*, **14**(1), 107–119.

Genitourinary Conditions

Benitz, K.F. and Kramer, A.W. Jr. (1965) Spontaneous tumors in the Mongolian gerbil. *Laboratory Animal Care*, **15**(5), 281–294.

Ringel, S.A. (1995) Pathologic findings in an aging Mongolian gerbil (*Meriones unguiculatus*) colony. *Laboratory Animal Science*, **45**(5), 597–600.

Custodia, A.M.G, Santos, F.C.A., Campos, S.G.P., et al. (2008) Aging effects on the Mongolian gerbil female prostate (Skene's paraurethral glands), Structural, ultrastructural, quantitative, and hormonal evaluations. *Anatomical Record*, **291**(4), 463–474.

de la Puente-Redondo, V.A., Gutiérrez-Martín, C.B., Pérez-Martínez, C., et al. (1999) Epidemic infection caused by *Citrobacter rodentium* in a gerbil colony. *Veterinary Record*, **145**(14), 400–403.

Fisher, P.G. (2006) Exotic mammal renal disease: causes and clinical presentation. *Veterinary Clinics of North America: Exotic Animal Practice*, **9**(1), 33–67.

Greenacre, C.B. (2004) Spontaneous tumors of small mammals. *Veterinary Clinics of North America: Exotic Animal Practice*, **7**(3), 627–51, vi.

Guzmán-Silva, M.A, and Costa-Neves, M. (2006) Incipient spontaneous granulosa cell tumour in the gerbil, *Meriones unguiculatus*. *Laboratory Animals (UK)*, **40**(1), 96–101.

Meckley, P.E, and Zwicker, G.M. (1979) Naturally-occurring neoplasms in the Mongolian gerbil, Meriones unguiculatus. *Laboratory Animals (UK)*, **13**(3), 203–6.

Norris, M.L., and Adams, C.E. (1972) Incidence of cystic ovaries and reproductive performance in the Mongolian gerbil, *Meriones unguiculatus*. *Laboratory Animals (UK)*, **6**(3), 337–42.

Oliveira, S.M., Santos, F.A.C., Corradi, L.S., et al. (2011) Microscopic evaluation of proliferative disorders in the gerbil female prostate: Evidence of aging and the influence of multiple pregnancies. *Micron*, **42**, 712–717.

Port, C.D., Baxter, D.W., Richter, W.R. (1974) The Mongolian gerbil as a model for lead toxicity. I. Studies of acute poisoning. *American Journal of Pathology*, **76**(1), 79–94.

Port, C.D., Baxter, D.W., and Righter, W.R. (1975) The Mongolian gerbil as a model for chronic lead toxicity. *Journal of Comparative Pathology*, **85**(1), 119–131.

Port, C.D. (1976) Animal model of human disease: acute and chronic lead nephropathy. *American Journal of Pathology*, **85**(2), 519–522.

Rowe, S.E., Simmons, J.L., Ringler, D.H., and Lay, D.M. (1974) Spontaneous neoplasms in aging Gerbillinae. A summary of forty-four neoplasms. *Veterinary Pathology*, **11**(1), 38–51.

Vincent, A.L., Porter, D.D., and Ash, L.R. (1975) Spontaneous lesions and parasites of the Mongolian gerbil, *Meriones unguiculatus*. *Laboratory Animal Science*, **25**(6), 711–22.

Vincent, A.L., Rodrick, G.E., and Sodeman, W.A. Jr. (1979) The pathology of the Mongolian Gerbil (*Meriones unguiculatus*), a review. *Laboratory Animal Science*, **29**(5), 645–51.

Wagner, J.E., and Farrar, P.L. (1987) Husbandry and medicine of small rodents. *Veterinary Clinics of North America: Exotic Animal Practice*, **17**(5), 1061–1087.

Wexler, B.C., Judd, J.T., Lutmer, R.F., and Saroff, J. (1971) Spontaneous arteriosclerosis in male and female gerbils (*Meriones unguiculatus*). *Atherosclerosis*, **14**(1), 107–119.

White, M.R. (1990) Ovarian cysts in an aged gerbil. *Laboratory Animals (UK)*, **19**, 20–22.

Yahr, P. and Kessler, S. (1975) Suppression of reproduction in water-deprived Mongolian gerbils (*Meriones unguiculatus*). *Biology of Reproduction*, **12**(2), 249–254.

General Urogenital

Bucher, O.M. and Krstić, R.V. (1979) Pericapsular smooth muscle cells in renal corpuscles of the Mongolian gerbil. *Cell Tissue Research*, **199**(1), 75–81.

Oliveira, S.M., Santos, F.A.C., Corradi, L.S., et al. (2011) Microscopic evaluation of proliferative disorders in the gerbil female prostate: Evidence of aging and the influence of multiple pregnancies. *Micron*, **42**, 712–717.

Santos, F.C.A., Leite, R.P., Custódio, A.M.G., et al. (2006) Testosterone stimulates growth and secretory activity of the adult female prostate of the gerbil (*Meriones unguiculatus*). *Biology of Reproduction*, **75**, 370–379.

Santos, F.C.A., Carvalho, H.F., Góes, R.M., and Taboga, S.R. (2003) Structure, histochemistry and ultrastructure of the epithelium and stroma in the gerbil (*Meriones unguiculatus*) female prostate. *Tissue Cell*, **35**, 447–457.

Nervous Conditions

Bingel, S.A. (1995) Pathologic findings in an aging Mongolian gerbil (*Meriones unguiculatus*) colony. *Laboratory Animal Science*, **45**(5), 597–600.

Guzmán-Silva, M.A., Rossi, M.I., and Guimarães, J.S. (1988) Craniopharyngioma in the Mongolian gerbil (*Meriones unguiculatus*): a case report. *Laboratory Animals (UK)*, **22**(4), 365–368.

Heatley, J.J. (2009) Cardiovascular anatomy, physiology, and disease of rodents and small exotic mammals. *Veterinary Clinics of North America: Exotic Animal Practice*, **12**(1), 99–113.

Kaplan, H. and Miezejeski, C. (1972) Development of seizures in the mongolian gerbil (*Meriones unguiculatus*). *Journal of Comparative Physiology and Psychology*, **81**(2), 267–273.

Laidley, D.T., Colbourne, F., and Corbett, D. (2005) Increased behavioral and histological variability arising from changes in cerebrovascular anatomy of the Mongolian gerbil. *Current Neurovascular Research*, **2**(5), 401–407.

Laming, P.R., Cosby, S.L., and O'Neill, J.K. (1989) Seizures in the Mongolian gerbil are related to a deficiency in cerebral glutamine synthetase. *Comparative Biochemistry and Physiology, Part C*, **94**(2), 399–404.

Loskota, W.J., Lomax, P., Rich, S.T. (1974) The gerbil as a model for the study of the epilepsies. Seizure patterns and ontogenesis. *Epilepsia*. **15**(1), 109–119.

Veazey, R.S., Paulsen, D.B., Schaeffer, D.O. (1992) Encephalitis in gerbils due to naturally occurring infection with Bacillus piliformis (Tyzzer's Disease). *Laboratory Animal Science*, **42**(5), 516–518.

Hematopoietic and Lymphoid Conditions

Benitz, K.F., and Kramer, A.W. Jr. (1965) Spontaneous tumors in the Mongolian gerbil. *Laboratory Animal Care*, **15**(5), 281–94.

Bingel, S.A. (1995) Pathologic findings in an aging Mongolian gerbil (*Meriones unguiculatus*) colony. *Laboratory Animal Science*, **45**(5), 597–600.

Chen, H.C., Slone, T.W. Jr, and Frith, C.H. (1992) Histiocytic sarcoma in an aging gerbil. *Toxicologic Pathology*, **20**(2), 260–263.

Dillon, W.G. and Glomski, C.A. (1975) The Mongolian gerbil: qualitative and quantitative aspects of the cellular blood picture. *Laboratory Animals (UK)*, **9**(4), 283–7.

Guzman-Silva, M.A. (1997) Systematic mast cell disease in the Mongolian gerbil, *Meriones unguiculatus*: case report. *Laboratory Animals (UK)*, **31**, 373–378.

Rembert, M.S., Coleman, S.U., Klei, T.R., and Goad, M.E. (2000) Neoplastic mass in an experimental Mongolian gerbil. *Contemporary Topics in Laboratory Animal Science*, **39**(3), 34–6.

Ringle, D.A., and Dellenback, R.J. (1963) Age changes in plasma proteins of the Mongolian gerbil. *American Journal of Physiology*, **204**, 275–278.

Rowe, S.E., Simmons, J.L., Ringler, D.H., Lay, D.M. (1974) Spontaneous neoplasms in aging Gerbillinae. A summary of forty-four neoplasms. *Veterinary Pathology*, **11**(1), 38–51.

Troup, G.M., Smith, G.S., Walford, R.L. (1969) Life span, chronologic disease patterns, and age-related changes in relative spleen weights for the Mongolian gerbil (*Meriones unguiculatus*). *Experimental Gerontology*, **4**(3), 139–143.

Vincent, A.L., Porter, D.D., and Ash, L.R. (1975) Spontaneous lesions and parasites of the Mongolian gerbil, *Meriones unguiculatus*. *Laboratory Animal Science*, **25**(6), 711–22.

Vincent, A.L., and Ash, L.R. (1978) Further observations on spontaneous neoplasms in the Mongolian gerbil *Meriones unguiculatus*. *Laboratory Animal Science* **28**(3), 297–300.

Vincent, A.L., Rodrick, G.F., and Sodeman, W.A. Jr. (1979) The pathology of the Mongolian gerbil (*Meriones unguiculatus*): A review. *Laboratory Animal Science*, **29**(5), 645–651.

Ophthalmic Conditions

Bauck, L. (1989) Ophthalmic conditions in pet rabbits and rodents. *Comparative Cont Education*, **258**(11), 259.

Bihun, C. (2004) Basic anatomy, physiology, husbandry, and clinical techniques. In: *Ferrets, Rabbits and Rodents: Clinical Medicine and Surgery* (eds. K.E. Quesenberry and J.W. Carpenter), 2nd edn. Saunders, St. Louis, MO, pp. 286–298.

Kirschner, S.E. (1997) Ophthalmologic diseases in small mammals. In: *Ferrets, Rabbits and Rodents: Clinical Medicine and Surgery* (eds. E.V. Hillyer and K.E. Quesenberry), 1st edn. Saunders, St. Louis, MO, pp. 339–345.

Ortiz, G.G., Feria-Velasco, A., Falcón-Franco, M.A., et al. (2001) Different patterns in the histology and autofluorescence of the Harderian glands of the Syrian Hamster, rat, mouse, Mongolian gerbil and guinea pig. *Anatomia, Histologia, Embryologia*, **30**(2), 107–115.

Sakai, T. and Yohro, T. (1981) A histological study of the Harderian gland of Mongolian gerbils, *Meriones meridianus. Anatomical Record*, **200**(3), 259–270.

Thiessen, D.D. (1988) Body temperature and grooming in the Mongolian gerbil. *Annals of the New York Academy of Sciences*, **525**, 27–39.

Thiessen, D.D. and Kittrell, E.M. (1980) The Harderian gland and thermoregulation in the gerbil (*Meriones unguiculatus*). *Physiology & Behavior*, **24**(3), 417–424.

Thiessen, D.D. and Pendergrass, M. (1982) Harderian gland involvement in facial lesions in the Mongolian gerbil. *Journal of the American Veterinary Medical Association*, **181**(11), 1375–1377.

8

Mice

8.1   Introduction

Of the pet species covered in this book, mice are least likely to be presented for veterinary care and pathologic examination. Despite this, mice are the most frequently used mammalian species in biomedical research, with tens of millions used globally on an annual basis. There is an enormous body of scientific literature available characterizing their anatomy and physiology, as well as detailed information regarding diseases, neoplasia, and the pathophysiology of aging in laboratory mice. Most laboratory mice kept for research use in North America and Europe are of very high health status and are purchased from large commercial breeders. The aim of many commercial laboratory mouse breeders is to eliminate all known primary viral, bacterial, fungal, and parasitic pathogens that may interfere with research. Many opportunistic pathogens also have been eradicated from these colonies. These mice may be highly inbred for specific characteristics and are housed using methods that minimize their exposure to environmental pathogens and contaminants. This is very different from the ways that pet, show or feeder mice are traditionally kept. The clinician or pathologist seeking information about conditions seen specifically in laboratory mice is advised to seek references from the laboratory mouse pathology literature. This chapter will focus on spontaneous conditions seen in conventionally raised mice, conditions that often differ from those seen in laboratory mice.

Mice may be kept as pets or for show or hobby purposes. There are many fancy mouse breeders and clubs in North America and Europe. Fancy mice bred for show tend to be larger overall with a sleeker body type than typical laboratory mice, and they have larger ears and a longer tail. Mice are bred also for use as feeder rodents for reptile hobbyists and breeders, raptor and wildlife rehabilitation centers, and zoos. Because they are small, mice breed well in captivity, and can be raised successfully in small spaces, and it can be common for commercial feeder breeders to keep tens of thousands of mice in relatively close quarters. This type of operation requires modest capital investment and usually receives minimal veterinary oversight, if any. A moderate (e.g., 20%) mortality level induced by background disease may be accepted by breeders using this type of conventional housing, which would not be tolerated by commercial laboratory mouse breeders or research facilities. Whereas high density housing makes for efficiency in managing animal breeding, this situation can lead to animal welfare issues and explosive disease outbreaks with very high morbidity and mortality when significant infections are present. Disease prevalence can be reduced significantly in most operations but requires more intensive management and early culling of affected animals, and, for specific diseases, cessation of all breeding activities for several months.

When providing information regarding treatment for murine cases, it is critical for the veterinarian to consider the numbers of animals involved, whether neonates are present and may be impacted adversely by therapeutic agents prescribed, whether new animals are added to the colony on a regular basis, the effect of therapeutic agents on prey species (if the mice are being used as feed), the ability of the client to sanitize and disinfect the environment adequately as part of the treatment plan, and the likelihood that wild rodents may be able to access and re-infect colony animals. Conditions that are potentially zoonotic should receive high priority, and emphasizing regular hand washing measures in client reports or discussions to minimize disease transmission is always appropriate.

8.2   Integument Conditions

Fancy mice come in a wide variety of possible coat colors and markings, controlled by over 130 different genes and 1,000 alleles. Similar to other small mammal species, skin conditions are one of the most commonly reported signs in mice because the coat appearance is highly prized by clients, changes in hair coat are observed readily, and because hair or skin irregularities in feeder mice can lead purchasers to refuse animals. There are many possible etiologies for skin diseases in mice. Ectoparasites are very common in pet and feeder mice and should be included as a differential diagnosis in most dermatopathies. A poor, staring, or ruffled coat is often a nonspecific sign of ill-thrift in mice, and a complete post-mortem examination is warranted.

It is important to note that epidermal thickness and hypodermal fat stores change as a consequence of the hair growth cycle, being thickest in anagen. Similarly, sebaceous gland size and density change with age and hair cyclicity. Because hair growth cycles occur as waves over the length of the body, control sections of skin for histopathology should be collected close to affected areas to permit appropriate comparisons.

8.2.1 Alopecia

Congenitally hairless mice are sometimes bred for the pet and fancy mouse markets. These animals have a different genetic defect than athymic hairless mice used in research and are fully immunocompetent.

Nonpruritic hair loss in pet or feeder mice may be due to several etiologies. Common noninfectious causes include mechanical trauma from rough surfaces in the cage, such as the cage floor, lid, feeder, any cage furniture, and occasionally from coarse bedding material. The location of hair loss and whether it is accompanied by other cutaneous abrasions may be helpful in determining an etiology. Barbering, hair chewing or overgrooming are very common in certain strains of mice. Hair or whiskers are chewed at the level of the skin, leaving hairless patches, and usually the skin itself is intact. Hair chewing is a learned behavior that may be performed by any animal in the social hierarchy and is generally indicative of a problem in the cage, or the social or physical environment. Significant self-chewing, self-mutilation, and autophagy may be indicative of chronic pain and distress and should be investigated further.

Mild alopecia with scaling can occasionally be seen with fur mite infestations (see Section 8.2.4.1) as well as with dermatophytoses. Generally, multiple colony animals are affected. Persistent or complex cases of alopecia should be investigated with a diligent search for ectoparasites, a skin scraping, and skin biopsy.

8.2.2 Bacterial Dermatitis and Abscesses

Causes and signs of bacterial dermatitis in mice are similar to those seen for rats and other small mammal pets. There are a few conditions that occur commonly in mice.

8.2.2.1 Ulcerative Dermatitis

Ulcerative dermatitis, characterized by moist, focal to locally extensive exudative lesions, is seen commonly in certain strains (e.g., those of C57BL/6 background) and lines of mice (Figure 8.1). Histologically, ulcerated areas may be covered with a serocellular crust containing scant to numerous bacterial colonies, and moderate to marked mixed inflammatory cell infiltrates are present in the surrounding dermis, depending on the duration and severity of the wound. Partial or complete healing may occur with extensive dermal fibrosis. Lesions are initiated by fighting, mechanical injury, or self-trauma, often in response to ectoparasite infestation, with secondary opportunistic bacterial infection. *Staphylococcus aureus*, *S. xylosus*, and *Streptococcus* spp. are common isolates. In C57BL/6 mice, the condition is often considered idiopathic and is more common in older females and during warm, humid months.

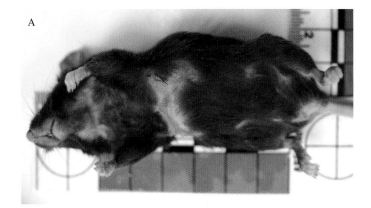
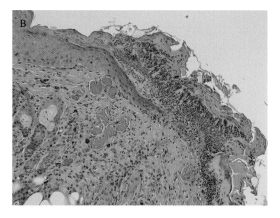

Figure 8.1 A: Ulcerative dermatitis is common in mice, especially those with a C57BL/6 genetic background. The etiopathogenesis is incompletely understood. B: The affected skin is ulcerated with a dense serocellular crust and there is a moderate, predominantly neutrophilic, infiltrate within the superficial dermis and epidermis. Dermal fibrosis may be present in chronic cases and secondary infection with *Staphylococcus aureus* is common.

8.2.2.2 Abscesses and Other Bacterial Skin Conditions

Subcutaneous abscesses and bacterial dermatitis may occur in mice (Figure 8.2) and presentation, causes, and diagnoses are similar to those discussed for the rat (see Chapter 5). Abscesses have been reported occasionally in association with the use of ear tags for identification. Suppurative adenitis involving the preputial or clitoral glands is seen in some animals, often in association with fighting. Opportunistic bacteria, including *Staphylococcus* spp., *Streptococcus* spp., *Pasteurella pneumotropica*, and *Corynebacterium* spp. may be cultured from abscesses and moist dermatitis in mice.

8.2.3 Dermatophytosis

Fungal diseases of mice are similar to those described for rats (see Chapter 5). The overall incidence of infection is low and *Trichophyton mentagrophytes* is the most common fungal agent isolated from skin lesions. Pruritus is usually mild and areas of alopecia and scaling in mice are found more frequently on the head, tail, and neck. Cytology, culture, or histopathology may be used to definitively diagnose fungal infections.

8.2.4 External Parasites

Mice are susceptible to a number of external parasites, which are found commonly in both asymptomatic and pruritic pet and feeder animals.

8.2.4.1 Fur Mites

Most mites affecting mice are from the suborders *Astigmata* and *Prostigmata*, which are surface dwellers with mouthparts adapted for sucking and ingesting superficial secretions and cellular debris. The most

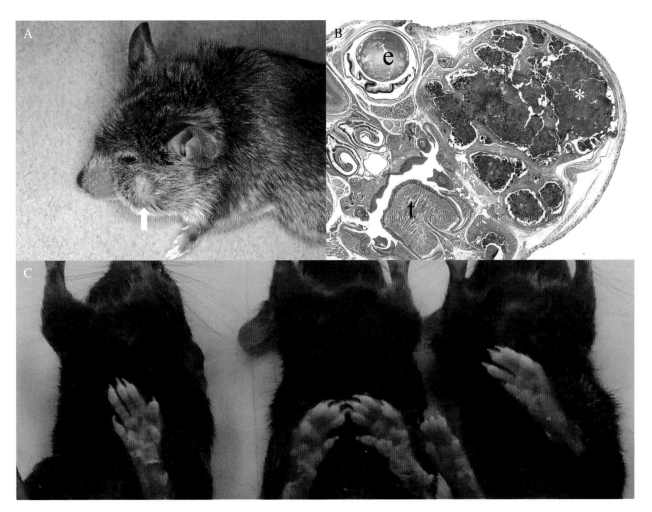

Figure 8.2 A: Facial botryomycosis in a mouse involving the whisker pad (arrow). B: Head section from this mouse demonstrating dense staphylococcal bacterial colonies in grape-like clusters surrounded by bright eosinophilic Splendore-Hoeppli material (*). There is a marked neutrophilic infiltrate. The eye (e) and tongue (t) are labeled for orientation. C: Staphylococcal pododermatitis in several young mice. The condition occurs more frequently during hot and humid ambient conditions. Mice with this condition must be euthanized to avoid development of gangrenous pododermatitis induced by bacterial exotoxins.

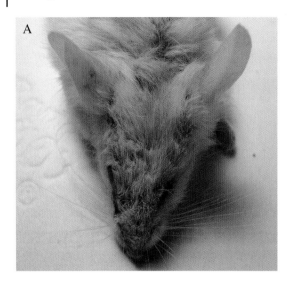
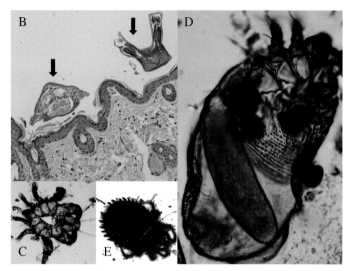

Figure 8.3 A: Mouse with heavy fur mite infestation. Note the patchy alopecia around the head and ears and signs of recent excoriation. B: Photomicrograph of skin from a mouse infested with fur mites (arrows). Mites are in close apposition to the epithelium and are recognizable by their chitinous exoskeleton, jointed appendages, skeletal muscle, and internal digestive tract. Fur mites are surface feeders and minimal inflammation may be induced in the superficial epithelium. C: Mixed infestations with *Myobia musculi* and *Myocoptes musculinus* are common. Shown is a male specimen of *Myocoptes* sp. Mites can be detected readily by applying cellophane tape to the head and neck area and examining microscopically, by histology, and by PCR. D: A gravid female *Myocoptes musculinus*. Eggs, once laid, are readily seen at the base of hairs. E: An example of an *Ornithonyssus bacoti* mite. These are long-legged, highly motile mites and are often gone when the cadaver is examined. The bedding and cadaver packaging material should be checked carefully for mites when infestations are suspected.

common fur mites are *Myobia musculi*, *Myocoptes musculinus*, and *Radfordia affinis*, and mixed infections are common. The entire life cycle is spent on the skin of the host and in the majority of infections, pruritus is mild, and patchy scaling and thinning of the hair coat may be seen at the back of the neck or around the ears, where mites are most numerous (Figure 8.3). Despite their surface-dwelling nature, a strong IgE response may be elicited following infestation in some breeds and strains of mice with marked resultant pruritus and development of ulcerative dermatitis. These mites do not infest humans.

Mesostigmid mites, including the tropical rat mite, *Ornithonyssus bacoti* (Figure 8.3), and the house mouse mite, *Liponyssoides sanguineus*, are highly motile blood-sucking mites found on wild rodents and occasionally on mice obtained from pet stores and feeder colonies. These mites may cause decreased reproductive efficiency, anemia, and death in mice and also may bite humans and other warm-blooded animals, such as cats and dogs. *Liponyssoides sanguineus* can transmit a rickettsial agent, *Rickettsia akari*, which can induce an acute self-limiting febrile disease with hepatitis in humans that clinically can be confused with cutaneous anthrax or smallpox. Morphology distinguishes these mites from *Astigmata* and *Prostigmata* mites.

8.2.4.2 Lice, Fleas and Ticks
Polyplax serrata is a sucking louse found occasionally on pet and feeder mice. They can transmit *Eperythrozoon*

coccoides, a rickettsial agent of mice, but the lice do not bite human handlers. All life cycle phases occur on the host, with eggs attached to the base of the hairs and visible to the unaided eye. Heavy infestations can induce severe pruritus and anemia, with localized excoriations, crusting, edema, and mixed, predominantly neutrophilic superficial epithelial infiltrates (Figure 8.4).

Fleas are uncommon in pet mice and tick infestations are only reported anecdotally.

Laboratory Diagnostics Ectoparasites of mice can often be visualized and identified by pressing a piece of cellophane tape firmly on the pelage, and viewing the tape on a glass slide under the microscope. Parasites can be identified in histologic sections of skin. More mobile mites may move off the host after death and be seen within the shipping container or bag.

Colony Management Although the majority of ectoparasites seen on mice are nonpathogenic, they can be a source of irritation and discomfort to animals, can transmit diseases, and should be eliminated from colonies. Concurrent environmental sanitation and treatment are important to minimize opportunities for re-infestation. Additionally, wild animals must be excluded from breeding operations.

8.2.5 Mousepox

Mousepox is caused by ectromelia virus, an orthopoxvirus related to the causative agents of smallpox, cowpox, and

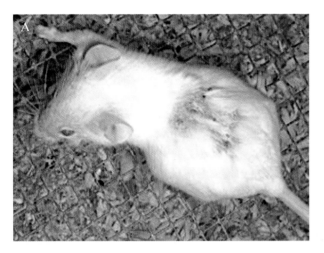
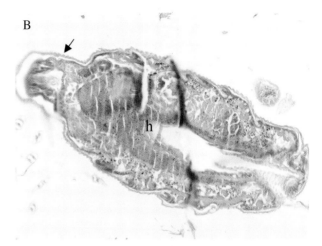

Figure 8.4 A: Mouse from a 10,000-mouse feeder-breeder colony with a heavy *Polyplax serrata* infestation, demonstrating patchy areas of excoriations and serocellular crusting on the back. B: *Polyplax serrata* are sucking lice (Anoplura) with a narrow head and mouthparts (arrow). The central hemocoel (h) is filled with blood and these lice may induce anemia and death in young animals.

monkeypox. Ectromelia virus has been eradicated largely from laboratory mouse colonies in North America and Europe but the virus is still thought to be enzootic in wild mouse populations around the world. The virus is highly contagious and is spread by aerosol or direct contact of microabraded skin with infected material or contaminated fomites. Animals present with depression and inactivity and a primary localized swelling may occur at the site of cutaneous inoculation. From the epidermis, the virus is transmitted to lymphoid tissue and then disseminates throughout the body, with secondary viremia developing from infection of the spleen, liver, and bone marrow. Infected macrophages localize in dermal capillaries, leading to an exanthematous cutaneous rash with later crusting and vasculitis with ischemic necrosis of distal appendages and the tail. The severity of the disease depends upon the strain of mouse and virus, the route of inoculation, and the viral load. In some infections, animals will die within 7–10 days, whereas infections in other strains may be subclinical and cleared incompletely by the host.

Histologically, dermal lesions may initially appear edematous with a marked lymphocytic epithelial infiltrate. Large, eosinophilic intracytoplasmic inclusion bodies may be seen in infected epithelial cells before necrosis and sloughing occur. A serocellular crust forms over the ulcerated area and the local lymph nodes are markedly enlarged and edematous. In animals that survive the primary viremia, a secondary generalized cutaneous rash with conjunctivitis may occur within the following 7–10 days. Lesions resolve with permanent fibrosis and alopecia in survivors. Multifocal splenic and hepatic necrosis may be seen in some animals and splenic scarring occur in those surviving the infection. Animals shed virus into the environment within days of infection and continue shedding until all the skin crusts have fallen off. The virus can remain infective in the environment for months, and thorough environmental disinfection is imperative. Immunity is long-lasting but not lifelong in survivors.

8.2.6 Cutaneous Masses and Neoplasia

Mice develop the same range of cutaneous tumors as seen in other species (Figures 8.5, 8.6, and 8.7). However, other than mammary tumors, epithelial tumors are relatively uncommon spontaneous lesions in pet mice. Preputial gland ectasia can be seen in aging mice as well as in some specific strains as a congenital lesion.

8.2.6.1 Mammary Gland Tumors

Mammary tumors are the most common tumor in sexually mature female mice, with estimated prevalence up to 70% in some strains. As for rats, mammary gland tissue is distributed widely over the ventrum and up the sides, flanks, and neck. Mouse mammary tumors are sensitive to prolactin and estrogen levels, although, unlike rats, most mammary tumors in mice are adenocarcinomas. Masses can be very large and may ulcerate. Most mice carry one or more endogenous oncogenic mammary retroviruses (mouse mammary tumor viruses, MMTV), which determine susceptibility to and malignancy of tumors. Retroviruses may be transmitted both horizontally via the milk and vertically between generations of mice. Mammary gland tumors are thought to arise in terminal ductules and alveoli.

Microscopically, masses may be single or multiple, are generally unencapsulated, and may have a solid, acinar or papillary pattern, with or without central necrosis and local invasion (Figure 8.8). Metastases tend to occur late in the disease with nodules noted primarily in the lungs.

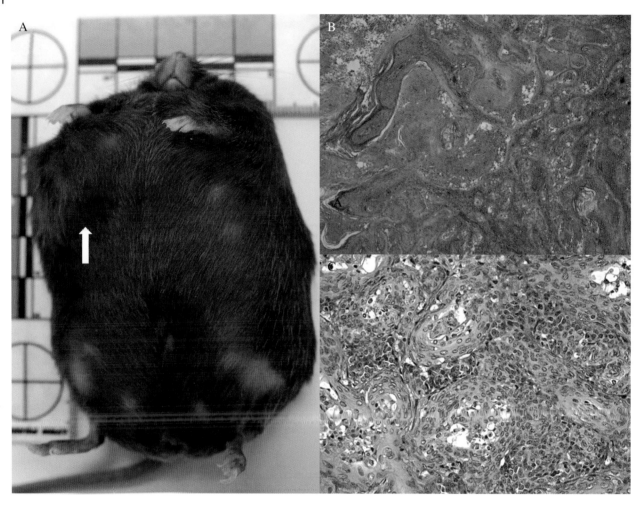

Figure 8.5 A: Keratoacanthoma (arrow) in an obese mouse. B: Masses are well differentiated and overlain by a hyperplastic epithelium. C: Whorls of epithelial cells within the dermis surround central cavities filled with keratin. Sometimes a single central pore exists and keratinaceous material may be extruded. Contrast this with Figure 8.6.

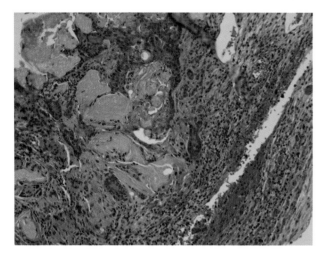

Figure 8.6 Squamous cell carcinoma excised from the neck of a mouse. In contrast to Figure 8.5, this mass is poorly circumscribed and small clusters of basophilic neoplastic cells have penetrated into the underlying hypodermis, accompanied by a mixed inflammatory cell infiltrate.

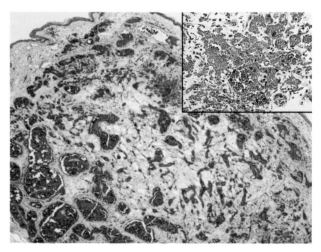

Figure 8.7 Cutaneous hemangioma in a mouse. The raised mass appeared red grossly, and is well circumscribed and composed of blood-filled channels lined by flattened endothelial cells (inset). No mitoses are present.

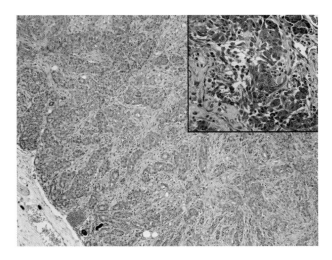

Figure 8.8 Mammary tumors are common in female mice. This mass has an acinar pattern with moderate fibrovascular tissue. While much of this tumor is well circumscribed, clusters of less well differentiated neoplastic cells are seen at the periphery (inset), consistent with an adenocarcinoma.

8.2.6.2 Preputial Gland Ectasia

Uni- or bilateral fluctuant nonpainful subcutaneous masses may occasionally be observed on either side of the penis in aging male mice. In some animals, these may rupture with ulceration of the overlying skin. Histologically, these correspond to cystic dilatation of the preputial glands, with attenuation of the lining epithelium and fluid

and keratinaceous debris within the lumena (Figure 8.9). The incidence of this lesion may be moderately high within certain breeds and strains of mice. The etiopathogenesis is unknown but likely reflects a degenerative change. Differential diagnoses for this condition include abscesses, cystic dilatation of the bulbourethral glands, and preputial gland neoplasia.

8.2.7 Other Skin Conditions

8.2.7.1 Ringtail

Ringtail, which is recognized by annular constrictions of the tail with distal swelling and ischemic necrosis of the tail, may occur in infant and weanling mice under conditions of low humidity and temperature, as in rats. The condition is seasonal, with increased incidence in the winter. The exact pathogenesis of the condition is unknown, although recent studies have suggested primary or secondary cornification disorders as an underlying etiology.

8.2.7.2 Auricular Chondritis

Auricular chondritis, characterized by bilateral nodular thickening and granulomatous inflammation of the ear cartilage with necrosis and osseous metaplasia, is reported as both a rare spontaneous condition of older mice and following the use of ear tags for identification of mice. It has been hypothesized that metal ions in the ear tags induce an autoimmune response, leading to chronic inflammation.

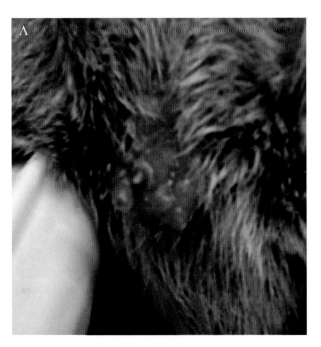

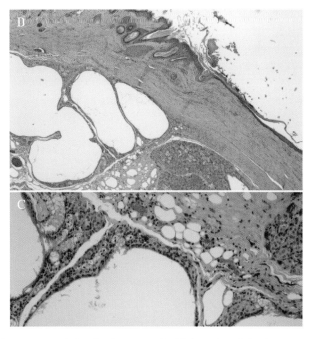

Figure 8.9 A: Cystic preputial glands in a mouse with recurrent paraphimosis. B: Multifocally, there is marked, bilateral, multifocal dilatation of the preputial glands with mild orthokeratotic hyperkeratosis, acanthosis, and loss of adnexal structures in the overlying epidermis. C: Glands are lined by attenuated epithelium. *Source:* A: Courtesy of K. Nielsen.

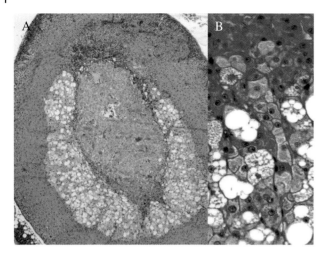

Figure 8.10 A: Adrenal gland depicting X-zone between cortex and medulla. B: The X zone spontaneously regresses in male mice at puberty and in female mice following their first pregnancy.

8.3 Endocrine Conditions

Although mice are used frequently as induced models of diabetes mellitus, spontaneous endocrine conditions and related tumors are rarely reported in pet mice.

There is sexual dimorphism in adrenal gland size and function, with female mice displaying larger glands and increased levels of circulating ACTH, aldosterone, and corticosterone. Mice also demonstrate a unique transitory layer (X zone) of vacuolated cells surrounding the inner cortex, which spontaneously regresses in male mice at puberty and in female mice at their first pregnancy (Figure 8.10). The function of this cellular layer is unknown. Spontaneous changes are noted commonly in the adrenal glands of aging mice, but are generally interpreted as incidental. This includes adrenocortical atrophy or hypertro-

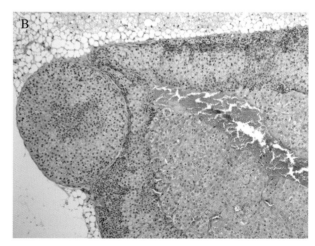

Figure 8.11 Pituitary adenoma from an aged mouse. The tumors compress surrounding brain structures, which may result in clinical signs, depending on the rate of growth and the degree of compensation. Neoplastic epithelial cells are arranged in cords, within a fine fibrovascular stroma (inset).

phy, nodular hyperplasia (generally subcapsular), pigment deposition, and extramedullary hematopoiesis.

Pituitary adenomas are only reported sporadically (Figure 8.11). Amyloid deposition may occur in the thyroid gland of aged mice. Thyroid gland hyperplasia is often seen in mice exposed to environmental contaminants. Thyroid gland ectasia is common in aging mice as is adrenal cortical hyperplasia (Figure 8.12).

8.4 Respiratory Conditions

Mice have high respiratory rates because of their rapid metabolism, inspiring up to 35 L of air per day. Because

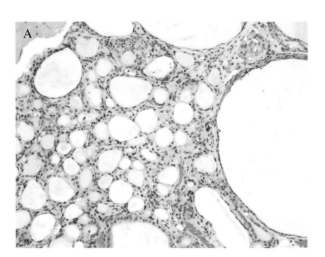

Figure 8.12 A: Thyroid gland ectasia in an aged mouse demonstrating variable dilatation of follicles, which are lined by flattened epithelium. B: Adrenocortical nodule formation; nodules may or not be associated with clinical signs of hyperadrenocorticism.

of this, mice are very sensitive to changes in relative humidity, which will alter hydration of their mucous membranes, as well as to levels of irritating particulates and volatile contaminants within their environment. Poor husbandry conditions leading to increased levels of ammonia and carbon dioxide may exacerbate the deleterious effects of opportunistic and pathogenic respiratory microorganisms.

Mice are obligate nose breathers and the nasal architecture is relatively complex, suited for functions of respiration, filtering of various respiratory pathogens and particulates, and finely tuned olfaction. Mice have a sensitive vomeronasal organ located in the rostral nasal passages that detects chemosensory cues and it is linked to a large olfactory bulb.

The relative size of nasal- and bronchus-associated lymphoid tissue is variable, and based on antigenic stimulation. Hyaline droplets may be extruded into the lumen of the nasal passages by respiratory epithelium, and extrusion may increase when mice are exposed to respiratory irritants. Mice have no intrapulmonary cartilaginous rings to support bronchioles and have a single left lung lobe and four lobes on the right.

8.4.1 Bacterial Diseases

8.4.1.1 Mycoplasmosis

Mycoplasma pulmonis, an important agent of chronic murine respiratory disease, has been eradicated largely from laboratory mouse colonies but remains a very important infection of mice raised and housed under conventional conditions. The organism is small and pleiomorphic, lacking a cell wall.

Presenting Clinical Signs Subclinical infections are common with *M. pulmonis*, and signs may not manifest until late in the course of the disease. Clinical signs in infected animals may include staring hair coat, weight loss, lethargy, and reduced reproductive performance, as well as dyspnea, chattering, sneezing, oculonasal discharge, head tilt, and chromodacryorrhea. Animals may be found dead with few prodromal signs.

Pathology Grossly, there may be chronic suppurative rhinitis, suppurative otitis media, tracheitis, and patchy bronchopneumonia with abscessation (Figure 8.13). Microscopically, pulmonary lesions are characterized by marked suppurative to pyogranulomatous to lymphoplasmacytic peribronchiolar inflammation with squamous metaplasia or loss of ciliated bronchiolar epithelial lining, necrosis of peribronchiolar smooth muscle, and accumulation of mature and degenerate neutrophils, mucus, and sloughed cellular debris within airways. Affected airways may be collapsed and inflammation may extend into the surrounding parenchyma. In chronic cases, there may be marked peribronchiolar and perivascular lymphoid aggregates.

Laboratory Diagnostics Whereas serology is used commonly for colony surveillance, it can take several months for individual animals to develop antibodies to the organism and seroconvert, therefore serology is not a reliable tool for diagnosis of an acute infection. Both PCR assay and culture can be used to confirm suspected cases. *M. pulmonis* is a fastidious organism and may grow slowly in culture. There are several strains of *M. pulmonis*, with varying pathogenicity.

Disease/Colony Management *M. pulmonis* is highly contagious and spread by aerosol or direct contact. Infection may be widespread within a colony by the time it is detected. Chronic infections are difficult to treat, and, in breeding colonies, affected animals should be culled to minimize environmental contamination. The disease may be transmitted between mice and rats, and feral animals should always be excluded from breeding colonies. Complete eradication from an infected colony may require depopulation and repopulation with known negative stock. New colony introductions should be quarantined and observed for clinical respiratory signs. Donor colony serology surveillance reports, if available, should be reviewed before accepting new stock from other breeders.

Differential Diagnoses Co-infections with cilia-associated respiratory bacillus (CARB) are very common, and the two infections are indistinguishable without special histologic staining (see Section 8.4.1.2). Infection with *Corynebacterium kutscheri* may induce pulmonary abscesses and can be distinguished on culture and by microscopic examination, and by the presence of abundant Gram-positive coccobacilli in and around the necrosuppurative lesions. *Pasteurella pneumotropica* may induce rhinitis, otitis media, and pneumonia with anteroventral consolidation but tends to be less suppurative and more localized than *M. pulmonis*. *Streptococcus pneumonia* may induce otitis media, rhinitis, and a fibrinosuppurative pleuropneumonia in mice. Other bacterial pathogens may be distinguished from *M. pulmonis* infection by histopathology and bacterial culture. Common viral agents inducing pneumonia in mice, including Sendai virus and pneumonia virus of mice, can be differentiated microscopically and by serology. Subclinical viral infection may predispose animals to secondary bacterial disease by *M. pulmonis* or other agents.

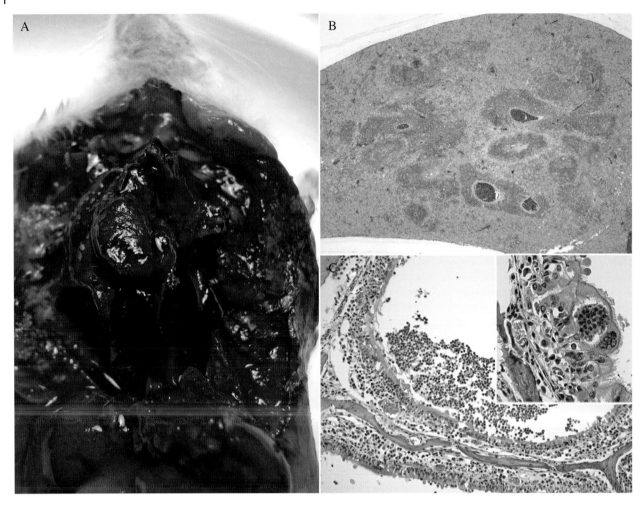

Figure 8.13 Suppurative bronchopneumonia and rhinitis in a feeder-breeder mouse infected with *Mycoplasma pulmonis*. A: Multifocal pulmonary abscesses are present throughout the lungs. B: Photomicrograph of the lung demonstrating marked peribronchiolar and perivascular lymphoid aggregates. C: Marked suppurative rhinitis is present with marked lumenal accumulation of mature and degenerate neutrophils admixed with cellular debris and desquamated respiratory epithelium, intraepithelial pustules (inset) and multinucleated giant cells consistent with chronic infection.

8.4.1.2 Cilia-Associated Respiratory Bacillus Infections (CARB)

Cilia-associated respiratory bacilli (CARB) are gliding, filamentous bacteria that are capable of infecting the respiratory tract of mice. CARB may be transmitted between rats and mice but generally require direct nose-to nose contact for transmission. Rabbits also may harbor CARB; however, the murine and leporid strains are species-specific and rarely, if ever, cross-infect other species. The presenting signs and pathology for CARB are identical to those described for *Mycoplasma pulmonis*, and infections with one or both agents are common within pet populations. CARB is agyrophillic and induces pathology by intercalating between cilia on respiratory mucosa, interfering with beating patterns, and predisposing to secondary bacterial or viral infections. The organism cannot be cultured by traditional techniques and is best

demonstrated histologically using a Warthin-Starry stain or by polymerase chain reaction (PCR) of affected tissue. Serologic testing is non-specific. Early treatment of affected pets or colonies with antimicrobials may eradicate the disease; however, treatment of chronically infected animals is usually intermittent and palliative.

8.4.1.3 Other Bacterial Infections

Pasteurella pneumotropica is a Gram-negative, nonmotile coccobacillus and is an opportunistic pathogen for rodents and rabbits. Whereas subclinical infections with the bacteria are moderately to highly common in laboratory and pet mice, clinical disease is uncommon. The bacterium may colonize the middle ear, lacrimal glands, upper and lower respiratory tract, and urogenital tract, leading to corresponding signs of head tilt, suppurative conjunctivitis, and lymphadenitis, sneezing, rhinitis, pneumonia, reproductive

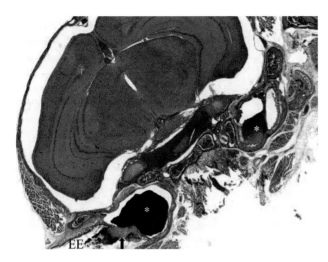

Figure 8.14 Bilateral otitis media in a mouse infected with *Pasteurella pneumotropica*. The middle ears (*) are filled with dense mats of mature and degenerate neutrophils. Unilaterally, there is inflammation of the tympanic membrane (arrow) with exudation into the external ear (EE) canal.

failure, and abortion (Figure 8.14). In severe cases, abscesses may be apparent grossly in the lungs. The agent is transmitted by direct contact, and exclusion of feral rodents from breeding operations is important in its eradication. Detection is best performed by PCR or culture.

Although mice may be infected experimentally with *Bordetella bronchiseptica*, a Gram-negative rod, natural infection or even isolation is uncommon and it is not considered a primary respiratory pathogen of mice. *B. hinzi* has recently been reported as a low prevalence bacterial contaminant of laboratory mouse colonies, and signs noted in affected animals included sneezing, chattering, and acute bronchopneumonia.

Streptococcus pneumoniae is a Gram-positive, alpha-hemolytic bacterium that is carried within the oropharynx of mice and other rodents. Clinical disease is uncommon in immunocompetent animals, but, when it occurs, lesions may consist of fibrinopurulent otitis media, rhinitis, pleuropneumonia, pericarditis, or meningitis. The disease is transmitted by aerosol or in oculonasal secretions, and the bacteria can be cultured readily from infected animals. Coccoid bacteria can be visualized in lesions, often forming pairs or short chains. Humans frequently carry this organism in their oropharynx and may transmit the bacterium to mice and other small mammal pets.

Klebsiella pneumoniae and *Corynebacterium kutscheri* are infrequently isolated from clinical respiratory conditions in mice. These organisms, when present, may be cultured from the oropharynx. *Francisella tularensis* infections are enzootic amongt wild mice (including house mice) and other rodents in the United States, Canada, and parts of Europe and Asia. Infected animals may display signs and lesions consistent with a necrotizing pneumonia. Increased human cases of tularemia have been correlated with epizootics of *F. tularensis* infections in wild mice. Wild mice should be excluded from mouse holding and breeding areas, and human caregivers and others handling contaminated cages, equipment, and cadavers should wash hands carefully afterwards.

8.4.2 Pneumocystosis

Pneumocystis murina is a ubiquitous ascomycete fungal agent that is associated with pneumonia in immunodeficient strains of mice. Immunocompetent animals clear the infection within 2–6 weeks of infection but shed abundant infective organisms into the environment until immunity develops. Pups are protected initially by colostral antibodies. Affected immunodeficient mice may waste and die of a chronically progressive pneumonia. Grossly, lungs appear inflated and pale, and an interstitial alveolitis is present microscopically, with thickening of septa, interstitial lymphohistiocytic or pyogranulomatous infiltrates, and aggregates of alveolar macrophages containing foamy intracytoplasmic material. Cyst forms are usually readily apparent in immunodeficient mice by using a Gomori methenamine-silver (GMS) stain on affected tissue. Specific lesions may not be present grossly or microscopically in immunocompetent mice and intrapulmonary cyst forms cannot be visualized using a GMS stain, as in immunodeficient mice. The organism may be detected by PCR, regardless of host immune status. It is difficult to know the prevalence of pneumocystosis in pet mice but it is assumed to be high, as per wild mice.

8.4.3 Viral Respiratory Diseases

Sendai virus and pneumonia virus of mice (PVM) are two different mouse paramyxoviruses that historically have been very important as causes of murine respiratory disease in laboratory settings. Neither has been isolated recently from pet or wild mice. PVM is a member of the respiratory syncytial virus family and causes an acute, mild, and self-limiting infection in mice that is subclinical in immunocompetent animals. Severe, nonsuppurative interstitial pneumonia with wasting and death may be seen in immunodeficient animals. Viral diagnosis is achieved typically via serology or PCR.

Sendai virus is a member of the P-1 parainfluenza virus family and the disease is highly contagious and transmitted by aerosol. The infection is acute and, in immunocompetent animals, the disease is usually subclinical, although some strain variations are seen in susceptibility. For example, DBA/2 mice are highly susceptible to Sendai virus infection and subsequent disease, as these mice mount a delayed immune response, allowing the virus to become deeply seated within the respiratory tree. Pulmonary damage is largely mediated by the host immune response. In affected animals, plum-colored consolidation of the anteroventral lobes may be seen grossly, with patchy, nonsuppurative, necrotizing bronchiolitis seen microscopically (Figure 8.15). Diagnosis is by serology or PCR. Although it is sporadically reported with low prevalence in wild rats, it is not reported in wild mice.

Polyomavirus and cytomegalovirus infections may occur in mice and can involve the respiratory tract, but infections are often subclinical, except in neonates, in which infections can occasionally be fatal. Both viruses may induce distinctive and species-typical intranuclear inclusion bodies; however, cytomegalovirus inclusions are more common in salivary glands whereas polyomavirus inclusions are more common in pulmonary endothelial cells or elsewhere in the body. Prevalence of cytomegalovirus infection approaches 100% in wild mouse populations, and wild mice should always be excluded from pet or mouse feeder breeding colonies.

Hantaviruses, enveloped DNA viruses in the Bunyaviridae family, were first reported in 1993 as the cause of hantaviral pulmonary syndrome and hemorrhagic fever with renal syndrome in humans exposed to infected rodent urine in the southwest United States. They since have been linked to human disease in most continents, and all exposures have been linked to rodent transmission. The virus is found in the saliva, urine, and feces of rodent hosts and may be transmitted by aerosolization or direct bites. Infections are subclinical in the rodent host for which the virus is specifically adapted; however, experimentally challenged laboratory mice develop severe pulmonary disease with pleural effusion, lymphoid depletion, and endothelial cell necrosis. Suspicious deaths and outbreaks

of disease in pet, fancy, or feeder mouse breeding colonies should always be investigated to determine whether potentially zoonotic agents are present. In North America, viruses typically are carried by deer mice (*Peromyscus maniculatus*), white-footed mice (*P. leucopus*), various voles (*Microtus* spp.), cotton rats (*Sigmodon hispidus*), rice rats (*Oryzomys palustris*), and other wild rats (*Rattus* spp.). Viral prevalence may exceed 50% in the rodent host, and diagnosis is based on serology or PCR findings. Whereas they are not common pathogens of laboratory mice, hantaviruses may cause serious zoonotic disease with mortality. For this reason, wild rodents should be excluded from captive rodent breeding colonies. Caregivers should always wash hands thoroughly after touching rodents or their cages, and rescued feral or semiferal rodents should always be quarantined away from other rodent pet or breeding colony animals to ensure that they are free of apparent disease before introducing them to colony animals.

8.4.4 Pulmonary Neoplasia

Pulmonary hyperplasia and subsequent tumor formation are very common in older mice, with marked strain-specific prevalence and higher incidence in females. Tumors are thought to arise from Clara cells or type II pneumocytes. While generally benign, they grow by compressing normal parenchyma and may induce respiratory compromise with signs of dyspnea and hunched posture in some animals. Murine lung tumors metastasize rarely and are often an incidental finding at necropsy. Pulmonary tumors are classified simply as adenomas or carcinomas. Carcinomas may be categorized further, according to histologic appearance, including papillary, solid, or mixed.

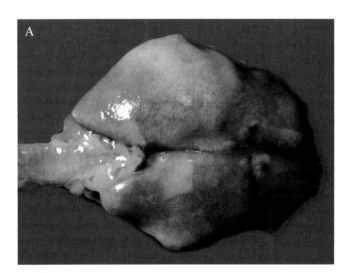
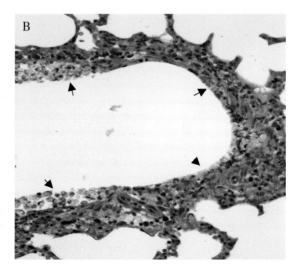

Figure 8.15 Sendai virus infection in a mouse. A: Multifocal plum-colored areas of consolidation are noted. B: Airways are predominantly affected with desquamation of necrotic ciliated bronchiolar epithelium and leukocytic infiltrate (arrows). *Source:* A: Courtesy of J.H. Park.

In animals with leukemia or thymic lymphosarcoma, neoplastic lymphocytes may be present on the pleural surfaces, within alveolar interstitia or as perivascular aggregates. These neoplasms must be differentiated from perivascular mononuclear cell aggregates seen in conventionally housed mice that form in response to environmental antigen exposure or secondary to pulmonary infections. The latter can be large and coalescing and generally have a mixed population of lymphocytes, plasma cells, and histiocytes, compared with more monomorphic neoplastic aggregates. Mammary and hepatic carcinomas may metastasize to the lungs. Other tumors involving pulmonary parenchyma, such as squamous cell carcinoma and mesothelioma, are uncommon.

8.4.5 Other Respiratory Conditions

Rhinitis, necrosis of the olfactory and respiratory epithelium, and nasal turbinate atrophy may occur in mice exposed to high ammonia levels (e.g., those exceeding 50 ppm), as may occur when mice are overcrowded or when cages become heavily soiled.

Intracellular aggregations of amorphous eosinophilic material may be seen within the nasal epithelium of mice, as well as in the glandular stomach, gall bladder, esophagus, and other tissues. The proteins have been identified as YM1/2 chitinases and may play a role in allergy sensitization.

Subpleural and alveolar histiocytosis may be seen in older mice and consists of aggregates of macrophages, some of which may contain intracytoplasmic hemosiderin, foamy material or cholesterol clefts. Without other signs of inflammation, these aggregates are interpreted as incidental.

Mild, patchy pulmonary congestion and hemorrhage are seen commonly in mice euthanatized by CO_2 inhalation.

8.5 Musculoskeletal Conditions

As for other rodents, mice have no Haversian systems within their bones and growth plates remain open for life. Spontaneous musculoskeletal problems are uncommon in pet mice.

Paresis or paralysis with deep cellulitis and myositis may occur in mice secondarily to fighting injuries (Figure 8.16). Paralysis may also occur secondary to fibro-osseous hyperplasia (see Section 8.10), neoplastic infiltration of musculature or following development of other conditions inducing neuronal degeneration (Figure 8.17). Animals that are malnourished or suffering from inanition from many different potential causes may present with apparent ataxia or weakness. Other systemic conditions should be explored if no apparent underlying musculoskeletal conditions are detected.

Idiopathic eosinophilic myositis involving cardiac and skeletal muscle has been reported in one group of mice presenting with ataxia, weakness, and difficulty in righting when placed on their backs. Sarcocystosis of skeletal muscles is a common finding in field mice but is not reported in pet mice. Severe vitamin E and selenium deficiencies in the diet may induce myopathy of both skeletal and cardiac muscle, secondary to peroxidative injury.

Although numerous mouse models exist for spontaneous and induced arthritis in laboratory mice, only anecdotal reports exist for the development of spontaneous arthritis in pet mice. Infection with Streptobacillus mon-

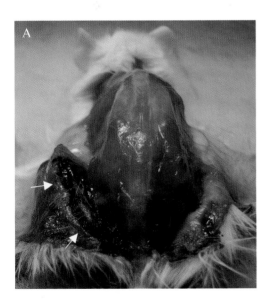
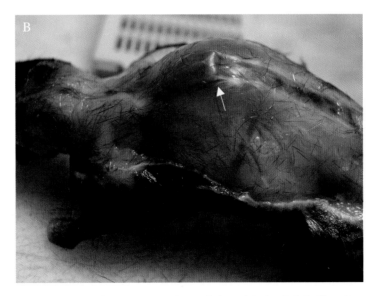

Figure 8.16 A: Myositis and cellulitis (arrows) with subsequent paresis in a male mouse, secondary to fighting injuries. B: Spinal luxation (arrow) in a mouse with hemiparalysis secondary to an inappropriate restraint technique.

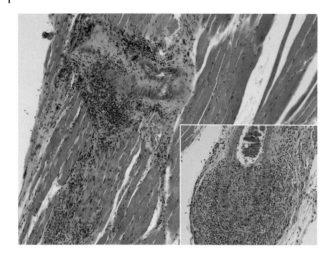

Figure 8.17 Multifocal polyarteritis with secondary myodegeneration in a 1.25 year-old mouse with bilateral hind limb paresis. Polyarteritis may develop as a result of antigen-antibody complex deposition with subsequent complement activation, mixed leukocytic infiltration and fibrinoid necrosis of the tunica muscularis, with partial lumenal occlusion (inset).

iliformis can lead to joint swelling and fibrinosuppurative polyarthritis.

Trauma with subsequent luxation or bony fracture of the legs and vertebrae are common in mice (Figure 8.16). These may occur in animals that are not restrained properly, are inadvertently dropped, or when animals' legs are caught between cage bars or spokes of exercise wheels. Pathologic

fractures may also occur secondary to neoplastic infiltration of bone, leading to paresis or paralysis, depending on the fracture site. Pathologic fractures occur commonly with osteosarcomas and lymphosarcoma.

Osteosarcomas (Figure 8.18) and rhabdomyosarcomas are reported sporadically in older mice. Chondroma, ossifying fibromas, and hemangiomas are very rare. Potential differentials for firm fast-growing masses include peripheral nerve sheath tumors (Figure 8.18).

8.6 Gastrointestinal Conditions

Mice are monophydont coprophagic omnivores. Similar to many other rodents, they have constantly growing incisors and fixed molars, with a dental formal of 1/1, 0/0, and 3/3, for a total of 16 teeth. The occlusal surfaces of the molar teeth are normally flat. Some independent movement of the lower incisors can be seen because of the split mandibular symphysis. Renin is produced in the sublingual and submaxillary salivary glands of mice, as well as in the coagulating glands. There is sexual dimorphism of salivary glands in mice, and mature male mice have larger acini lined by columnar cells containing abundant secretory granules, whereas acini of female mice are smaller and lined by cuboidal cells.

Mice have a single, simple stomach divided into a thin-walled, keratinized, nonglandular portion and a glandular

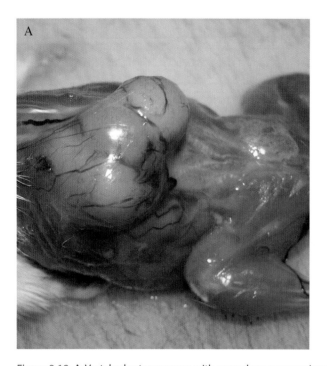

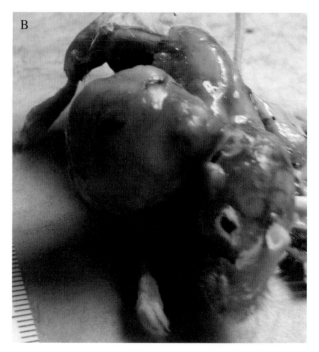

Figure 8.18 A: Vertebral osteosarcoma with secondary compression of the spinal cord and paresis. B: Peripheral nerve sheath tumor on the shoulder of a mouse. This mass was very fast-growing achieving the depicted size within a week. The animal demonstrated rapid onset of forelimb paralysis.

portion. The lamina propria of the glandular portion contains simple tubular gastric glands and the mucosa consists of columnar epithelial cells. Similar to other rodents, mice are unable to vomit. Small intestinal villi are finger-shaped, similar to villi of humans and dogs. Mice have significantly higher β-glucuronidase activity throughout their intestinal tract compared with other mammals, accounting in part for their high rate of metabolism of many chemical substances. Regional expression of various proteins throughout the digestive tract is highly dependent upon the specific bacterial flora. Flora becomes established shortly after birth and remains relatively stable throughout the life of an animal, although this depends on a constant diet and the use of antimicrobial agents. The rectum of mice is short and not enveloped in serosa, making it very susceptible to prolapse under conditions of rectal inflammation, irritation, obstipation, or tenesmus.

The mouse liver has four main lobes, although some variability may be seen in lobation. They also have a gall bladder. Histologically, anisokaryosis, cytomegaly, and binucleate hepatocytes are common, with the incidence increasing with age. Depending on when animals are euthanatized or die in relation to eating, there may be marked perinuclear hepatocellular rarefaction, indicative of glycogen accumulation. Generalized hepatocellular macrovesiculation is common in obese animals.

8.6.1 Oral Conditions

Overgrowth and malocclusion of the incisors are commonly seen in mice. These teeth may subsequently fracture or grow and penetrate the surrounding soft tissue or oral mucosa, leading to pain, local inflammation, cheilitis, or ulceration. Loss of dental pulp, enamel, and odontoblasts is present microscopically in maloccluded incisors, with replacement by fibrous mesenchymal tissue and inflammatory cells. The pathogenesis of incisor malocclusion may be related to insufficient wear of elodont incisors or may be due to primary incisor malformation. Intrapulpal denticles and calcified pulp material (pulp stones) are reported in mice, both of which may interfere with inductive epithelium and tooth growth, and lead to dental dysplasias. Supernumerary incisors may be seen occasionally within or beside fractured incisors.

Impacted hair fragments with secondary foreign body gingivitis, stomatitis, and glossitis are common in mice (Figure 8.19) and may predispose animals to anorexia. Fragments of hair may be found anywhere in the oral cavity but are common around the gingival sulci and periodontal ligaments of the third maxillary molars. An intense, localized, mixed, predominantly neutrophilic infiltrate may be seen in association with moderate edema. In more chronic cases, accompanying erosion of the tooth or underlying alveolar bone may be seen, with a marked local and responsive myelopoiesis in nearby marrow spaces.

Dental caries are reported sporadically in pet mice (Figure 8.19). Odontogenic or other oral tumors are rare with only sporadic reports of odontomas in mice.

Salivary gland infection with cytomegalovirus is common in wild and pet mice, although infections are usually mild and subclinical. Large, characteristic eosinophilic intracytoplasmic and intranuclear inclusion bodies may be seen in the salivary glands of infected animals with accompanying mild lymphocytic infiltrates. Rarely, the virus may reactivate inducing systemic disease, including multifocal hepatic, splenic, and adrenocortical necrosis. Mouse thymic virus (murid herpesvirus-3), another herpesvirus, but one that causes marked thymic necrosis in

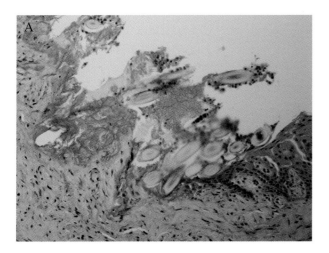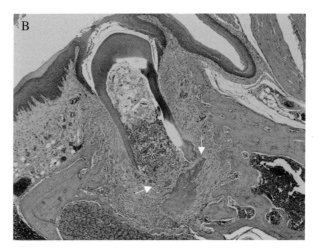

Figure 8.19 A: Foreign body stomatitis in a mouse with anorexia. Embedded hair fragments and bacteria are seen. This condition is common in C57BL/6 mice that barber or overgroom, but may also be seen in other strains of mice. B: Tooth root lysis with bony fragmentation and associated inflammation (arrows) in a mouse presenting with anorexia.

newborn mice, can also be isolated commonly from the salivary glands of chronically infected mice. This virus is also common in wild mice.

Cervical swelling due to sialoadenitis and necrosis may be seen sporadically associated with foreign body penetration of the esophagus with subsequent inoculation of subtending tissues with bacteria. Coarse food, bedding, and enrichment materials have all been associated with this condition in mice.

8.6.2 Gastric Conditions

Situs inversus and other congenital gastrointestinal anomalies are rarely seen in mice.

Mice with reduced food intake often have secondary orthokeratotic hyperkeratosis of the nonglandular stomach with overgrowth of commensal lactobacilli and yeast.

Spontaneous gastric or intestinal erosions and ulcers with profuse acute hemorrhage and death can be seen sporadically in acutely stressed mice (Figure 8.20). Stressors may include recent transportation, inability to access food or water, or recent management changes. Discontinuities in the gastric mucosal surface may be focal and may be seen grossly or after formalin fixation. Intestinal erosions may be more difficult to visualize, although affected segments can sometimes be identified by their dilated, black content.

Gastric stasis and dilatation with spontaneous death has been reported in mice exposed to high levels of environmental *E. coli* contamination. Affected animals also had elevated gastrin levels and severe chronic nephropathy.

Dilatation of gastric glands is seen commonly in aging mice. Glands may contain debris or exfoliated cells. Dystrophic calcification of the gastric muscularis and tongue may also be seen in some strains of mice with age.

Squamous cell papillomas and carcinomas may be found rarely in the forestomach and esophagus of aged mice. A single report of gastric carcinoid exists for mice. These tumors display neuroendocrine differentiation and can be characterized further using neuron-specific enolase or synaptophysin immunohistochemistry.

8.6.3 Bacterial Enteritis

Subclinical enteric disease is common in conventionally housed mouse colonies but may be managed if animals are provided with good environmental hygiene, including regular disinfection of their housing space and cleaning and disinfection of food and water containers. Explosive outbreaks of bacterial and viral enteric disease can occur under conditions of poor hygiene, overcrowding or when animals from outside sources are mixed with current breeding stock without sufficient quarantine periods. Before seeking veterinary assistance, breeders may attempt to treat colonies via the food or water using readily available antimicrobials for enteritis in poultry or other food animal species, and microbiologic culture of feces or fresh tissue samples from affected animals may be unrewarding. A complete history, including application of extra-label antimicrobials or other treatments, is important when evaluating cases.

8.6.3.1 Helicobacter-Associated Typhlocolitis

Helicobacter spp. are fastidious, microaerophilic, curved to spiral Gram-negative bacteria. They are the most prevalent opportunistic bacterial pathogens isolated from laboratory and pet mice. They are also commonly isolated from wild mice. There are many species of *Helicobacter*; however, *H. bilis* and *H. hepaticus* are most important in immunocompetent mice. Bacteria may be found within cecal and

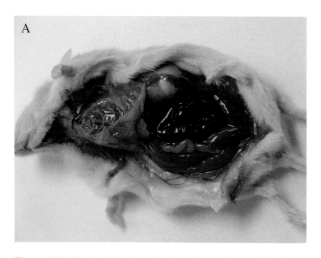
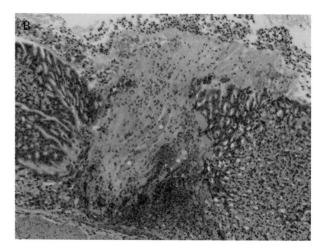

Figure 8.20 Acute gastrointestinal erosion or ulceration with subsequent bleed-out and death are common in mice and may be related to management stress, lack of access to food or water, intercurrent disease or other stressors. A: Colonic hemorrhage and bleed-out in a mouse. B: Deep gastric mucosal erosion and bleed-out in a found dead mouse.

colonic glands as well as in the liver (see below). In immunocompetent mice, enteric infections are usually asymptomatic, but co-infection with other enteric pathogens may induce clinical disease, including mild diarrhea. In immunodeficient mice, a proliferative typhlocolitis may occur with diarrhea, proctitis, and rectal prolapse. Abundant bacteria may be visualized on the mucosal surface and deep within colonic glands in Giemsa or Warthin-Starry stains of tissues (Figure 8.21), although these stains are not specific for *Helicobacter* spp. *H. bilis* may be transmitted from mice to rats and other rodents via feces or contaminated bedding. Bacterial presence can be confirmed by conducting PCR on fecal pellets. Serology may be used to detect antibodies; however, it can take up to 12 weeks for mice to seroconvert following *Helicobacter* spp. infection.

8.6.3.2 Salmonellosis

Salmonella spp. are rod-shaped, Gram-negative bacteria that are classified into serovars based on O antigen phenotypes. Typical species isolated from mice include *Salmonella enterica* serovars Enteritidis and Typhimurium. Infections are sporadic in pet and feeder mice but have significant public health implications when they occur because of the zoonotic potential. Murine salmonellosis may vary widely in terms of impact on individual and colony animals, and can be asymptomatic or mild in enzootically infected colonies with low mortality or severe with high mortality in acute outbreaks. Animals may present with hunched posture, rough hair coat, weight loss, dehydration, and death can occur peracutely with few prodromal signs. Microscopic findings include multifocal, suppurative hepatic, splenic, and lymphoid necrosis with necrotizing typhlocolitis. Fecal culture may be used to confirm infection. Co-infection with other bacterial or viral agents may exacerbate the severity of the infection, and transmission occurs by fecal-oral contamination.

Several highly publicized cases of human salmonellosis have occurred recently in the United States, Canada, and the United Kingdom, all thought to arise from human handling of *Salmonella*-contaminated frozen feeder rodents or mice (thought to have become infected from other rodents held in multi-species animal distribution centers). Some strains isolated from these rodents have been found to have multiple antibiotic resistance. For this reason, veterinarians and clients handing live or dead mice should always wash hands thoroughly with soap after handling to prevent inadvertent disease transmission. Wild rodents should be excluded from breeding colonies to minimize contamination.

8.6.3.3 Other Bacterial Conditions

Citrobacter rodentium may induce a proliferative colitis with diarrhea sporadically and as enzootics with high morbidity in laboratory mice, but infection is not reported in pet mice. *C. rodentium* has attaching and effacing properties, similar to enteropathogenic strains of *E. coli*, but is difficult to isolate from affected animals. Infections are often self limiting in older animals. Similarly, *E. coli* may induce diarrhea and proliferative typhlocolitis in young mice co-infected with rotavirus or coronavirus; however, the prevalence of pathogenic *E. coli* in pet and feeder mouse colonies has not been examined. Work-up for diarrhea cases should include histologic evaluation of gut sections. Fecal or tissue culture for bacterial pathogens may be warranted, depending on histologic findings. Any condition causing chronic diarrhea or rectal irritation and inflammation may result in rectal prolapse, which should be interpreted as a nonspecific finding (Figure 8.22).

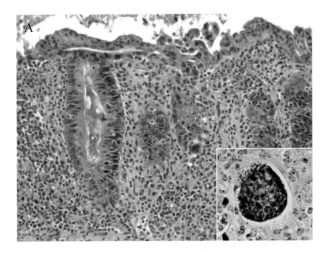
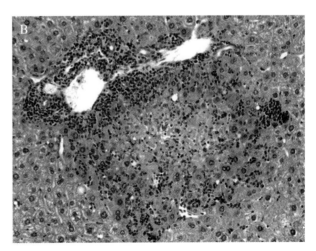

Figure 8.21 A: Marked colitis with mucosal hyperplasia, attenuation and sloughing of overlying epithelium, and marked, mixed, predominantly lymphoplasmacytic mucosal and submucosal infiltrates. This mouse was infected with *Helicobacter hepaticus*. Inset: abundant spiral-shaped bacteria are noted in the colonic glands with a Warthin-Starry stain. B: Multifocal hepatic necrosis secondary to *H. hepaticus* infection. Hepatic lesions are nonspecific and other etiologic agents must be considered.

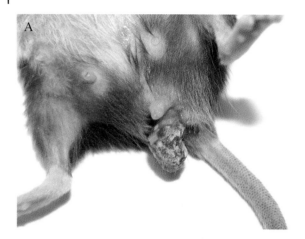
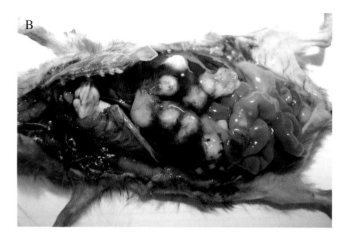

Figure 8.22 A: Rectal prolapse is a very common presentation in mice. Possible etiologies include pinworm infestation, mouse hepatitis virus infection, salmonellosis, and helicobacteriosis. B: Intra-abdominal abscesses in a feeder-breeder colony mouse. Culture of lesions demonstrated growth of *Corynebacterium kutscheri*.

Corynebacterium kutscheri, *Proteus mirabilis*, and *Streptobacillus moniliformis* are opportunistic bacteria that are isolated commonly from the oropharynx or intestinal tract of pet or feeder mice. Under conditions of poor hygiene, adverse stress, overcrowding, or following co-infection with other pathogenic bacteria or viruses, these infections may become systemic, leading to multi-organ abscessation, septicemia, or polyarthritis (*S. moniliformis*) (Figure 8.22).

Clostridium piliforme, the etiologic agent causing Tyzzer's disease, is rarely reported in pet or feeder mice. A triad of lesions may be seen when clinical signs are present, including myocarditis, necrotizing typhlocolitis and hepatitis. For further information, see Section 8.6.8.

8.6.4 Viral Enteritis

A number of enteric viral agents are known to infect mice and are routinely monitored in laboratory rodent colonies, including mouse adenovirus-2, rotavirus, and coronavirus (mouse hepatitis virus). Murine norovirus, parvovirus, and astrovirus also are internalized from specific receptors in the gut and may be detected serologically in mice. Despite very high seroprevalence of some of these agents in wild and pet mouse population surveys, they may cause acute subclinical infection and are either cleared readily from immunocompetent hosts or persist as latent, asymptomatic infections (e.g., some parvovirus strains). The enteric viruses of primary concern for pet or feeder colonies include murine coronavirus and rotavirus.

8.6.4.1 Coronaviral Enteritis
Mouse hepatitis virus (MHV) remains one of the most common viral infections of wild and domestic mice, and consists of a group of coronavirus strains that may exhibit more enterotropic versus polytropic tendencies, although infection patterns may be mixed. Like other coronaviruses, MHV is a single-stranded, enveloped RNA virus with a high propensity for mutation. Immunity is short-lived and strain-specific, and colony re-infection can occur rapidly. Different strains exhibit tropism for epithelial cells in the intestinal or respiratory tracts, hepatocytes, neurons, lymphocytes, or macrophages. The manifestations of disease depend on host age, mouse strain, and viral biotype and pathogenicity. Enterotropic strains may cause diarrhea, dehydration, reduced weight gains, and rapid death in neonatal and suckling mouse pups. The virus infects less-differentiated crypt progenitor cells, leading to an inability to adequately replenish sloughed enterocytes, subsequent loss of surface area, and a severe malabsorptive diarrhea. Animals older than 2 weeks of age may survive infection and exhibit runting. Depending on the viral strain, pathogenic effects in mice may be caused by the virus alone or may be due to synergistic interactions with other opportunistic pathogens, such as coccidia or *E. coli*. Older mice are less susceptible to the disease following infection with enterotropic strains because of more rapid intestinal epithelial cell kinetics, which permit faster cell turnover and repair. Viral immunity may be transferred to pups in utero, and postnatally, by IgG in the milk.

On gross examination, loops of small or large intestine may be distended and filled with watery content. No signs may be seen in older animals with clinically inapparent infections. Typical microscopic findings in affected animals include segmental villus atrophy, blunting, and fusion, crypt hyperplasia, desquamation of necrotic enterocytes, edema, and lymphocytic infiltrates. Epithelial cell syncytia may be present (Figure 8.23). Viral dissemination to mesenteric lymph nodes and other organs such as liver and brain may occur. Acute hepatocellular coagulation necrosis with multinucleated giant

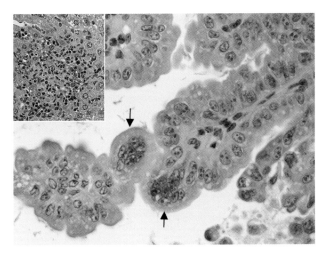

Figure 8.23 Enterotropic mouse hepatitis virus (MHV) infection in a pre-weaned mouse from a feeder-breeder mouse colony. The colony had a history of significant production losses and a preweaning mortality rate exceeding 35%. Syncytial cells are present at the tips of villi (arrows) and large tufts of epithelial cells are pinching off villi, contributing to villus blunting, maldigestion, and diarrhea. Inset: adult animals had evidence of multifocal hepatic necrosis. Both feces and hepatocytes were positive for MHV by PCR assay.

cells occurs rarely in immunocompetent mice following polytropic virus infection.

Once an outbreak of disease has occurred in a breeding colony, the virus may become enzootic and is maintained by mild self-limiting infections of young animals once passive maternal immunity has waned or when new naïve animals are introduced into the colony. MHV is highly infectious and contagious and readily transmitted by direct contact, aerosol, and by fecal fomites. It is diagnosed by serology, tissue or fecal PCR assay, and histopathology. MHV can be eradicated from conventional colonies but the process is difficult and requires strict cessation of all breeding and colony introductions for at least 8 weeks with concurrent environmental decontamination. Wild mice commonly harbor the virus and can readily transmit it to colony animals. They should be excluded from access to the colony.

8.6.4.2   Rotaviral Enteritis

Rotaviral enteritis (also known as epizootic diarrhea of infant mice or EDIM) is less prevalent and usually induces less severe disease than does MHV but rotavirus can contribute to reduced weight gain, diarrhea, runting, and rarely death of preweaning animals. Infection is caused by a nonenveloped double-stranded RNA virus in the Reoviridae family. The virus only infects more terminally differentiated enterocytes, resulting in less villus atrophy and cell sloughing. Affected pups often continue to nurse, but may demonstrate fecal staining, lethargy, and a distended abdomen.

Gross examination of affected pups may reveal segmentally dilated loops of small or large intestine with watery content. Histologically, there is hydropic swelling and vacuolation of terminal enterocytes with sloughing, mild lamina proprial inflammation, and lymphatic dilatation. Disease severity may be augmented by co-infection with pathogenic strains of *E. coli*. Virus can be detected in other tissues, but, generally, no lesions are present outside of the gastrointestinal tract.

Partial and incomplete passive mucosal immunity is afforded from ingestion of milk by pups from seropositive dams. The virus persists in the environment for days and is transmitted by direct contact or fecal contamination. Diagnosis can be made by histopathology, serology, and PCR of feces or tissues.

8.6.5   Parasitic Enteric Infections

Enteric parasitic infections are common in pet and wild mice. Some agents, such as pinworms, may be difficult to eradicate completely from colonies. Good hygiene, good nutrition, and colony management can help to reduce the severity of signs seen because infections are transmitted by ingestion of eggs, infective cysts, or larvae found in the environment. A nutritionally complete diet should be offered as vitamin E deficiencies may make mice more susceptible to enteric parasite infections. For protozoal infections, clinical signs are usually seen in weanling animals and may be exacerbated by concurrent infections with enteric viruses or bacteria. Some protozoal infections may be self-limiting; as immune resistance develops with age. Wild rodents should be eliminated from colony rooms, wherever possible, to reduce further parasite exposure.

8.6.5.1   Enteric Oxyuriasis

Pinworm infections are very common in pet, feeder, and wild mouse populations. There are two species seen regularly in mice, *Aspiculuris tetraptera* and *Syphacia obvelata*, although a third species, *Syphacia muris*, has occasionally been reported. These nematodes have a simple, direct life cycle and infection occurs via ingestion of embryonated eggs (that is, fecal-oral transmission). Adult female pinworms reside in the cecum or proximal colon. *Syphacia* spp. migrate to the anus to lay eggs (ovoid and flattened on one side) on the perianal skin where they become infective within hours. Eggs and hatched larvae can be detected by pressing cellophane tape on the perianal skin and evaluating it microscopically (Figure 8.24). *Aspiculuris* sp. lay eggs (ovoid, bilaterally symmetrical) in the distal colon that are shed in the feces, becoming infective within 5–8 days. These eggs can be detected using fecal flotation. The prepatent period for pinworms varies from approximately 11 (*Syphacia* spp.) to

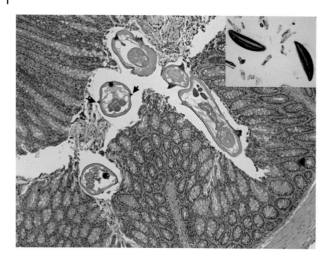

Figure 8.24 Adult female pinworm sections in the colon of a mouse. Sections demonstrate lateral alae (arrows), polymyarium musculature, internal digestive tract, and uterus. There is minimal mucosal reaction. Inset: Pinworm eggs are often readily detected following application of cellophane tape to the anus. *Syphacia* spp. (depicted) eggs are flattened on one side.

25 (*Aspiculuris* sp.) days. PCR assays conducted on murine bedding material or fecal pellets are a highly sensitive method to detect low-level infections.

Pinworm infections rarely result in clinical signs, even with heavy adult worm burdens. Occasionally, rectal prolapse and poor hair coat have been associated with severe pinworm infection in mice. Sections of adult worms and larvae can be seen microscopically in the cecum and colon and demonstrate typical features of nematodes, with lateral alae, platymyarian musculature, and a true coelom with intestinal and reproductive tracts. Eggs of both species are light and sticky, readily aerosolized, and are distributed widely in the environment, making complete eradication challenging in conventionally housed mice, even with repeated parasiticide treatment of colony animals. Environmental decontamination is critically important when attempting colony eradication. Humans are dead end hosts for murine pinworms, which are unable to reproduce in the human gastrointestinal tract.

8.6.5.2 Murine Coccidiosis

Several *Eimeria* species can be isolated from pet and wild mice. Coccidiosis can result in diarrhea, runting, and even death in severely infected colonies. Infective oocysts can be recovered with fecal flotation, and asexual and sexual protozoal stages can be seen microscopically as segmental infections within the intestinal tract (Figure 8.25). The severity of infection may be augmented by co-infection with other enteric bacteria or viruses.

8.6.5.3 Other Enteric Parasitic Conditions

Many other gastric or enteric protozoa can be isolated from mice; however, most are considered commensal and are interpreted as incidental when observed. Several other opportunistic protozoa, including *Cryptosporidium muris*, *Giardia muris*, and *Spironucleus muris* may be associated with diarrhea in young animals, especially those with concurrent viral or bacterial disease (Figure 8.26). Organisms are best detected by direct smears of intestinal contents or microscopic evaluation of intestinal sections.

Several cestodes may be seen in mice, including *Rodentolepis nana* and *Hymenolepis diminuta*. Cross-sections of tapeworms are found in the small intestine and are rarely associated with clinical signs (Figure 8.27B).

8.6.6 Other Enteric Conditions

Marked intestinal dilatation and stasis with death is seen sporadically in mice, particularly primiparous mice in early lactation. Animals present as off-feed with a massively distended abdomen and may or not have concurrent mild diarrhea. Dilated stomach and intestinal sections may contain food, fluid or both. Occasionally, inspissated fecal pellets are noted in the distal colon. Histologically, lesions vary from markedly dilated gastric, intestinal, and colonic sections with attenuated mucosa and mild to moderate submucosal edema to fibrinonecrotizing enteritis. Lymphocytolysis may be seen in Peyer's patches and mesenteric lymph nodes. The pathogenesis of this condition is unknown. *Clostridium perfringens* type A has been isolated from some cases. Whether a dysbiosis event occurs with secondary clostridial overgrowth has not been determined. Increasing dietary fat for lactating mice may help to minimize the occurrence of this condition (Figure 8.27 (a)).

Intestinal amyloidosis can be seen in aging mice (see Section 8.6.8.2) (Figure 8.28).

Intestinal leiomyoma, leiomyosarcoma, and **adenocarcinoma** are rarely seen as spontaneous tumors of pet mice.

8.6.7 Exocrine Pancreatic Conditions

Spontaneous pancreatitis is not commonly seen in mice and may be an indication of an underlying autoimmune disorder. Depletion of exocrine pancreatic zymogen granules is a common finding in mice with concurrent inanition.

Congenital exocrine pancreatic hypoplasia with steatorrhea and runting has been reported in mice. Affected mice have microscopically normal pancreatic islets as well as normal serum insulin levels. Fatty infiltration of the pancreas may be seen in older mice.

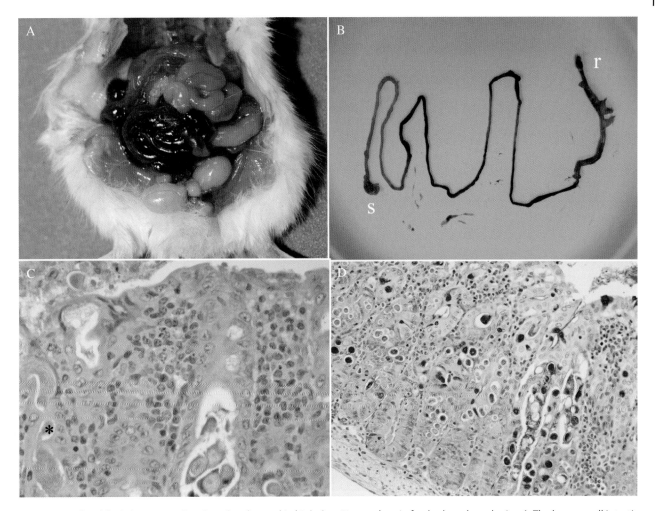

Figure 8.25 Coccidiosis is common in mice when housed in high densities, such as in feeder-breeder colonies. A: The lower small intestine of this young mouse contains partially digested bloody content. B: Gastrointestinal tract removed to demonstrate areas of coccidial replication and damage (s = stomach, r = rectum). C: Co-infections with other protozoa are common. In addition to *Eimeria* sp. replication, mats of *Spironucleus* organisms (*) are seen in adjacent crypts. D: All coccidial life cycle phases occur in the intestinal mucosa. PAS.

8.6.8 Hepatobiliary Conditions

Extramedullary hematopoiesis and myelopoiesis are commonly seen in adult mice and may be increased under conditions of physiologic stress or chronic infection. Islands of myelopoiesis must be distinguished from microgranulomas.

Heterotopic hepatocytes are found occasionally within the lamina propria of the gallbladder and stomach in rodents. Similarly, ectopic pancreatic and renal tissue may be seen on rare occasion within the liver and gallbladder.

A number of aging changes are commonly seen in the livers of mice. Mild to moderate hepatocellular changes, including cytomegaly, karyomegaly, anisocytosis, anisokaryosis, polyploidy, and intranuclear cytoplasmic indentations, are common and may be seen in young adult animals. Binucleate cells are commonly seen and increase in number from 4% at 4 weeks of age in mice to 30% by 36 months. The timing of these changes and ploidy changes are strain-specific. Nuclei may contain up to eight times the usual complement of nuclear DNA. This appears to be due to chromosome duplication without nuclear division. There is reduced cell turnover in aged animals and decreased numbers of hepatocytes per microscopic field. To compensate, the cytoplasmic volume increases as liver:body weight ratios are maintained relatively consistently throughout life. Dietary protein restriction retards hepatic polyploidy in mice.

Intranuclear "inclusions" are seen occasionally in the hepatocyte nuclei of mice. These represent cytoplasmic invaginations of the nuclear membrane, and appear as round, eosinophilic, eccentric membrane-bound structures occupying less than one-third of the nucleus.

Various pigments may also be seen as an incidental finding within the hepatocytes and the Kupffer cells of aging

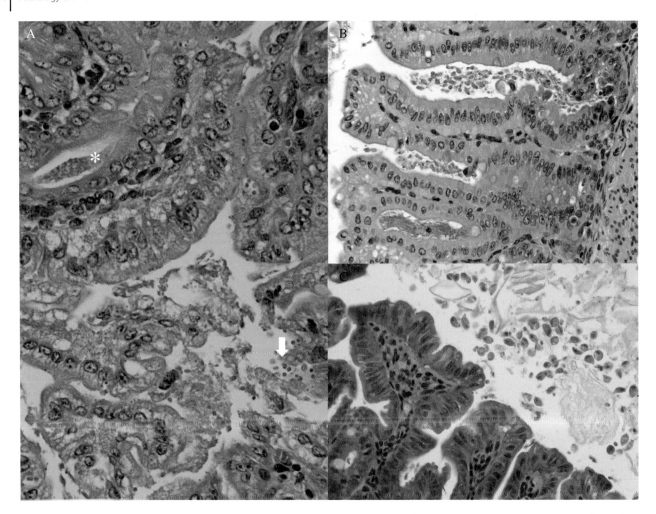

Figure 8.26 Other protozoal species are seen on occasion and overgrowth and signs of diarrhea may occur in conjunction with *E. coli* or MHV infections. A: *Spironucleus* sp. (*) densely aggregated in small intestinal crypts and *Cryptosporidium* sp. (arrow) in preweaned mice co-infected with MHV. B: Giardiasis in a feeder-breeder colony mouse. Trophozoites are found near the mucosa. C: *Tritrichomonas* sp. and *Cryptosporidium* sp. infection in a feeder mouse. *Tritrichomonas* sp. trophozoites are commonly found within the colonic lumen closely associated with the mucosa but rarely are associated with a mucosal inflammatory reaction, even in very large numbers.

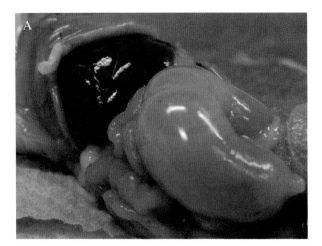

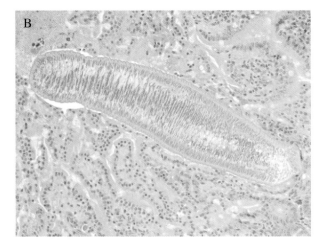

Figure 8.27 A: Clostridial typhlocolitis with marked cecal dilatation and sudden death. B: *Hymenolepis diminuta* in the small intestine of a mouse, an incidental finding in a feeder mouse colony. *Source:* A: Courtesy of J. Sunohara-Neilson.

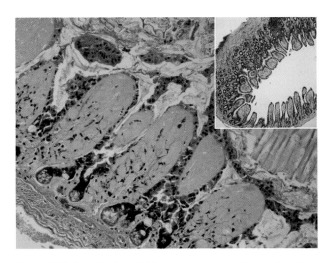

Figure 8.28 Intestinal amyloidosis can cause wasting and death in aging mice. Inset: Application of a Congo red stain will confirm the presence of amyloid proteins. Apple-green birefringence is noted under polarized light.

animals. These include lipofuscin, hemosiderin, and small amounts of bile pigments.

8.6.8.1 Bacterial Hepatitis

Helicobacter spp. infections are very common in wild and pet mice. Although many species have been isolated from mice, pathology in immunocompetent mice is largely associated with *H. bilis* or *H. hepaticus* infection. *Helicobacter* spp. infections may be cleared acutely or may result in chronic cholangiohepatitis. Typical microscopic findings include focal necrosis with hepatocytomegaly, ductular cell hyperplasia, and pericholangitis with mixed, predominantly lymphoplasmacytic inflammatory infiltrates. Bacteria are best demonstrated in bile canaliculi with a Warthin-Starry stain or by PCR of tissues.

Tyzzer's disease occurs sporadically in mice and is caused by *Clostridium piliforme*, a Gram-negative spore-forming bacterial rod. The bacterium may be carried as an inapparent infection or acquired and cleared acutely. Infected animals tend to be younger and may appear runted with poor haircoats. Acute disease may be seen following stress or under conditions of poor husbandry. Grossly, the disease may appear as multifocal hepatic necrosis, with or without accompanying typhlocolitis and myocarditis. Histologically, abundant intracytoplasmic aggregates of rod-like bacteria may be seen surrounding the areas of hepatocellular necrosis. Spores are resistant to killing and may persist for months in the environment. Serology is not specific and false positives are common. Histopathology of lesions and PCR of tissues or feces may be used to confirm infected animals.

Microgranulomas are very common as an incidental finding within the livers of mice at necropsy. These consist of focal to multifocal aggregates of mixed leukocytic infiltrates surrounding a few degenerate or necrotic hepatocytes. The pathogenesis of these lesions is unknown but may be related to sporadic bacterial showering of the liver from the portal vasculature. Larger necrotic or inflammatory foci are not interpreted as incidental and may be related to viral or bacterial hepatitis or septicemia. Examples of bacterial agents that may cause these lesions include *Proteus mirabilis*, *Salmonella* spp., *Corynebacterium* spp., and *Pseudomonas* spp. Other differential diagnoses for multifocal hepatic necrosis in mice include ectromelia virus, *Helicobacter* spp. infection, mouse hepatitis virus, *Clostridium piliforme*, *Staphylococcus* spp., and reovirus infection.

8.6.8.2 Amyloidosis

This condition is common in both wild and domestic mice and is caused by extracellular deposition of amyloid fibrils and serum amyloid P, an acute phase protein of mice. There are significant variations in susceptibility to the condition between strains, as well as variations in the age of onset. Both primary and secondary amyloidosis can occur in mice. The incidence of amyloidosis may be increased by a variety of factors including stress, such as overcrowding and fighting, and chronic parasitism, for example, cutaneous acariasis. Tissue amyloid distribution varies by mouse strain but the most frequently involved sites are liver, nasal submucosa, renal glomeruli, lamina propria of small and large intestine, and myocardium. The condition is commonly associated with cardiac atrial thrombosis and renal papillary necrosis. It can be difficult to distinguish primary from secondary amyloidosis. Secondary amyloidosis has been associated with chronic infections and fighting, and tends to be seen in the liver and spleen, whereas these sites are minimally affected with primary amyloidosis. Tumor-associated amyloidosis is seen also, particularly with pulmonary adenomas. In the liver, amyloid deposition (serum amyloid P protein) usually is seen underlying the sinusoids and within portal vessel walls. A diagnosis can be made by applying a Congo red stain and looking for apple-green birefringence of the eosinophilic material under polarized light.

8.6.8.3 Other Hepatic Conditions

Cyst forms (strobilicerci) of *Taenia taeniformis* may be found occasionally on the capsule of the liver at necropsy. This is usually the result of bedding or feed contamination by cat feces and is interpreted as an incidental finding.

Hepatocellular adenoma and **adenocarcinomas** occur rarely as spontaneous tumors in pet mice (Figures 8.29 and 8.30). **Histiocytic sarcomas** involving the liver are relatively common in aged mice (see Section 8.10).

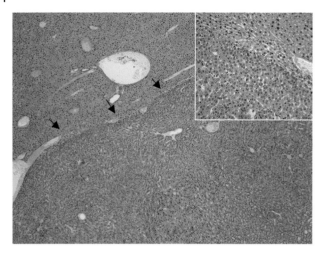

Figure 8.29 Hepatic adenoma in an aging mouse. A large mass of well differentiated hepatocytes is seen compressing the normal hepatic tissue (arrows). Portal triads are absent in the adenoma. Inset: Differential staining characteristics are also visible between the adenoma cells (lower left) and the normal hepatocytes (upper left).

8.7 Cardiovascular Conditions

Cardiovascular conditions of mice are not appreciated widely ante mortem and are often an incidental finding at necropsy. In cases of severe disease, animals may present with dyspnea, wasting, and hunched posture.

Myocardial degeneration is moderately common in aged mice but is often asymptomatic. Typical microscopic findings include myofiber vacuolation, fragmentation, hypereosinophilia, and loss of cross striations with mild dissecting myocardial fibrosis and scattered mononuclear leukocytic infiltrates (Figure 8.31).

Epicardial and myocardial mineralization can occur as spontaneous lesions in several strains of mice, such as BALB/C, DBA, and C3H, and may be related to a recessive mutation in some lines. The lesion may vary widely in severity and distribution, and in severe cases, hearts may be enlarged with pale streaking evident on the epicardial surface and extending throughout the epicardium. Histologically, there are patchy to coalescing foci of mineralization involving myofibres and connective tissue, with minimal inflammatory response and fibrosis. Mineralized foci may also be present in other tissues including the muscles of the tongue and sclera.

Myocarditis and endocarditis can occur as sporadic cases or outbreaks in colonies. Patchy to locally extensive myocardial necrosis may be seen with marked neutrophilic infiltrates (Figure 8.31B). Suppurative endocarditis with thrombus formation can be seen at times and bacterial colonies may be abundant. Differential diagnoses for acute myocardial necrosis include infection with *Streptococcus* spp., *Salmonella* spp., Tyzzer's disease, *Pseudomonas* sp., *C. kutscheri*, or ectromelia virus infection.

Atrial thrombosis may be seen spontaneously in some strains of mice and may be associated with **amyloidosis**. The left ventricle is more commonly affected (Figure 8.32).

Polyarteritis nodosa occurs in mice, as in rats, and is characterized by nodular vascular swellings of small arterioles in the mesentery, heart base, pancreas, testis, and elsewhere. Microscopically, affected vessels are enlarged with total to subtotal lumenal occlusion, medial fibrinoid necrosis and a variable mixed inflammatory

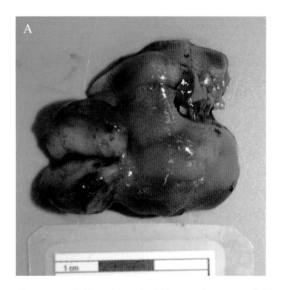

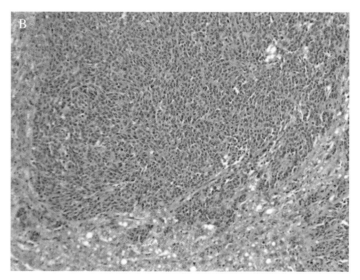

Figure 8.30 A: Hepatic carcinoid in an aging mouse. B: Neoplastic cells are pleomorphic and are arranged in cords, nests, packets, and densely cellular sheets with areas of swirling and herringbone patterns, with a neuroendocrine appearance. Contrast the appearance with Figure 8.29.

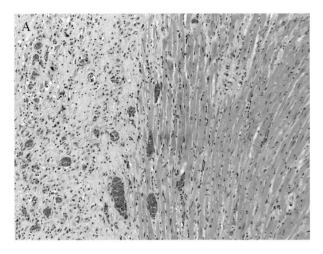 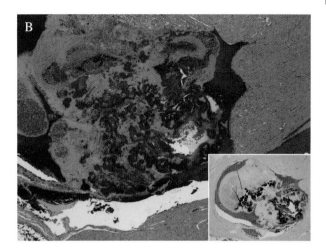

Figure 8.31 A: Myocardial degeneration and fibrosis is a common incidental finding in aged mice. B: Suppurative endocarditis with ventricular thrombosis can occur sporadically. Inset: Dense aggregates of Gram-positive bacteria are seen. *Staphylococcus aureus* was cultured from the heart.

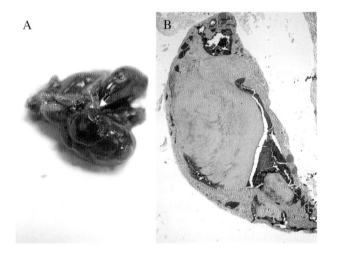

Figure 8.32 A: Atrial thrombosis (arrow) in a 1-year-old mouse that was found dead. B: Photomicrograph of atrium from this mouse. No other microscopic lesions were noted.

cell infiltrate (Figure 8.33). These lesions are thought to arise from antigen-antibody complex deposition and subsequent inflammation.

Hemangiomas and hemangiosarcomas are rarely reported in mice (Figure 8.34).

8.8 Genitourinary Conditions

Similar to other rodents, mice have unipapillate kidneys and a single major calyx. In male mice, the parietal layer of cells lining Bowman's capsule may have a cuboidal appearance. Mild proteinuria is present in normal mice and may be increased in sexually mature male mice. Major urinary proteins are produced by hepatocytes and excreted by the kidneys and likely play a role in pheromone signaling. Exposure to these proteins from male

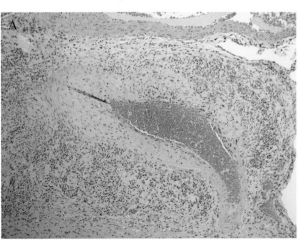 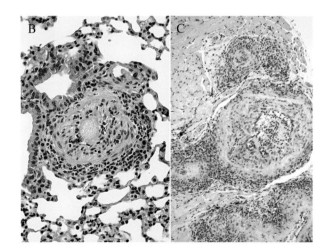

Figure 8.33 Polyarteritis in a coronary vessel (A), lung section (B), and tongue (C) of aging mice. This is a common and often incidental lesion in older mice and can be found in almost any organ or tissue.

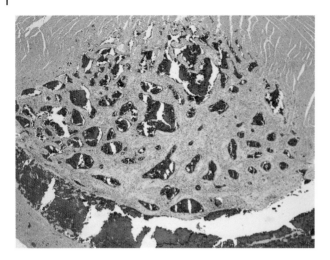

Figure 8.34 Ventricular hemangiosarcoma in an 8-month-old mouse. Tumor characteristics are similar to other mammals.

mice is important for onset of puberty, maintenance of pregnancy, and the stimulation of estrus in female mice. The extent of urinary protein excretion in male mice is related to dietary restriction and ad lib feeding.

Vaginal cytology may be used to accurately stage the estrous cycle of female mice.

8.8.1 Urinary Tract Conditions

8.8.1.1 Chronic Renal Disease

Chronic renal disease is a common finding with up to 100% prevalence in some strains of mice. The condition occurs more commonly in aging males and the pathogenesis is unknown although some suggest that it may be related to ad libitum feeding as well as types and amount of protein in the diet. Affected animals may show

increased drinking and urination, weight loss, urine scalding, and a ruffled hair coat. Clinical chemistry may indicate marked proteinuria, hypoproteinemia, and anemia. Kidneys may appear granular and pitted on the cortical surface. Microscopically, there are multifocal dilated tubules in the cortical and outer medullary zones with evidence of tubular degeneration and regeneration, proteinaceous casts, and a mild interstitial and perivascular lymphoplasmacytic infiltrate (Figure 8.35A).

In some animals, there is concurrent glomerular enlargement with thickening of mesangial tufts and glomerular capillary basement membranes by dense amorphous to fibrillar proteinaceous deposits, and glomerular hypercellularity. Differential diagnoses include renal amyloidosis and membranoproliferative glomerulonephritis with antigen-antibody deposition. A Congo red stain can be used to distinguish renal amyloidosis, which may be localized or systemic.

8.8.1.2 Cystitis, Pyelonephritis, and Nephritis

Ascending and hematogenous bacterial renal infections are commonly seen in older mice and may be uni- or bilateral. Grossly, kidneys may appear swollen and hemorrhagic, and may be adherent to other structures within the retroperitoneal space by means of fibrous or fibrinous attachments. Affected animals may have a nonspecific history of inanition, dehydration, and ruffled hair coat. Overgrooming of the genital area and paraphimosis may also be seen. Acute hematogenous infections may appear as dense bacterial colonies within the glomeruli with minimal inflammatory cell infiltrate. Subsequent involvement of surrounding tubules and interstitial infiltrates and fibrosis may be seen with chronic infections. Pyelonephritis may appear initially as suppurative

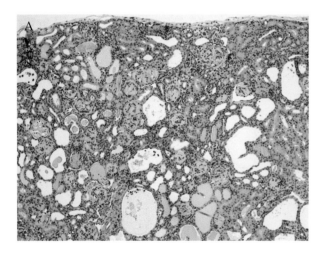

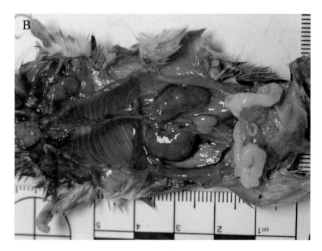

Figure 8.35 A: Chronic renal disease in an aging male mouse characterized by tubular degeneration and regeneration, glomerulosclerosis, multifocal lymphoplasmacytic interstitial infiltrates, and marked renal tubular dilatation with lumenal protein casts. B: Pale, raised areas on these kidneys corresponded to marked suppurative nephritis.

inflammation in the renal pelvis that extends into the overlying parenchyma, with necrosis and collapse of renal tissue in severe cases (Figure 8.35B). Ureteritis and involvement of the prostate gland are common. Common bacterial isolates include *E. coli, Klebsiella* spp., *Corynebacterium kutscheri, S. aureus, Proteus mirabilis,* and *Streptococcus* spp.

Pet or wild mice may be chronically infected with *Leptospira ballum* but the infection is generally subclinical in mice. Leptospirosis has been reported in an adult human who owned pet mice, and who subsequently developed pyrexia, gastroenteritis, and orchitis. The mice were asymptomatic, but were later found to be shedding *Leptospira* organisms in the urine. Diagnosis can be confirmed by urine or tissue culture or histologic evaluation of the tissue and demonstration of spirochetes by silver staining. Hands should always be washed with soap and water after handling mice or their cages, and mice should not share utensils, plates, or other objects that might enter the owner's mouth.

8.8.1.3 Other Renal Conditions

Klossiella muris is a coccidial parasite of mice and can be found sporadically in pet and wild mice as an asymptomatic infection. Sporocysts are shed in the urine and are ingested by other animals. The organism has tropism for renal tissue, and schizogony and gametogony occur largely within glomeruli and renal tubular epithelial cells. Microscopically, developmental protozoal stages can be seen with in glomeruli and tubules. There may be mild tubular necrosis and a localized lymphohistiocytic inflammatory cell infiltrate. Intratubal spores and sporozoites convey a honeycomb appearance to tissue sections. Infection may be accompanied by a mild lymphoplasmacytic infiltrate, and the parasite is not zoonotic.

Single or multiple **congenital renal cysts** may be seen sporadically as spontaneous autosomal recessive conditions in mice. In addition to tubular cysts, pancreatic and biliary ducts may also be dilated.

Congenital **unilateral renal agenesis** and **congenital hydronephrosis** are seen sporadically. Both conditions likely result from inherited mesonephric duct defects, and breeding pairs should be culled. Congenital hydronephrosis must be distinguished from **acquired hydronephrosis**, which may accompany severe urolithiasis or urethral blockage by a protein coagulum. Acquired hydronephrosis is often bilateral and bilateral hydroureter and urinary bladder dilatation may be seen concurrently (Figure 8.36). Single or multiple **proteinaceous coagula** are found commonly within the urethra of male mice at necropsy, and the urinary bladder should be evaluated for patency. In cases of true **urethral *obstruction***, there is often marked suppurative inflammation with suppurative prostatitis and cystitis at and around the site of obstruction. Ketamine/medetomidine anesthesia has been associated with urinary coagula formation and urethral obstruction in male mice, with subsequent death. The pathogenesis of this effect is unknown.

Both histiocytic sarcoma and lymphosarcoma may result in **hyaline droplet accumulation** within renal tubules of mice. Composition of the protein droplets varies depending on the tumor type. Histiocytic sarcomas typically produce an excess of lysozyme, which is excreted by the kidneys and reabsorbed by the proximal tubules. The actual tumors may or not be present within the kidneys and the effect of tubular protein accumulation on renal function is unknown.

Urolithiasis is uncommon in mice. When present, calculi can be seen within the kidney or urinary bladder

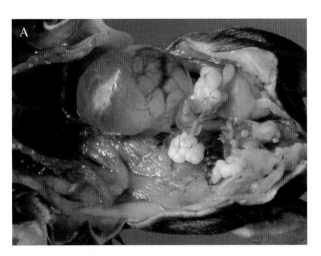
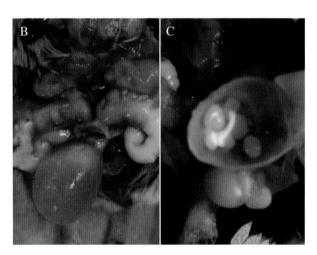

Figure 8.36 Renal and urinary tract lesions are common in aging mice of all strains and both sexes. A: Unilateral hydronephrosis in a male mouse. The condition is commonly acquired secondary to urinary bladder obstruction (B) and urolithiasis (C).

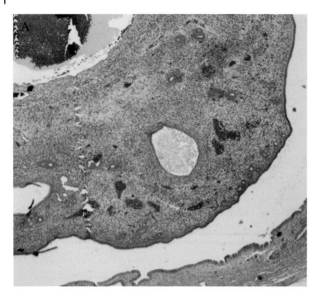 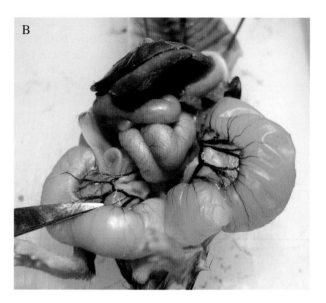

Figure 8.37 A: Cystic endometrial hyperplasia and stromal polyps are common incidental findings in aging mice. B: Marked hydrometra in a young female mouse kept for breeding. The animal had a progressively enlarging abdomen.

(see Figure 8.36). Renal tubular adenomas and carcinomas occur sporadically in mice.

8.8.2 Reproductive Tract Conditions

8.8.2.1 Reproductive Masses

Uterine stromal polyps are very common in older female mice and consist of benign, often pedunculated, proliferative masses of largely fibrous tissue lined by differentiated endometrial cells (Figure 8.37). Occasional glands may be entrapped within the stromal mass. These should be differentiated from leiomyomas and leiomyosarcomas, which are both much less common and occur as single masses. Leiomyomas consist of well differentiated smooth muscle cells, whereas leiomyosarcomas are less well differentiated and poorly circumscribed. Uterine adenocarcinoma occurs sporadically in mice.

Ovarian carcinomas, teratomas, and granulosa cell tumors occur sporadically (Figure 8.38) and have microscopic characteristics similar to other mammals. Local seeding and metastases may occur. Testicular teratomas and interstitial cell tumors are uncommon in mice.

8.8.2.2 Other Reproductive Conditions

Cystic endometrial hyperplasia is seen commonly in aged female mice. Glands are dilated, may contain low

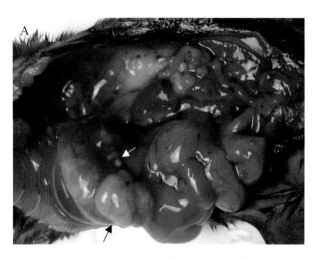 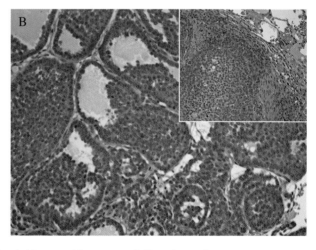

Figure 8.38 A: Ovarian carcinoma (black arrow) with peritoneal seeding (white arrow) in a mouse. B: Granulosa cell tumors occur sporadically in aging female mice and have similar microscopic characteristics to those of other companion animals, including round nuclei, moderate, granular cytoplasm, and a microfollicular pattern. Pulmonary metastases (inset) may be present.

protein material, and are increased in number (see Figure 8.37).

Hydrometra is seen occasionally in female mice and is characterized by massively dilated uterine horns, which may be noted clinically as an enlarging abdomen (see Figure 8.37). Horns are filled with a low protein mucoid material. This condition is congenital and inherited, related to an imperforate hymen, and breeding pairs should be culled.

Uterine inertia and death can be seen in breeding mice with prolonged delivery times. Retained placentas and subsequent metritis occur also, usually in aging breeders. **Abortions** have been associated with infection with *Pasteurella pneumotropica* and *Staphylococcus aureus*. Chronically infected male breeders may transmit these infections to breeding females. Culling breeding animals at 6–8 months of age may help minimize bacterial transmission within colonies.

Prolapsed uterus may be seen sporadically in mice. The cause is unknown but most females in which this occurs are not pregnant. The condition may be related to any process inducing obstipation or severe tenesmus, such as diarrhea or urinary tract disease, and other systems should be evaluated when this condition is seen.

Fetal loss and fetal malformations have been seen experimentally in female mice receiving an excess of dietary vitamin A. Most commercial diets contain appropriate levels of nutrients as long as diets are used within one year of milling and are stored in a dark, cool place. Nutrient imbalances are seen sometimes with homemade diets and diets that are past their expiry dates or that have been stored improperly.

Ovarian atrophy is a common degenerative change in older mice. Interstitial tissue may be mildly expanded, although the overall ovary size is decreased and there may be scant to no follicles present. Ectatic blood vessels may be present. **Parovarian cysts** are also seen commonly. Cysts are lined by ciliated epithelium and may severely compress normal ovarian tissue, leading to atrophy (Figure 8.39).

Prostatitis may occur in sexually mature male mice housed under conventional conditions. Lesions involve mixed, predominantly neutrophilic infiltrates within the prostate gland with initial reactive hyperplasia, followed by necrosis of acinar cells, interstitial edema and congestion, and aggregation of cellular debris and degenerate neutrophils within the lumena. Bacterial colonies are often abundant. Infections may involve other secondary sex glands and result from bite wounds (Figure 8.40A). *S. aureus* and *E. coli* are the most commonly isolated bacteria in spontaneous cases.

Seminal vesicle impaction and dilatation may be seen in older male mice and also may present as abdominal distension. Distension may become so severe that the tissues are mistaken for uterine horns (Figure 8.40B). Bulbourethral glands may become ectatic and filled with pale, acellular eosinophilic material. Gland secretion is required for semen survival, and the condition may result in infertility in a breeding colony. This condition should be differentiated from cystic or infected bulbourethral glands.

Generalized, **bilateral testicular atrophy** occurs in aging males and is interpreted as incidental. Prostatic tumors are rare.

8.9 Nervous System Conditions

The mouse brain is lissencephalic, as for other rodents, and has a very large olfactory bulb. There is sexual dimorphism of brain size, with male brains being marginally

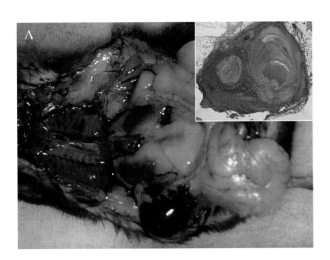
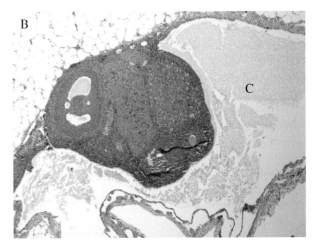

Figure 8.39 A: Hemorrhagic ovarian cyst in an aged mouse. Cystic tissue may become blood-filled (inset). B: Parovarian cyst. lumen (C) contains low protein fluid and the cyst lining is markedly attenuated. Mice may present off feed with hunched posture and signs of abdominal pain.

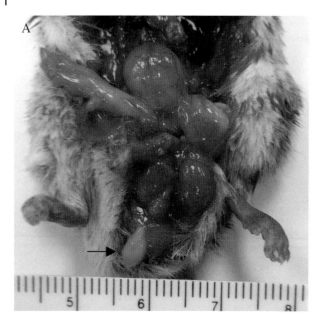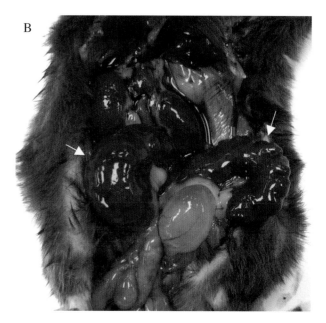

Figure 8.40 A: Peritesticular abscesses (arrow) may occur in group-housed male mice following fighting. B: Seminal vesicle impaction (arrows) is a common incidental finding in aging male mice.

larger. Regional differences in size of certain structures and nuclei are seen between male and female mice.

Although head tilt, ataxia, circling, and seizures are seen routinely in some strains of mice, brain histologic correlates are uncommon, and the pathogenesis of many of these conditions remains a mystery. A thorough work-up of peripheral tissues is warranted to rule out other conditions, such as otitis media, trauma, underlying systemic disease and inanition, fracture, and neoplastic cell infiltrate. Other causes for these conditions may include polyarteritis, spontaneous brainstem infarction, abscess, or tumor. Epilepsy in FVB mice has been linked to parenchymal necrosis within the hippocampus, thalamus, and cerebral cortex, although the underlying cause of this is unknown. Affected animals may present in intractable status epilepticus and die.

Congenital hydrocephalus occurs sporadically in mice and is caused by an accumulation of fluid with the cerebral ventricles, resulting in pressure-induced necrosis of the surrounding parenchyma. Doming of the skull may be observed in young animals as fluid accumulates and animals may survive to early adulthood, although rarely beyond (Figure 8.41). Severity of clinical signs is proportional to the loss of parenchyma and the rate of accumulation of fluid. The defect may be transmitted as a recessive mutation and affected breeding pairs should be culled.

Lymphocytic choriomeningitis virus (LCMV) is an enveloped arenavirus that is enzootic among wild mice. The virus typically causes asymptomatic infections in mice and can be transmitted to other rodents and humans via aerosolization of contaminated saliva, urine, drop-

pings and nesting material. Antibodies in mice persist post-infection for many months and are thus not necessarily indicative of active infection. In most humans, LCMV infection leads to mild, self-limiting, influenza-like symptoms but LCMV can cause fetal ocular defects, hydrocephalus, and abortions in pregnant women. Wild mice should be excluded from breeding colonies and pregnant women should avoid contact with rodent urine and soiled bedding. Appropriate hand hygiene should be conducted after handling mice.

Prolactin-secreting pituitary hyperplasia of the pars distalis and adenoma are both seen commonly in some strains of mice, such as FVB, and may be associated with mammary gland hyperplasia. Other central nervous system tumors are very uncommon in mice (Figure 8.42).

The extent of *Toxoplasma gondii* infection in pet or feeder mice is unknown. Similarly, mice and other rodents are considered reservoirs for *Encephalitozoon cuniculi*; however, infections are generally subclinical in mice.

8.10 Hematopoietic and Lymphoid Conditions

Extramedullary hematopoiesis (EMH) occurs very commonly in mice and appears as small clusters of hematopoietic cells with characteristics typical of either erythroid or myeloid populations within the liver, spleen, adrenal glands or other tissues. As for other mammals, the rodent liver is the primary site of hematopoiesis for the first half of gestation, but the spleen and bone marrow

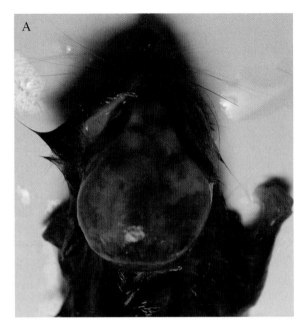 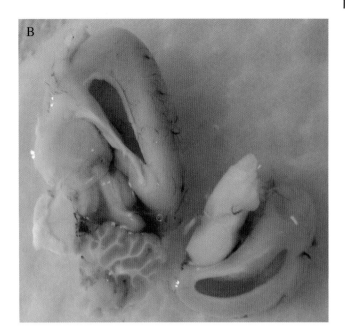

Figure 8.41 A: Skin reflected to demonstrate doming of the calvarium in a young mouse with congenital hydrocephalus. B: Brain removed and opened demonstrating markedly expanded ventricles in an animal with congenital hydrocephalus.

become the primary hematopoietic organs after birth. Recently, stem cells with characteristics of bone-marrow-derived hematopoietic stem cells have been isolated from the livers of mature mice, which may help to explain the restriction of post-natal EMH to the liver. Proliferation is regulated in part by hepatocyte growth factor. Typically, hematopoiesis is extravascular, occurring within the sub-endothelial space, whereas granulopoiesis tends to occur

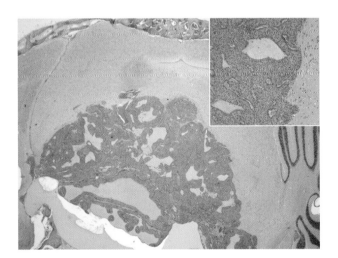

Figure 8.42 Benign choroid plexus tumor in an unthrifty mouse. The mass is compressing the adjacent neuropil and is composed of polygonal cells arranged in anastomosing cords (inset) and lining up to form variably-sized cavities filled with eosinophilic granular matrix. Excessive fluid is present within the fourth ventricle.

in periportal areas. Both erythropoiesis and granulopoiesis can occur in the same liver; however, clusters do not contain mixed populations. Megakaryocytes can be seen, although less commonly. EMH within the spleen and liver are seen in animals undergoing physiologic stress (e.g., pregnancy, anemia, neoplasia, systemic or local inflammation, necrosis, and infarction). Differential diagnoses for this condition include inflammation and necrosis, in which mixed populations of leukocytes are typically seen, or neoplasia, e.g., myeloid leukemia.

The normal myeloid:erythroid ratio within the bone marrow is approximately 2–3:1 and relative changes in approximate cell line ratios may be seen with chronic systemic infection or blood loss. The sternebrae is a convenient site to evaluate bone marrow in mice as it often does not require decalcification before trimming and embedding, even in mature animals.

Normal peripheral lymph nodes in mice are usually inapparent at postmortem, and focal to multifocal lymph node enlargement is indicative of neoplasia or systemic disease.

8.10.1 Infectious Hematopoietic and Lymphoid Conditions

Multifocal to coalescing splenic necrosis can be seen with ectromelia virus infection, as well as infection with various bacterial agents, such as *Salmonella* spp., *C. kutscheri*, and *S. pneumoniae*. Diagnostic investigation should include bacterial culture and histopathology. Intracytoplasmic inclusion bodies may be seen with ectromelia virus infection and rarely, concurrent lymph node or Peyer's patch necrosis. Serology or PCR of affected tissue may be used to confirm viral infection.

Although mouse parvoviruses, and mouse minute virus in particular, have a tropism for hematopoietic and lymphoid tissues, and viral prevalence is moderate to high in wild and pet mice, no clinical or microscopic signs are typically associated with infection.

8.10.2 Hematopoietic and Lymphoid Neoplasia

Lymphosarcoma occurs commonly in mice and is related to strain, stock, age, and retroviral infection (Figures 8.43 and 8.44). Both T and B cell lymphomas may be seen and can be classified based on tissue distribution, cell morphology and immunohistochemistry. B cell lymphomas often involve the spleen, mesenteric lymph node and intestinal Peyer's patches and may be somewhat pleiomorphic in appearance. Patterns include follicular center cell (CD45 positive), plasma cell (CD138 positive), and lymphoblastic. T cell lymphomas primarily involve the thymus (CD3 positive) and may have a lymphoblastic pattern. Generalized distribution with a lymphoid leukemia is commonly seen in the final stages of T cell lymphoma.

Histiocytic sarcomas are common in mice and frequently involve the hepatic sinusoids and uterus, with secondary metastasis to the lungs (Figure 8.45). Tumors may be seen in the spleen, mesenteric lymph nodes, and, less commonly, the bone marrow. Neoplastic cells are large, round to spindle-shaped with a pleiomorphic nucleus and abundant pale eosinophilic cytoplasm, which is often positive for lysozyme, MAC-2, and CD11, confirming a mononuclear cell origin. The pattern may be more sarcomatous or histiocytic. Multinucleated giant cells may be scattered

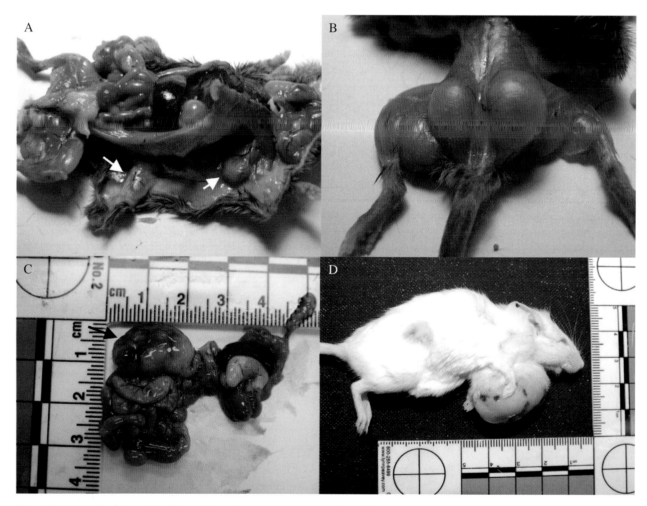

Figure 8.43 Manifestations of multicentric lymphosarcoma in mice. A: Any enlargement of peripheral lymph nodes in mice is abnormal. Axillary and inguinal lymph nodes (arrows) are enlarged as well as the spleen. B: This animal presented with hemiparesis of the hind end. Neoplastic lymphocytes had infiltrated the spinal cord and dorsal nerve roots. C: Markedly enlarged mesenteric lymph node (arrow). D: This ulcerated mass had its anatomical roots in the submandibular lymph node. Differential diagnoses at necropsy included mammary gland adenocarcinoma and fibrosarcoma.

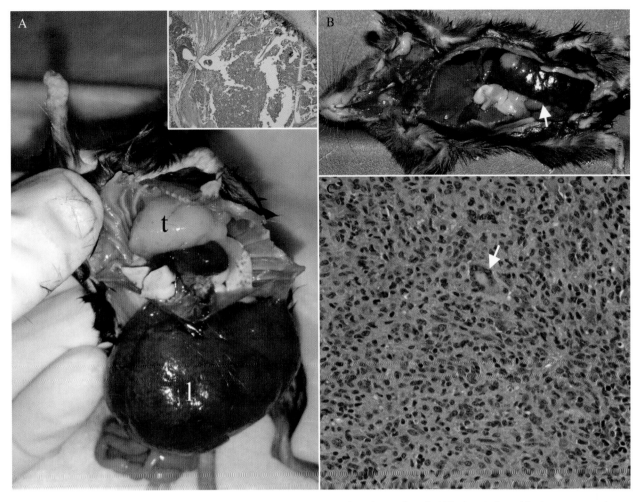

Figure 8.44 A: Thymic lymphoma (t) and hepatomegaly (l) in a mouse with end stage lymphoid leukemia. Inset: The bone marrow is replaced by neoplastic round cells and dense neoplastic infiltrates were present in most tissues. B: Splenic histiocytic sarcoma (arrow). C: Microscopically, the mass is composed of an admixture of round and spindloid cells with scattered multinucleated giant cells (arrow).

throughout, particularly in the liver, as well as islands of EMH. Renal tubular epithelial cells may contain dense hyaline droplets, which are lysozyme-positive, although these are less common in mice than in rats with histiocytic sarcoma.

Myeloid leukemia (myeloperoxidase positive) occurs much less commonly. Other forms of hematopoietic tumors are rare in mice.

8.10.3 Other Hematopoietic Conditions

Fibro-osseous hyperplasia is a condition seen occasionally in older mice, predominantly in females. The lesion may be seen in the sternebrae and long bones and consists of partial to complete replacement of normal hematopoietic cells of the marrow by dense infiltrates of fibroblasts, multinucleate giant cells, and collagenous matrix with stimulation of bony trabecula formation.

The infiltrates can extend outside of the marrow cavity into surrounding muscle, which may induce hemiparesis or paralysis in mice and it may also involve surrounding nerves.

8.11 Ophthalmic Conditions

The eyelids of newborn mice are closed and open between 12–14 days after birth. Mice have three pairs of lacrimal glands: infraorbital, extraorbital, and Harderian. The Harderian gland secretes lipids, porphyrin, melatonin, and various pheromones, and has a foamy appearance, histologically. Rarely, the Harderian gland can become inflamed or hyperplastic, resulting in exophthalmos.

Anophthalmia and microphthalmia are common in certain strains of mice and may be uni- or bilateral. The

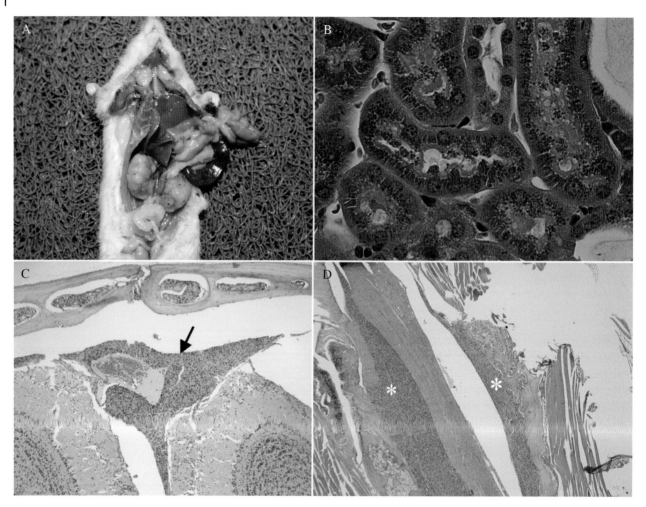

Figure 8.45 A: Bilateral renal histiocytic sarcoma. B: Photomicrograph of kidneys from animal in (A) demonstrating hyaline droplets in the apical cytoplasm of renal tubular epithelial cells. The droplets are composed of lysozyme produced by the neoplastic histiocytes. C: Infiltration of the meninges and extension into the skull cavity is common. Depicted are histiocytic sarcoma infiltrates (arrow) surrounding the olfactory bulbs. This animal presented hunched, lethargic, and anorectic. (D) Histiocytic sarcoma infiltrates may also extend from the vertebral marrow along and within the spinal cord (*) and within vertebral bodies causing microfractures and leading to paresis and paralysis.

condition may be acquired following trauma, or, more commonly, is inherited.

For the lesions described below, no sex predilection has been identified.

8.11.1 Conditions of the Eyelid and Conjunctiva

Conjunctivitis and keratoconjunctivitis are seen commonly in pet mice (Figure 8.46) and may be caused by infection with *Pasteurella pneumotropica*, *Mycoplasma pulmonis*, *Staphylococcus aureus*, *Streptococcus* spp., *Salmonella* spp., *Corynebacterium* spp., ectromelia virus, or lymphocytic choriomeningitis virus. Infections may be exacerbated by volatile oils in softwood bedding or other particulates or ocular irritants in the environment. Ulcers with crusting may be seen in severe cases with marked neutrophilic infiltrates. Lesions may be exacerbated by self-excoriations.

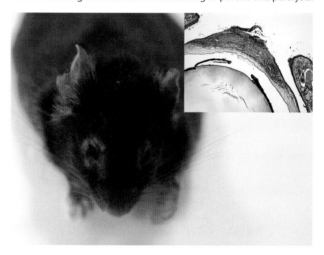

Figure 8.46 Bilateral conjunctivitis in a feeder-breeder colony mouse co-infected with *Pasteurella pneumotropica* and *Mycoplasma pulmonis*. Inset: Focal ulcerative keratitis can result from self-excoriation.

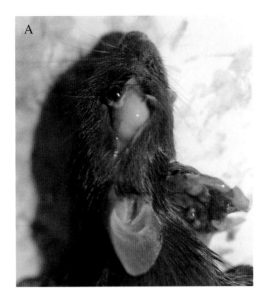 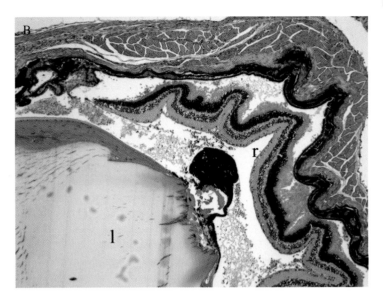

Figure 8.47 A: Retrobular abscess in a young mouse. B: Ocular melanoma on the posterior surface of the lens capsule (l) in a mouse.

8.11.2 Conditions of the Cornea and Anterior Chamber

Corneal dystrophy is common in mice and increases with age, presenting clinically as focal to multifocal punctate white opacities on the corneal surface. The pathogenesis is unknown although a positive correlation has been made with decreased environmental air quality and increased ammonia levels. Microscopically, there may be focal stromal mineralization with neovascularization and stromal edema.

8.11.3 Uveal and Lenticular Conditions

Iris colobomas are occasionally reported. Partial to complete cataracts are common in mice and may be strain- and age-dependent, although the pathogenesis of this defect is unknown. Persistent pupillary membranes can be seen with moderate frequency in certain strains of mice.

8.11.4 Retinal Conditions

Retinal degeneration is common in mice and may be heritable with early onset or develop secondary to phototoxic retinopathy. In the latter case, long-term exposure of photoreceptors to moderate intensity light leads to permanent photoreceptor damage. Retinal folds and fundic coloboma are less common.

Ocular tumors are uncommon but may result in exophthalmos (Figure 8.47B). A single case of intraocular teratoma has been reported. Retrobulbar abscesses may be seen sporadically and can be associated with foreign bodies (Figure 8.47A).

Bibliography

Alopecia

Bechard, A., Meagher, R., and Mason, G. (2011) Environmental enrichment reduces the likelihood of alopecia in adult C57BL/6J mice. *Journal of the American Association for Laboratory Animal Science*, **50**(2), 171–174.

Garner, J.P., Weisker, S.M., Dufour, B., and Mench, J.A. (2004) Barbering (fur and whisker trimming) by laboratory mice as a model of human trichotillomania and obsessive-compulsive spectrum disorders. *Comparative Medicine*, **54**(2), 216–224.

Tynes, V.V. (2013) Behavioral dermatopathies in small mammals. *Veterinary Clinics of North America: Exotic Animal Practice*, **16**, 801–820.

Bacterial Dermatitis

Cover, C.E., Keenan, C.M., and Bettinger, G.E. (1989) Ear tag induced *Staphylococcus* infection in mice. *Laboratory Animals (UK)*, **23**(3), 229–233.

Kastenmayer, R.J., Fain, M.A., and Perdue, K.A. (2006) A retrospective study of idiopathic ulcerative dermatitis in mice with a C57BL/6 background. *Journal of the American Association for Laboratory Animal Science*, **45**(6), 8–12.

Radaelli, E., Manarolla, G., Pisoni, G., et al. (2010) Suppurative adenitis of preputial glands associated with *Corynebacterium mastitidis* infection in mice. *Journal of the American Association for Laboratory Animal Science*, **49**(1), 69–74.

Stewart, D.D., Buck, G.E., McConnell, E.E., and Amster, R.L. (1975) An epizootic of necrotic dermatitis in laboratory mice caused by Lancefield group G streptococci. *Laboratory Animal Science*, **25**(3), 296–302.

Weisbroth, S.H., Scher, S., and Boman, I. (1969) *Pasteurella pneumotropica* abscess syndrome in a mouse. *Journal of the American Veterinary Medical Association*, **155**(7), 1206–1210.

Wilson, P. (1976) *Pasteurella pneumotropica* as the causal organism of abscesses in the masseter muscle of mice. *Laboratory Animals (UK)*, **10**(2), 171–172.

Dermatophytoses

Lane, R.F. (2003) Diagnostic testing for fungal diseases. *Veterinary Clinics of North America: Exotic Animal Practice*, **6**, 301–314.

Pollock, C. (2003) Fungal diseases of laboratory rodents. *Veterinary Clinics of North America: Exotic Animal Practice*, **6**(2), 401–413.

Parasitic Dermatitis

Baker, D.G. (ed.) (2007) *Flynn's Parasites of Laboratory Animals*, 2nd edn. Wiley-Blackwell, Ames, IA.

Cole, J.S., Sabol-Jones, M., Karolewski, B., and Byford, T. (2005) *Ornithonyssus bacoti* infestation and elimination from a mouse colony. *Contemporary Topics in Laboratory Animal Science*, **44**(5), 27–30.

Madison, G., Kim-Schluger, L., Braverman, S., Nicholson, W.L., and Wormser, G.P. (2008) Hepatitis in association with rickettsialpox. *Vector Borne Zoonotic Diseases*, **8**(1), 111–115.

Pochanke, V., Hatak, S., Hengartner, H., Zinkernagel, R.M., and McCoy, K.D. (2006) Induction of IgE and allergic-type responses in fur mite-infested mice. *European Journal of Immunology*, **36**(9), 2434–2345.

Reeves, W.K. and Cobbs, A.D. (2005) Ectoparasites from house mice (*Mus musculus*) obtained from pet stores in South Carolina, USA. *Comparative Parasitology*, **72**(2), 193–195.

Cutaneous Masses and Neoplasia

Cardiff, R.D., Anver, M.R., Gusterson, B.A., et al. (2000) The mammary pathology of genetically engineered mice: the consensus report and recommendations from the Annapolis meeting. *Oncogene*, **19**(8), 968–988.

Greenacre, C.B. (2004) Spontaneous tumors of small mammals. *Veterinary Clinics of North America: Exotic Animal Practice*, **7**(3), 627–651.

NIH (n.d.) *Histology Atlas of the Mouse Mammary Gland*. http://mammary.nih.gov/atlas/ (accessed January 25, 2012).

Ross, S.R. (2010) Mouse mammary tumor virus molecular biology and oncogenesis. *Viruses.* **2**(9), 2000–2012.

Welsch, C.W. and Nagasawa, H. (1977) Prolactin and murine mammary tumorigenesis: a review. *Cancer Research*, **37**(4), 951–963.

Other Information

Donnelly, T.M. (2011) What's your diagnosis? Enlarged mouse preputial glands. *Laboratory Animals (NY)*. **40**(3), 69–71.

Esteban, D.J. and Buller, R.M. (2005) Ectromelia virus: the causative agent of mousepox. *Journal of General Virology*, **86**(Pt 10), 2645–2659.

Fenner, F. (1948) The clinical features and pathogenesis of mouse-pox (infectious ectromelia of mice). *Journal of Pathology and Bacteriology*, **60**(4), 529–562.

Hill, L.R., Coghlan, L.G., and Baze, W.B. (2002) Perineal swellings in two strains of mice. *Contemporary Topics in Laboratory Animal Science*, **41**(1), 51–53.

Kitagaki, M. and Hirota, M. (2007) Auricular chondritis caused by metal ear tagging in C57BL/6 mice. *Veterinary Pathology*, **44**(4), 458–466.

Labelle, P., Hahn, N.E., Fraser, J.K., et al. (2009) Mousepox detected in a research facility: case report and failure of mouse antibody production testing to identify Ectromelia virus in contaminated mouse serum. *Comparative Medicine*, **59**(2), 180–186.

Lipman, N.S., Perkins, S., Nguyen, H., Pfeffer, M., and Meyer, H. (2000) Mousepox resulting from use of ectromelia virus-contaminated, imported mouse serum. *Comparative Medicine*, **50**(4), 426–435.

Recordati, C., Basta, S.M., Benedetti, L., et al. (2015) Pathologic and environmental studies provide new pathogenetic insights into ringtail of laboratory mice. *Veterinary Pathology*, **52**(4), 700–711.

Taylor, D.K., Rogers, M.M., and Hankenson, F.C. (2006) Lanolin as a treatment option for ringtail in transgenic rats. *Journal of the American Association for Laboratory Animal Science*, **45**(1), 83–87.

General Information

Chase, H.B., Montagna, W., and Malone, J.D. (1953) Changes in the skin in relation to the hair growth cycle. *Anatomical Record*, **116**(1), 75–81.

Harkness, J.E., Turner, P.V., VandeWoude, S. and Wheler, C.L. (2010) *Harkness and Wagner's Biology and Medicine of Rabbits and Rodents*, 5th edn. Wiley-Blackwell, Ames, IA.

Hoppmann, E. and Wilson Barron, H. (2007) Rodent dermatology. *Journal of Exotic Pet Medicine*, **16**(4), 238–255.

Steingrímsson, E., Copeland, N.G. and Jenkins, N.A. (2006) Mouse coat color mutations: from fancy mice to functional genomics. *Developmental Dynamics*, **235**(9), 2401–2411.

Sundberg, J.P. and Silva, K.A. (2012) What color is the skin of a mouse? *Veterinary Pathoogy*, **49**(1), 142–145.

Endocrine Conditions

Collins, B.R. (2008) Endocrine diseases of rodents. *Veterinary Clinics of North America: Exotic Animal Practice*, **11**, 153–162.

El Wakil, A., Mari, B., Barhanin, J. and Lalli, E. (2013) Genomic analysis of sexual dimorphism of gene expression in the mouse adrenal gland. *Hormone and Metabolic Research*, **45**(12), 870–873.

Petterino, C., Naylor, S., Mukaratirwa, S. and Bradley, A. (2015) Adrenal gland background findings in CD-1 (Crl:CD-1(ICR)BR) mice from 104-week carcinogenicity studies. *Toxicologic Pathology*, **43**(6), 816–824.

Thorson, L. (2014) Thyroid diseases in rodent species *Veterinary Clinics of North America: Exotic Animal Practice*, **17**, 51–67.

Bacterial Respiratory Infections

Bemis, D.A., Shek, W.R., and Clifford, C.B. (2003) *Bordetella bronchiseptica* infection of rats and mice. *Comparative Medicine*, **53**(1), 11–20.

Brennan, P.C., Fristz, T.E., and Flynn, R.J. (1969) Murine pneumonia: A review of etiologic agents. *Laboratory Animal Care*, **19**(3), 360–371.

Ellis, J., Oyston, P.C., Green, M., and Titball, R.W. (2002) Tularemia. *Clinical Microbiology Reviews*, **15**(4), 631–646.

Fallon, M.T., Reinhard, M.K., Gray, B.M., Davis, T.W., and Lindsey, J.R. (1988) Inapparent *Streptococcus pneumoniae* type 35 infections in commercial rats and mice. *Laboratory Animal Science*, **38**(2), 129–132.

Goto, K., Nozu, R., Takakura, A., Matsushita, S., and Itoh, T. (1995) Detection of cilia-associated respiratory bacillus in experimentally and naturally infected mice and rats by the polymerase chain reaction. *Experimental Animals*, **44**(4), 333–336.

Hayashimoto, N., Morita, H., Yasuda, M., et al. (2011) Prevalence of *Bordetella hinzii* in mice in experimental facilities in Japan. *Research in Veterinary Science*, **93**, 624–626.

Hayashimoto, N., Yasuda, M., Goto, K., Takakura, A., and Itoh, T. (2008) Study of a *Bordetella hinzii* isolate from a laboratory mouse. *Comparative Medicine*, **58**(5), 440–446.

Kawamoto, E., Sasaki, H., Okiyama, E., et al. (2011) Pathogenicity of *Pasteurella pneumotropica* in immunodeficient NOD/ShiJic-scid/Jcl and immunocompetent Crlj:CD1 (ICR) mice. *Experimental Animals*, **60**(5), 463–70.

Lindsay, J.R., Baker, H.J., Overcash, R.G., Cassell, G.H., and Hunt, C.E. (1971) Murine chronic respiratory disease. *American Journal of Pathology*, **64**(3), 675–708.

Matsushita, S. and Suzuki, E. (1995) Prevention and treatment of cilia-associated respiratory bacillus in mice by use of antibiotics. *Laboratory Animal Science*, **45**(5), 503–507.

Origgi, F.C., König, B., Lindholm, A.K., Mayor, D., and Pilo, P. (2015) Tularemia among free-ranging mice without infection of exposed humans, Switzerland, 2012. *Emerging Infectious Diseases*, **21**(1), 133–135.

Ueno, Y., Shimizu, R., Nozu, R., et al. (2002) Elimination of *Pasteurella pneumotropica* from a contaminated mouse colony by oral administration of enrofloxacin. *Experimental Animals*, **51**(4), 401–405.

van der Linden, M., Al-Lahham, A., Nicklas, W., and Reinert, R.R. (2009) Molecular characterization of pneumococcal isolates from pets and laboratory animals. *PLoS ONE*. **4**(12), e8286.

Fungal Infections

Aliouat-Denis, C.M., Chabé, M., et al. (2008) *Pneumocystis* species, co-evolution and pathogenic power. *Infection, Genetics and Evolution*, **8**(5), 708–726.

Hernandez-Novoa, B., Bishop, L., et al. (2008) Immune responses to *Pneumocystis murina* are robust in healthy mice but largely absent in CD40 ligand-deficient mice. *Journal of Leukocyte Biology*, **84**(2), 420–430.

Weisbroth, S.H. (2006) *Pneumocystis*: newer knowledge about the biology of this group of organisms in laboratory rats and mice. *Laboratory Animals (NY)*, **35**(9), 55–61.

Viral Respiratory Diseases

Becker, S.D., Bennett, M., Stewart, J.P., and Hurst, J.L. (2007) Serological survey of virus infection among wild house mice (*Mus domesticus*) in the UK. *Laboratory Animals*, **41**(2), 229–238.

Easterbrook, J.D., Kaplan, J.B., Glass, G.E., Watson, J., and Klein, S.L. (2008) A survey of rodent-borne pathogens carried by wild-caught Norway rats: a potential threat to laboratory rodent colonies. *Laboratory Animals* **42**(1), 92–98.

Easton, A.J., Domachowske, J.B., and Rosenberg, H.F. (2004) Animal pneumoviruses: molecular genetics and pathogenesis. *Clinical Microbiology Reviews*, **17**(2), 390–412.

Jay, M., Ascher, M.S., Chomel, B.B., et al. (1997) Seroepidemiologic studies of hantavirus infection among wild rodents in California. *Emerging Infectious Diseases*, **3**(2), 183–190.

Kashuba, C., Hsu, C., Krogstad, A., and Franklin, C. (2005) Small mammal virology. *Veterinary Clinics of North America: Exotic Animal Practice* **8**(1), 107–122.

Rosenberg, H.F. and Domachowske, J.B. (2008) Pneumonia virus of mice: severe respiratory infection in a natural host. *Immunology Letters*, **118**(1), 6–12.

Seto, T., Nagata, N., Yoshikawa, K., et al. (2012) Infection of Hantaan virus strain AA57 leading to pulmonary disease in laboratory mice. *Virus Research*, **163**(1), 284–290.

Smith, A.L., Singleton, G.R., Hansen, G.M., and Shellam, G. (1993) A serologic survey for viruses and *Mycoplasma pulmonis* among wild house mice (*Mus domesticus*) in southeastern Australia. *Journal of Wildlife Diseases*, **29**(2), 219–229.

Zeier, M., Handermann, M., Bahr, U., et al. (2005) New ecological aspects of hantavirus infection: a change of a paradigm and a challenge of prevention-a review. *Virus Genes.* **30**(2), 157–180.

Pulmonary Masses and Neoplasia

Greenacre, C.B. (2004) Spontaneous tumors of small mammals. *Veterinary Clinics of North America: Exotic Animal Practice*, **7**(3), 627–651.

Nikitin, A.Y., Alcaraz, A., Anver, M.R., et al. (2004) Classification of proliferative pulmonary lesions of the mouse: recommendations of the mouse models of human cancers consortium. *Cancer Research*, **64**(7), 2307–2316.

Prejean, J.D., Peckham, J.C., Casey, A.E., et al. (1973) Spontaneous tumors in Sprague-Dawley rats and Swiss mice. *Cancer Research*, **33**(11), 2768–2773.

General Information

Dammann, P., Hilken, G., Hueber, B., et al. (2011) Infectious microorganisms in mice (*Mus musculus*) purchased from commercial pet shops in Germany. *Laboratory Animals (UK)*, **45**(4), 271–275.

DiVincenti, L. Jr., Moorman-White, D., Bavlov, N., Garner, M., and Wyatt, J. (2012) Effects of housing density on nasal pathology of breeding mice housed in individually ventilated cages. *Laboratory Animals (NY)*, **41**(3), 68–76.

Harkema, J.R., Carey, S.A., and Wagner, J.G. (2006) The nose revisited: a brief review of the comparative structure, function, and toxicologic pathology of the nasal epithelium. *Toxicologic Pathology*, **34**(3), 252–269.

Kelliher, K.R. and Wersinger, S.R. (2009) Olfactory regulation of the sexual behavior and reproductive physiology of the laboratory mouse: effects and neural mechanisms. *ILAR Journal*, **50**(1), 28–42.

Kling, M.A. (2011) A review of respiratory system anatomy, physiology, and disease in the mouse, rat, hamster, and gerbil. *Veterinary Clinics of North America: Exotic Animal Practice*, **14**(2), 287–337.

Pritchett-Corning, K.R., Cosentino, J., and Clifford, C.B. (2009) Contemporary prevalence of infectious agents in laboratory mice and rats. *Laboratory Animals (UK).* **43**(2), 165–173.

Vogelweid, C.M., Zapien, K.A., Honigford, M.J., et al. (2011) Effects of a 28-day cage-change interval on intracage ammonia levels, nasal histology, and perceived welfare of CD1 mice. *Journal of the American Association for Laboratory Animal Science*, **50**(6), 868–878.

Ward, J.M., Yoon, M., Anver, M.R., et al. (2001) Hyalinosis and Ym1/Ym2 gene expression in the stomach and respiratory tract of 129S4/SvJae and wild-type and CYP1A2-null B6, 129 mice. *American Journal of Pathology*, **158**, 323–332.

Musculoskeletal Conditions

Albassam, M.A. and Courtney, C.L. (1996) Nonneoplastic and neoplastic lesions of the bone. In: *Pathobiology of the Aging Mouse*, vol. **2**. (eds. D.L. Dungworth, C.C. Capen, et al.). ILSI Press: Washington, DC, pp. 425–437.

Bagi, C.M., Berryman, E., and Moalli, M.R. (2011) Comparative bone anatomy of commonly used laboratory animals: Implications for drug discovery. *Comparative Medicine*, **61**(1), 76–85.

Ceccarelli, A.V. and Rozengurt, N. (2002) Outbreak of hind limb paralysis in young CFW Swiss Webster mice. *Comparative Medicine*, **52**(2), 171–175.

Davis, J.A., Miller, G.F. and St Claire, M.F. (1997) Spontaneous rhabdomyosarcomas in (A/J x CBA/J)Fl mice. *Contemporary Topics in Laboratory Animal Science*, **36**(1), 87–89.

Gardner, M.B. (1985) Retroviral spongiform polioencephalomyelopathy. *Review of Infectious Diseases*, **7**(1), 99–110.

Gardner, M.B. (1993) Genetic control of retroviral disease in aging wild mice. *Genetica*, **91**(1–3), 199–209.

Glastonbury, J.R., Morton, J.G., and Matthews, L.M. (1996) *Streptobacillus moniliformis* infection in Swiss white mice. *Journal of Veterinary Diagnostic Investigation*, **8**(2), 202–209.

Huang, P. and Suit, H.D. (1996) Spontaneous osteosarcoma in a severe combined immunodeficient (SCID/Sed) mouse. *Contemporary Topics in Laboratory Animal Science*, **35**(6), 75–77.

Kavirayani, A.M., Sundberg, J.P., and Foreman, O. (2012) Primary neoplasms of bones in mice: retrospective study and review of literature. *Veterinary Pathology*, **49**(1), 182–205.

Krugner-Higby, L.A., Gendron, A., Garland, T. Jr., et al. (1998) Eosinophylic polymyositis in a mouse. *Contemporary Topics in Laboratory Animal Science*, **37**, 94–97.

Salminen, A., Kainulainen, H., Arstila, A.U., and Vihko, V. (1984) Vitamin E deficiency and the susceptibility to lipid peroxidation of mouse cardiac and skeletal muscles. *Acta Physiologica Scandinavica*, **122**(4), 565–570.

Tamano, S., Hagiwara, A., Shibata, M.A., et al. (1988) Spontaneous tumors in aging (C57BL/6N x C3H/HeN) F1 (B6C3F1) mice. *Toxicologic Pathology*, **16**(3), 321–326.

Oral and Salivary Gland Conditions

Capello, V. (2008) Diagnosis and treatment of dental disease in pet rodents. *Journal of Exotic Pet Medicine*, **17**(2), 114–23.

Chen, H.C. and Cover, C.E. (1988) Spontaneous disseminated cytomegalic inclusion disease in an ageing laboratory mouse. *Journal of Comparative Pathology*, **98**(4), 489–493.

Cross, S.S., Parker, J.C., Rowe, W.P., and Robbins, M.L. (1979) Biology of mouse thymic virus, a herpesvirus of mice, and the antigenic relationship to mouse cytomegalovirus. *Infection and Immunity*, **26**(3), 1186–1195.

Dayan, D., Waner, T., Harmelin, A., and Nyska, A. (1994) Bilateral complex odontoma in a Swiss (CD-1) male mouse. *Laboratory Animals (UK)*, **28**(1), 90–92.

Legendre, L.F. (2003) Oral disorders of exotic rodents. *Veterinary Clinics of North America: Exotic Animal Practice*, **6**(3), 601–628.

Long, P.H. and Herbert, R.A. (2002) Epithelial-induced intrapulpal denticles in B6C3F1 mice. *Toxicologic Pathology*, **30**(6), 744–748.

Losco, P.E. (1995) Dental dysplasia in rats and mice. *Toxicologic Pathology*, **23**(6), 677–688.

Mannini, A. and Medearis, D.N. Jr. (1961) Mouse salivary gland virus infections. *American Journal of Hygiene*, **73**, 329–343.

Morse, S.S. (1987) Mouse thymic necrosis virus: a novel murine lymphotropic agent. *Laboratory Animal Science*, **37**(6), 717–725.

Robins, M.W. and Rowlatt, C. (1971) Dental abnormalities in aged mice. *Gerontologia*, **17**(5), 261–272.

Gastric Conditions

García, A., Erdman, S., Sheppard, B.J., Murphy, J.C., and Fox, J.G. (2001) Gastric dilatation syndrome associated with chronic nephropathy, hypergastrinemia, and gastritis in mice exposed to high levels of environmental antigens. *Comparative Medicine*, **51**(3), 262–267.

Hummel, K.P. and Chapman, D.B. (1959) Visceral inversion and associated anomalies in the mouse. *Journal of Heredity*, **50**(1), 9–13.

Miyajima, R., Kihara, T., Hosoi, M., Yamamoto, S., Mikami, S., Yamakawa, S., Iwata, H. and Enomoto, M. (1999) A congenital ciliated epithelial cyst on the stomach of a B6C3F1 mouse. *Toxicologic Pathology*, **27**(5), 600–603.

Okimoto, K., Matsumoto, I., Kuoki, K. and Tanaka, K. (2003) Spontaneous gastric carcinoid tumor in a male B6C3F1 mouse. *Journal of Toxicologic Pathology*, **16**, 175–178.

Tamano, S., Hagiwara, A., Shibata, M.A., Kurata, Y., Fukushima, S. and Ito, N. (1988) Spontaneous tumors in aging (C57BL/6N x C3H/HeN)F1 (B6C3F1) mice. *Toxicologic Pathology*, **16**(3), 321–326.

Enteric Conditions

Amao, H., Komukai, Y., Sugiyama, M., et al. (1995) Natural habitats of *Corynebacterium kutscheri* in subclinically infected ICGN and DBA/2 strains of mice. *Laboratory Animal Science*, **45**(1), 6–10.

Au Yeung, K.J., Smith, A., Zhao, A., et al. (2005) Impact of vitamin E or selenium deficiency on nematode-induced alterations in murine intestinal function. *Experimental Parasitology*, **109**(4), 201–208.

Barthold, S.W., Beck, D.S., and Smith, A.L. (1993) Enterotropic coronavirus (mouse hepatitis virus) in mice: influence of host age and strain on infection and disease. *Laboratory Animal Science*, **43**(4), 276–284.

Becker, S.D., Bennett, M., Stewart, J.P., and Hurst, J.L. (2007) Serological survey of virus infection among wild house mice (*Mus domesticus*) in the UK. *Laboratory Animals (UK)*, **41**(2), 229–38.

Cartwright, E.J., Nguyen, T., Melluso, C., et al. (2016) A multistate investigation of antibiotic-resistant *Salmonella enterica* Serotype I4,[5],12:i:-infections as part of an international outbreak associated with frozen feeder rodents. *Zoonoses Public Health*, **63**(1), 62–71.

Casebolt, D.B., Qian, B., and Stephensen, C.B. (1997) Detection of enterotropic mouse hepatitis virus fecal excretion by polymerase chain reaction. *Laboratory Animal Science*, **47**(1), 6–10.

Casebolt, D.B. and Schoeb, T.R. (1988) An outbreak in mice of salmonellosis caused by *Salmonella enteritidis* serotype enteritidis. *Laboratory Animal Science*, **38**(2), 190–192.

CDC (2005) Outbreak of multidrug-resistant *Salmonella* typhimurium associated with rodents purchased at retail pet stores – United States, December 2003–October 2004. *Morbidity and Mortality Week Reports*, **54**(17), 429–433.

Dagnaes-Hansen, F., Moser, J.M., Smith-John, T. and Aarup, M. (2010) Sudden death in lactating mice. *Laboratory Animals (NY)*, **39**(7), 205–207.

Dammann, P., Hilken, G., Hueber, B., et al. (2011) Infectious microorganisms in mice (*Mus musculus*) purchased from commercial pet shops in Germany. *Laboratory Animals (UK)*, **45**(4), 271–275.

Dyson, M.C., Eaton, K.A., and Chang, C. (2009) *Helicobacter* spp. in wild mice (*Peromyscus leucopus*) found in laboratory animal facilities. *Journal of the American Association for Laboratory Animal Science*, **48**(6), 754–756.

Easterbrook, J.D., Kaplan, J.B., Glass, G.E., Watson, J., and Klein, S.L. (2008) A survey of rodent-borne pathogens carried by wild-caught Norway rats: a potential threat to laboratory rodent colonies. *Laboratory Animals (UK)*, **42**(1), 92–98.

Feinstein, R.E., Morris, W.E., Waldemarson, A.H., Hedenqvist, P., and Lindberg, R. (2008) Fatal acute intestinal pseudoobstruction in mice. *Journal of the American Association for Laboratory Animal Science*, **47**(3), 58–63.

Fernández, P.E., Carbone, C., and Gimeno, E.J. (1996) Cryptosporidiosis in mice in Argentina. *Laboratory Animal Science*, **46**(6), 685–686.

Fuller, C.C., Jawahir, S.L., Leano, F.T., et al. (2008) A multi-state *Salmonella* Typhimurium outbreak associated with frozen vacuum-packed rodents used to feed snakes. *Zoonoses and Public Health*, **55**(8–10), 481–487.

Glastonbury, J.R., Morton, J.G., and Matthews, L.M. (1996) *Streptobacillus moniliformis* infection in Swiss white mice. *Journal of Veterinary Diagnostic Investigation*, **8**(2), 202–209.

Haberkorn, A., Friis, C.W., Schulz, H.P., Meister, G., and Feller, W. (1983) Control of an outbreak of mouse coccidiosis in a closed colony. *Laboratory Animals (UK)*, **17**(1), 59–64.

Harker, K.S., Lane, C., De Pinna, E., and Adak, G.K. (2011) An outbreak of *Salmonella* typhimurium DT191a associated with reptile feeder mice. *Epidemiology and Infection*, **139**(8), 1254–1261.

Hill, W.A., Randolph, M.M., and Mandrell, T.D. (2009) Sensitivity of perianal tape impressions to diagnose pinworm (*Syphacia* spp.) infections in rats (*Rattus norvegicus*) and mice (*Mus musculus). Journal of the American Association for Laboratory Animal Science*, **48**(4), 378–380.

Homberger, F.R. (1997) Enterotropic mouse hepatitis virus. *Laboratory Animals*, **31**(2), 97–115.

Jones, J.B., Estes, P.C., and Jordan, A.E. (1972) *Proteus mirabilis* infection in a mouse colony. *Journal of the American Veterinary Medical Association*, **161**(6), 661–664.

Kjeldsberg, E. and Hem, A. (1985) Detection of astroviruses in gut contents of nude and normal mice. Brief report. *Archives of Virology*, **84**(1–2), 135–140.

Krugner-Higby, L., Girard, I., Welter, J., et al. (2006) Clostridial enteropathy in lactating outbred Swiss-derived (ICR) mice. *Journal of the American Association for Laboratory Animal Science*, **45**(6), 80–87.

Kunstýr, I. (1986) Paresis of peristalsis and ileus lead to death in lactating mice. *Laboratory Animals (UK)*, **20**(1), 32–35.

Lee, K.M., McReynolds, J.L., Fuller, C.C., et al. (2008) Investigation and characterization of the frozen feeder rodent industry in Texas following a multi-state *Salmonella* Typhimurium outbreak associated with frozen vacuum-packed rodents. *Zoonoses and Public Health*. **55**(8–10), 488–496.

Little, L.M. and Shadduck, J.A. (1982) Pathogenesis of rotavirus infection in mice. *Infection and Immunity*, **38**(2), 755–763.

Macnish, M.G., Morgan, U.M., Behnke, J.M., and Thompson, R.C. (2002) Failure to infect laboratory rodent hosts with human isolates of *Rodentolepis* (= *Hymenolepis*) *nana*. *Journal of Helminthology*, **76**(1), 37–43.

Mumphrey, S.M., Changotra, H., Moore, T.N., et al. (2007) Murine norovirus 1 infection is associated with histopathological changes in immunocompetent hosts, but clinical disease is prevented by STAT1-dependent interferon responses. *Journal of Virology*, **81**(7), 3251–3263.

Mundy, R., MacDonald, T.T., Dougan, G., Frankel, G., and Wiles, S. (2005) *Citrobacter rodentium* of mice and man. *Cellular Microbiology*, **7**(12), 1697–1706.

Newsome, P.M. and Coney, K.A. (1985) Synergistic rotavirus and *Escherichia coli* diarrheal infection of mice. *Infection and Immunity*, **47**(2), 573–574.

Parker, S.E., Malone, S., Bunte, R.M., and Smith, A.L. (2009) Infectious diseases in wild mice (*Mus musculus*) collected on and around the University of Pennsylvania (Philadelphia) Campus. *Comparative Medicine*, **59**(5), 424–430.

Perdue, K.A., Green, K.Y., Copeland, M., et al. (2007) Naturally occurring murine norovirus infection in a large research institution. *Journal of the American Association for Laboratory Animal Science*, **46**(4), 39–45.

Pritchett-Corning, K.R., Cosentino, J., and Clifford, C.B. (2009) Contemporary prevalence of infectious agents in laboratory mice and rats. *Laboratory Animals (UK)*. **43**(2), 165–173.

Pritchett, K.R. and Johnston, N.A. (2002) A review of treatments for the eradication of pinworm infections from laboratory rodent colonies. *Contemporary Topics in Laboratory Animal Science*, **41**(2), 36–46.

Reavill, D. (2014) Pathology of the exotic companion mammal gastrointestinal system. *Veterinary Clinics of North America: Exotic Animal Practice*, **17**, 145–164.

Rollman, C., Olshan, K., and Hammer, J. (1998) Abdominal distension in lactating mice. *Laboratory Animals (NY)*, **7**(1), 19–20.

Smith, A.L., Singleton, G.R., Hansen, G.M., and Shellam, G. (1993) A serologic survey for viruses and *Mycoplasma pulmonis* among wild house mice (*Mus domesticus*) in southeastern Australia. *Journal of Wildlife Diseases*, **29**(2), 219–229.

Swanson, S.J., Snider, C., Braden, C.R., et al. (2007) Multidrug-resistant *Salmonella enterica* serotype Typhimurium associated with pet rodents. *New England Journal of Medicine*, **356**(1), 21–28.

Taffs, L.F. (1976) Pinworm infections in laboratory rodents: a review. *Laboratory Animals*, **10**(1), 1–13.

Taylor, J.D., Stephens, C.P., Duncan, R.G., and Singleton, G.R. (1994) Polyarthritis in wild mice (*Mus musculus*) caused by *Streptobacillus moniliformis*. *Australian Veterinary Journal*, **71**(5), 143–145.

Whary, M.T. and Fox, J.G. (2004) Natural and experimental Helicobacter infections. *Comparative Medicine*, **54**(2), 128–158.

Exocrine Pancreatic Conditions

Cheeseman, M.T., Chrobot, N., Fray, M.D., and Deeny, A.A. (2007) Spontaneous exocrine pancreas hypoplasia in specific pathogen-free C3HeB/FeJ and 101/H mouse pups causes steatorrhea and runting. *Comparative Medicine*, **57**(2), 210–216.

Hepatobiliary Conditions

Dyson, M.C., Eaton, K.A., and Chang, C. (2009) *Helicobacter* spp. in wild mice (*Peromyscus leucopus*) found in laboratory animal facilities. *Journal of the American Association for Laboratory Animal Science*, **48**(6), 754–756.

Fox, J.G., Rogers, A.B., Whary, M.T. et al. (2004) *Helicobacter bilis*-associated hepatitis in outbred mice. *Comparative Medicine*, **54**(5), 571–577.

Ganaway, J.R., Allen, A.M., and Moore, T.D. (1971) Tyzzer's disease. *American Journal of Pathology*, **64**(3), 717–730.

Lipman, R.D., Gaillard, E.T., Harrison, D.E., and Bronson, R.T. (1993) Husbandry factors and the prevalence of age-related amyloidosis in mice. *Laboratory Animal Science*, **43**, 439–444.

Livingston, R.S. and Riley, L.K. (2003) Diagnostic testing of mouse and rat colonies for infectious agents. *Laboratory Animals (UK)*, **32**, 44–51.

Parker, S.E., Malone, S., Bunte, R.M., and Smith, A.L. (2009) Infectious diseases in wild mice (*Mus musculus*) collected on and around the University of Pennsylvania (Philadelphia) Campus. *Comparative Medicine*, **59**(5), 424–430.

Riley, L.K., Franklin, C.L., Hook, R.R. Jr., and Besch-Williford, C. (1996) Identification of murine helicobacters by PCR and restriction enzyme analyses. *Journal of Clinical Microbiology*, **34**, 942–946.

Smith, A.L., Singleton, G.R., Hansen, G.M., and Shellam, G. (1993) A serologic survey for viruses and Mycoplasma pulmonis among wild house mice (*Mus domesticus*) in southeastern Australia. *Journal of Wildlife Diseases*, **29**(2), 219–229.

Tyzzer, E.E. (1917) A fatal disease of the Japanese waltzing mouse caused by a spore-bearing bacillus (*Bacillus piliformis*, N. Sp). *Journal of Medical Research*, **37**, 307–388.

Ulhar, C.M. and Whitehead, A.S. (1999) Serum amyloid A, the major vertebrate acute-phase reactant. *European Journal of Biochemistry*, **265**, 501–523.

Whary, M.T. and Fox, J.G. (2004) Natural and experimental *Helicobacter* infections. *Comparative Medicine*, **54**(2), 128–158.

General Gastrointestinal References

Bates, M.D., Erwin, C.R., Sanford, L.P., et al. (2002) Novel genes and functional relationships in the adult mouse gastrointestinal tract identified by microarray analysis. *Gastroenterology*, **122**(5), 1467–1482.

Becker, S.D., Bennett, M., Stewart, J.P., and Hurst, J.L. (2007) Serological survey of virus infection among wild house mice (*Mus domesticus*) in the UK. *Laboratory Animals (UK)*, **41**(2), 229–238.

Capello, V. (2008) Diagnosis and treatment of dental disease in pet rodents. *Journal of Exotic Pet Medicine*, **17**(2), 114–123.

Johnson-Delaney, C.A. (2006) Anatomy and physiology of the rabbit and rodent gastrointestinal system. In: *AEMV Proceedings*, 2006, pp. 9–17.

Kararli, T.T. (1995) Comparison of the gastrointestinal anatomy, physiology, and biochemistry of humans and commonly used laboratory animals. *Biopharmaceutics and Drug Disposition*, **16**(5), 351–380.

Kon, Y. and Endoh, D. (1999) Renin in exocrine glands of different mouse strains. *Anatomia, Histologia, Embryologia*, **28**(4), 239–242.

Schaedler, R.W., Dubos, R., and Costello, R. (1965) The development of bacterial flora in the gastrointestinal tract of mice. *Journal of Experimental Medicine*, **122**, 59–66.

Cardiovascular Conditions

Booth, C.J. and Sundberg, J.P. (1995) Hemangiomas and hemangiosarcomas in inbred laboratory mice. *Laboratory Animal Science*, **45**(5), 497–502.

Duignan, P.J. and Percy, D.H. (1992) Diagnostic exercise: unexplained deaths in recently acquired C3H3 mice. *Laboratory Animal Science*, **42**(6), 610–611.

Eaton, G.J., Custer, R.P, Johnson, F.N., and Stabenow, K.T. (1978) Dystrophic cardiac calcinosis in mice: genetic, hormonal, and dietary influences. *American Journal of Pathology*. **90**(1), 173–186.

Heatley, J.L. (2009) Cardiovascular anatomy, physiology, and disease of rodents and small exotic mammals. *Veterinary Clinics of North America Exotic Animal Practice*, **12**, 99–113.

Van Vleet, J.F and Ferrans, V.J. (1986) Myocardial diseases of animals. *American Journal of Pathology*, **124**(1), 98–178.

Renal Conditions

Decker, J.H., Dochterman, L.W., Niquette, A.L., and Brej, M. (2012) Association of renal tubular hyaline droplets with lymphoma in CD-1 mice. *Toxicologic Pathology*, **40**(4), 651–655.

Fischer, E., Gresh, L., Reimann, A., and Pontoglio, M. (2004) Cystic kidney diseases: learning from animal models. *Nephrology Dialysis Transplantation*, **19**(11), 2700–2702.

Friedmann, C.T., Spiegel, E.L., Aaron, E., and McIntyre, R. (1973) *Leptospirosis ballum* contracted from pet mice. *California Medicine*, **118**(6), 51–52.

Frith, C.H. and Ward, J.M. (1988) *Color Atlas of Neoplastic and Non-neoplastic Lesions in Aging Mice.* Elsevier. Adapted for the Web by: The Jackson Laboratory, Bar Harbor, Maine, August 2010. http://www.informatics.jax.org/frithbook/index.shtml Last accessed March 2, 2010.

Geistfeld, J.G., Weisbroth, S.H., Jansen, E.A., and Kumpfmiller, D. (1998) Epizootic of group B *Streptococcus agalactiae* serotype V in DBA/2 mice. *Laboratory Animal Science*, **48**(1), 29–33.

Giller, K., Huebbe, P., Doering, F., Pallauf, K., and Rimbach, G. (2013) Major urinary protein 5, a scent communication protein, is regulated by dietary restriction and subsequent re-feeding in mice. *Proceedings of the Royal Society, B: Biological Sciences*, **280**(1757), 20130101.

Hard, G.C. and Snowden, R.T. (1991) Hyaline droplet accumulation in rodent kidney proximal tubules: an association with histiocytic sarcoma. *Toxicologic Pathology*, **19**(2), 88–97.

Pettan-Brewer, C. and Treuting, P. (2011) Practical pathology of aging mice. *Pathobiology of Aging & Age-related Diseases, North America*, May 1. Available at: http://www.pathobiologyofaging.net/index.php/pba/article/view/7202>. Last accessed: March 2, 2012.

Rand, M.S. (1994) Hantavirus: an overview and update. *Laboratory Animal Science*, **44**(4), 301–304.

Taylor, J.Y., Wagner, J.E., Kusewitt, D.K., and Mann, P.C. (1979) *Klossiella* parasites of animals: a literature review. *Veterinary Parasitology*, **5**, 137–144.

Wells, S., Trower, C., Hough, T.A., Stewart, M., and Cheeseman, M.T. (2009) Urethral obstruction by seminal coagulum is associated with medetomidine-ketamine anesthesia in male mice on C57BL/6J and mixed genetic backgrounds. *Journal of the American Association for Laboratory Animal Science*, **48**(3), 296–299.

Yang, Y.H. and Grice, H.C. (1964). *Klossiella muris* parasitism in laboratory mice. *Canadian Journal of Comparative Medicine and Veterinary Science*, **28**(3), 63–66.

Renal and Reproductive Masses

Davis, B. (2012) Endometrial stromal polyps in rodents: Biology, etiology and relevance to disease in women. *Toxicologic Pathology*, **40**(3).

Greenacre, C.B. (2004) Spontaneous tumors of small mammals. *Veterinary Clinics of North America: Exotic Animal Practice*, **7**, 627–651.

Locklear, J., Mahler, J., Thigpen, J.E., Goelz, M.F., and Forsythe, D. (1995) Spontaneous vulvar carcinomas in 129/J mice. *Laboratory Animal Science*, **45**(5), 604–606.

Meier, H., Myers, D.D., Fox, R.R., and Laird, C.W. (1970) Occurrence, pathological features, and propagation of gonadal teratomas in inbred mice and in rabbits. *Cancer Research*, **30**(1), 30–34.

Other Reproductive Conditions

Byers, S.L., Wiles, M.V., Dunn, S.L,. and Taft, R.A. (2012) Mouse estrous cycle identification tool and images. *PLoS One*, **7**(4), e35538.

Cora, M.C., Kooistra, L., and Travlos, G. (2015) Vaginal cytology of the laboratory rat and mouse: Review and criteria for the staging of the estrous cycle using stained vaginal smears. *Toxicologic Pathology*, **43**(6), 776–793.

Kalter, H. and Warkany, J. (1961). Experimental production of congenital malformations in strains of inbred mice by maternal treatment with hypervitaminosis A. *American Journal of Pathology*, **38**, 1–21.

Myles, M.H., Foltz, C.J., Shinpock, S.G., Olszewski, R.E., and Franklin, C.L. (2002) Infertility in CFW/R1 mice associated with cystic dilatation of the bulbourethral gland. *Comparative Medicine*, **52**(3), 273–276.

Ward, G.E., Moffatt, R., and Olfert, E. (1978) Abortion in mice associated with *Pasteurella pneumotropica*. *Journal of Clinical Microbiology*, **8**(2), 177–180.

General Urinary Tract

Finlayson, J.S. and Baumann, C.A. (1957) Mouse proteinuria. *American Journal of Physiology*, **192**, 67–72.

Fisher, P.G. (2006a) Exotic mammal renal disease: Causes and clinical presentation. *Veterinary Clinics of North America: Exotic Animal Practice*, **9**, 33–67.

Fisher, P.G. (2006b) Exotic mammal renal disease: Diagnosis and treatment. *Veterinary Clinics of North America: Exotic Animal Practice*, **9**, 69–96.

Kelliher, K.R. and Wersinger, S.R. (2009) Olfactory regulation of the sexual behavior and reproductive physiology of the laboratory mouse: effects and neural mechanisms. *ILAR Journal*, **50**(1), 28–42.

Yamada, E. (1955) The fine structure of the renal glomerulus of the mouse. *Journal of Biophysical and Biochemical Cytology*, **1**(6), 551–566.

Nervous System Conditions

Barton, L.L. and Hendron, N.J. (2000) Lymphocytic choriomeningitis virus: reemerging central nervous system pathogen. *Pediatrics*, **105**(3), e35.

Goelz, M.F., Mahler, J., Harry, J., et al. (1998) Neuropathologic findings associated with seizures in FVB mice. *Laboratory Animal Science*, **48**(1), 34–37.

Knust, B., Ströher, U., Edison, L. et al. (2014) Lymphocytic choriomeningitis virus in employees and mice at multipremises feeder-rodent operation, United States, 2012. *Emerging Infectious Diseases*, **20**(2), 240–247.

Krinke, G.J., Kaufmann, W., Mahrous, A.T., and Schaetti, P. (2000) Morphologic characterization of spontaneous nervous system tumors in mice and rats. *Toxicologic Pathology*, **28**(1), 178–192.

Meredith, A.L. and Richardson, J. (2015) Neurological diseases of rabbits and rodents. *Journal of Exotic Pet Medicine*, **24**, 21–33.

Radaelli, E., Arnold, A., Papanikolaou, A., et al. (2009) Mammary tumor phenotypes in wild-type aging female FVB/N mice with pituitary prolactinomas. *Veterinary Pathology*, **46**(4), 736–745.

Southard, T. and Brayton, C.F. (2011) Spontaneous unilateral brainstem infarction in Swiss mice. *Veterinary Pathology*, **48**(3), 726–729.

Spring, S., Lerch, J.P., and Henkelman, R.M. (2007) Sexual dimorphism revealed in the structure of the mouse brain using three-dimensional magnetic resonance imaging. *Neuroimagery*, **35**(4), 1424–1433.

Wakefield, L.M., Thordarson, G., Nieto, A.I., et al. (2003) Spontaneous pituitary abnormalities and mammary hyperplasia in FVB/NCr mice: Implications for mouse modeling. *Comparative Medicine*, **53**(4), 424–432.

Infectious Hematopoietic and Lymphoid Conditions

Becker, S.D., Bennett, M., Stewart, J.P., and Hurst, J.L. (2007) Serological survey of virus infection among wild house mice (*Mus domesticus*) in the UK. *Laboratory Animals (UK)*, **41**(2), 229–238.

Dick, E.J. Jr., Kittell, C.L., Meyer, H., et al. (1996) Mousepox outbreak in a laboratory mouse colony. *Laboratory Animal Science*, **46**(6), 602–611.

Jacoby, R.O., Ball-Goodrich, L.J., Besselsen, D.G., et al. (1996) Rodent parvovirus infections. *Laboratory Animal Science*, **46**(4), 370–380.

Kashuba, C., Hsu, C., Krogstad, A., and Franklin, C. (2005) Small mammal virology. *Veterinary Clinics of North America: Exotic Animal Practice* **8**(1), 107–122.

Lindstrom, N.M, Moore, D.M., Zimmerman, K., and Smith, S.A. (2015) Hematologic assessment in pet rats, mice, hamsters, and gerbils: blood sample collection and blood cell identification. *Veterinary Clinics of North America: Exotic Animal Practice* **18**(1), 21–32.

Hematopoietic and Lymphoid Neoplasia

Frith, C.H., Ward, J.M., and Chandra, M. (1993) The morphology, immunohistochemistry, and incidence of hematopoietic neoplasms in mice and rats. *Toxicologic Pathology*, **21**(2), 206–218.

Hard, G.C. and Snowden, R.T. (1991) Hyaline droplet accumulation in rodent kidney proximal tubules: an association with histiocytic sarcoma. *Toxicologic Pathology*, **19**(2), 88–97.

Lacroix-Triki, M., Lacoste-Collin, L., Jozan, S., et al. (2003) Histiocytic sarcoma in C57Bl/6 female mice is associated with liver hematopoiesis: review of 41 cases. *Toxicologic Pathology*, **31**, 304–309.

Luz, A. and Murray, A.B. (1991) Hyaline droplet accumulation in kidney proximal tubules of mice with histiocytic sarcoma. *Toxicologic Pathology*, **19**(4 Pt 2), 670–671.

Rehg, J.E., Rahija, R., Bush, D., Bradley, A., and Ward, J.M. (2015) Immunophenotype of spontaneous hematolymphoid tumors occurring in young and aging female CD-1 mice. *Toxicologic Pathology*, **43**(7), 1025–1034.

Ward, J.M. (2006) Lymphomas and leukemias in mice. *Experimental Toxicologic Pathology*, **57**(5–6), 377–381.

Ward, J.M., Erexson, C.R., Faucette, L.J., et al. (2006) Immunohistochemical markers for the rodent immune system *Toxicologic Pathology*, **34**(5), 616–630.

General Hematopoietic

Albassam, M.A., Wojcinski, Z.W., Barsoum, N.J., and Smith, G.S. (1991) Spontaneous fibro-osseous proliferative lesions in the sternums and femurs of B6C3F1 mice. *Veterinary Pathology*, **28**(5), 381–388.

Cardier, J.E. and Barbera-Guillam, E. (1997) Extramedullary hematopoiesis in the adult mouse liver is associated with specific hepatic sinusoidal endothelial cells. *Hepatology*, **26**, 165–175.

Kotton, D.N., Fabian, A.J., and Mulligan, R.C. (2005) A novel stem cell population in adult liver with potent hematopoietic-reconstitution activity. *Blood*, **106**, 1574–1580.

Nishino, T., Hisha, H., Nishino, N., Adachi, M., and Ikehara, S. (1995) Hepatocyte growth factor as a hematopoietic regulator. *Blood*, **11**, 3093–3100.

Pilny, A.A. (2008) Clinical hematology of rodent species. *Veterinary Clinics of North America: Exotic Animal Practice* **11**(3), 523–533.

Conditions of the Conjunctiva and Cornea

McWilliams, T.S., Waggie, K.S., Luzarraga, M.B., French, A.W., and Adams, R.J. (1993) *Corynebacterium* species-associated keratoconjunctivitis in aged male C57BL/6J mice. *Laboratory Animal Science*, **43**(5), 509–512.

Needham, J.R. and Cooper, J.E. (1975) An eye infection in laboratory mice associated with *Pasteurella pneumotropica. Laboratory Animals (UK)*, **9**, 197–200.

Conditions of the Uveal Tract and Retina

Hubert, M-F., Gerin, G. and Durand-Cavagna, G. (1999) Spontaneous ophthalmic lesions in young Swiss mice. *Laboratory Animal Science*, **49**(3), 232–240.

Smith, R.S., Miller, J.V. and Sundberg, J.P. (2002) Intraocular teratoma in a mouse. *Comparative Medicine*, **52**(1), 68–72.

Van Winkle, T.J. and Balk, M.W.B. (1986) Spontaneous corneal opacities in laboratory mice. *Laboratory Animal Science*, **36**(3), 248–255.

General Ophthalmic Conditions

Beaumont, S.L. (2002) Ocular disorders of pet mice and rats. *Veterinary Clinics of North America: Exotic Animal Practice*, **5**(2), 311–324.

Kern, T.J. (1997) Rabbit and rodent ophthalmology. *Seminars in Avian and Exotic Pet Medicine*, **6**(3), 138–145.

Mukaratirwa, S., Petterino, C., Naylor, S.W., and Bradley, A. (2015) Incidences and range of spontaneous lesions in the eye of Crl:CD-1(ICR)BR mice used in toxicity studies. *Toxicologic Pathology*, **43**(4), 530–535.

Pettan-Brewer, C. and Treuting, P. (2011) Practical pathology of aging mice. *Pathobiology of Aging & Age-related Diseases, North America*. May 1. Available at: http://www.pathobiologyofaging.net/index.php/pba/article/view/7202 (accessed March 2, 2012).

Williams, D. (2007) Rabbit and rodent ophthalmology. *European Journal of Comparative Animal Practice*, **17**(3), 242–252.

9

Hedgehogs

9.1 Introduction

All hedgehogs are members of the subfamily Erinaceinae of the family Erinaceidae, which is comprised of 17 species in five genera. The European hedgehog, *Erinaceus europaeus*, is the best-known member of the family. This species is found throughout Britain; in northern, western, and central Europe; and in New Zealand where it was introduced in the 1890s. In the early 1900s, the European hedgehog was used considerably in research involving fundamental mechanisms of temperature control, hibernation, and reproduction, and infectious disease. The European hedgehog is not commonly kept as a pet; it is protected and its keeping is regulated in many European countries. While the European hedgehog has been exhibited in zoological parks around the world, the majority of information regarding its care and diseases derives from wildlife rehabilitation and rescue programs, particularly in the United Kingdom, where up to several thousand animals are cared for each year, and from surveys of disease in free-ranging animals.

The African hedgehog became popular as an exotic pet in North America in the 1980s, and the species is also kept as a display animal in zoological collections. Animals were initially imported from Africa, but the need for this was rapidly replaced by captive breeding. In addition, importation of African hedgehogs into the United States was banned in 1991 when it became more widely known that they can be subclinically infected with foot-and-mouth disease virus. The veterinary literature is somewhat inconsistent with regards to taxonomy; most sources refer to the pet hedgehog as *Atelerix albiventris*, also known as the African pygmy hedgehog, the white-bellied hedgehog, and the four-toed hedgehog (on the basis of its vestigial or absent hallux). Other sources state that lesser numbers of North African or Algerian hedgehogs (*A. algirus*) were also imported and were cross-bred with *A. albiventris*, creating hybrids. Ownership of pet hedgehogs is illegal in certain U.S. states, and may require a permit in others. The popularity of these animals as pets seems to have

waned in North America in recent years, but has increased in Central America and Asia. In some parts of Europe, the long-eared hedgehog (*Hemiechinus auritus*) is more commonly kept as a pet.

A. albiventris is nocturnal and found naturally in a broad band across central Africa, where it inhabits a wide range of ecosystems, including grassland, savannah, scrub, and suburban gardens. The general range of body weight is 250–700 g, with males weighing more than females. The upper range of weight likely reflects obese captive animals. The life span of captive animals has been reported to range from 4–6 years, with occasional reports of up to 10 years. The average life span of 39 animals in an inbred zoo population was only 3.4 ± 1.1 years.

Although taxonomically an insectivore, *A. albiventris* is omnivorous, feeding on meat, eggs, and vegetable matter, as well as insects. These animals can digest 64–68% of dietary chitin, as compared to only 38% of fiber presented as cellulose. In captivity, hedgehogs can be maintained on a non-insect-based diet, such as commercial cat or dog food, which is high in protein and moderate in fat. Insects, earthworms, and chopped fruits and vegetables may be added. Hedgehogs are prone to obesity, regardless of diet, and, if fed primarily on unsupplemented insects, are at risk of developing metabolic bone disease as a result of low dietary calcium. Diseases seen in obligate carnivores, such as taurine or specific fatty acid deficiencies, have not been described in the African pygmy hedgehog.

A review of the literature can be confusing, as reference only to conditions in "hedgehogs" is common, without any further explanation of species or context. Diseases seen in the wild are very different than those in captive-bred animals, and it may not be appropriate to assume that disease susceptibility in the African hedgehog species parallels that in the European animal. The focus of this chapter will be on the diseases of the pet African hedgehog, considered here to be *Atelerix albiventris*, but information pertaining to other hedgehog species will be included where relevant.

Pathology of Small Mammal Pets, First Edition. Patricia V. Turner, Marina L. Brash and Dale A. Smith.
© 2018 John Wiley & Sons, Inc. Published 2018 by John Wiley & Sons, Inc.

Published information on the diseases of the African pygmy hedgehog tends toward case reports of a specific disease in a small number of animals or review articles on the captive care and veterinary management of the species. Only a few publications summarize the types of disease and their prevalence in the larger hedgehog population and many of these are summaries of necropsy findings, with little related clinical information. African hedgehogs are like many small exotic mammals in that chronic conditions often present to the veterinarian in the guise of acute problems. Clinical signs are often cryptic, and generally nonspecific, including anorexia, weight loss, and reduced activity regardless of the actual disease condition. At necropsy, multiple processes are often discovered incidental to the main clinical problem. There is a very high rate of neoplasia in the captive African pygmy hedgehog and retrospective studies report neoplasia in 29%–53% of animals examined. Males and females are equally affected, other than for neoplasia of the reproductive tract, and animals frequently have more than one type of neoplasm. The incidence of neoplasia is higher in older animals, involving up to 69% of hedgehogs over 3 years of age in one study, with malignant tumors predominating. Oral squamous cell carcinoma, soft tissue sarcomas, and lymphoma are the three most common neoplastic processes in African pygmy hedgehogs.

9.2 Integument Conditions

The spines of the hedgehog are its most defining feature. The crown of the head and dorsum of the body are densely covered in thousands of smooth, unbarbed, sharply pointed spines 0.5–2 cm in length. In the African pygmy hedgehog, there is a linear spineless track 0.5 cm in width running approximately 2 cm in length cranially to caudally along the crown of the head. The natural color of the spines is brown with white ticking but hedgehog color variants exist, the most common being the white, or snowflake. The spines are modified hairs composed of keratin and have a fibrous cortex and a spongy, complex internal structure that allows them to be light and strong. Spines are predominantly in telogen and at the base they narrow just before a bulbous expansion at the follicle, which prevents them from being easily plucked. On traction the quill is more likely to break mid-shaft, and on pressure the spine will bend through the narrowed area rather than pressing into the skin of the animal. Spines are replaced individually at up to 18-month intervals. The underlying skin has a thin epidermis, a loose layer of thick, poorly vascularized fibrous dermis, and subcutaneous fat, and is without sebaceous glands. Brown fat is present and used during periods of

torpor or, in some species, hibernation. The face, legs, and ventrum of the hedgehog are spine-free and, in the African pygmy hedgehog, covered in pale fur from which originates the common name of "white-bellied" hedgehog. Sweat glands and sebaceous glands are present in haired areas and on the soles of the feet. Both male and female hedgehogs have up to 10 nipples in two mammary chains. The toenails are round and highly curved.

Young hedgehogs are born with the spines underneath the dorsal skin, which is edematous and swollen. The excess fluid is absorbed within the first day of birth, allowing the spines to emerge and then stiffen. The initial spines are unpigmented, flattened, and shorter than those of the adult. A second set of spines, which more closely resembles those of the adult, emerges within 2–3 days of birth.

The hedgehog is able to roll into a ball as a protective behavior, literally tucking its entire body within an outer covering of erect spines. The hedgehog can remain in this position for hours, if necessary. Hedgehog spines are sharp and can easily scratch or puncture human skin if the animal is not properly handled. Skin punctures from spines can turn septic since hedgehogs normally roll in their own fecal material.

A wide variety of diseases of the integumentary system are seen, but the most common are mite infestation, dermatomycosis, and neoplasia. Traumatic lesions can result from entanglement of toes and limbs in carpet or other fibers or in wire caging or exercise wheels, and from interactions with other hedgehogs or other domestic animals. Hedgehogs will self-mutilate after surgery. Poor management can lead to considerable overgrowth of the toenails and to dermatitis of the feet and toes from soiled wet bedding and dirty cages (Figure 9.1A).

9.2.1 Dermatitis and Quill Loss

Clinical signs of integumentary disease include poor spine and hair condition, spine loss, excessive scaling of the skin and ear margins, and cutaneous ulceration. Examination of the skin and quills with a hand lens for ectoparasites, skin scraping and cytology, and skin or quill biopsy and histology are all useful methods in differentiating the causes of dermatitis. Cultures should also be taken for bacteria and, particularly, for dermatophytes and other fungal agents. Differential diagnoses include poor diet or husbandry, and immune, infectious, and parasitic diseases. Bacterial dermatitis caused by *Staphylococcus aureus* occurs in European hedgehogs.

9.2.2 Allergic and Immune-Mediated Dermatitis

Allergic or immune-mediated disease is seen in African pygmy hedgehogs. Microscopic examination of biopsies

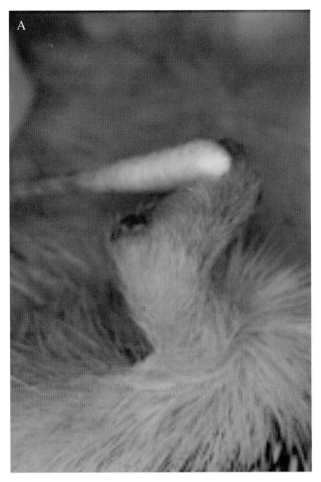

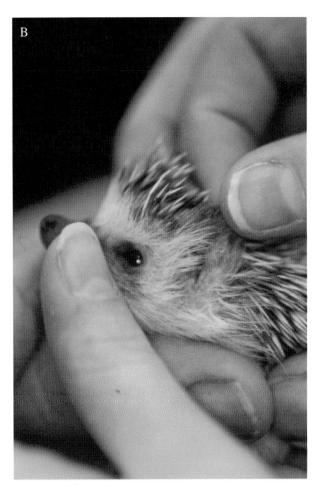

Figure 9.1 A: Pododermatitis in an African pygmy hedgehog; B: Exudative otitis externa in a hedgehog. *Source:* A and B: Courtesy of C. Wheler.

is consistent with allergic disease and lesions respond to corticosteroid treatment, but often no trigger is identified. In one report, a hedgehog developed progressive alopecia, pruritis, and facial swelling. Mild, diffuse, lymphoplasmacytic, lichenoid dermatitis with focal epithelial dysplasia and diffuse subacute dermatitis was diagnosed on a biopsy. The animal reacted to a number of items on serologic testing for allergies, and was treated with dietary change, antihistamines, and eventually glucocorticoids. Food hypersensitivity is also suspected in some cases of dermal erythema with an allergic dermatitis on the ventrum. A single case of pemphigus foliaceous-like disease has been reported in an African pygmy hedgehog. Clinical signs included dry flaking skin, loss of spines, moist inflammation on the legs, ears, chin, and anus, and epidermal collarettes on the ventral abdomen and limbs. Microscopic changes, including orthokeratotic hyperkeratosis, subcorneal pustules with eosinophils and acanthocytes in the epidermis and follicular openings, and a superficial dermatitis, were strongly suggestive of pemphigus foliaceous.

9.2.3 Otitis Externa

Otitis externa is frequently reported, with clinical signs including a purulent discharge and ear odor (see Figure 9.1B). Differential diagnoses include yeast or bacterial infection, secondary to or exacerbated by the presence of mites. Otic infestation by *Notoedres cati* has been described and occurs more commonly in European than in African pygmy hedgehogs. Clinical signs include an accumulation of waxy otic debris and pruritis; mites were identified in a smear of ear contents. Pinnal dermatitis is a non-specific finding seen in both pet and wild African pygmy hedgehogs. Affected ears have ragged edges, an accumulation of secretions along the margins, and superficial crusts. Etiologies include dermatophytosis, acariasis, nutritional deficiencies, dry skin, and non-specific seborrhea with hyperkeratosis.

9.2.4 Cutaneous Dermatophytosis

Dermatophytosis is frequently reported in wild European hedgehogs and, with increasing frequency, in pet African pygmy hedgehogs. *Trichophyton erinacei* (previously *Trichophyton mentagrophytes* var *erinacei*) is the most common fungus identified. Observations from naturally infected hedgehogs suggest that although subclinical infection is common, lesions include a crusting and usually non-pruritic dermatitis, particularly at the edges of the pinnae, on the face, or at the base of the spines. Spine breakage and loss can occur and the skin may have a powdery or cracked appearance. The head is most frequently affected, spread to the rest of the body is slow, but there is no evidence of self-cure, and the infection is not highly transmissible. Simultaneous infection with *Caparinia tripilis* mites is common. Histologically, *T. erinacei* infection results in a neutrophilic dermal infiltrate in association with superficial exudation and hyperkeratosis. Mycelia and arthrospores can be found invading the stratum corneum between hairs, and are present in a characteristic pattern in the medullae of the spines.

There are numerous cases of human dermatophytosis resulting from contact, sometimes quite minimal, with clinically or subclinically infected hedgehogs, as well as with a contaminated environment or with dogs that have been in contact with European hedgehogs. Multiple cases of mycotic dermatitis in pet African pygmy hedgehogs and their owners have been described in Asia, Europe, and South America. In Japan, dermatophytes were cultured from 7 of 18 (39%) pet *A. albiventris*. The fungus isolated from these cases has been identified, by molecular work and mating tests, as *Arthroderma benhamiae* in teleomorph and *T. mentagrophytes* var. *erinacei* in anamorph. It was suggested that the hedgehog isolates compose a unique genotype (genotype III) that originated in Africa and was imported into Japan with the species. It is surprising that there have been no descriptions of the fungus or of zoonotic disease from North America.

Microsporum sp. has also been found in both species of hedgehog.

9.2.5 Other Causes of Mycotic Dermatitis

Several single case reports describe other causes of mycotic dermatitis in African pygmy hedgehogs. Infection by *Paecilomyces variotii* in an otherwise healthy 3-month-old African pygmy hedgehog resulted in a non-pruritic hyperkeratosis on one side of its face; the hair and quills in the area could easily be epilated. *Paecilomyces* species are saprophytic filamentous fungi that rarely cause disease in animals. The same authors described a 1-year-old hedgehog with a 3-week history of a well-circumscribed area of alopecia, scaling, and pinpoint hemorrhages on its back. Scrapings of the lesion revealed septate hyphae and, on culture, conidial heads resembling those of an *Aspergillus* sp. were present. Gene sequencing confirmed the organism to be *Neosartorya*

hiratsukae, a rare opportunistic pathogen in immuno-compromised humans that had not been previously described from a natural infection in an animal.

9.2.6 External Parasites

9.2.6.1 Acariasis

Acariasis is very common in pet African pygmy hedgehogs and clinical signs include erythema, pruritis, excessive flaking and crusting of the skin, and quill loss. The pinnae and face are most often affected, followed by the back, and then the ventrum. Self-trauma, secondary bacterial infection, and mortality can result. Diagnosis is made by microscopic examination of scrapings or superficial debris (Figure 9.2). A *Caparinia* sp. psoroptid mite (*C. tripilis*) is often responsible. Mites from African pygmy hedgehogs have also been identified as *Chorioptes* sp. It is likely that *Caparinia* mites were misidentified as *Chorioptes*, which they resemble. These mites are not considered to be transmissible to humans.

In one case, dermatitis resulted from a dual infection by *Notoedres cati* and *Trichophyton erinacei* in a captive-bred African pygmy hedgehog. Thick, hard, yellow and white crusts were present on the head, ears, carpus, and footpads. The mite was identified on the basis of its morphology; no source of infection was found. Treatment with antiparasitic and antifungal medications resolved the lesions. Both these infectious agents can cause zoonotic disease. *Ornithonyssus bacoti*, the tropical rat mite, is associated with flaky skin and quill loss in African pygmy hedgehogs. This mite can affect a variety of species, including humans.

Sarcoptes scabiei has been reported in *Atelerix albiventris* in West Africa.

9.2.6.2 Other Ectoparasites

Ectoparasites other than mites are not common on pet African pygmy hedgehogs. These animals may act as transient hosts for fleas of other species, but do not appear to become colonized by the fleas of dogs or cats.

9.2.7 Foot and Mouth Disease

African hedgehogs are susceptible to infection by the foot and mouth disease virus, and can be subclinically affected, spreading the disease to cattle. This resulted in a ban on their importation into the United States in 1991.

9.2.8 Nodular and Neoplastic Conditions

Nodular lesions can result from infection and abscessation, and nodular or ulcerative lesions from neoplasia. Fine needle aspiration followed by cytology or excisional biopsy and histopathology, combined with culture for infectious agents, is necessary for a specific diagnosis. Mycobacterial

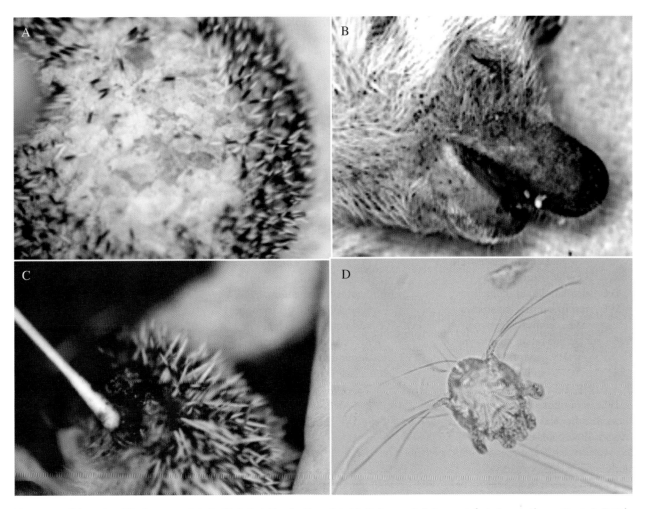

Figure 9.2 Skin and quill lesions associated with infestation by *Caparinia tripilis* (mange). A: Severe infestation on the ventrum. B: Facial mange. C: Ear infestation with eosinophilic granuloma formation. D: *Caparinia tripilis* mite from skin scraping. *Source:* A: and C: Courtesy of C. Wheler.

infection (*M. marinum*) has been described in a captive European hedgehog with granulomatous subcutaneous nodules and lymphadenitis.

In terms of neoplastic cutaneous lesions, papillomas, squamous cell carcinoma, epitheliotrophic lymphoma, mast cell tumors, sebaceous gland carcinomas, hemangiosarcoma, various stromal tumors, and mammary gland tumors are all reported.

9.2.8.1 Cutaneous Papillomatosis

Cutaneous papillomatosis is seen in African pygmy hedgehogs, with lesions ranging from single nodules to widely disseminated masses over most of the integument. A viral etiology has been proposed, but microscopic lesions have not been described.

9.2.8.2 Squamous Cell Carcinoma

Squamous cell carcinomas of the skin are seen sporadically. In one animal, severe abscessation and necrosis of the abdominal skin and underlying musculature at the junction of the quilled and non-quilled areas were associated with the presence of a squamous cell carcinoma. Generalized cutaneous squamous cell carcinoma was diagnosed on biopsy and necropsy of a 5 year-old male African pygmy hedgehog with a four-year history of dermatitis poorly responsive to a variety of treatments administered over a two-year period. Gram-negative bacterial infection, *Caparinia* sp. mite infestation, and *Trichophyton* sp. dermatophytosis had all been diagnosed clinically. See also Section 9.7.2.

9.2.8.3 Sebaceous Gland Carcinomas

Sebaceous gland carcinomas are diagnosed sporadically, and pulmonary metastases have been reported. A recurring highly aggressive sebaceous carcinoma was present in a 1.5 year-old male. The initial firm, non-movable, subcutaneous lesion, located on the ventral chest area, was surgically removed. On cut section, the mass oozed purulent exudate from necrotic areas and infiltrated adjacent soft tissue. On microscopic examination, the tumor was unencapsulated and composed of neoplastic cells with distinct borders and abundant vacuolated cytoplasm forming trabeculae and lobules. Nuclei were large and pleomorphic with 1–3 prominent nucleoli; there were high numbers of sometimes atypical mitotic figures. Immunohistochemistry was used to make the final diagnosis. Three months after surgery the neoplasm recurred and the animal was euthanized.

9.2.8.4 Mast Cell Tumor

Cutaneous mast cell tumors occur sporadically in hedgehogs and are generally benign, although one invasive mast cell tumor has been reported. Tumors can be single or multiple, and are often present on the head, neck, or axilla. Metachromatic granules and accompanying eosinophils are characteristic features, as in other species. Mast cell tumors of hedgehogs have been described as most closely resembling the canine grade 2 mast cell tumor.

9.2.8.5 Hemangiosarcoma

Cutaneous hemangiosarcoma is seen sporadically in African pygmy hedgehogs. One report details a poorly differentiated epithelioid variant hemangiosarcoma in the skin of a 4 year-old female African pygmy hedgehog. A cutaneous mass initially appeared after trauma, was surgically removed, and reoccurred approximately 7 months later, at which time the animal was euthanized. At necropsy the mass was large, multilobulated and exophytic with ulcerated areas. It was regionally dark red to black. On microscopic examination, the mass was composed of neoplastic endothelial cells lining serpiginous vascular channels. These cells were positive for factor VIII-related antigen on immunohistochemistry. Neoplastic foci were also present in lung, liver, and kidney.

9.2.8.6 Cutaneous Stromal Tumors

Cutaneous stromal tumors seen in hedgehogs, include lipoma, fibroma and fibrosarcoma, soft tissue sarcoma, and myxoma and myxosarcoma. While invasive, these tumors are slow to metastasize.

There are several reports of malignant peripheral nerve sheath tumors. One report describes cutaneous stromal tumors from two female African pygmy hedgehogs with consistent microscopic features. The identity of the neoplastic masses was investigated using histology, immunohistochemistry, and electron microscopy. A second case report describes the surgical amputation of the forelimb of a 6 year-old African pygmy hedgehog as a result of the presence of a mass on the lateral aspect of the shoulder. Cytology was consistent with the diagnosis of a sarcoma, although moderate numbers of eosinophils

and mast cells were also present. The mass was initially biopsied, and the presence of infiltrative pleomorphic neoplastic cells resulted in a diagnosis of poorly differentiated soft tissue sarcoma, likely a peripheral nerve sheath tumor. A peripheral nerve sheath tumor was also diagnosed in a 3 year-old female African pygmy hedgehog with a raised, red skin lump, which had been increasing in size for 3 weeks. Microscopic examination of the excised mass showed the dermis was expanded by a well-circumscribed, non-encapsulated mass of spindle cells arranged in short, interlacing bundles that were randomly oriented (neuroid differentiation). The mass was limited to the dermis, and the underlying panniculus was not affected. Nuclei were euchromatic, with small nucleoli, marked anisokaryosis, and there were 1–2 mitotic figures/400x field.

9.2.8.7 Mammary Gland Conditions

Mammary gland neoplasia is frequently seen in African pygmy hedgehogs. Tumors can be single subcutaneous nodules or multiple masses, and are more often malignant than benign. Metastasis to lymph nodes can occur. In one survey of biopsy tissue from eight reproductively active female hedgehogs, there was one papillary adenoma and eight carcinomas: one papillary, two tubular, and four solid. In three cases there was invasion of lymphatics, and in one of these where additional tissue was available, actual lymph node metastasis. Cases of primary inflammatory disease are rare, with one mammary gland abscess listed in a review of husbandry and reproduction of the African pygmy hedgehog.

9.3 Endocrine Conditions

9.3.1 Adrenal Gland Neoplasia

Unilateral adrenal cortical carcinomas have been described in several African pygmy hedgehogs. In most cases, clinical signs were associated with other intercurrent problems and there was no evidence of endocrine-related disease. In one case; however, clinical signs included alopecia, pendulous abdomen, polyuria, polydypsia, and polyphagia. On gross examination the tumors were large and in two animals there was seeding of the peritoneal serosa, liver, spleen and lung, sometimes accompanied by a serosanguinous effusion. The neoplasms were multilobulated with neoplastic cells arranged in cords and perivascular rosettes with a fine fibrovascular stroma. Cells were round to polyhedral with pale basophilic or eosinophilic cytoplasm, large round or indented nuclei, and mild nuclear pleomorphism and anisokaryosis. Mitotic figures were rare in two cases and common in the third.

Pheochromocytomas have rarely been reported in African pygmy hedgehogs.

9.3.2 Neoplasia of the Endocrine Pancreas

Three islet cell tumors have been reported; however, endocrine-associated clinical disease was not seen in two cases where clinical information was provided. A 4 year-old male African pygmy hedgehog had multiple fibrinous adhesions between the liver, omentum, peritoneum, and a 3-cm, dark red, friable neoplastic mass located at the hepatic hilus. On microscopic examination, the neoplastic cells were polyhedral, and arranged in cords and ribbons separated by fine fibrous stroma and there was local extension into the liver with a final diagnosis of pancreatic islet cell carcinoma.

9.3.3 Neoplasia of the Parathyroid Gland

A parathyroid adenoma was identified as an incidental finding in a 3 year-old female African pygmy hedgehog with multiple other pathologic processes, including a thyroid follicular adenoma and multicentric skeletal sarcomas associated with a retroviral infection.

9.3.4 Neoplasia of the Thyroid Gland

A unilateral thyroid adenocarcinoma was described in an adult African pygmy hedgehog. The tumor enlarged and effaced the gland. Clinical signs were referable to cellulitis in the associated cervical area; there was no evidence of tumor-associated endocrine disease. Bilateral thyroid adenocarcinoma with multiple organ metastasis has been diagnosed in a 3 year-old African pygmy hedgehog. Additional thyroid neoplasms reported as incidental findings include a thyroid follicular carcinoma and a thyroid follicular adenoma.

A parafollicular C-cell tumor was described in a 3 year-old male African pygmy hedgehog with a clinical history of dysphagia, weight loss, and tetraparesis. On gross examination, there was a palpable mass on the ventral neck. The thyroid gland was replaced by infiltrating neoplastic cells forming lobules separated by fine fibrovascular stroma. The diagnosis was based on consistent histology, intracytoplasmic staining for neuron-specific enolase, and the electron microscopic appearance of the tumor cells, including the presence of numerous neurosecretory granules. Two other C-cell carcinomas are reported in African pygmy hedgehogs.

9.4 Respiratory Conditions

Clinical signs of respiratory infection reported in hedgehogs include nasal discharge, sneezing, epistaxis, rhinitis, increased respiratory noise, dyspnea, lethargy, and inappetence. Death may occur acutely or after a period of clinical illness.

Suboptimal environmental temperature is suggested as a predisposing factor to respiratory infection through reduced immune function, and cedar shavings are likely a respiratory irritant, as in other species.

9.4.1 Bacterial Pneumonia

Pneumonia is a common disease of African pygmy hedgehogs. In one case of necrosuppurative bronchopneumonia with pulmonary abscesses and suppurative pericarditis and myocarditis in a young African pygmy hedgehog, *Corynebacterium* sp. was isolated. Other bacteria important in respiratory infections of hedgehogs include *Pasteurella* spp. and *Bordetella bronchiseptica*. *B. bronchiseptica* was associated with contagious catarrhal rhinitis and bronchopneumonia in one colony of captive hedgehogs (species not stated). Clinical signs included purulent nasal discharge, sneezing, and dyspnea.

9.4.2 Respiratory Parasites

The only report of parasitic infection of the respiratory system in the African pygmy hedgehog is the presence of *Armillifer* (a pentastome) larvae.

9.4.3 Respiratory Neoplasia

Neoplasms of the respiratory system of the African pygmy hedgehog are infrequent. Pulmonary carcinomas and adenocarcinomas are rarely described. A pulmonary adenoma was found incidentally during necropsy of a 2 year-old male African hedgehog.

9.4.4 Other Causes of Respiratory Disease

Viral causes of respiratory disease are largely unknown for African pygmy hedgehogs. Mycotic pulmonary disease also appears rare. Granulomatous pneumonia with intralesional *Aspergillus* sp. and associated mediastinal lymphadenitis was described in 7 of 98 wild European hedgehogs that were culled in New Zealand.

Chronic interstitial pneumonia, consistent with exposure to toxic fumes or gases, was described in an 18 month-old African pygmy hedgehog that was euthanized due to mite infestation. Microscopic lesions included alveolar hyaline membranes, type II pneumocyte hyperplasia, syncytial cell formation, and occasional hemosiderin-laden macrophages.

A 5 year-old male hedgehog was diagnosed with severe, acute fibrinous pneumonia due to aspiration of a small fragment of bone with subsequent mixed bacterial infection.

Hemothorax can occur as a result of trauma to the anterior vena cava, a common venipuncture site.

9.5 Musculoskeletal Conditions

The skeleton of the hedgehog is generally unremarkable, with the exception of a short tail and neck. *Atelerix albiventris* lacks a hallus and thus has only four toes on its hind foot, unlike all other members of the family Erinaceidae that have five. There are five toes on the front foot. The tibia and fibula are united distally. The age of a hedgehog can be determined by counting the number of periosteal growth lines in a decalcified section of the mandible taken at the level of the last molar tooth.

9.5.1 Trauma

Traumatic lesions, including skeletal fracture, are most frequently the result of falls, entanglement in cage wire or wire running wheels, or fighting with another hedgehog. Osteomyelitis, myositis, and cellulitis can result from injury and subsequent infection.

9.5.2 Degenerative Lesions

Osteoarthritis and intervertebral disc disease resulting in spinal cord compression are seen infrequently (see Section 9.9). A mandibular bone cyst has been described in one animal, consisting of reactive chondro osseous tissue intermingled with connective tissue, at the center of which was necrotic bone. Differential diagnoses for the cyst included trauma, infection, and neoplasia. Vertebral spondylosis is common in older animals.

9.5.3 Metabolic Bone Disease

Invertebrates contain little calcium, thus animals fed on a largely insect diet can develop metabolic bone disease. Feeding a broader range of foodstuffs and calcium supplementation is required to prevent this condition.

9.5.4 Musculoskeletal Neoplasia

One case of a disseminated rhabdomyosarcoma is reported from an African pygmy hedgehog.

Several cases of osteosarcoma have been seen in African pygmy hedgehogs. Affected animals ranged from 2–5 years of age and tumors were found on the ribs, vertebral column, mandible, hind leg, and extraskeletal sites. Tumors have characteristics as seen in other cases of mammalian osteosarcoma.

Parosteal sarcomas have been described in two 3-year-old sibling hedgehogs, a male and a female. Clinical signs in the male included anorexia, incoordination, weakness, and diarrhea. Firm swellings were palpable over the maxilla, and radiographs revealed exostoses there and in multiple other locations. The animal was euthanized and at necropsy multiple hard bony swellings were identified on the zygomatic arch, maxilla, ribs, and lumbar vertebrae.

The female died several weeks after surgery to remove an abnormal uterus. Similar gross lesions were present on the ribs, including the costochondral junctions. Microscopically, the tumors were composed of nodules of spindle cells with an outer periosteum-like layer. Cells showed chondroid and osteogenic differentiation with areas of mineralization and varying degrees of anaplasia. Large numbers of enveloped viral particles morphologically similar to type-C retroviruses were identified in neoplastic tissue from both animals. There are similarities between these cases and the retrovirus-induced feline osteochondromatosis associated with feline leukemia virus (FeLV) infection; however, immunoperoxidase staining for FeLV in the male was negative.

A chondroma with osseous differentiation of the ribs was diagnosed in a 3 year-old female African pygmy hedgehog that had experienced unilateral hind leg lameness, which progressed to bilateral hind leg paresis 2 weeks later. The tumor was present adjacent to the vertebral column, and in focal intercostal spaces. Microscopically, the mass was well delineated, and contiguous with the periosteum of the ribs. It bulged into the vertebral space, severely compressing the spinal cord but remaining extradural. It consisted of a central core of dense, partially necrotic lamellar bone surrounded by trabeculae of variably differentiated woven bone and lakes of poorly differentiated cartilage. The bone trabeculae were lined by numerous well-differentiated osteoblasts. At the site of compression, the right spinal ganglion and the right side of the spinal cord were displaced and had collapsed but had no significant morphological changes.

A soft tissue mass associated with severe lysis of the tibia and fibula in an adult male African pygmy hedgehog was diagnosed as an anaplastic fibrosarcoma. The affected leg had been amputated, but there was no follow-up on the case.

9.6 Gastrointestinal Conditions

Hedgehogs have broad skulls with muscular attachments on the pronounced cheek bones arranged to facilitate shearing. Hedgehogs are brachydont, i.e., have closed rooted teeth, and the dental formula is 2(I 3/2, C 1/1, P 3/2, M 3/3) for a total of 36 teeth. Dental variation in African pygmy hedgehogs kept as pets likely exists, but has not been frequently described. The upper first incisors are long, project slightly forward, and are widely spaced leaving a gap into which the mandibular first incisors can fit. This is considered useful in capturing and spearing insects. The deciduous teeth erupt at approximately 3 weeks of age, and are without molars. They are replaced by permanent dentition at between 7–9 weeks of age.

Hedgehogs have a simple stomach and can vomit. They have no cecum; the small intestine is continuous with the simple colon. Gastrointestinal transit time is approximately 12–16 hours. Droppings vary from soft to pellet-like. Hedgehogs do not rely on hindgut bacterial fermentation and thus do not show antibiotic sensitivities, as do rabbits and many rodents.

Clinical signs of gastrointestinal disease are similar to those in other species and are often non-specific.

Hedgehogs can ingest foreign bodies, particularly hair, carpet fibres, and rubber. Intestinal accidents such as torsion can occur. There is one report of gastroesophageal intussusception associated with megaesophagus and severe esophagitis and esophageal ulceration in a 3 month-old African pygmy hedgehog. Congenital megaesophagus was considered likely; the most significant clinical sign was vomiting.

9.6.1 Oral Conditions

9.6.1.1 Dental Disease

Tartar accumulation, gingivitis, periodontitis, gingival recession, fractured and loose teeth, excessive wear of the teeth, and dental abscesses are all common. Feeding dry food and hard-bodied insects is felt to help in the prevention of these conditions. Food objects, such as nuts and grains, can wedge between the teeth or against the hard palate. One case of mandibular osteomyelitis and severe local cellulitis resulting from infection by *Actinomyces naeslundii*, presumed to have originated from the oral flora, is described in an adult African pygmy hedgehog. The animal died, despite a period of antibiotic treatment, and at necropsy had severe pyogranulomatous lesions containing characteristic colonies of clumped, elongate bacilli present in the mandible and surrounding soft tissues, and in the lung. Acute interstitial pneumonia, and suppurative and lymphocytic inflammation in the heart, kidneys, and liver were also present, leading to a diagnosis of death due to systemic bacterial infection.

9.6.2 Neoplasia of the Oral Cavity

Oral squamous cell carcinomas are relatively common and are usually invasive to soft tissue and bone; however, metastases to lung or regional lymph node have been seen in a few cases (Figure 9.3). Clinical signs can mimic those of dental disease and associated epithelial hyperplasia, inflammation, and osteomyelitis, but in more advanced cases marked local swelling, oral ulceration, bone destruction, and extension into the nasal cavity and sinuses can occur. Histologic and cytologic findings are characteristic of squamous cell carcinomas of other mammals.

An oral papilloma was diagnosed from a biopsy in a 4-year-old male African hedgehog. The mass was a papillary structure covered by well-differentiated keratinizing stratified squamous epithelium exhibiting pseudocarcinomatous hyperplasia. Occasional foci of hydropic and vacuolar epithelial degeneration affected the superficial epithelial layers. There was approximately one mitotic figure per high power field in the stratum basale and only occasionally in the stratum spinosum. Another gingival biopsy in a 3 year-old female African hedgehog was diagnosed as an acanthomatous ameloblastoma (acanthomatous epulis) with pyogranulomatous gingivitis. Hyperplastic epithelium was seen in cords and projections throughout the mass, with spongiosis and prominent intercellular bridges within the cords, bordered by pallisading cuboidal to columnar epithelial cells. Between the resulting islands was a fine fibrovascular stroma, with a mixed inflammatory cell population.

An invasive oral fibrosarcoma was reported in a 5 year-old African pygmy hedgehog.

9.6.3 Salivary Gland Conditions

One case of a salivary carcinoma and one case of a mucoepidermoid carcinoma of the parotid gland, with extension to the neck, have been reported in African pygmy hedgehogs.

9.6.4 Enteric Salmonellosis

Although salmonellosis is listed in the reviews of diseases of *Atelerix albiventris*, actual case reports and surveys of disease refer to the European hedgehog. The prominent exceptions to this are two Centers for Disease Control reports of human salmonellosis in association with direct or indirect contact with pet African pygmy hedgehogs in North America. In 1994, *S.* Tilene was first isolated in the United States from a 10 month-old girl with enteritis. The family of the patient raised African pygmy hedgehogs. The same organism was isolated from the feces of one of three hedgehogs sampled from the household. Since then at least 11 additional cases have been described in the United States and Canada. The majority of affected individuals have been young children. All except two cases were associated with ownership or handling of hedgehogs, particularly breeding herds. In several instances the affected person did not directly handle the hedgehog, but other family members did. In 2011–2013, an outbreak of an unusual subtype of *S.* Typhimurium affected 26 people; eight were hospitalized and one died. Investigation revealed contact with apparently healthy hedgehogs in 20/25 people, and the same outbreak strain was isolated from hedgehogs in the homes of affected individuals. No single source of

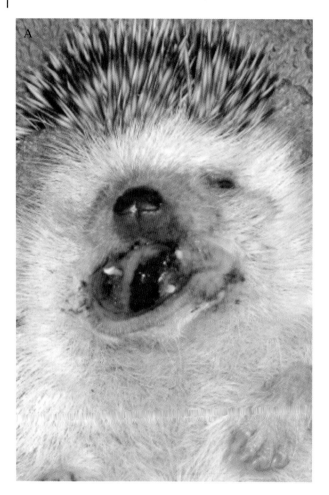
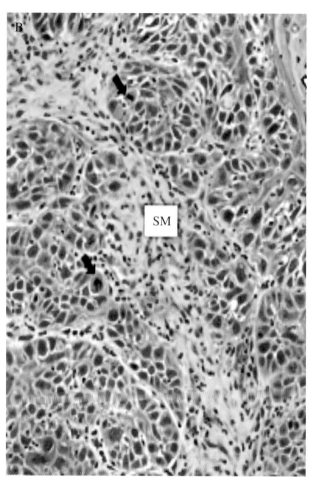

Figure 9.3 A: Oral squamous cell carcinoma with gingival proliferation, incisor malalignment, and mucosal ulceration. B: Oral squamous cell carcinoma invading underlying submucosa (SM), which contains many inflammatory cells. Keratinization, keratin pearl formation, and mitotic figures (black arrows) are present. *Source:* A: Courtesy of The Links Road Animal and Bird Clinic.

animals was identified. The extent of infection of African pygmy hedgehogs with other species of *Salmonella* is unknown.

9.6.5 Other Enteric Infectious Conditions

Diarrhea can result in African pygmy hedgehogs following dietary indiscretion, and has been reported to occur with the feeding of milk and bread.

Candida albicans was identified by cytology and culture from the feces of an African pygmy hedgehog whose clinical signs included weight loss, depression, and melena. Malnourishment was thought to be a predisposing factor.

Infection with *Mycobacterium marinum*, *M. avium* type 2, and *M. avium intracellulare* have been reported in European hedgehogs. *M. avium* type 2 has been cultured from the mesenteric lymph nodes of apparently healthy wild animals. Severe granulomatous facial and otic dermatitis due to *M. marinum* occurred in an adult animal

that originated from a pet store but was held in a zoo. The hedgehog died after a prolonged clinical course, and, at necropsy, mycobacteriosis was diagnosed in the skin lesions, lymph nodes, and lung. It was hypothesized that the bacterium had been acquired from a fish tank in which the animal had been held in the pet store. *M. marinum* had not been previously identified as a cause of disease in a homeothermic vertebrate; the lower body temperature of the hedgehog may have facilitated infection.

9.6.6 Enteric Parasitism

It is difficult to find reports of any enteric parasites of African pygmy hedgehogs. Species of nematodes, cestodes, and protozoa likely occur in wild *Atelerix albiventris*; however, few seem to have survived the transition to domestically bred animals. Stronglyoides-type eggs were identified in the feces of two animals imported from Africa which had blood-stained diarrhea, but no adult nematodes were identified at necropsy. Spirurid-type nematodes were identified in the stomachs of these animals, numbering from few to many.

A single case of cryptosporidiosis is described in a neonatal African pygmy hedgehog in a zoo. The diagnosis was based on histopathology; the animal had shown no clinical signs prior to death. The entire intestinal tract was filled with clear fluid and organisms were present in the jejunum, where up to 75% of the epithelial cells were affected, and in the ileum and colon. Villous atrophy and mucosal hyperplasia were present in the affected small intestine and colon, respectively. A commercial fluorescent diagnostic test for the detection of *C. parvum* was strongly positive; however, cross-reactions with other mammalian cryptosporidia occurred, thus the zoonotic potential of the infection could not be confirmed.

9.6.7 Gastrointestinal Neoplasia

Lymphosarcoma is the most common neoplastic process in the gastrointestinal tract of the African pygmy hedgehog. One case of a colonic plasmacytoma has also been described (see Hematopoietic and Lymphoid Conditions). Single reports are published for gastric, small intestinal, and colonic adenocarcinoma, and intestinal neuroendocrine tumor. The gastric carcinoma occurred in a 4 year-old male with clinical signs including respiratory difficulty, hematuria, and hematochezia. At necropsy, there was extensive metastasis to the lung with the replacement of entire lobes, as well as to the liver, spleen, and pancreas.

9.6.8 Hepatic Lipidosis

Hepatic lipidosis is an extremely common finding in African pygmy hedgehogs and may accompany a range of other disease processes or simply reflect inanition in a species that is frequently obese. Icterus may also be present, and is most easily noted in the skin of the inguinal area.

9.6.9 Herpesvirus Hepatitis

Hepatitis associated with herpes simplex virus infection has been described in one African pygmy hedgehog. The animal was placed on corticosteroid therapy for a prolapsed intervertebral disc, but two weeks later became anorectic and died. On gross post-mortem examination, there were multiple pale foci which, microscopically, correlated to areas of necrosis with neutrophils and cellular debris at the periphery. Eosinophilic intranuclear inclusion bodies with marginated chromatin were present in many hepatocytes adjacent to the lesions, and there were also syncytial cells. Immunohistochemistry and virus isolation confirmed the presence of a herpes simplex virus type 1. Members of the owner's family periodically suf-

fered from cold sores, and this was assumed to be the source of the infection.

9.6.10 Other Hepatic Conditions

Degenerative and proliferative lesions such as periportal hepatitis, bile duct hyperplasia, and fibrosis/cirrhosis can occur. Cirrhosis is commonly seen in association with hepatic lipidosis. The use of cedar chips or scented bedding has been described anecdotally as being associated with liver disease. Iron accumulation in the liver (and spleen) in association with other disease processes has been described.

Primary and metastatic neoplasias occur in the liver but prevalence estimates and pathology are not well detailed. Single cases, each of hepatic adenoma and cholangiocarcinoma, and three cases of hepatocellular carcinoma, two with widespread metastases, are reported.

9.6.11 Exocrine Pancreatic Conditions

There are few reports of exocrine pancreatic disease in African pygmy hedgehogs. A single case each of pancreatitis and pancreatic carcinoma exist.

9.7 Cardiovascular Conditions

The anatomy of the heart of *Atelerix albiventris* has not been specifically described, but in the European hedgehog the heart valves are mainly muscular, the inter-atrial septum is composed of a very thin layer of fibrous tissue, and there is cartilage in the heart base. Incidental foci of myocardial mineralization are seen sporadically. Cardiac insufficiency as a result of myocardial mineralization is commonly seen in association with chronic renal failure in African pygmy hedgehogs.

9.7.1 Cardiac Insufficiency

Congestive heart failure due to endocardiosis of the mitral valves has been reported in an adult African pygmy hedgehog. The animal had a 2-week history of lethargy, reduced appetite, and weakness. Severe cardiomegaly, left atrial and ventricular dilation, and nodular thickening of the mitral valve leaflets were noted on gross examination. Microscopic changes in the valves included hyalinization and fragmentation, and increased fibroblasts and basophilic myxoid matrix. Concurrent vacuolation of the white matter in the brain and spinal cord, consistent with wobbly hedgehog syndrome, may have contributed to the animal's clinical signs.

9.7.2 Cardiomyopathy

Cardiomyopathy is moderately common in aging hedgehogs and animals may die without premonitory signs.

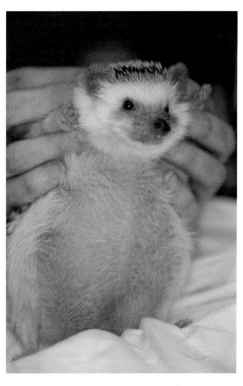

Figure 9.4 Ascites in a hedgehog with underlying heart disease. *Source:* Courtesy of C. Wheler.

On gross examination, cardiomegaly, hepatomegaly with rounded nutmeg livers, pulmonary congestion and edema, and ascites may be seen (Figure 9.4). Microscopically, myocardial degeneration with myonecrosis and mineralization are noted. Acute renal tubular necrosis resulting from poor renal perfusion is also common. No specific cause for cardiomyopathy has been determined, although genetic and nutritional factors may underlie some cases.

9.7.3 Myocarditis

Myocarditis has been reported in several cases, two from Texas, subsequent to *Trypanosoma cruzi* infection. A mild zoonotic risk is present as blood from infected animals may be infectious to humans. In both animals, infection was proposed to result from ingestion of infected *Triatoma* sp. insects.

9.7.4 Other Cardiovascular Conditions

Severe, bilateral cardiac mural thrombosis was diagnosed in a 4 year-old African pygmy hedgehog with clinical signs of depression, weakness, and bilateral hind leg paralysis. Gross post-mortem examination revealed an animal in good body condition, with a markedly enlarged, globular heart caused by bilateral atrial thrombosis. Although a specific cause for the hind leg paralysis was

not found, it may have been due to emboli lodging in the hind limb vessels.

Myocardial necrosis and mineralization were described in a 1 year-old female African pygmy hedgehog, with a 1-week history of decreased appetite and lack or energy, culminating in death. Microscopic examination of the heart showed multifocal necrosis and severe mineralization of the left ventricle. Both kidneys exhibited focal depressed areas on their surfaces which correlated with wedge-shaped areas of necrosis and fibrosis of the cortex. Although the etiology of the myocardial necrosis was not discovered, selenium or vitamin E deficiency was suggested as a cause. Renal lesions were thought to be due to hypoxia from impaired cardiac function.

A hemangioma in the apex of the left ventricular free wall has been described as an incidental finding in 3.5 year-old female African pygmy hedgehog.

9.8 Genitourinary Conditions

African pygmy hedgehogs breed throughout the year in captivity. Sexual maturity can be reached as early as 2–3 months of age for females, and 5–8 months of age for males. Castration and ovariohysterectomy can be performed, but are not done routinely.

In the male, the prepuce and penis are located on the ventral mid-abdomen. There is no scrotum, the inguinal rings are open, and the testes are located in subcutaneous para-anal recesses and may or not be palpable. The testes and vas deferens are normally surrounded by fat. The penis is spineless with lateral horns on either side of the meatus.

In the female, the opening of the urogenital tract is only a few mm ventral (cranial) to the anus. The vagina is long and always open, and the bicornuate uterus begins immediately at the single muscular cervix; there is no common uterine body. A fan-shaped gland homologous to Cowper's gland lies on either side of the vagina. The short (7.5 mm) and simple Fallopian tubes emerge terminally from the side of each uterine horn and extend back along the horn. There are no sperm storage glands, as are present in some other insectivores. The mesosalpinx and ovarian bursa generally contain large amounts of fat. The ovaries are held within a tough peritoneal capsule. The placenta is discoid, lies on the antimesometrial side of the uterus and is hemochorial.

9.8.1 Urinary Tract Conditions

Renal disease is common in African pygmy hedgehogs, with a prevalence of up to 50%. Clinical signs include polyuria and polydypsia, lethargy, and weight loss. On gross examination, affected kidneys are often small and have a

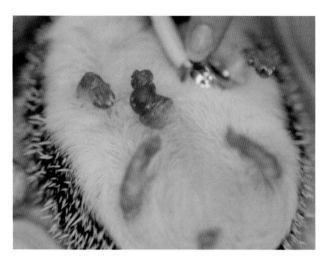

Figure 9.5 Penile prolapse in an African pygmy hedgehog. *Source:* Courtesy of C. Wheler.

roughened, pitted appearance with an adherent capsule. Pale wedge-shaped lesions, linear streaks and foci, and a granular appearance may be seen in the cortex on gross examination of cut sections. Polycystic kidney disease occurs sporadically. A wide range of pathologic processes are seen including tubulointerstitial nephritis with a lymphoplasmacytic interstitial infiltrate, linear cortical interstitial fibrosis; nephrosis, tubular necrosis, and tubular regeneration; membranoproliferative glomerulonephritis or glomerulopathy with tubular dilation and hyaline renal casts, and glomerular sclerosis; subacute to chronic renal cortical infarction, nephrocalcinosis; and focal osseous metaplasia. There is no general consensus on the reasons for the development of renal disease.

Cystitis, crystalluria, and urolithiasis, and renal nephroliths, including bilateral staghorn calculi in the renal pelvis, may occur. It has been suggested that these processes may be linked to cat food diets. Urethral obstruction can occur in the male, and penile prolapse is seen sporadically (Figure 9.5). Reported renal neoplasms include transitional cell carcinomas of the bladder, adenocarcinomas, hemangioma, and hemangiosarcoma.

9.8.2 Reproductive Tract Conditions

Abortion, stillbirth, uterine rupture and dystocia can occur in African pygmy hedgehogs, but dystocia is rare.

Young hedgehogs can be aged to some degree by development: as a rough guideline for African pygmy hedgehogs, spines erupt within 24 hours after birth, ears open at 14–18 days of age, eyes remain closed until 15–24 days of age. The hair on the ventrum and face develops by 3 weeks of age, deciduous teeth erupt at 3–4 weeks of age, and permanent dentition emerges at 7–9 weeks of age. Weaning generally takes place 4–6 weeks after birth and full adult size is reached at approximately 2–3 months of age.

Few conditions of the male reproductive system have been described. These include posthitis associated with substrate trapped in the prepuce and paraphimosis associated with a swollen penis. Neoplastic conditions include one Sertoli cell tumor in an undescended testicle. A periurogenital neurofibrosarcoma was seen in one male African pygmy hedgehog.

9.8.2.1 Neonatal Mortality

Maternal desertion and cannibalism of the young by either parent can occur, especially with animals that are not well socialized. Failure of lactation is considered a common cause of unexplained neonatal deaths. Based on data from European hedgehogs, the main colostral transfer of maternal antibodies is thought to take place over the first 24–72 hours after birth; however, transmission of maternal immunoglobulins appears to continue through the suckling period. Lack of colostrum has been associated with increased susceptibility to infectious disease. Bacterial infections can lead to bacteremia, septicemia, and death.

9.8.2.2 Uterine Conditions

Causes of uterine discharge include pyometra and metritis, endometrial polyps, endometrial venous aneurysms, diffuse endometrial hyperplasia with cysts, uterine stromal hyperplasia, and neoplasia (Figure 9.6). The discharge is frequently bloody and can be confused with hematuria.

Uterine disease, both neoplastic and non-neoplastic, is common in the African pygmy hedgehog with multiple pathological processes frequently present in the same uterus.

One case series described proliferative lesions in the uteri of 15 African pygmy hedgehogs, all of which presented with vaginal bleeding or hematuria. All uteri had numerous small and ill-defined areas of stromal cell hyperplasia restricted to the superficial endometrium with no cellular atypia or increased mitoses. These findings suggest that ovariohysterectomy may prolong survival of hedgehogs with uterine tumors.

Other reported uterine lesions include adenomatosis, endometrial polyps, uterine adenocarcinoma, cervicouterine squamous cell carcinoma, stromal cell sarcoma, leiomyoma, and leiomyosarcoma. In most cases, the uterus is grossly distorted by the presence of the neoplasm and there is often a history of vaginal bleeding.

9.8.2.3 Ovarian Conditions

Ovarian disease is seen much less frequently. Granulosa cell tumors have been reported twice with microscopic characteristics as seen in other mammals. One case of a malignant ovarian teratoma has been described in a 1.4 year-old African pygmy hedgehog. The mass incorporated both ovaries and a portion of one uterine horn. On microscopic

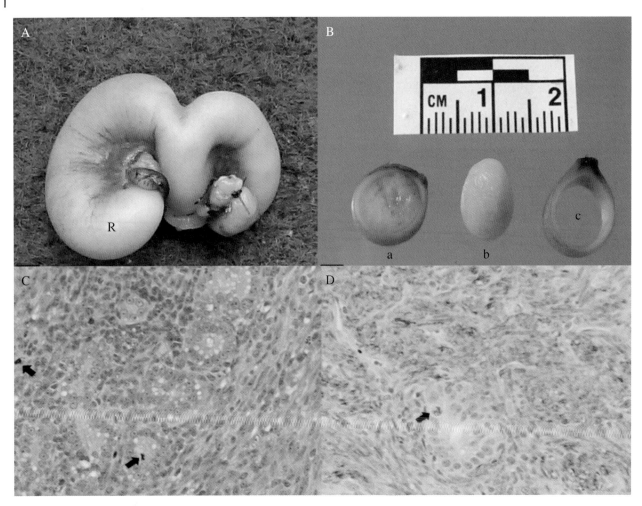

Figure 9.6 A: Formalin fixed uterus, removed surgically. Right horn (R) is larger than the left due to the presence of a hyperplastic endometrial polyp. B: Right horn transversely sectioned at the point of attachment of the polyp (a), the rounded free end of a section of polyp (b) that was freely moveable in the distended lumen of the adjacent uterus (c). C: Photomicrograph of uterine stromal tumor. Glandular epithelial profiles are embedded in solid sheets of fusiform, streaming endometrial stromal cells. Mitotic figures are present (arrows). D: Widespread positive immunolabeling of stromal cells for alpha smooth-muscle actin.

evaluation, tissues of all three germ layers and embryonic (immature) cells were noted and neoplastic cells were also present in lymphatics and a peritoneal metastasis.

9.9   Nervous System Conditions

The olfactory lobe and vomeronasal organ of the hedgehog are well developed, reflecting the importance of the sense of smell.

Differential diagnoses for clinical signs suggesting nervous system involvement include trauma, intervertebral disc disease and spinal cord compression, vertebral osteosarcoma, wobbly hedgehog syndrome, otitis media, infection, hepatic encephalopathy secondary to hepatic lipidosis, and neoplasia. Hedgehogs are also susceptible to neurologic disease caused by migration of *Baylisascaris*

species and to polioencephalomalacia; a nutritional deficiency causing degeneration of the white matter of the brain. Hypocalcemia, responsive to calcium supplementation, has been reported anecdotally in association with postpartum eclampsia, malnutrition, and as an idiopathic condition. Animals in torpor must be differentiated from those with true neurological disease. Lumbar polyradiculopathy, characterized by ballooning myelin sheaths and axonal distortion in the dorsal and ventral intradural nerve rootlets, was described as an age-related change in a 1 year-old hedgehog of undescribed species.

9.9.1   Intervertebral Disc Disease and Spinal Compression

Clinical signs of intervertebral disk disease include progressive hind limb ataxia, proprioceptive loss, lameness, and urinary stasis. Cases involving the cervical and lumbar vertebrae are reported and survey radiographs may demonstrate spondylosis and narrowing of the cervical intervertebral spaces. Microscopically, intervertebral discs show features of chondrodystrophic breed-associated disc disease in canids, including degeneration and mineralization of the nucleus pulposus and annulus fibrosis, and dorsal protrusion into the vertebral canal. Bridging osteophytes may be seen. In one case, a fibrocartilaginous embolus was present within a longitudinal venous sinus.

9.9.2 Wobbly Hedgehog Syndrome

This condition may affect up to 10% of African pygmy hedgehogs in North America. The cause is unknown, but there is no evidence for transmission of the condition, no gender bias, and reported cases are restricted to certain family lineages. Hence, an inherited condition is suspected. Initial clinical signs include an inability to pull the quills (the 'hood') over the face, and mild ataxia and incoordination, particularly related to hindlimb function. Progressive paralysis ensues with the hedgehogs eventually being unable to even lift their heads. Although animals remain alert, problems develop with dysphagia and an inability to prehend and masticate food. Other clinical signs include tremors, seizures, falling consistently to one side, exophthalmos, self-mutilation, and problems regulating body temperature. Clinical signs may wax and wane and the onset generally occurs in animals less than 2 years of age, with most animals developing complete paralysis within 9–15 months. No treatment has been effective in slowing the disease progression. Diagnosis is based on histopathology; gross lesions reflect secondary changes such as emaciation, neurogenic muscle atrophy, secondary scoliosis, and fatty liver. The hallmark lesions include vacuolation of the white matter of the cerebrum, cerebellum, brainstem, and spinal cord; the condition is not inflammatory (Figure 9.7). Myelin loss is followed by axonal and then neuronal degeneration. Gliosis and the presence of gemistocytic astrocytes develop with time. Lower motor neurons in the spinal cord may also be affected, but dorsal rootlets, spinal and peripheral ganglia, and peripheral nerves are not.

9.9.3 Other Encephalitides

Rabies has been diagnosed in wild European hedgehogs. There is little reason to suspect that African pygmy hedgehogs would not also be susceptible.

Severe meningoencephalitis was diagnosed in an orphaned young European hedgehog. Eosinophilic intranuclear inclusion bodies were present in the neurons and the glial cells, and immunohistochemical labeling was positive for herpes simplex virus 1 and 2 antigens. The

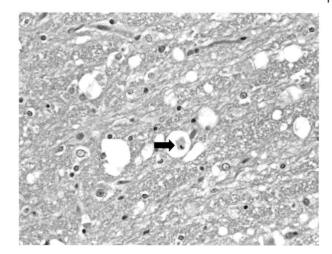

Figure 9.7 Vacuolation of white matter tracts in the brainstem of a hedgehog with wobbly hedgehog syndrome. A gitter cell is present (arrow).

animal was assumed to have acquired the infection from a human carrier.

Chronic diffuse lymphoplasmacytic meningoencephalitis was described in a 1 year-old male African pygmy hedgehog with clinical neurologic signs. No etiologic diagnosis was made. The animal had a concurrent mild suppurative otitis interna.

Nonsuppurative encephalitis was described in an approximately 6 month-old African pygmy hedgehog in Japan with clinical signs consistent with wobbly hedgehog syndrome. Microscopic lesions consisted of a nonsuppurative encephalitis, with lymphohistiocytic meningitis, perivascular cuffs, lymphocytic infiltration of the neuropil, reactive microgliosis and scattered neuronal degeneration and necrosis. The cerebrum, cerebellum, thalamus, and brainstem were all affected. Vacuolation associated with demyelination and Wallerian degeneration were particularly prominent in the cerebellum. There was also a mild cardiomyopathy. RNA reads from the brain were highly homologous (96.5% on whole genome sequencing) with pneumonia virus of mice (PVM) strain 15, a paramyxovirus; PVM antigen was also identified by IHC in brain and lung.

9.9.4 Neoplasia of the Nervous System

Neoplasia of the central nervous system is more common in the African pygmy hedgehog than in other mammalian species. Tumors reported include astrocytoma, microglioma, and fibroblastic meningioma, and no metastases were identified. Ganglioneuromas also occur sporadically.

Two cases of anaplastic astrocytoma have been described in African pygmy hedgehogs that were approximately 2 years old; both animals showed clinical signs of progressive hind limb to forelimb paresis. The first case involved a tumor in the spinal cord and immunohistochemical labeling of neoplastic cells was strongly positive with GFAP and S-100. In the second case, the tumor occurred in the medulla oblongata and spinal cord and GFAP labeling was strongly positive in some tumor cells. In both cases, the clinical picture could be confused with that of wobbly hedgehog syndrome.

A single case of an oligoastrocytoma was identified in a 3.5 year-old female African pygmy hedgehog with a 6-month clinical history of circling, progressing to falling to one side. At necropsy, neoplastic cells had infiltrated large portions of the cerebrum, cerebellum, and brain stem. Morphologic features reflected two distinct populations of neoplastic cells, which was further supported by immunohistochemical testing. One cell population was positive for GFAP and vimentin, while the other was positive for isoform A of the neuritic outgrowth inhibitor (Nogo-A) and oligodendrocyte transcription factor Olig-2, indicating the presence of a mixed astrocytic and oligodendroglial neoplasm.

9.10 Hematopoietic and Lymphoid Conditions

Hematologic and biochemical reference intervals for the African pygmy hedgehog have been published. General interpretation of parameters is no different than for other mammalian species.

Splenic extramedullary hematopoiesis and associated splenic enlargement are very common in both male and female African pygmy hedgehogs. Affected spleens are diffusely red brown and over 50% of the splenic parenchyma can be diffusely or multifocally replaced by a combination of erythroid, myeloid, and platelet lineages. This condition is likely a nonspecific finding, rather than a reflection of clinical disease and increased demand.

9.10.1 Hereditary Congenital Erythropoietic Porphyria

Hereditary congenital erythropoietic porphyria was described in a 6 month-old African pygmy hedgehog. The animal had pink teeth, and urine, which fluoresced under ultraviolet light. Spectrophotometric and thin layer chromatography of urine and feces from the affected animal, its dam, and control animals were used to make the diagnosis.

9.10.2 Histoplasmosis

A single case of histoplasmosis has been described in a 2 year-old African pygmy hedgehog living indoors in an area endemic for the disease. Clinical signs over an approximately 6-week clinical course included inappetence, lethargy, weight loss, and splenomegaly. The animal was anemic with decreased white blood cells and platelets. It died and at post-mortem examination, there was severe splenomegaly, with the spleen weighing 2.4% of body weight, and mild hepatomegaly. Granulomatous inflammation with multinucleated giant cells was present in multiple organs including the spleen, the liver, the kidney, the myocardium, the lung, and the gastric and enteric lamina propriae. Intralesional yeasts were diagnosed as *Histoplasma capsulatum* var *capsulatum* based on morphology. The source of infection was assumed to be dust in the air or bedding.

9.10.3 Lymphosarcoma

Lymphosarcoma is commonly seen in African pygmy hedgehogs and affected animals are typically over 3 years of age. The tumor can occur in any tissue and it is generally multicentric in distribution, although a number of gastrointestinal cases have been reported with metastasis to mesenteric lymph nodes.

Only one report describes hematologic findings in conjunction with histopathology. A 4 year-old male African pygmy hedgehog with a history of decreased appetite, weight loss, and intermittent tarry stool had a marked lymphocytosis (48×10^9/L) with abnormal lymphocytes in circulation. At necropsy, lymphosarcoma was diagnosed with neoplastic cells in the stomach, intestines, the pancreas, and the regional lymph nodes. The bone marrow was unaffected.

9.10.4 Myelogenous Leukemia

Multiple cases of myelogenous leukemia have been reported in African pygmy hedgehogs. A complete blood count may demonstrate marked leukocytosis (100×10^9/L) and neutrophilia (84×10^9/L) with a profound left shift, including cells as early as myelocytes. A substantial number of circulating undifferentiated blast cells may be seen in addition to anemia. Numerous mature and immature granulocytes with eosinophilic granules and round to ovoid, sometimes indented and hyperchromatic, nuclei are seen in the blood vessels and the heart as well as the spleen, lymph nodes, renal glomeruli, the bone marrow, and the liver.

9.10.5 Other Hematopoietic Neoplasms

Splenic hemangiosarcoma is seen sporadically in hedgehogs. A plasmacytoma was identified in the large intestine of a 3 year-old male African pygmy hedgehog. The animal had a brief history of anorexia and weight loss

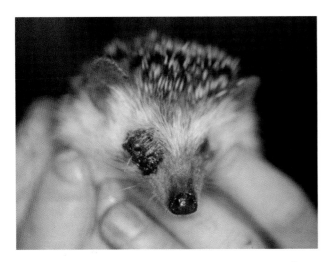

Figure 9.8 Ocular trauma in a hedgehog. *Source:* Courtesy of C. Wheler.

before death. Neoplastic round cells with plasmacytoid features diffusely infiltrated the lamina propria and submucosa, with extension to the muscularis and mesocolon with few mitotic figures and occasional multinucleated giant cells. Diagnosis was based on the light and electron microscopic examination of the neoplastic cells.

9.11 Ophthalmic Conditions

Animals have been trained to discriminate between certain colors, particularly in good light. A retro-orbital sinus is present in the African pygmy hedgehog.

African pygmy hedgehogs have a wide palpebral fissure and a shallow orbit which can predispose to proptosis or injury, particularly in animals with large amounts of retrobulbar fat, periocular inflammation, or other causes of peri- or retro-orbital swelling (Figure 9.8). Lesions may be far advanced before they are identified due the small eye size and the shy nature of some individuals. Reported ocular lesions include corneal ulceration and perforation, hyphema and vitreous hemorrhage, and panophthalmitis. Cataracts occur sporadically and Meibomian cysts have been described.

Intraocular hemangioma, acinic cell carcinoma, and lacrimal gland carcinoma have all been described as single case reports in African pygmy hedgehogs.

Bibliography

Introduction

Allen, M. (1992) The nutrition of insectivorous mammals. *Proceedings of the American Association of Zoo Veterinarians*, Oakland, CA, pp. 113–115.

Clarke, D.E. (2003) Oral biology and disorders of chiroptera, insectivores, monotremes, and marsupials. *Veterinary Clinics: Exotic Animal Practice*, **6**, 523–564.

Dierenfeld, E. (2009) Feeding behaviour and nutrition of the African pygmy hedgehog (*Atelerix albiventris*). *Veterinary Clinics: Exotic Animal Practice*, **12**, 335–337.

Done, L.B., Dietze, M., Cranfield, M., and Ialeggio, D. (1992) Necropsy lesions by body systems in African hedgehogs (*Atelerix albiventris*): clues to clinical diagnosis, in *Proceedings of the Joint Meeting of the American Association of Zoo Veterinarians/American Association of Wildlife Veterinarians*, Oakland, CA, pp. 100–112.

Garner, M. (2011) Diseases of pet hedgehogs, chinchillas, and sugar gliders, in *Proceedings of the Association of Avian Veterinarians*, Seattle, WA, pp. 405–412.

Graffam, W.S., Fitzpatrick, M.P., and Dierenfeld, E. (1998) Fiber digestion in the African white-bellied hedgehog (*Atelerix albiventris*): preliminary evaluation. *Journal of Nutrition*, **128**, 2671S–2673S.

Heatley, J. (2009) Hedgehogs. In: *Manual of Exotic Pet Practice* (eds. M.A. Mitchell and T.N. Tulley). Saunders, St. Louis, MO, pp. 433–455.

Heatley, J.J., Mauldin, G.E., and Cho, D.Y. (2005) A review of neoplasia in the captive African hedgehog (*Atelerix albiventris*). *Seminary of Avian and Exotic Pet Medicine*, **14**(3), 182–192.

Hsieh, P.-C., Yu, J.-F., and Wang, L. (2015) A retrospective study of the medical status on 63 African hedgehogs (*Atelerix albiventris*) at the Taipei Zoo from 2003–2011. *Journal of Exotic Pet Medicine*, **24**, 105–111.

Ivey, E. and Carpenter, J.W. (2004) African hedgehogs, in *Ferrets, Rabbits and Rodents Clinical Medicine and Surgery* (eds. K.E. Quesenberry and J.W. Carpenter), Saunders, St Louis, MO, pp. 339–353.

Johnson, D. (2010) African pygmy hedgehogs, in *BSAVA Manual of Exotic Pets* (eds. A. Meredith and C. Johnson-Delaney). BSAVA, Gloucester, pp. 139–147.

Morris, P. (1994) *Hedgehogs*. Whittet Books, London.

Nowak, R.M. (1999) *Walker's Mammals of the World*, 6th edn, Johns Hopkins University Press, Baltimore, MD, vol. **1**, pp. 168–178.

Ramos-Vara, J.A. (2001) Soft tissue sarcomas in the African hedgehog (*Atelerix albiventris*), microscopic and immunohistologic study of three cases. *Journal of Vet Diagnostic Investigation*, **13**(5), 442–445.

Raymond, J.T. and Garner, M.M. (2001a) Spontaneous tumors in captive African hedgehogs (*Atelerix albiventris*): a retrospective study. *Journal of Comparative Pathology*, **124**(2), 128–133.

Raymond, J.T. and Garner, M.M. (2001b) Spontaneous tumors in hedgehogs: a retrospective study of fifty cases. In *Proceedings of the American Association of Zoo Veterinarians*, Orlando, FL, pp. 326–327.

Raymond, J.T. and White, M.R. (1999) Necropsy and histopathologic findings in 14 African hedgehogs (*Atelerix albiventris*): a retrospective study. *Journal of Zoo and Wildlife Medicine*, **30**(2), 273–277.

Reeve, N. (1994) *Hedgehogs*. T&AD Poyser Natural History, London.

Santana, E.M., Jantz, H., and Best, T.L. (2010) *Atelerix albiventris (Erinaceomorpha: Erinaceidae). Mammal Species*, **42**(857), 99–110.

Smith, A.J. (1999) Husbandry and nutrition of hedgehogs. *Veterinary Clinics: Exotic Animal Practice*, **2**(1), 127–141.

Smith, J.M.B. (1968) Diseases of hedgehogs. *Veterinary Bulletin Journal*, **38**(7), 425–430.

Stocker, L. (1987) *The Complete Hedgehog*. Chatto & Windus, London.

Anatomy and Physiology

Elliott, M.W., Dunstan, R.W., and Slocombe, R.F. (1996) A comparative study of the morphologic features of porcupine, hedgehog, and echidna quills and quill follicles. *12th Proceedings of the AAVD/ACVD Meeting*, Las Vegas, NV, pp. 59–60.

Fairley, J.A., Suchniak, J., and Paller, A.S. (1999) Hedgehogs hives. *Archives of Dermatology*, **135**, 561–563.

Hentley, J. (2009) Hedgehogs, in *Manual of Exotic Pet Practice* (eds. M.A. Mitchell and T.N. Tulley). Saunders, St. Louis, MO, pp. 433–455.

Slavin, R.G. (2008) The tale of the allergist's life: A series of interesting case reports. *Allergy and Asthma Proceedings*, **29**, 417–420.

Overview

Done, L.B., Dietze, M., Cranfield, M., and Ialeggio, D. (1992) Necropsy lesions by body systems in African hedgehogs (*Atelerix albiventris*): clues to clinical diagnosis, in *Proceedings of the Joint Meetings of American Association of Zoo Veterinarians/American Association of Wildlife Veterinarians*, Oakland, CA, pp. 100–112.

Ellis, C. and Mori, M. (2001) Skin diseases of rodents and small exotic mammals. *Veterinary Clinics: Exotic Animal Practice*, **4**(2), 493–542.

Tappe, J.P., Weitzman, I., Liu, S., Dolensek, E.P., and Karp, D. (1983) Systemic *Mycobacterium marinum* infection in a European hedgehog. *Journal of American Veterinary Medical Association*, **183**(11), 1280–1281.

Allergic/Immune-Mediated Dermatitis

Ellis, C. and Mori, M. (2001) Skin diseases of rodents and small exotic mammals. *Veterinary Clinics of North America: Exotic Animal Practice*, **4**(2), 493–542.

Lightfoot, T. (1998) Dermatopathy in hedgehogs. *Exotic DVM*, **1**(1), 11–12.

Wack, R. (2000) Pemphigus foliaceus in an African hedgehog, in *Proceedings of the North American Veterinarians Conference*, p. 1023.

Otitis

Hoefer, H.L. (1999) Clinical approach to the African hedgehog, in *Proceedings of the North American Veterinarians Conference*, pp. 836–837.

Johnson, D. African pygmy hedgehogs, in *BSAVA Manual of Exotic Pets* (eds. A. Meredith A. and C. Johnson-Delaney), BSAVA, Gloucester, pp. 139–147.

Larsen, S.R. and Carpenter, J.W. (1999) Husbandry and medical management of African hedgehogs. *Veterinary Medicine*, **94**(10), 877–888.

Pantchev, N. and Hofman, T. (2006) Notoedric mange caused by *Notoedres cati* in a pet African pygmy hedgehog (*Atelerix albiventis*). *Veterinary Record*, **158**, 59–60.

Robinson, I. and Routh, A. (1999) Veterinary care of the hedgehog. *In Practice*, **21**(3), 128–137.

Smith, A.J. (1999) Husbandry and nutrition of hedgehogs. *Veterinary Clinics of North America: Exotic Animal Practice*, **2**(1), 127–141.

Smith, A.J. (2000) General husbandry and medical care of hedgehogs in *Kirk's Current Veterinary Therapy*, Vol. **XIII**, *Small Animal Practice* (ed. J.D. Bonagura), W.B. Saunders Company, Philadelphia, PA, pp. 1128–1133.

Cutaneous Dermatophytosis and Mycotic Dermatitis

Carman, M.G., Rush-Munro, F.M., and Carter, M.E. (1979) Dermatophytes isolated from domestic and feral animals. *New Zealand Veterinary Journal*, **27**(7), 136–144.

Ellis, C. and Mori, M. (2001) Skin diseases of rodents and small exotic mammals. *Veterinary Clinics of North America: Exotic Animal Practice*, **4**(2), 493–542.

Han, J.I. and Na, K.J. (2008) Dermatitis caused by *Neosartorya hiratsukae* infection in a hedgehog. *Journal of Clinical Microbiology*, **46**, 3119–3123.

Han, J.I. and Na, K.J. (2010) Cutaneous paecilomycosis caused by *Paecilomyces variotii* in an African pygmy hedgehog (*Atelerix albiventris*). *Journal of Exotic Pet Medicine*, **19**(4), 309–312.

Hsieh, C., Sun, P.L. and Wu, Y.H. (2010) *Trichophyton erinacei* infection from a hedgehog: a case report from Taiwan. *Mycopathologia*, **170**, 417–421.

Kano, R., Sano, A., Makimura, K., Watanabe, S., et al. (2008) A new genotype of *Arthroderma benhamiae*. *Medical Mycology*, **46**(7), 739–744.

Kuttin, E.S., Beemer, A.M., and Gerson, U. (1976) A dermatitis in a hedgehog associated with *Sarcoptes scabiei* and fungi. *Mykosen*, **20**(2), 51–53.

Marples, M.J. and Smith, J.M.B. (1960) The hedgehog as a source of human ringworm. *Nature*, **4753**, 867–868.

Robinson, I. and Routh, A. (1999) Veterinary care of the hedgehog. *In Practice*, **21**(3), 128–137.

Rosen, T. (2000) Hazardous hedgehogs. *South African Medical Journal*, **93**, 936–938.

Smith, J.M.B. and Marples, M.J. (1964) *Trichophyton mentagrophytes* var. *erinacei. Sabouraudia*, **3**,1–10.

Takahashi, Y., Haritani, K., Sano, A., et al. (2002) An isolate of *Arthroderma benhamiae* with *Trichophyton mentagrophytes* var. *erinacei* anamorph isolated from a four-toed hedgehog (*Atelerix albiventris*) in Japan. *Japanese Journal of Medical Mycology*, **43**, 249–255.

Takahashi, Y., Sano, A., Takizawa, K., et al. (2003) The epidemiology and mating behavior of *Arthroderma benhamiae* var. *erinacei* in household four-toed hedgehogs (*Atelerix albiventris*) in Japan. *Japanese Journal of Medical Mycology*, **44**(1), 31–38.

Ectoparasites

Ellis, C. and Mori, M. (2001) Skin diseases of rodents and small exotic mammals. *Veterinary Clinics of North America: Exotic Animal Practice*, **4**(2), 493–542.

Gerson, L. and Boever, W.J. (1963) Acariasis (*Caparinia sp.*) in hedgehogs (*Erinaceus spp.*), diagnosis and treatment. *Journal of Zoo Animal Medicine*, **14**(1), 17–19.

Gregory, M.W. and Stocker, L. (1991) Hedgehogs, in *BSAVA Manual of Exotic Pets* (eds. P.H. Beynon, and J.E. Cooper), BSAVA, Shurdington, pp. 63–68.

Heatley, J. (2009) Hedgehogs, in *Manual of Exotic Pet Practice* (eds. M.A. Mitchell and T.N. Tulley). Saunders, St Louis, MO, pp. 433–455.

Hoefer, H.L. (1994) Hedgehogs. *Veterinary Clinics of North America: Exotic Animal Practice*, **24**(1), 113–119.

Ivey, E. and Carpenter, J.W. (2004) African hedgehogs, in *Ferrets, Rabbits and Rodents Clinical Medicine and Surgery* (eds. K.E. Quesenberry and J.W. Carpenter), Saunders, St Louis, MO, pp. 339–353.

Johnson-Delaney, C.A. (2002) Other small mammals, in *BSAVA Manual of Exotic Pets*, 4th edn (eds. A. Meredith and S. Redrobe), BSAVA, Quedgeley, UK, pp. 108–112.

Johnson-Delaney, C.A. and Harrison, L. (1996) Hedgehogs, in *Exotic Companion Medicine Handbook for Veterinarians*, Wingers Publishing, Lake Worth, FL, pp. 1–14.

Kim, D-H., Oh, D-S., Ahn, K-S. and Shin, S-S. (2012) An outbreak of *Caparinia tripilis* in a colony of African pygmy hedgehogs (*Atelerix albiventris*) from Korea. *Korean Journal of Parasitology*, **50**(2), 151–156.

Leonatti, S.R. (2007) *Ornithonyssus bacoti* mite infestation in an African pygmy hedgehog. *Exotic DVM*, **9**(2), 3–4.

Letcher, J.D. (1988) Amitraz as a treatment for acariasis in African hedgehogs (*Atelerix albiventris*). *Journal of Zoo Animal Medicine*, **19**, 4–29.

Lightfoot, T.L. (2003) Therapeutics of African pygmy hedgehogs and prairie dogs. *Veterinary Clinics of North America: Exotic Animal Practice*, **3**(1), 155–72.

Moreira, A, Troyo, A., and Calderón-Arguedas, O. (2013) First report of acariasis by *Caparinia tripilis* in African hedgehogs, (*Atelerix albiventris*), in Costa Rica. *The Revista Brasileira de Parasitologia Veterinária*, **22**(1), 155–158.

Mori, M. and O'Brien, S.E. (1997) Husbandry and medical management of African hedgehogs. *Iowa State University Veterinarians*, **59**(2), 64–71.

Pantchev, N. and Hofman, T. (2006) Notoedric mange caused by *Notoedres cati* in a pet African pygmy hedgehog (*Atelerix albiventis*). *Veterinary Record*, **158**, 59–60.

Foot and Mouth Disease

Hulse, E.C. and Edwards, J.T. (1937) Foot-and-mouth disease in hibernating hedgehogs. *Journal of Comparative Pathology*, **50**, 421–430.

Smith, J.M.B. (1968) Diseases of hedgehogs. *Veterinary Bulletin*, **38**(7), 425–430.

Proliferative and Neoplastic Diseases

Buergelt, C.D. (2001) Neoplasms in captive hedgehogs. *Veterinary Medicine*, **96**(7), 524–527.

Chung, T-H., Kim, H-J., and Choi, U-S. (2014) Multicentric epitheliotropic T-cell lymphoma in an African hedgehog (*Atelerix albiventris*). *Veterinary Clinical Pathology*, **43**(4), 601–604.

Done, L.B. (1999) What you don't know about hedgehog diseases, in *Proceedings of the North American Veterinarians Conference*, pp. 824–825.

Finkelstein, A., Hoover, J.P., Caudell, D., and Confer, A.W. Cutaneous epithelioid variant hemangiosarcoma in a captive African hedgehog (*Atelerix albiventris*). *Journal of Exotic Pet Medicine*, **17**(1), 49–53.

Garner, M. (2011) Diseases of pet hedgehogs, chinchillas, and sugar gliders, in *AEMV Proceedings*, Seattle, WA, pp. 405–412.

Ghadially, F.N. (1960) Carcinogenesis in the skin of the hedgehog. *British Journal of Cancer*, **14**, 212–217.

Heatley, J.J., Mauldin, G.E., and Cho, D.Y. (2005) A review of neoplasia in the captive African hedgehog (*Atelerix albiventris*). *Seminars in Avian and Exotic Pet Medicine*, **14**(3), 182–192.

Hruban, Z., Vardiman, J., Meehan, T., Frye, F., and Carter, W.E. (1992) Haematopoietic malignancies in zoo animals. *Journal of Comparative Pathology*, **106**(1), 15–24.

Huang, J., Eshar, D., Andrews, G., and Delk, K. (2014) Diagnostic challenge. *Journal of Exotic Pet Medicine*, **23**, 418–420.

Juan-Sallés, C. and Garner, M.M. (2007) Cytologic diagnosis of diseases of hedgehogs. *Veterinary Clinics of North America: Exotic Animal Practice*, **10**(1), 51–59.

Juan-Salles, C., Raymond, J.T., Garner, M.M., and Paras, A. (2006) Adrenocortical carcinoma in three captive African hedgehogs (*Atelerix albiventris*). *Journal of Exotic Pet Medicine*, **15**(4), 278–280.

Kim, H-J., Kim, Y-B., Park, J-W., et al. (2007) Recurrent sebaceous carcinoma in an African hedgehog (*Atelerix albiventris*). *Journal of Veterinary Medical Science*, **72**(7), 947–949.

Lightfoot, T. (1998) Dermatopathy in hedgehogs. *Exotic DVM*, **1**(1), 11–12.

Martin, K.K. and Johnston, M.S. (2006) Forelimb amputation for treatment of a peripheral nerve sheath tumor in an African pygmy hedgehog. *Journal of the American Veterinary Medical Association*, **229**, 706–710.

Mikaelian, I. and Reavill, D.R. Spontaneous proliferative lesions and tumors of the uterus of captive African hedgehogs (*Atelerix albiventris*). *Zoo and Wildlife Medicine*, **35**(2), 216–220.

Ramirez, J., Chávez, L.A., Aburto, E., and Aurora Ramos, L. (2008) Carcinoma de glandulas sebaceas en un erizo africano (*Atelerix albiventris*) Sebaceous gland carcinoma in an African hedgehog (*Atelerix albiventris*). *Veterinaría México*, **39**(1), 91–96.

Ramos-Vara, J.A. (2001) Soft tissue sarcomas in the African hedgehog (*Atelerix albiventris*), microscopic and immunohistologic study of three cases. *Journal of Veterinary Diagnostic Investigation*, **13**(5), 442–445.

Raymond, J.T. and Garner, M.M. (2000) Mammary gland tumors in captive African hedgehogs. *Journal of Wildlife Diseases*, **36**(2), 405–408.

Raymond, J.T. and Garner, M.M. (2001) Spontaneous tumors in captive African hedgehogs (*Atelerix albiventris*): a retrospective study. *Journal of Comparative Pathology*, **124**(2), 128–133.

Raymond, J.T. and White, M.R. (1999) Necropsy and histopathologic findings in 14 African hedgehogs (*Atelerix albiventris*): a retrospective study. *Journal of Zoo and Wildlife Medicine*, **30**(2), 273–277.

Raymond, J.T., White, M.R., and Janovitz, E.B. (1997) Malignant mast cell tumor in an African hedgehog (*Atelerix albiventris*). *Journal of Wildlife Diseases*, **33**(1), 140–142.

Reyes Matute, A., Bernal, A.M., Lezama, J.R., Guadalupe, M.P.L., and Antonio, G.A.M. (2014) Sebaceous gland carcinoma and mammary gland carcinoma in an African hedgehog. *Journal of Zoo and Wildlife Medicine*, **45**(3), 682–685.

Spugnini, E.P., Pagotto, A., Zazzera, F., et al. (2008) Cutaneous T-cell lymphoma in an African hedgehog (*Atelerix albiventris*). *In Vivo*. **22**, 43–46.

Wellehan, J.F.X., Southorn, E., Smith, D.A., and Taylor, W.M. (2003) Surgical removal of a mammary adenocarcinoma and a granulosa cell tumor in an African pygmy hedgehog. *Canadian Veterinary Journal*, **44**(4), 235–237.

Endocrine Conditions

Campbell, D.J. and Smith, W.T. (1966) A pituitary adenoma in a hedgehog (*Erinaceus europaeus*). *Endocrinology*, **79**(4), 842–844.

Done, L.B. (1999) What you don't know about hedgehog diseases, in *Proceedings of the North American Veterinary Conference*, pp. 824–825.

Done, L.B., Dietze, M., Cranfield, M., and Ialeggio, D. (1992) Necropsy lesions by body systems in African hedgehogs (*Atelerix albiventris*), clues to clinical diagnosis, in *Proceedings of the Joint Meeting of the American Association of Zoo Veterinarians/American Association of Wildlife Veterinarians*, Oakland, CA, pp. 100–112.

Garner, M. (2011) Diseases of pet hedgehogs, chinchillas, and sugar gliders, in *AEMV Proceedings*, Seattle, WA, pp. 405–412.

Heatley, J.J., Mauldin, G.E., and Cho, D.Y. (2005) A review of neoplasia in the captive African hedgehog (*Atelerix albiventris*). *Seminars in Avian and Exotic Pet Medicine*, **14**(3), 182–192.

Hsieh, P-C., Yu, J-F., and Wang, L. (2015) A retrospective study of the medical status on 63 African hedgehogs (*Atelerix albiventris*) at the Taipei Zoo from 2003–2011. *Journal of Exotic Pet Medicine*, **24**, 105–111.

Johnson-Delaney, C.A. (2002) Other small mammals, in *BSAVA Manual of Exotic Pets*, 4th edn (eds. A. Meredith and S. Redrobe), BSAVA, Quedgeley, UK, pp. 108–112.

Juan-Sallés, C. and Garner, M.M. (2007) Cytologic diagnosis of diseases of hedgehogs. *Veterinary Clinics of North America: Exotic Animal Practice*, **10**(1), 51–59.

Juan-Sallés, C., Raymond, J.T., Garner, M.M., and Paras, A. (2006) Adrenocortical carcinoma in three captive African hedgehogs (*Atelerix albiventris*). *Journal of Exotic Pet Medicine*, **15**(4), 278–280.

Miller, D.L., Styer, E.L., Stobaeus, J.K., and Norton, T.M. (2002) Thyroid C-cell carcinoma in an African pygmy hedgehog (*Atelerix albiventris*). *Journal of Zoo and Wildlife Medicine*, **33**(4), 392–396.

Peauroi, J.R., Lowenstine, L.J., Munn, R.J., and Wilson, D.W. (1994) Multicentric skeletal sarcomas associated with probable retrovirus particles in two African hedgehogs (*Atelerix albiventris*). *Veterinary Pathology.* **31**(4), 481–484.

Raymond, J.T. and Garner, M.M. (2001) Spontaneous tumors in captive African hedgehogs (*Atelerix albiventris*): a retrospective study. *Journal of Comparative Pathology,* **124**(2), 128–133.

Bacterial Pneumonia

Keymer, I.F., Gibson, E.A., and Reynolds, D.J. (1991) Zoonoses and other findings in hedgehogs (*Erinaceus europaeus*): a survey of mortality and review of the literature. *Veterinary Record,* **128**(11), 245–249.

Raymond, J.T., Williams, C., and Wu, C.C. (1998) Corynebacterial pneumonia in an African hedgehog. *Journal of Wildlife Diseases,* **34**(2), 397–399.

Wallach, J.D. and Boever, W.J. (1983) *Diseases of Exotic Animals. Medical and Surgical Management.* Saunders: Philadelphia, PA, pp. 653–663.

Respiratory Parasites

Gregory, M.W. and Stocker, L. (1991) Hedgehogs, in *BSAVA Manual of Exotic Pets* (eds. P.H. Beynon and J.E. Cooper), BSAVA Shurdington, pp. 63–68.

Isenbugel, E. and Baumgartner, R.A. (1993) Insectivora: diseases of the hedgehog, in *Zoo and Wild Animal Medicine: Current Therapy,* vol. **3** (ed. M.E. Fowler), Saunders: Toronto, pp. 294–302.

Reeve, N. (1994) *Hedgehogs.* T&AD Poyser Natural History, London.

Robinson, I. and Routh, A. (1999) Veterinary care of the hedgehog. *In Practice,* **21**(3), 128–137.

Smith, J.M.B. (1968) Diseases of hedgehogs. *Veterinary Bulletin,* **38**(7), 425–430.

Sweatman, G.K. (1971) Mites and pentastomes, in *Parasitic Diseases of Wild Mammals* (eds. J.W. Davis and R.C. Anderson). Iowa State University Press: Ames, pp. 3–64.

Respiratory Neoplasia

Greenacre, C.B. (2004) Spontaneous tumors of small mammals. *Veterinary Clinics of North America: Exotic Animal Practice,* **7**(3), 627–651.

Heatley, J.J., Mauldin, G.E., and Cho, D.Y. (2005) A review of neoplasia in the captive African hedgehog (*Atelerix albiventris*). *Seminars in Avian and Exotic Pet Medicine,* **14**(3), 182–192.

Hsieh, P.-C., Yu, J.-F., and Wang, L. (2015) A retrospective study of the medical status on 63 African hedgehogs (*Atelerix albiventris*) at the Taipei Zoo from 2003–2011. *Journal of Exotic Pet Medicine,* **24**, 105–111.

Wallach, J.D. and Boever, W.J. (1983) *Diseases of Exotic Animals. Medical and Surgical Management.* Saunders: Philadelphia, PA, pp. 653–663.

General Information

Buergelt, C.D. (2002) Histopathologic findings in pet hedgehogs with nonneoplastic conditions. *Veterinary Medicine,* **97**(9), 660–665.

Done, L.B., Dietze, M., Cranfield, M., and Ialeggio, D. (1992) Necropsy lesions by body systems in African hedgehogs (*Atelerix albiventris*): clues to clinical diagnosis, in *Proceedings of the Joint Meeting of the American Association of Zoo Veterinarians/American Association of Wildlife Veterinarians,* Oakland, CA, pp 100–112.

Johnson, D.H. (2011) Hedgehogs and sugar gliders: respiratory anatomy, physiology, and disease. *Veterinary Clinics of North America: Exotic Animal Practice,* **14**:267–285.

Raymond, J.T. and White, M.R. (1999) Necropsy and histopathologic findings in 14 African hedgehogs (*Atelerix albiventris*): a retrospective study. *Journal of Zoo and Wildlife Medicine,* **30**(2), 273–277.

Vizoso, A.D. and Thomas, W.E. (1981) Paramyxoviruses of the morbilli group in the wild hedgehog *Erinaceus europeus. British Journal of Experimental Pathology,* **62**(1), 79–86.

Musculoskeletal Neoplasia

Benoit-Biancamano, M.O., d'Anjou, M.A., Girard, C., and Langlois, I. (2006) Rib osteoblastic osteosarcoma in an African hedgehog (*Atelerix albiventris*). *Journal of Veterinary Diagnostic Investigation,* **18**(4), 415.

Buergelt, C.D. (2002) Histopathologic findings in pet hedgehogs with nonneoplastic conditions. *Veterinary Medicine,* **97**(9), 660–665.

Done, L.B. (1999) What you don't know about hedgehog diseases, in *Proceedings of the North American Veterinary Conference,* pp. 824–825.

Greenacre, C.B. (2004) Spontaneous tumors of small mammals. *Veterinary Clinics of North America: Exotic Animal Practice,* **7**(3), 627–651.

Heatley, J.J., Mauldin, G.E., and Cho, D.Y. (2005) A review of neoplasia in the captive African hedgehog (*Atelerix albiventris*). *Seminars in Avian and Exotic Pet Medicine,* **14**(3), 182–192.

Peauroi, J.R., Lowenstine, L.J., Munn, R.J., and Wilson, D.W. (1994) Multicentric skeletal sarcomas associated with probable retrovirus particles in two African hedgehogs (*Atelerix albiventris*). *Veterinary Pathology,* **31**(4), 481–484.

Phair, K., Carpenter, J.W., Marrow, J., Andrews, G., and Bawa, B. (2011). Management of an extraskeletal osteosarcoma in an African hedgehog (*Atelerix albiventris*). *Journal of Exotic Pet Medicine,* **20**(2), 151–155.

Raymond, J.T. and Garner, M.M. (2001). Spontaneous tumors in captive African hedgehogs (*Atelerix albiventris*): a retrospective study. *Journal of Comparative Pathology,* **124**(2), 128–133.

Rhody, J.L. and Schiller, C.A. (2006). Spinal osteosarcoma in a hedgehog with pedal self-mutilation. *Veterinary Clinics of North America: Exotic Animal Practice*, **9**(3), 625–631.

Traumatic, Degenerative and Nutritional Diseases

Allen, M. (1992) The nutrition of insectivorous mammals, in *Proceedings of the American Association of Zoo Veterinarians*, Oakland, CA, pp. 113–115.

Heatley, J. (2009) Hedgehogs, in *Manual of Exotic Pet Practice* (eds. M.A. Mitchell and T.N. Tulley). Saunders, St. Louis, MO, pp. 433–455.

Johnson, D. (2010) African pygmy hedgehogs, in *BSAVA Manual of Exotic Pets* (eds. A. Meredith and C. Johnson-Delaney), BSAVA, Gloucester, pp. 139–147.

Johnson-Delaney, C.A. (1998) Jaw swelling in an African pygmy hedgehog. *Exotic Pet Practice*, **3**(8), 63.

Johnson-Delaney, C.A. and Harrison, L. (1996) Hedgehogs, in *Exotic Companion Medicine Handbook for Veterinarians*. Wingers Publishing, Lake Worth, FL, pp. 1–14.

Robinson, I. and Routh, A. (1999) Veterinary care of the hedgehog. *In Practice*, **21**(3), 128–137.

Wallach, J.D. (1970) Nutritional diseases of exotic animals. *Journal of the American Veterinary Medical Association*, **157**(5), 583–599.

General Information

Morris, P.A. (1970) A method for determining absolute age in the hedgehog. *Notes from the Mammal Society*, **20**, 277–281.

Nowak, R.M. (1999) *Walker's Mammals of the World*, 6th edn. Johns Hopkins University Press, Baltimore, MD, pp. 168–178.

Reeve, N. (1994) *Hedgehogs*. T&AD Poyser Natural History, London.

Dental Disease

Clarke, D.E. (2003) Oral biology and disorders of chiroptera, insectivores, monotremes, and marsupials. *Veterinary Clinics: Exotic Animal Practice*, **6**(3), 523–564.

Gregory, M.W. (1985) Hedgehogs, in *BSAVA Manual of Exotic Pets* (eds. J.E. Cooper, M.F. Hutchinson, O.F. Jackson, and R.J. Maurice), BSAVA, Cheltenham, pp. 54–58.

Hoefer, H. L. (1999) Clinical approach to the African hedgehog, in *Proceedings of the North American Veterinarians Conference*, pp. 836–837.

Isenbugel, E. and Baumgartner, R.A. (1993) Insectivora: Diseases of the hedgehog, in *Zoo and Wild Animal Medicine: Current Therapy* III (ed. M.E. Fowler) Saunders: Toronto, pp. 294–302.

Martinez, L.S., Juan-Sallés, C., Cucchi-Stefanoni, K., and Garner, M.M. (2005) *Actinomyces naeslundii* infection in an African hedgehog (*Atelerix albiventris*) with mandibular osteomyelitis and cellulitis. *Veterinary Records*, **157**(15), 450–451.

Mori, M. and O'Brien, S.E. (1997) Husbandry and medical management of African hedgehogs. *Iowa State University Veterinary Journal*, **59**(2), 64–71.

Smith, A.J. (2000) General husbandry and medical care of hedgehogs, in *Kirk's Current Veterinary Therapy, XIII Small Animal Practice* (ed. J.D. Bonagura) W.B. Saunders Company, Philadelphia, PA, pp. 1128–1133.

Neoplasia of the Oral Cavity

Buergelt, C.D. (2001) Neoplasms in captive hedgehogs. *Veterinary Medicine*, **96**(7), 524–527.

Done, L.B. (1999) What you don't know about hedgehog diseases, in *Proceedings of the North American Veterinary Conference*, pp. 824–825.

Heatley, J.J., Mauldin, G.E., and Cho, D.Y. (2005) A review of neoplasia in the captive African hedgehog (*Atelerix albiventris*). *Seminars in Avian and Exotic Pet Medicine*, **14**(3), 182–192.

Johnson-Delaney, C.A. (1998) Jaw swelling in an African pygmy hedgehog. *Exotic Pet Practice*, **3**(8), 63.

Juan-Sallés, C. and Garner, M.M. (2007) Cytologic diagnosis of diseases of hedgehogs. *Veterinary Clinics of North America: Exotic Animal Practice*, **10**(1), 51–59

Juan-Sallés, C., Raymond, J.T., Garner, M.M., and Paras, A. (2006) Adrenocortical carcinoma in three captive African hedgehogs (*Atelerix albiventris*). *Journal of Exotic Pet Medicine*, **15**(4), 278–280.

Raymond, J.T. and Garner, M.M. (2001) Spontaneous tumors in hedgehogs: a retrospective study of fifty cases, in *Proceedings of the American Association of Zoo Veterinarians*, Orlando, FL, pp. 326–327.

Raymond, J.T. and Garner, M.M. (2000) Mammary gland tumors in captive African hedgehogs. *Journal of Wildlife Diseases*, **36**(2), 405–408.

Raymond, J.T. and Garner, M.M. (2001) Spontaneous tumors in captive African hedgehogs (*Atelerix albiventris*): a retrospective study. *Journal of Comparative Pathology*, **124**(2), 128–133.

Reams Rivera, R.Y. and Janovitz, E.B. (1992) Oronasal squamous cell carcinoma in an African hedgehog (*Erinaceidae albiventris*). *Journal of Wildlife Diseases*, **28**(1), 148–150.

Salivary Gland Disease

Brunnert, S.R., Hensley, G.T., Citino, S.B., Herron, A.J., and Altman, N.H. (1991) Salivary gland oncocytes in African hedgehogs (*Atelerix albiventris*) mimicking cytomegalic inclusion disease. *Journal of Comparative Pathology*, **105**(1), 83–91.

Done, L.B. (1999) What you don't know about hedgehog diseases, in *Proceedings of the North American Veterinary Conference*, pp. 824–825.

Enteric Salmonellosis

Borczyk, A.I. and Styliadis, S. (1997) Pet hedgehogs and *Salmonella*. *Public Health and Epidemiology Report, Ontario*, **8**(2), 28.

Centers for Disease Control and Prevention. (2013) Multistate outbreak of human *Salmonella* Typhimurium infections linked to pet hedgehogs (final update). http://www.cdc.gov/salmonella/typhimurium-hedgehogs-09-12/. Accessed January 3, 2015.

Craig, C., Styliadis, S., Woodward, D., and Werker, D. (1997) African pygmy hedgehog-associated *Salmonella tilene* in Canada. *Canada Communicable Disease Report*. **23**(17), 129–131.

Isenbugel, E. and Baumgartner, R.A. (1993) Insectivora: diseases of the hedgehog, in *Zoo and Wild Animal Medicine: Current Therapy*, vol.3 (ed. M.E. Fowler), Saunders: Toronto, pp. 294–302.

Lipsky, S. and Tanino, T. (1995) African pygmy hedgehog-associated salmonellosis: Washington, 1994. *Morbidity and Mortality Weekly Report*, **44**(24), 462–463.

Marsden-Haug, N., Meyer, S., Bidol, S.A., et al. (2013) Multistate outbreak of human *Salmonella* Typhimurium infections linked to contact with pet hedgehogs, United States, 2011–2013. *Morbidity and Mortality Weekly Report*, **62**(4), 4.

Nastasi, A. and Mammina Villafrate, M.R. (1993) Epidemiology of *Salmonella* Typhimurium: ribosomal DNA analysis of strains from human and animal sources. *Epidemiology and Infection*, **110**(3), 553–565.

Robinson, I. and Routh, A. (1999) Veterinary care of the hedgehog. *In Practice*, **21**(3), 128–137.

Woodward, D.L., Khakhria, R., and Johnson, W.M. (1997) Human salmonellosis associated with exotic pets. *Journal of Clinical Microbiology*, **35**(11), 2786–2790.

Other Enteritides

Campbell, T. (1997) Intestinal candidiasis in an African hedgehog (*Atelerix albiventris*). *Exotic Pet Practice*, **2**(10), 79.

Gregory, M.W. and Stocker, L. (1991) Hedgehogs, in *BSAVA Manual of Exotic Pets* (eds. P.H. Beynon and J.E. Cooper), BSAVA: Shurdington, pp. 63–68.

Riley, P.Y. and Chomel, B.B. (2005) Hedgehog zoonoses. *Emerging Infectious Diseases*, **11**(1), 1–5.

Smith, J.M.B. (1968) Diseases of hedgehogs. *Veterinary Bulletin*, **38**(7), 425–430.

Enteric Parasitism

Brunnert, S.R., Hensley, G.T., Citino, S.B., Herron, A.J., and Altman, N.H. (1991) Salivary gland oncocytes in African hedgehogs (*Atelerix albiventris*) mimicking cytomegalic inclusion disease. *Journal of Comparative Pathology*, **105**(1), 83–91.

Epe, C., Coati, N. and Schnieder, T. (2004) Results of parasitological examinations of faecal samples from horses, ruminants, pigs, dogs, cats, hedgehogs and rabbits between 1998 and 2002. *Deutsche tierärztliche Wochenschrift*, **111**(6), 243–246.

Graczyk, T.K., Cranfield, M.R., Dunning, C., and Strandberg, J.D. (1998) Fatal cryptosporidiosis in a juvenile captive African hedghehog (*Atelerix albiventris*). *Journal of Parasitology*, **84**(1), 178–180.

Gregory, M.W. and Stocker, L. (1991) Hedgehogs, in *BSAVA Manual of Exotic Pets* (eds. P.H. Beynon and J.E. Cooper), BSAVA, Shurdington, pp. 63–68.

Isenbugel, E. and Baumgartner, R.A. (1993) Insectivora: diseases of the hedgehog, in *Zoo and Wild Animal Medicine: Current Therapy* (ed. M.E. Fowler), vol. **3**. Saunders: Toronto, pp. 294–302.

Lightfoot, T.L. (2000) Therapeutics of African pygmy hedgehogs and prairie dogs. *Veterinary Clinics of North America: Exotic Animal Practice*, **3**(1), 155–72.

Robinson, I. and Routh, A. (1999) Veterinary care of the hedgehog. *In Practice* **21**(3), 128–137.

Smith, J.M.B. (1968) Diseases of hedgehogs. *Veterinary Bulletin* **38**(7), 425–430.

Sweatman, G.K. (1971) Mites and pentastomes, in *Parasitic Diseases of Wild Mammals* (eds. J.W. Davis and R.C. Anderson), Iowa State University Press, Ames, pp. 3–64.

Gastrointestinal Neoplasia

Heatley, J.J., Mauldin, G.E., and Cho, D.Y. (2005) A review of neoplasia in the captive African hedgehog (*Atelerix albiventris*). *Seminars in Avian and Exotic Pet Medicine*, **14**(3), 182–192.

Raymond, J.T. and Garner, M.M. (2001) Spontaneous tumors in hedgehogs: a retrospective study of fifty cases, in *Proceedings of the American Association of Zoo Veterinarians*, Orlando, FL, pp. 326–327.

Raymond, J.T. and Garner, M.M. (2001) Spontaneous tumors in captive African hedgehogs (*Atelerix albiventris*): a retrospective study. *Journal of Comparative Pathology*, **124**(2), 128–133.

Hepatic Lipidosis

Graesser, D., Spraker, T.R., Dressen, P., et al. (2006) Wobbly hedgehog syndrome in African pygmy hedgehogs (*Atelerix* spp.). *Journal of Exotic Pet Medicine*, **15**(2), 59–65.

Raymond, J.T. and White, M.R. (1999) Necropsy and histopathologic findings in 14 African hedgehogs (*Atelerix albiventris*): a retrospective study. *Journal of Zoo and Wildlife Medicine*, **30**(2), 273–277.

Herpesvirus Hepatitis

Allison, N., Chang, T.C., Steele, K.E., and Hilliard, J.K. (2002) Fatal herpes simplex infection in a pygmy African hedgehog (*Atelerix albiventris*). *Journal of Comparative Pathology*, **126**, 76–78.
Stack, M.J., Higgins, R.J., Challoner, D.J., and Gregory, M.W. (1990) Herpesvirus in the liver of a hedgehog (*Erinaceus europaeus*). *Veterinary Record*, **127**(25/26), 620–621.
Widén, F., Gavier-Widén, D., Nikiila, T., and Mörner, T. (1996) Fatal herpesvirus infection in a hedgehog (*Erinaceus europaeus*). *Veterinary Record*, **139**(10), 237–238.

Other Hepatic Conditions

Beckman, K.B. and Norton, T.M. (1992) Disseminated hemangiosarcoma in an African hedgehog, in *Proceedings of the Joint Conference of American Association of Zoo Veterinarians/American Association of Wildlife Veterinarians*, Oakland, CA. pp. 195–198.
Done, L.B. (1999) What you don't know about hedgehog diseases, in *Proceedings of the North American Veterinary Conference*, pp. 824–825.
Garner, M. (2011) Diseases of pet hedgehogs, chinchillas, and sugar gliders, in *AEMV Proceedings*, Seattle, WA, pp. 405–412.
Helmer, P. (2000) Abnormal hematologic findings in an African hedgehog (*Atelerix albiventris*) with gastrointestinal lymphosarcoma. *Canadian Veterinary Journal*, **41**(6), 489–490.
Keahey, K.K. (1968) Incidence and classification of exotic animal diseases, in *Proceedings of the American Association of Zoo Veterinarians*, East Lansing, MI, pp. 1–6.
Raymond, J.T. and Garner, M.M. (2001) Spontaneous tumors in captive African hedgehogs (*Atelerix albiventris*): a retrospective study. *Journal of Comparative Pathology*, **124**(2), 128–133.
Smith, A.J. (2000) General husbandry and medical care of hedgehogs, in *Kirk's Current Veterinary Therapy, XIII Small Animal Practice* (ed. J.D. Bonagura), W.B. Saunders Company: Philadelphia, PA. pp. 1128–1133
Wadsworth, P.F., Jones, D.M., and Pugsley, S.L. (1985) A survey of mammalian and avian neoplasms at the Zoological Society of London. *Journal of Zoo and Wildlife Medicine*, **16**(2), 73–80.

Exocrine Pancreatic Conditions

Buergelt, C.D. (2001) Neoplasms in captive hedgehogs. *Veterinary Medicine*, **96**(7), 524–527.
Keahey, K.K. (1968) Incidence and classification of exotic animal diseases, in *Proceedings of the American Association of Zoo Vets*, East Lansing, MI, pp. 1–6.

General Information

Buergelt, C.D. (2002) Histopathologic findings in pet hedgehogs with nonneoplastic conditions. *Veterinary Medicine*, **97**(9), 660–665.
Clarke, D.E. (2003) Oral biology and disorders of chiroptera, insectivores, monotremes, and marsupials. *Veterinary Clinics of North America: Exotic Animal Practice*, **6**(3), 523–564.
Done, L.B., Dietze, M., Cranfield, M. and Ialeggio, D. (1992) Necropsy lesions by body systems in African hedgehogs (*Atelerix albiventris*): clues to clinical diagnosis, in *Proceedings of the Joint Meeting of the American Association of Zoo Veterinarians/American Association of Wildlife Veterinarians*, Oakland, CA, pp. 100–112.
Hsieh, P-C., Yu, J-F., and Wang, L. (2015) A retrospective study of the medical status on 63 African hedgehogs (*Atelerix albiventris*) at the Taipei Zoo from 2003–2011. *Journal of Exotic Pet Medicine*, **24**, 105–111.
Ivey, E. and Carpenter, J.W. (2004) African hedgehogs, in *Ferrets, Rabbits and Rodents. Clinical Medicine and Surgery* (eds. K.E. Quesenberry and J.W. Carpenter). Saunders: St Louis, MO, pp. 339–353.
Johnson, D. (2010) African pygmy hedgehogs, in *BSAVA Manual of Exotic Pets* (eds. A. Meredith and C. Johnson-Delaney). BSAVA, Gloucester. pp. 139–147.
Johnson-Delaney, C.A., and Harrison, L. (1996) Hedgehogs, in *Exotic Companion Medicine Handbook for Veterinarians*, Wingers Publishing, Lake Worth, FL, pp. 1–14.
Lee, S-Y. and Park, H-M. (2012) Gastroesophageal intussusception with megaesophagus in a hedgehog. *Journal of Exotic Pet Medicine*, **21**(2), 168–171.
Lightfoot, T.L. (2000) Therapeutics of African pygmy hedgehogs and prairie dogs. *Veterinary Clinics of North America: Exotic Animal Practice*, **3**(1), 155–172.
McColl, I. (1967) The comparative anatomy and pathology of anal glands. *Annals of the Royal College of Surgeons, England*, **40**(1), 36–37.
Reeve, N. (1994) *Hedgehogs*. T&AD Poyser Natural History, London.
Smith, A.J. (1992) Husbandry and medicine of African hedgehogs (*Atelerix albiventris*). *Journal of Small Exotic Animal Medicine*, **2**(1), 21–28.
Smith, A.J. (1999) Husbandry and nutrition of hedgehogs. *Veterinary Clinics of North America: Exotic Animal Practice*, **2**(1), 127–141.

Stevens, C.E. (1988) *Comparative Physiology of the Vertebrate Digestive System*, Cambridge University Press, Cambridge.

Cardiomyopathy

Juan-Sallés, C. and Garner, M.M. (2007) Cytologic diagnosis of diseases of hedgehogs. *Veterinary Clinics of North America: Exotic Animal Practice*, **10**(1), 51–59.

Raymond, J.T. and Garner, M.M. (2000) Cardiomyopathy in captive African hedgehogs (*Atelerix albiventris*). *Journal of Veterinary Diagnostic Investigations*, **12**, 468–472.

Myocarditis

deMaar, T.W., Kassell, N.L., and Blumer, E.S. (1994) Chagas' disease in an African hedgehog, in *Proceedings of the Joint Meeting of the American Association of Zoo Veterinarians/Association of Reptilian and Amphibian Veterinarians*, Pittsburgh, PA, pp. 132–133.

Latas, P., Reavill, D., and Nicholson, D. (2004) Trypanosoma infection in sugar gliders (*Petaurus breviceps*) and a hedgehog (*Atelerix albiventris*) from Texas, in *Proceedings of the Joint Meeting of the American Association of Zoo Veterinarians/American Association of Wildlife Veterinarians/Wildlife Disease Association*, San Diego, CA, pp 183–184.

Raymond, J.T. and White, M.R. (1999) Necropsy and histopathologic findings in 14 African hedgehogs (*Atelerix albiventris*): a retrospective study. *Journal of Zoo and Wildlife Medicine*, **30**(2), 273–277.

Schmidt, R.E. and Hubbard, G.B. (1987) *Atlas of Zoo Animal Pathology*, vol. **I** *Mammals*. CRC Press, Boca Raton, FL.

Hemangioma

Peauroi, J.R., Lowenstine, L.J., Munn, R.J. and Wilson, D.W. (1994) Multicentric skeletal sarcomas associated with probable retrovirus particles in two African hedgehogs (*Atelerix albiventris*). *Veterinary Pathology*, **31**(4), 481–484.

General Information

Allison, N. (2003) A hyperplastic endometrial polyp and vascular thrombosis in a hedgehog. *Veterinary Medicine*, **98**(4), 298–303.

Black, P.A., Marshall, C., Seyfield, A.W., and Bartin, A.M. (2011) Cardiac assessment of African hedgehogs (*Atelerix albiventris*). *Journal of Zoo and Wildlife Medicine*, **42**(1), 49–53.

Buergelt, C.D. (2002) Histopathologic findings in pet hedgehogs with nonneoplastic conditions. *Veterinary Medicine*, **97**(9), 660–665.

Delk, K.W., Eshar, D., Garcia, E. and Harkin, K. (2013) Diagnosis and treatment of congestive heart failure secondary to dilated cardiomyopathy in a hedgehog. *Journal of Small Animal Practice*, **55**(3), 174–177.

Done, L.B., Dietze, M., Cranfield, M. and Ialeggio, D. (1992) Necropsy lesions by body systems in African hedgehogs (*Atelerix albiventris*): clues to clinical diagnosis, *Proceedings of the Joint Meeting of the American Association of Zoo Veterinarians/American Association of Wildlife Veterinarians*, Oakland, CA, pp. 100–112.

Garner, M. (2011) Diseases of pet hedgehogs, chinchillas, and sugar gliders, in *AEMV Proceedings*, Seattle, WA, pp. 405–412.

Heatley, J.J. (2009) Cardiovascular anatomy, physiology, and disease of rodents and small exotic mammals. *Veterinary Clinics of North America: Exotic Animal Practice*, **12**(1), 99–113.

Hedley, J., Benato, L., Fraga, G., Palgrave, C., and Eatwell, K. (2013) Congestive heart failure due to endocardiosis of the mitral valves in an African pygmy hedgehog. *Journal of Exotic Pet Medicine*, **22**(2), 212–217.

Hsieh, P-C., Yu, J-F., Wang, L. (2015) A retrospective study of the medical status on 63 African hedgehogs (*Atelerix albiventris*) at the Taipei Zoo from 2003–2011. *Journal of Exotic Pet Medicine*, **24**, 105–111.

Diseases of the Urinary System

Buergelt, C.D. (2002) Histopathologic findings in pet hedgehogs with nonneoplastic conditions. *Veterinary Medicine*, **97**(9), 660–665.

Done, L.B. (1999) What you don't know about hedgehog diseases, in *Proceedings of the North American Veterinary Conference*, pp. 824–825.

Done, L.B., Dietze, M., Cranfield, M., and Ialeggio, D. (1992) Necropsy lesions by body systems in African hedgehogs (*Atelerix albiventris*): clues to clinical diagnosis. In: *Proceedings of the Joint Meeting of the American Association of Zoo Veterinarians/American Association of Wildlife Veterinarians*, Oakland, CA, pp. 100–112.

Fisher, P.G. (2006) Exotic mammal renal disease: causes and clinical presentation. *Veterinary Clinics of North America: Exotic Animal Practice*, **9**(1), 33–67.

Garner, M. (2011) Diseases of pet hedgehogs, chinchillas, and sugar gliders, in *AEMV Proceedings*, Seattle, WA. Pp. 405–412.

Graesser, D., Spraker, T.R., Dressen, P., et al. (2006) Wobbly hedgehog syndrome in African pygmy hedgehogs (*Atelerix* spp.). *Journal of Exotic Pet Medicine*, **15**(2), 59–65.

Heatley, J.J., Mauldin, G.E., and Cho, D.Y. (2005) A review of neoplasia in the captive African hedgehog (*Atelerix albiventris*). *Seminars in Avian and Exotic Pet Medicine*, **14**(3), 182–192.

Helmer, P. (2000) Abnormal hematologic findings in an African hedgehog (*Atelerix albiventris*) with gastrointestinal lymphosarcoma. *Canadian Veterinary Journal*, **41**(6), 489–490.

Johnson, D.H. (2001) Hedgehog with suspected bilateral renal calculi. *Exotic DVM*, **3**(1), 5.

Raymond, J.T. and White, M.R. (1999) Necropsy and histopathologic findings in 14 African hedgehogs (*Atelerix albiventris*): a retrospective study. *Journal of Zoo and Wildlife Medicine*, **30**(2), 273–277.

Rhody, J.L. and Schiller, C.A. (2006) Spinal osteosarcoma in a hedgehog with pedal self-mutilation. *Veterinary Clinics: Exotic Animal Practice*, **9**(3), 625–631.

Wheler, C.L., Grahn, B.H., and Pocknell, A.M. (2001) Unilateral proptosis and orbital cellulitis in eight African hedgehogs (*Atelerix albiventris*). *Journal of Zoo and Wildlife Medicine*, **32**(2), 236–241.

Female Reproductive Conditions

Allison, N. (2003) A hyperplastic endometrial polyp and vascular thrombosis in a hedgehog. *Veterinary Medicine*, **98**(4), 298–303.

Campbell, T. (1999) Uterine neoplasia in two African hedgehogs. *Exotic Pet Practice*, 4, 51.

Chu, P.Y., Zhuo, Y.X., Wang, F.I., et al. (2012) Spontaneous neoplasms in zoo mammals, birds, and reptiles in Taiwan: a 10-year survey. *Animal Biology*, **62**(1), 95–110.

Done, L.B. (1999) What you don't know about hedgehog diseases. in *Proceedings of the North American Veterinary Conference*, pp. 824–825.

Done, L.B., Deem, S.L., and Fiorello, C.V. (2007) Surgical and medical management of a uterine spindle cell tumor in an African hedgehog (*Atelerix albiventris*). *Journal of Zoo and Wildlife Medicine*, **38**(4), 601–603.

Done, L.B., Dietze, M., Cranfield, M., and Ialeggio, D. (1992) Necropsy lesions by body systems in African hedgehogs (*Atelerix albiventris*): clues to clinical diagnosis, in *Proceedings of the Joint Meeting of the American Association of Zoo Veterinarians/American Association of Wildlife Veterinarians*, Oakland, CA, pp. 100–112.

Garner, M. (2011) Diseases of pet hedgehogs, chinchillas, and sugar gliders, in *AEMV Proceedings*, Seattle, WA, pp. 405–412.

Greenacre, C.B. (2004) Spontaneous tumors of small mammals. *Veterinary Clinics of North America: Exotic Animal Practice*, **7**(3), 627–651.

Hoefer, H.L. (1999) Clinical approach to the African hedgehog. in *Proceedings of the North American Veterinary Conference*, pp. 836–837.

Juan-Sallés, C., Raymond, J.T., Garner, M.M., and Paras, A. (2006) Adrenocortical carcinoma in three captive African hedgehogs (*Atelerix albiventris*). *Journal of Exotic Pet Medicine*, **15**(4), 278–280.

Larsen, S.R. and Carpenter, J.W. (1999) Husbandry and medical management of African hedgehogs. *Veterinary Medicine*, **94**(10), 877–888.

Peauroi, J.R., Lowenstine, L.J., Munn, R.J., and Wilson, D.W. (1994) Multicentric skeletal sarcomas associated with probable retrovirus particles in two African hedgehogs (*Atelerix albiventris*). *Veterinary Pathology*, **31**(4), 481–484.

Phair, K., Carpenter, J.W., Marrow, J., Andrews, G., and Bawa, B. (2011) Management of an extraskeletal osteosarcoma in an African hedgehog (*Atelerix albiventris*). *Journal of Exotic Pet Medicine*, **20**(2), 151–155.

Phillips, I.D., Taylor, J.J., and Allen, A.L. (2005) Endometrial polyps in 2 African pygmy hedgehogs. *Canadian Veterinary Journal*, **46**(6), 514–527.

Ramos-Vara, J.A. (2001) Soft tissue sarcomas in the African hedgehog (*Atelerix albiventris*), microscopic and immunohistologic study of three cases. *Journal of Veterinary Diagnostic Investigation*, **13**(5), 442–445.

Raymond, J.T. and Garner, M.M. (2001) Spontaneous tumors in captive African hedgehogs (*Atelerix albiventris*): a retrospective study. *Journal of Comparative Pathology*, **124**(2), 128–133.

Song, S-H., Park, N-W., Jung, S-K., Kim, J-H., and Eom, K-D. (2014) Bilateral malignant ovarian teratoma with peritoneal metastasis in a captive African pygmy hedgehog (*Atelerix albiventris*). *Journal of Exotic Pet Medicine*, **23**(4), 403–408.

Vuolo, S. and Whittington, J.K. (2008) Dystocia secondary to a perianal fetal hernia in an African hedgehog. *Exotic DVM*, **10**(3), 10–12.

Wellehan, J.F.X., Southorn, E., Smith, D.A. and Taylor, W.M. (2003) Surgical removal of a mammary adenocarcinoma and a granulosa cell tumor in an African pygmy hedgehog. *Canadian Veterinary Journal* **44**(4), 235–237.

Neonatal Mortality

Brodie, E.D., Brodie, E.D. and Johnson, J.A. (1982) Breeding the African hedgehog *Atelerix pruneri* in captivity. *International Zoo Yearbook*, **22**, 195–198.

Gregory, M.W. and Stocker, L. (1991) Hedgehogs, in *BSAVA Manual of Exotic Pets* (eds. P.H. Beynon, and J.E. Cooper), BSAVA, Shurdington, pp. 63–68.

Meritt, D.A. (1981) Husbandry, reproduction and behaviour of the West African hedgehog at Lincoln Park Zoo. *International Zoo Yearbook*, **21**(1), 128–131.

Morris, B. and Rudge, G. (1970) Serum proteins in young hedgehogs. *Journal of Zoology*, **162**(4), 461–468.

Reeve, N. (1994) *Hedgehogs*. T&AD Poyser Natural History, London.

Robinson, I. and Routh, A. (1999) Veterinary care of the hedgehog. *In Practice*, **21**(3), 128–137.

Smith, A.J. (1995) Neonatology of the hedgehog (*Atelerix albiventris*). *Journal of Small Exotic Animal Medicine*, **3**(1), 15–18.

Smith, A.J. (1999) Husbandry and nutrition of hedgehogs. *Veterinary Clinics of North America: Exotic Animal Practice*, **2**(1), 127–141.

Male Reproductive Conditions

Garner, M. (2011) Diseases of pet hedgehogs, chinchillas, and sugar gliders. *AEMV Proceedings*, Seattle, WA, pp. 405–412.

Heatley, J.J., Mauldin, G.E., and Cho, D.Y. (2005) A review of neoplasia in the captive African hedgehog (*Atelerix albiventris*). *Seminars in Avian and Exotic Pet Medicine*, **14**(3), 182–192.

Johnson-Delaney, C. (2007) What veterinarians need to know about hedgehogs. *Exotic DVM*, **9**(1), 38–44.

General Information

Allanson, M. (1934) The reproductive processes of certain mammals, Part VII. Seasonal variation in the reproductive organs of the male hedgehog. *Philosophical Transactions of the Royal Society of London, Series B*, **223**, 277–303.

Bedford, J.M., Mock, O.B., Nagdas, S.K., Winfrey, V.P., and Olson, G.F. (2000) Reproductive characteristics of the African pygmy hedgehog, *Atelerix albiventris*. *Journal of Reproduction and Fertility*, **120**, 143–150.

Brodie, E.D., Brodie, E.D. and Johnson, J.A. (1982) Breeding the African hedgehog *Atelerix pruneri* in captivity. *International Zoo Yearbook*, **22**, 195–198.

Deanesly, R. (1934) The reproductive processes of certain mammals, Part VI. The reproductive cycle of the female hedgehog. *Philosophical Transactions of the Royal Society of London, Series B*, **223**, 239–276.

Heatley, J. (2009) Hedgehogs, in *Manual of Exotic Pet Practice* (eds. M.A. Mitchell and T.N. Tulley). Saunders, St. Louis, MO, pp. 433–455.

Hoyt, R. (1986) A review of the husbandry and reproduction of the African hedgehog (*Atelerix albiventris*). *AAZPA Annual Proceedings*, pp. 85–95.

Hruban, Z., Martan, J., and Mochizuki, Y. (1970) External prostate of the hedgehog. *Journal of Morphology*, **132**(2), 149–167.

Hsieh, P.-C., Yu, J.-F., Wang, L. (2015) A retrospective study of the medical status on 63 African hedgehogs (*Atelerix albiventris*) at the Taipei Zoo from 2003–2011. *Journal of Exotic Pet Medicine*, **24**, 105–111.

Ivey, E. and Carpenter, J.W. African hedgehogs, in *Ferrets, Rabbits and Rodents Clinical Medicine and Surgery* (eds. K.E. Quesenberry and J.W. Carpenter), Saunders: St Louis, MO, pp. 339–353

Johnson, D. (2010) African pygmy hedgehogs, in *BSAVA Manual of Exotic Pets* (eds. A. Meredith and C. Johnson-Delaney), BSAVA, Gloucester, pp. 139–147.

Johnson-Delaney, C.A. and Harrison, L. (1996) Hedgehogs, in *Exotic Companion Medicine Handbook for Veterinarians*. Wingers Publishing, Lake Worth, FL, pp. 1–14.

Morris, B. (1959) Transmission of passive immunity in an insectivore. *Nature*, **184**, 1151.

Reeve, N. (1994) *Hedgehogs*. T&AD Poyser Natural History, London.

Robinson, A. (1904) Lectures on the early stages in the development of mammalian ova and on the differentiation of the placenta in different groups of mammals: Lecture III, The placenta of the hedgehog. *Journal of Anatomy and Physiology*, **38**(Pt 4), 485–502.

Intervertebral Disc Disease and Spinal Compression

Allison, N., Chang, T.C., Steele, K.E., and Hilliard, J.K. (2002) Fatal herpes simplex infection in a pygmy African hedgehog (*Atelerix albiventris*). *Journal of Comparative Pathology*, **126**, 76–70.

Raymond, J.T., Aguilar, R., Dunker, F., et al. (2009) Intervertebral disc disease in African hedgehogs (*Atelerix albiventris*): four cases. *Journal of Exotic Pet Medicine*, **18**, 220–223.

Wobbly Hedgehog Syndrome

Benoit-Biancamano, M.O., d'Anjou, M.A., Girard, C., and Langlois, I. (2006) Rib osteoblastic osteosarcoma in an African hedgehog (*Atelerix albiventris*), *Journal of Veterinary Diagnostic Investigation*, **18**(4), 415.

Garner, M. and Graesser, D. (2006) Wobbly hedgehog syndrome. *Exotic DVM*, **8**(3), 57–59.

Hedley, J., Benato, L., Fraga, G., Palgrave, C., and Eatwell, K. (2013) Congestive heart failure due to endocardiosis of the mitral valves in an African pygmy hedgehog. *Journal of Exotic Pet Medicine*, **22**(2), 212–217.

Karkamo, V., Dillard, K., Schulman, K. and Anttila, M. (2012) The wobbly hedgehog syndrome: a clinical entity with variable CNS lesions, in *Proceedings of the European Society of Veterinary Pathologists/European College of Veterinary Pathologists*, Leon, Spain, p. 268.

Johnson, D. (2010) African pygmy hedgehogs, in *BSAVA Manual of Exotic Pets* (eds. A. Meredith and C. Johnson-Delaney), BSAVA, Gloucester, pp. 139–147.

Other Neurologic Conditions

Allison, N., Chang, T.C., Steele, K.E., and Hilliard, J.K. (2002) Fatal herpes simplex infection in a pygmy African hedgehog (*Atelerix albiventris*). *Journal of Comparative Pathology*, **126**, 76–78.

Buergelt, C.D. (2002) Histopathologic findings in pet hedgehogs with nonneoplastic conditions. *Veterinary Medicine*, **97**(9), 660–665.

Isenbugel, E. and Baumgartner, R.A. (1993) Insectivora: diseases of the hedgehog, in *Zoo and Wild Animal Medicine: Current Therapy*, vol. **3** (ed. M.E. Fowler), Saunders: Toronto, pp. 294–302.

Madarame, H., Ogihara, K., Kimura, M. et al. (2014) Detection of a pneumonia virus of mice (PVM) in an African hedgehog (*Atelerix arbiventris*) with suspected wobbly hedgehog syndrome (WHS), *Veterinary Microbiology*, **173**(1), 136–140.

Smith, J.M.B. (1968) Diseases of hedgehogs. *Veterinary Bulletin*, **38**(7), 425–430.

Cerebrospinal Neoplasia

Benneter, S.S., Summers, B.A., Schulz-Schaeffer, W.J., et al. (2014) Mixed glioma (oligoastrocytoma) in the brain of an African hedgehog (*Atelerix albiventris*). *Journal of Comparative Pathology*, **151**(4), 420–424.

Garner, M. (2011) Diseases of pet hedgehogs, chinchillas, and sugar gliders, in *AEMV Proceedings*, Seattle, WA, pp. 405–412.

Garner, M.M., Kiupel, M., and Munoz, J.F. (2010) Brain tumors in African hedgehogs (*Atelerix albiventris*), in *AEMV Proceedings*, San Diego, CA.

Gibson, C.J., Parry, N.M.A., Jakowski, R.M., and Eshar, D. (2008) Anaplastic astrocytoma in the spinal cord of an African pygmy hedgehog (*Atelerix albiventris*). *Veterinary Pathology*, **45**(6), 934–938.

Graesser, D., Spraker, T.R., Dressen, P., et al. (2006) Wobbly hedgehog syndrome in African pygmy hedgehogs (*Atelerix* spp.). *Journal of Exotic Pet Medicine*, **15**(2), 59–65.

Hoefer, H.L. (1999) Clinical approach to the African hedgehog, in *Proceedings of the North American Veterinary Conference*, pp. 836–837.

Nakata, M., Miwa, Y., Itou, T., et al. (2011) Astrocytoma in an African hedgehog (*Atelerix albiventris*) suspected wobbly hedgehog syndrome. *Japanese Society of Veterinary Science*, **73**(10), 1333–1335.

General Information

Anderson, W.I., Cummings, J.F., Steinberg, H., de Lahunta, A., and King, J.M. (1989) Subclinical lumbar polyradiculopathy in aged domestic, laboratory, and exotic mammalian species—a light and selected electron microscopic study. *Cornell Veterinary Journal*, **79**(4), 339–344.

Buergelt, C.D. (2002) Histopathologic findings in pet hedgehogs with nonneoplastic conditions. *Veterinary Medicine*, **97**(9), 660–665.

Done, L.B., Dietze, M., Cranfield, M. and Ialeggio, D. (1992) Necropsy lesions by body systems in African hedgehogs (*Atelerix albiventris*): clues to clinical diagnosis. *Proceedings of the Joint Meeting of American Association of Zoo Veterinarians/American Association of Wildlife Veterinarians*, Oakland, CA, pp. 100–112.

Graesser, D., Spraker, T.R., Dressen, P., et al. (2006) Wobbly hedgehog syndrome in African pygmy hedgehogs (*Atelerix* spp.), *Journal of Exotic Pet Medicine*, **15**(2), 59–65.

Heatley, J. (2009) Hedgehogs, in *Manual of Exotic Pet Practice* (eds. M.A. Mitchell and T.N. Tulley). Saunders, St. Louis, MO, pp. 433–455.

Herter, K. (1963) *Igel*, A. Ziemsen Verlag, Lutherstadt (*Hedgehogs*, English translation, JM Dent and Sons Ltd, 1965).

Ivey, E. and Carpenter, J.W. African hedgehogs, in *Ferrets, Rabbits and Rodents Clinical Medicine and Surgery* (eds K.E. Quesenberry and J.W. Carpenter), Saunders: St Louis, MO, pp. 339–353.

Johnson, D. (2010) African pygmy hedgehogs, in *BSAVA Manual of Exotic Pets* (eds. A. Meredith and C. Johnson-Delaney), BSAVA, Gloucester, pp. 139–147.

Lightfoot, T.L. (2003) Therapeutics of African pygmy hedgehogs and prairie dogs, *Veterinary Clinics of North America: Exotic Animal Practice*, **3**(1), 155–72.

Reeve, N. (1994) *Hedgehogs*. T&AD Poyser Natural History, London.

Hematopoietic and Lymphoid Conditions

Beckman, K.B. and Norton, T.M. (1992) Disseminated hemangiosarcoma in an African hedgehog, in *Proceedings of Joint Conference of American Association of Zoo Veterinarians/American Association of Wildlife Veterinarians*, Oakland, CA, pp. 195–198.

Rhody, J.L. and Schiller, C.A. (2006) Spinal osteosarcoma in a hedgehog with pedal self-mutilation. *Veterinary Clinics of North America: Exotic Animal Practice*, **9**(3), 625–631.

Lymphoid Neoplasia

Burballa, A., Martinez, J., and Martorell, J. (2012) A splenic lymphoma with cerebellar involvement in an African hedgehog (*Atelerix albiventris*). *Journal of Exotic Pet Medicine*, **21**(3), 255–259.

Chu, P.Y., Zhuo, Y.X., Wang, F.I., et al. (2012) Spontaneous neoplasms in zoo mammals, birds, and reptiles in Taiwan: a 10-year survey. *Animal Biology*, **62**(1), 95–110.

Done, L.B. (1999) What you don't know about hedgehog diseases, in *Proceedings of the North American Veterinary Conference*, pp. 824–825.

Graesser, D., Spraker, T.R., Dressen, P., et al. (2006) Wobbly hedgehog syndrome in African pygmy hedgehogs (*Atelerix* spp.). *Journal of Exotic Pet Medicine*, **15**(2), 59–65.

Greenacre, C.B. (2004) Spontaneous tumors of small mammals. *Veterinary Clinics: Exotic Animal Practice*, **7**(3), 627–651.

Heatley, J.J., Mauldin, G.E. and Cho, D.Y. (200). A review of neoplasia in the captive African hedgehog (*Atelerix albiventris*). *Seminars in Avian and Exotic Pet Medicine*, **14**(3), 182–192.

Helmer, P. (2000) Abnormal hematologic findings in an African hedgehog (*Atelerix albiventris*) with gastrointestinal lymphosarcoma. *Canadian Veterinary Journal*, **41**(6), 489–490.

Hruban, Z., Vardiman, J., Meehan, T., Frye, F., and Carter, W.E. (1992) Haematopoietic malignancies in zoo animals. *Journal of Comparative Pathology*, **106**(1), 15–24.

Hsieh, P.-C., Yu, J.-F. and Wang, L. (2015) A retrospective study of the medical status on 63 African hedgehogs (*Atelerix albiventris*) at the Taipei Zoo from 2003–2011. *Journal of Exotic Pet Medicine*, **24**, 105–111.

Juan Sallés, C. and Garner, M.M. (2007) Cytologic diagnosis of diseases of hedgehogs. *Veterinary Clinics: Exotic Animal Practice*, **10**(1), 51–59.

Ramos-Vara, J.A., Miller, M.A., and Craft, D. (1998) Intestinal plasmacytoma in an African hedgehog. *Journal of Wildlife Diseases*, **34**(2), 377–380.

Raymond, J.T., Clarke, K.A. and Schafer, K.A. (1998) Intestinal lymphosarcoma in captive African hedgehogs. *Journal of Wildlife Diseases*, **34**(4), 801–806.

Raymond, J.T. and Garner, M.M. (2001) Spontaneous tumors in hedgehogs: a retrospective study of fifty cases, in *Proceedings of the American Association of Zoo Veterinarians*, Orlando, FL, pp. 326–327.

Raymond, J.T. and Garner, M.M. (2001) Spontaneous tumors in captive African hedgehogs (*Atelerix albiventris*): a retrospective study. *Journal of Comparative Pathology*, **124**(2), 128–133.

Snider, T.A., Joyner, P.H., and Clinkenbeard, K.D. (2008) Disseminated histoplasmosis in an African pygmy hedgehog. *Journal of the American Veterinary Medical Association*, **232**(1), 74–76.

General Information

Ivey, E. and Carpenter, J.W. African hedgehogs, in *Ferrets, Rabbits and Rodents Clinical Medicine and Surgery* (eds. K.E. Quesenberry and J.W. Carpenter), Saunders: St Louis, MO, pp. 339–353.

Ness, R.D. (1999) Clinical pathology and sample collection of exotic small mammals. *Veterinary Clinics of North America: Exotic Animal Practice*, **2**(3), 591–620.

Raymond, J.T. and White, M.R. (1999) Necropsy and histopathologic findings in 14 African hedgehogs (*Atelerix albiventris*): a retrospective study. *Journal of Zoo and Wildlife Medicine*, **30**(2), 273–277.

Wolff, F.C., Corradini, P., and Cortés, G. (2005) Congenital erythropoietic porphyria in an African hedgehog (*Atelerix albiventris*). *Journal of Zoo and Wildlife Medicine*, **36**(2), 323–325.

Ophthalmic Conditions

Bridges, C.D.B. and Quilliam, T.A. (1973) Visual pigments of men, moles and hedgehogs. *Vision Research*, **13**(12), 2417–2421.

Done, L.B., Dietze, M., Cranfield, M., and Ialeggio, D. (1992) Necropsy lesions by body systems in African hedgehogs (*Atelerix albiventris*): clues to clinical diagnosis, in *Proceedings of the Joint Meeting of the American Association of Zoo Veterinarians/American Association of Wildlife Veterinarians*, Oakland, CA, pp. 100–112.

Fukuzawa, R., Fukuzawa, K., Abe, H., Nagai, T., and Kameyama, K. (2004) Acinic cell carcinoma in an African pygmy hedgehog (*Atelerix albiventris*). *Veterinary Clinical Pathology*, **33**(1), 39–42.

Garner, M.M., Kiupel, M., and Munoz, J.F. (2010) Brain tumors in African hedgehogs (*Atelerix albiventris*), in *AEMV Proceedings*, San Diego, CA, p. 65.

Hamlen, H. (1997) Retro-orbital blood collection in the African hedgehog (*Atelerix albiventris*). *Laboratory Animals (UK)*, **26**(7), 34–35.

Heatley, J. (2009) Hedgehogs, in *Manual of Exotic Pet Practice* (eds. M.A. Mitchell and T.N. Tulley). Saunders, St. Louis, MO, pp. 433–455.

Heatley, J.J., Mauldin, G.E. and Cho, D.Y. (2005) A review of neoplasia in the captive African hedgehog (*Atelerix albiventris*). *Seminars in Avian and Exotic Pet Medicine*, **14**(3), 182–192.

Herter, K. (1963) *Igel*. A. Ziemsen Verlag, Wittenberg (*Hedgehogs*, English translation J.M Dent and Sons, 1965).

Ivey, E. and Carpenter, J.W. (2000) African hedgehogs, in *Ferrets, Rabbits and Rodents Clinical Medicine and Surgery* (eds. K.E. Quesenberry and J.W. Carpenter), Saunders: St Louis, MO, pp. 339–353.

Johnson, D. (2010) African pygmy hedgehogs, in *BSAVA Manual of Exotic Pets* (eds. A. Meredith and C. Johnson-Delaney), BSAVA, Gloucester, pp. 139–147.

Johnson-Delaney, C.A. (2002) Other small mammals, in *BSAVA Manual of Exotic Pets*, 4th edn (eds. A. Meredith and S. Redrobe), BSAVA Quedgeley, pp. 108–12.

Kim, E., Kim, J., Jeong, J., et al. (2012) Primary epithelial tumor of the lacrimal gland in a African pygmy hedgehog (*Atelerix albiventris*). *Korean Society of Veterinary Clinics.* **1**, 154.

Wheler, C.L., Grahn, B.H., and Pocknell, A.M. (2001) Unilateral proptosis and orbital cellulitis in eight African hedgehogs (*Atelerix albiventris*). *Journal of Zoo and Wildlife Medicine*, **32**(2), 236–241.

Index

NOTE TO THE READER: Given the broad diversity of the different species covered in this book, a detailed species-specific approach has been followed in this index. We hope that this enhances the utility of the index for the student and practitioner alike.

Pathology of Small Mammal Pets, First Edition. Patricia V. Turner, Marina L. Brash and Dale A. Smith.
© 2018 John Wiley & Sons, Inc. Published 2018 by John Wiley & Sons, Inc.